SALEM HEALTH

COMPLEMENTARY & ALTERNATIVE MEDICINE

SALEM HEALTH

COMPLEMENTARY
& Alternative Medicine

Volume 3

Editors

Richard P. Capriccioso, M.D.
University of Phoenix

Paul Moglia, Ph.D.
South Nassau Communities Hospital

SALEM PRESS
A Division of EBSCO Publishing
Ipswich, Massachusetts   Hackensack, New Jersey

Note to Readers

The material presented in *Salem Health: Complementary and Alternative Medicine* is intended for broad informational and educational purposes. Readers who suspect that they or someone they know has any disorder, disease, or condition described in this set should contact a physician without delay. This set should not be used as a substitute for professional medical diagnosis. Readers who are undergoing or about to undergo any treatment or procedure described in this set should refer to their physicians and other health care providers for guidance concerning preparation and possible effects. This set is not to be considered definitive on the covered topics, and readers should remember that the field of health care is characterized by a diversity of medical opinions and constant expansion in knowledge and understanding.

Library of Congress Cataloging-in-Publication Data

Complementary & alternative medicine / editors, Richard P. Capriccioso, Paul Moglia.
    p. ; cm. — (Salem health)
Complementary and alternative medicine
Includes bibliographical references and indexes.
    ISBN 978-1-58765-870-9 (set : alk. paper) — ISBN 978-1-58765-871-6 (vol. 1) — ISBN 978-1-58765-872-3 (vol. 2) — ISBN 978-1-58765-873-0 (vol. 3) — ISBN 978-1-58765-874-7 (vol. 4)
    I. Capriccioso, Richard P. II. Moglia, Paul. III. Title: Complementary and alternative medicine. IV. Series: Salem health (Ipswich, Mass.)
    [DNLM: 1. Complementary Therapies–Encyclopedias–English. WB 13]
    LCclassification not assigned
    615.503–dc23

2011051023

Contents

Complete List of Contents ix

Lactose intolerance 781
Lady's slipper orchid 781
Laetrile 782
Lapacho 784
Larch arabinogalactan 785
Lavender 786
Lecithin 788
Lemon balm 789
Leukoplakia 791
Levodopa/carbidopa 792
Licensing and certification of CAM
   practitioners 793
Licorice 795
Life extension 797
Lignans 799
Ligustrum 800
Linden 801
Lipoic acid 802
Lithium 805
Liver disease 805
Lobelia 808
Lomatium 810
Loop diuretics 811
Low-carbohydrate diet 812
Low-glycemic-index diet 814
Lupus 819
Lust, Benedict 821
Lutein 821
Lycopene 823
Lysine 825
Maca 827
Macrobiotic diet 828
Macular degeneration 829
Magnesium 831
Magnet therapy 835
Mahesh Yogi, Maharishi 844
Maitake 845
Malic acid 846
Manganese 846
Manipulative and body-based practices 848
Mann, Felix 850
Mannose 851
Marshmallow 852
Massage therapy 853

Maté 856
Meditation 858
Medium-chain triglycerides 861
Melatonin 862
Memory and mental function
   impairment 867
Menopause 871
Men's health 876
Mental health 880
Meridians 884
Mesoglycan 885
Metabolic syndrome 887
Metamorphic technique 888
Methotrexate 890
Methoxyisoflavone 891
Methyldopa 892
Methyl sulfonyl methane 892
Migraines 894
Migraines: Homeopathic remedies 898
Milk thistle 899
Mind/body medicine 902
Mistletoe 903
Mitral valve prolapse 905
Molybdenum 907
Monoamine oxidase (MAO) inhibitors 908
Morning sickness 908
Motherwort 910
Muira puama 911
Mullein 912
Multiple sclerosis (MS) 913
Music therapy 916
Myrrh 919
N-acetyl cysteine 921
Nails, brittle 923
Narcotic addiction 925
National Center for Complementary and
   Alternative Medicine (NCCAM) 926
National Health Federation 929
Naturopathy 930
Nausea 932
Neck pain 934
Neem 936
Nettle 937
Nicotinamide adenine dinucleotide 939
Night vision, impaired 940
Nitrofurantoin 941

Nitroglycerin 941
Nitrous oxide.. 942
Nondairy milk 942
Noni 944
Nonsteroidal anti-inflammatory drugs
    (NSAIDs) 946
Nopal 950
Nosebleeds 951
Oak bark.. 953
Oat straw.. 954
Obesity and excess weight 955
Obsessive-compulsive disorder (OCD) 963
Office of Cancer Complementary and
    Alternative Medicine........................ 964
Office of Dietary Supplements.............. 965
Ohsawa, George 967
Oligomeric proanthocyanidins.............. 968
Olive leaf... 971
Optimal health 972
Oral contraceptives.............................. 973
Oral hypoglycemics.............................. 975
Oregano oil 977
Oregon grape....................................... 978
Ornithine alpha-ketoglutarate 979
Orthomolecular medicine..................... 981
Osha.. 983
Osteoarthritis 984
Osteoarthritis: Homeopathic remedies.............. 990
Osteopathic manipulation..................... 990
Osteoporosis.. 993
Oxerutins... 1000
PABA... 1003
Pain management 1004
Palmer, Daniel David 1007
Pancreatitis.. 1008
Pantothenic acid and pantethine 1009
Parasites, intestinal.............................. 1011
Parkinson's disease 1012
Parsley... 1016
Passionflower....................................... 1017
PC-SPES 1018
Pelargonium sidoides............................ 1019
Penicillamine....................................... 1021
Pennyroyal... 1021
Pentoxifylline 1022
Peppermint 1023
Peptic ulcer disease:
    Homeopathic treatment 1026
Perilla frutescens 1028

Periodontal disease 1029
Peyronie's disease................................. 1031
Phaseolus vulgaris................................ 1032
Phenobarbital....................................... 1033
Phenothiazines..................................... 1034
Phenylalanine....................................... 1036
Phenytoin 1038
Phlebitis and deep vein thrombosis................ 1041
Phosphatidylserine............................... 1043
Phosphorus 1046
Photosensitivity.................................... 1047
Phyllanthus 1049
Picrorhiza 1050
Placebo effect 1051
Plantain 1052
Pokeroot 1054
Policosanol 1055
Polycystic ovary syndrome 1057
Popular health movement..................... 1058
Popular practitioners............................ 1060
Potassium... 1063
Potassium-sparing diuretics................... 1064
Preeclampsia and pregnancy-induced
    hypertension.................................... 1065
Pregnancy support................................ 1067
Pregnenolone....................................... 1072
Premenstrual syndrome (PMS) 1073
Premenstrual syndrome (PMS):
    Homeopathic remedies 1076
Prickly ash.. 1076
Primidone... 1077
Probiotics... 1078
Progesterone 1085
Progressive muscle relaxation 1087
Prolotherapy... 1089
Prostatitis 1091
Protease inhibitors................................ 1092
Proteolytic enzymes 1094
Proton pump inhibitors......................... 1097
Pseudoscience....................................... 1098
Psoriasis 1100
Pulse diagnosis 1102
Pumpkin seed....................................... 1103
Pygeum 1104
Pyruvate 1105
Qigong... 1107
Quercetin 1110
Radiation therapy support:
    Homeopathic remedies 1113

Contents

Radionics 1113

Raw foods diet 1115

Raynaud's phenomenon........................ 1116

Red clover... 1116

Red raspberry...................................... 1118

Red tea.. 1119

Red yeast rice...................................... 1120

Reflexology.. 1122

Regulation of CAM 1126

Reiki.. 1128

Reishi 1131

Relaxation response............................. 1132

Relaxation therapies 1134

Restless legs syndrome 1138

Resveratrol.. 1139

Retinitis pigmentosa 1141

Reverse transcriptase inhibitors 1142

Rheumatoid arthritis 1142

Rheumatoid arthritis:
      Homeopathic remedies 1146

Rhodiola rosea.. 1147

Rhubarb... 1149

Ribose 1150

Rifampin.. 1151

Rolfing 1152

Rosacea 1153

Rose hips... 1154

Rosemary... 1155

Royal jelly.. 1157

Complete List of Contents

Volume 1

Contents v
Publisher's Note ix
Contributors xi
Complete List of Contents xiii

Acerola 1
Acetaminophen 1
Acne 2
Active hexose correlated compound 4
Acupressure 5
Acupuncture 7
Adenosine monophosphate 21
Adolescent and teenage health 22
Adrenal extract 26
Aging 27
Alcoholism 29
Alexander technique 32
Alfalfa 33
Allergies 35
Aloe 39
Alopecia 41
Alternative versus traditional medicine 43
Altitude sickness 44
Alzheimer's disease and non-Alzheimer's
        dementia 46
Amenorrhea 50
American Academy of Anti-Aging Medicine 51
Aminoglycosides 52
Amiodarone 52
Amoxicillin 53
Andrographis 54
Androstenedione 56
Angina 57
Angiotensin-converting enzyme (ACE)
        inhibitors 59
Antacids 61
Anthroposophic medicine 62
Antibiotics, general 64
Anti-inflammatory diet 65
Antioxidants 67
Anxiety and panic attacks 68
Applied kinesiology 71
Arginine 72
Arjun 76

Aromatherapy 77
Arrhythmia 81
Artichoke 83
Art therapy 84
Ashwagandha 86
Astaxanthin 87
Asthma 88
Aston-Patterning 94
Astragalus 95
Atherosclerosis and heart disease prevention 97
Athlete's foot 103
Attention deficit disorder 105
Atypical antipsychotics 108
Autism spectrum disorder 108
Autogenic training 110
Avicenna 112
Ayurveda 113
Bach flower remedies 121
Back pain 122
Balneotherapy 126
Barberry 127
Barrett, Stephen 129
Bates method 129
Beano 131
Bed-wetting 132
Bee pollen 133
Bee propolis 135
Bee venom therapy 136
Bell's palsy 137
Benign prostatic hyperplasia 138
Benzodiazepines 142
Beta-blockers 144
Beta-carotene 144
Beta-glucan 148
Betaine hydrochloride 150
Beta-sitosterol 151
Bilberry 152
Bile acid sequestrant drugs 153
Biochemic tissue salt therapy 153
Bioenergetics 154
Biofeedback 155
Biofeedback for the headache 158
Biologically based therapies 159
Biorhythms 160

Biotin 161
Bipolar disorder 163
Bitter melon 164
Black cohosh 165
Black tea 168
Bladder infection 170
Bladder infection: Homeopathic remedies 173
Bladderwrack 174
Blepharitis 175
Blessed thistle 176
Bloodroot 177
Blue cohosh 178
Blue flag 179
Boldo 179
Bone and joint health 181
Boron 184
Boswellia 186
Bowers, Edwin 187
Brahmi 188
Braid, James 189
Branched-chain amino acids 190
Breast engorgement: Homeopathic remedies 192
Breast enhancement 193
Breast-feeding support 195
Breast pain, cyclic 197
Bromelain 198
Bromocriptine 200
Bronchitis 200
Bruises 202
Bruises: Homeopathic remedies 204
Buchu 205
Bugleweed 206
Burdock 207
Burning mouth syndrome 208
Burns, minor 209
Burns, minor: Homeopathic remedies 211
Bursitis 212
Butcher's broom 212
Butterbur 214
Calcium 217
Calcium channel blockers 222
Calendula 223
CAM on PubMed 224
Cancer chemotherapy support:
    Homeopathic remedies 225
Cancer risk reduction 226
Cancer treatment support 233
Candida/yeast hypersensitivity syndrome 241
Candling 243

Candytuft 244
Canker sores 245
Caraway 246
Carbamazepine 247
Cardiomyopathy 251
Carnitine 252
Carnosine 257
Carob 258
Carotenoids 259
Carpal tunnel syndrome 260
Cartilage 262
Cataracts 263
Catnip 265
Cat's claw 266
Cavity prevention 268
Cayenne 269
Cephalosporins 272
Cervical dysplasia 272
Cetylated fatty acids 274
Chamomile 275
Chaparral 276
Charaka 277
Chasteberry 278
Chelation therapy 280
Cherries 281
Childbirth support: Homeopathic remedies 282
Childbirth techniques 283
Children's health 285
Chinese medicine 288
Chinese skullcap 290
Chiropractic 292
Chitosan 297
Chocolate 299
Cholesterol, high 301
Chondroitin 306
Chopra, Deepak 308
Chromium 310
Chronic fatigue syndrome 314
Chronic obstructive pulmonary disease
    (COPD) 316
Cinnamon 319
Cirrhosis 321
Cisplatin 324
Citrulline 325
Citrus aurantium 326
Citrus bioflavonoids 328
Cleavers 330
Clinical trials 331
Clomiphene 334

Clonidine 334
Codex Alimentarius Commission 335
Coenzyme Q₁₀ 336
Cola nut 340
Colchicine 341
Colds and flu 341
Coleus forskohlii 349
Colic 350
Color therapy 352
Colostrum 354
Coltsfoot 356
Comfrey 357
Common cold: Homeopathic remedies 359
Compulsive overeating 360
Congestive heart failure 362
Conjugated linoleic acid 365

Conjunctivitis 366
Constipation 367
Copper 369
Cordyceps 370
Coriolus versicolor 371
Corticosteroids 373
Corydalis 374
Cough 375
Cranberry 376
Creatine 379
Crohn's disease 382
Cryotherapy 384
Crystal healing 385
Cupping 386
Cyclosporine 388
Cystoseira canariensis 389

Volume 2

Contents v
Complete List of Contents ix

Damiana 391
Dance movement therapy 391
Dandelion 393
Dawkins, Richard 395
Deer velvet 396
Depression, mild to moderate 398
Detoxification 403
Devil's claw 404
Diabetes 406
Diabetes, complications of 412
Diabetes: Homeopathic remedies 414
Diarrhea 416
Diarrhea in children: Homeopathic remedies 420
Dietary Supplement Health and
    Education Act 421
Diet-based therapies 424
Digoxin 426
Diindolylmethane 427
Dioscorides, Pedanius 428
Diverticular disease 429
DMAE 431
Dong quai 432
Double-blind, placebo-controlled studies 434
Doxorubicin 436
Dupuytren's contracture 437
Dysmenorrhea 438

Dyspepsia 439
Ear infections 443
Ear infections: Homeopathic remedies 446
Eating disorders 447
Echinacea 448
Eczema 452
Edema 456
Education and training of CAM
    practitioners 456
Elderberry 459
Elder health 460
Elecampane 463
Electromagnetic hypersensitivity 464
Eleutherococcus senticosus 465
Endometriosis 466
Energy medicine 467
Engel, George Libman 469
Enzyme potentiated desensitization 470
Ephedra 471
Epilepsy 474
Epstein-Barr virus 478
Ernst, Edzard 480
Essential oil monoterpenes 480
Estriol 481
Estrogen 483
Ethambutol 484
Eucalyptus 484
Exercise 486
Exercise-based therapies 489

Eyebright 491
Faith healing 493
False unicorn 494
Fatigue 494
Feldenkrais method 496
Feng shui 497
Fennel 499
Fenugreek 500
Feverfew 502
Fibrate drugs 503
Fibromyalgia: Homeopathic remedies 504
Finsen, Niels Ryberg 505
Fish oil 506
Fitzgerald, William H. 513
5-Hydroxytryptophan 514
Flaxseed 517
Flaxseed oil 519
Fluoride 521
Fluoroquinolones 522
Folate 523
Folk medicine 527
Food allergies and sensitivities 530
Food and Drug Administration (FDA) 532
Fructo-oligosaccharides 535
Functional beverages 536
Functional foods: Introduction 537
Functional foods: Overview 539
GABA 543
Gallstones 544
Gamma-linolenic acid 545
Gamma oryzanol 549
Garlic 550
Gas, intestinal 554
Gastritis 555
Gastritis: Homeopathic remedies 558
Gastroesophageal reflux disease 558
Gastrointestinal health 560
Gattefossé, René-Maurice 563
Genistein 564
Gentian 567
Germander 567
Gerson, Max 568
Ginger 569
Ginkgo 571
Ginseng 577
Glaucoma 581
Glucomannan 583
Glucosamine 584
Glutamine 587

Glutathione 591
Glycine 592
Goldenrod 594
Goldenseal 595
Gotu kola 597
Gout 599
Grass pollen extract 600
Greater celandine 602
Green coffee bean extract 602
Green-lipped mussel 604
Green tea 605
Guarana 607
Guggul 608
Guided imagery 610
Gymnema 611
H_2 blockers 613
Hackett, George S. 613
Hahnemann, Samuel 614
Hawthorn 616
Headache, cluster 618
Headache, tension 619
Head injury: Homeopathic remedies 622
Health freedom movement 622
Hearing loss 624
Heart attack 626
Heart disease 630
Hellerwork 636
Hemorrhoids 637
Hemorrhoids: Homeopathic remedies 639
Heparin 639
Hepatitis, alcoholic 641
Hepatitis, viral 643
Herbal medicine 646
Herpes 648
He shou wu 650
Hibiscus 651
Histidine 652
History of alternative medicine 653
History of complementary medicine ... 656
HIV/AIDS support 659
HIV support: Homeopathic remedies 666
Hives 667
Home health 668
Homeopathy: Overview 670
Homocysteine, high 676
Honey 678
Hoodia 679
Hopkins, Frederick 680
Hops 681

Horehound.. 682
Horny goat weed 683
Horse chestnut 684
Horseradish 687
Horsetail 688
Hufeland, Cristoph Wilhelm............................ 689
Humor and healing 690
Huperzine A 691
Hydralazine 692
Hydrotherapy 693
Hydroxycitric acid.. 695
Hydroxymethyl butyrate 696
Hypertension.. 697
Hypertension: Homeopathic remedies 702
Hyperthyroidism 703
Hypnotherapy 704
Hypothyroidism 706
Hyssop.. 709
Immune support 711
Indigo 713
Indole-3-carbinol... 714
Infertility, female 715
Infertility, male 717
Influenza: Homeopathic remedies 719
Influenza vaccine 721
Injuries, minor 721
Innate intelligence 723
Inosine 725
Inositol 725
Insect bites and stings 727

Insect bites and stings:
    Homeopathic remedies 728
Insomnia... 729
Insulin 734
Insurance coverage 734
Integrative medicine 735
Intermittent claudication 740
The Internet and CAM.................................... 741
Interstitial cystitis 744
Iodine 746
Ipriflavone 747
Iridology 749
Iron 749
Irritable bowel syndrome 753
Irritable bowel syndrome:
    Homeopathic remedies 756
Ishizuka, Sagen... 756
Isoflavones.. 757
Isoniazid 762
Isotretinoin 763
Ivy leaf 764
Jensen, Bernard 765
Jet lag 765
Juniper berry... 767
Kava... 769
Kelp 772
Kidney stones 773
Kombucha tea 777
Krill oil 778
Kudzu... 779

Volume 3

Contents v
Complete List of Contents ix

Lactose intolerance.. 781
Lady's slipper orchid...................................... 781
Laetrile... 782
Lapacho 784
Larch arabinogalactan 785
Lavender... 786
Lecithin 788
Lemon balm 789
Leukoplakia... 791
Levodopa/carbidopa....................................... 792
Licensing and certification of CAM
    practitioners... 793

Licorice 795
Life extension.. 797
Lignans 799
Ligustrum 800
Linden 801
Lipoic acid 802
Lithium 805
Liver disease 805
Lobelia 808
Lomatium 810
Loop diuretics 811
Low-carbohydrate diet 812
Low-glycemic-index diet 814
Lupus 819
Lust, Benedict 821

Lutein 821
Lycopene 823
Lysine.. 825
Maca.. 827
Macrobiotic diet........................... 828
Macular degeneration 829
Magnesium.................................. 831
Magnet therapy 835
Mahesh Yogi, Maharishi................... 844
Maitake 845
Malic acid 846
Manganese.................................. 846
Manipulative and body-based practices.... 848
Mann, Felix................................. 850
Mannose 851
Marshmallow 852
Massage therapy 853
Maté 856
Meditation 858
Medium-chain triglycerides............... 861
Melatonin 862
Memory and mental function
    impairment............................ 867
Menopause 871
Men's health 876
Mental health 880
Meridians................................... 884
Mesoglycan 885
Metabolic syndrome 887
Metamorphic technique................... 888
Methotrexate............................... 890
Methoxyisoflavone 891
Methyldopa................................. 892
Methyl sulfonyl methane 892
Migraines................................... 894
Migraines: Homeopathic remedies....... 898
Milk thistle 899
Mind/body medicine...................... 902
Mistletoe 903
Mitral valve prolapse 905
Molybdenum................................ 907
Monoamine oxidase (MAO) inhibitors.... 908
Morning sickness 908
Motherwort 910
Muira puama 911
Mullein 912
Multiple sclerosis (MS) 913
Music therapy.............................. 916

Myrrh 919
N-acetyl cysteine 921
Nails, brittle 923
Narcotic addiction 925
National Center for Complementary and
    Alternative Medicine (NCCAM) 926
National Health Federation 929
Naturopathy 930
Nausea 932
Neck pain 934
Neem 936
Nettle 937
Nicotinamide adenine dinucleotide....... 939
Night vision, impaired 940
Nitrofurantoin.............................. 941
Nitroglycerin 941
Nitrous oxide............................... 942
Nondairy milk 942
Noni 944
Nonsteroidal anti-inflammatory drugs
    (NSAIDs) 946
Nopal 950
Nosebleeds 951
Oak bark 953
Oat straw 954
Obesity and excess weight 955
Obsessive-compulsive disorder (OCD) 963
Office of Cancer Complementary and
    Alternative Medicine.................. 964
Office of Dietary Supplements............ 965
Ohsawa, George 967
Oligomeric proanthocyanidins 968
Olive leaf.................................... 971
Optimal health 972
Oral contraceptives........................ 973
Oral hypoglycemics 975
Oregano oil 977
Oregon grape 978
Ornithine alpha-ketoglutarate 979
Orthomolecular medicine................. 981
Osha.. 983
Osteoarthritis 984
Osteoarthritis: Homeopathic remedies.... 990
Osteopathic manipulation................. 990
Osteoporosis................................ 993
Oxerutins................................... 1000
PABA 1003
Pain management 1004

Complete List of Contents

Palmer, Daniel David 1007
Pancreatitis 1008
Pantothenic acid and pantethine 1009
Parasites, intestinal.. 1011
Parkinson's disease 1012
Parsley 1016
Passionflower 1017
PC-SPES 1018
Pelargonium sidoides.. 1019
Penicillamine.. 1021
Pennyroyal.. 1021
Pentoxifylline 1022
Peppermint 1023
Peptic ulcer disease:
    Homeopathic treatment 1026
Perilla frutescens 1028
Periodontal disease 1029
Peyronie's disease.. 1031
Phaseolus vulgaris... 1032
Phenobarbital... 1033
Phenothiazines 1034
Phenylalanine... 1036
Phenytoin 1038
Phlebitis and deep vein thrombosis.................. 1041
Phosphatidylserine... 1043
Phosphorus 1046
Photosensitivity.. 1047
Phyllanthus 1049
Picrorhiza 1050
Placebo effect... 1051
Plantain.. 1052
Pokeroot 1054
Policosanol 1055
Polycystic ovary syndrome 1057
Popular health movement.................................. 1058
Popular practitioners... 1060
Potassium.. 1063
Potassium-sparing diuretics............................... 1064
Preeclampsia and pregnancy-induced
    hypertension 1065
Pregnancy support... 1067
Pregnenolone... 1072
Premenstrual syndrome (PMS) 1073
Premenstrual syndrome (PMS):
    Homeopathic remedies 1076
Prickly ash.. 1076
Primidone... 1077

Probiotics.. 1078
Progesterone 1085
Progressive muscle relaxation 1087
Prolotherapy... 1089
Prostatitis 1091
Protease inhibitors 1092
Proteolytic enzymes 1094
Proton pump inhibitors...................................... 1097
Pseudoscience 1098
Psoriasis 1100
Pulse diagnosis 1102
Pumpkin seed... 1103
Pygeum 1104
Pyruvate 1105
Qigong.. 1107
Quercetin 1110
Radiation therapy support:
    Homeopathic remedies 1113
Radionics 1113
Raw foods diet 1115
Raynaud's phenomenon..................................... 1116
Red clover... 1116
Red raspberry... 1118
Red tea 1119
Red yeast rice... 1120
Reflexology... 1122
Regulation of CAM 1126
Reiki 1128
Reishi.. 1131
Relaxation response... 1132
Relaxation therapies.. 1134
Restless legs syndrome 1138
Resveratrol.. 1139
Retinitis pigmentosa 1141
Reverse transcriptase inhibitors 1142
Rheumatoid arthritis 1142
Rheumatoid arthritis:
    Homeopathic remedies 1146
Rhodiola rosea... 1147
Rhubarb.. 1149
Ribose 1150
Rifampin 1151
Rolfing 1152
Rosacea 1153
Rose hips.. 1154
Rosemary.. 1155
Royal jelly... 1157

Volume 4

Contents v
Complete List of Contents vii

Saffron 1159
Sage 1160
Salacia oblonga 1161
Salt bush 1162
SAMe 1163
Sampson, Wallace 1166
Sandalwood 1166
Sarsaparilla 1167
Sassafras 1169
Saw palmetto 1169
Scar tissue 1171
Schisandra 1172
Schizophrenia 1173
Sciatica 1176
Scientific method 1177
Scleroderma 1178
Sea buckthorn 1180
Seasonal affective disorder 1181
Seborrheic dermatitis 1182
Selenium 1184
Self-care 1187
Senna 1188
Sexual dysfunction in men 1190
Sexual dysfunction in women 1193
Shiatsu 1195
Shiitake 1197
Shingles 1198
Sickle cell disease 1200
Silica hydride 1201
Silicon 1203
Silver 1205
Sjögren's syndrome 1206
Skin, aging 1207
Skullcap 1210
Slippery elm 1211
Smoking addiction 1212
Soft tissue pain 1214
Soy 1215
Spirituality 1219
Spirulina 1220
Spleen extract 1223
Sports and fitness support:
    Enhancing performance 1223

Sports and fitness support:
    Enhancing recovery 1231
Sports-related injuries:
    Homeopathic remedies 1234
SSRIs 1235
Stanols and sterols 1237
Statin drugs 1239
Stevia 1241
St. John's wort 1242
Strep throat 1247
Stress 1249
Strokes 1252
Strokes: Homeopathic remedies 1256
Strontium 1257
Sublingual immunotherapy 1258
Sulforaphane 1260
Suma 1261
Sunburn 1262
Superoxide dismutase 1264
Supplements: Introduction 1265
Surgery support 1266
Surgery support:
    Homeopathic remedies 1270
Sweet clover 1272
Swimmer's ear 1273
Tai Chi 1275
Tamoxifen 1277
Tardive dyskinesia 1277
Taurine 1279
Tea tree 1281
Temporomandibular joint
    syndrome (TMJ) 1283
Tendonitis 1284
Tetracyclines 1286
Theophylline 1287
Therapeutic touch 1287
Thiazide diuretics 1290
Thomson, Samuel 1291
Thymus extract 1292
Thyroid hormone 1293
Tiller, William A. 1295
Time to Talk campaign 1295
Tinnitus 1296
Tinnitus: Homeopathic remedies 1297
Tinospora cordifolia 1298
Tocotrienols 1299

Tongue diagnosis 1300
Traditional Chinese herbal medicine 1301
Traditional healing 1309
Tramadol 1313
Transcendental Meditation 1313
Tribulus terrestris 1315
Tricyclic antidepressants 1316
Triglycerides, high 1317
Trimethoprim/sulfamethoxazole 1319
Trimethylglycine 1319
Tripterygium wilfordii 1321
Turmeric 1322
Tylophora 1324
Tyrosine 1325
Ulcerative colitis 1327
Ulcers 1330
Unani medicine 1333
Usui, Mikao 1334
Uva ursi 1335
Uveitis 1337
Vaginal infection 1339
Valerian 1340
Valproic acid 1344
Varicose veins 1345
Vega test 1350
Vegan diet 1350
Vegetarian diet 1352
Venous insufficiency:
    Homeopathic remedies 1354
Vertigo 1355
Vertigo: Homeopathic remedies 1356
Vervain 1356
Vinpocetine 1357
Vitamin A 1359
Vitamin B$_1$ 1362
Vitamin B$_2$ 1363
Vitamin B$_3$ 1364
Vitamin B$_6$ 1368
Vitamin B$_{12}$ 1371
Vitamin C 1374
Vitamin D 1380
Vitamin E 1383
Vitamin K 1390
Vitamins and minerals 1393
Vitiligo 1396
Walking, mind/body 1399
Warfarin 1400
Warts 1404

Warts: Homeopathic remedies 1405
Weight loss, undesired 1406
Weil, Andrew T. 1408
Well-being 1409
Well-being: Homeopathic remedies 1411
Wellness therapies 1412
Wheat grass juice 1414
Whey protein 1416
White willow 1417
Whole medicine 1419
Wild cherry 1423
Wild indigo 1423
Wild yam 1424
Witch hazel 1425
Wolfberry 1426
Women's health 1427
Wormwood 1431
Wounds, minor 1433
Xylitol 1435
Yarrow 1437
Yellow dock 1438
Yerba santa 1438
Yoga 1439
Yohimbe 1442
Yucca 1444
Zinc 1445

Appendixes
Reference Tools
    Glossary 1453
    Homeopathic Remedies for Selected
        Conditions and Applications 1479
    Bibliography 1482
    Resources 1491
    Web Sites 1496

Historical Resources
    Timeline of Major Developments in
        Complementary and Alternative
        Medicine 1502
    Biographical Dictionary of Complementary
        and Alternative Medicine Practitioners
        and Critics 1512

Indexes
    Category 1523
    Personages 1533
    Subject 1535

SALEM HEALTH

COMPLEMENTARY
& Alternative Medicine

L

Lactose intolerance

CATEGORY: Condition
DEFINITION: Treatment of nonexisting levels of the lactose-digesting enzyme known as lactase in the digestive system.
PRINCIPAL PROPOSED NATURAL TREATMENT: Lactase
OTHER PROPOSED NATURAL TREATMENTS: Calcium, probiotics

INTRODUCTION

Sugar comes in many forms. One type of sugar, lactose, occurs primarily in milk. Young children have the ability to digest lactose, because they need to do so when they nurse. However, as a person grows up, he or she often loses the lactose-digesting enzyme known as lactase. The result is a condition called lactose intolerance. Symptoms of lactose intolerance include intestinal cramps, gas, and diarrhea following consumption of lactose-containing foods, such as milk and ice cream.

PRINCIPAL PROPOSED NATURAL TREATMENTS

Lactose intolerance is most prevalent in people of Hispanic, African, Asian, Middle Eastern, or Native American descent, although Caucasians can develop it too. Treatment consists primarily of avoiding foods containing lactose. The use of lactase supplements may help people who are lactose intolerant handle more lactose than otherwise. Also, special milk products (such as Lactaid) are available from which the lactose has been removed (often through the use of lactase).

OTHER PROPOSED NATURAL TREATMENTS

Aside from lactase, there are no effective natural treatments for lactose intolerance. Despite some positive anecdotes, scientific evidence suggests that the use of probiotics (friendly bacteria) such as *Lactobacillus acidophilus* will not improve symptoms. However, natural medicine does have one noted contribution to make to people who are lactose intolerant: reminding them to take calcium supplements. People who avoid lactose-containing foods often do not get enough calcium in their diets, and they may therefore be at increased risk of osteoporosis and other health problems. Calcium supplements, such as TUMS, should correct this problem.

Many people confuse milk allergy with lactose intolerance. The two conditions are not related. Milk allergy involves an allergic reaction to the protein component of milk, and lactase supplements will not help.

EBSCO CAM Review Board

FURTHER READING

Ojetti, V., et al. "The Effect of Oral Supplementation with *Lactobacillus reuteri* or Tilactase in Lactose Intolerant Patients." *European Review for Medical and Pharmacological Sciences* 14 (2010): 163-170.

Saltzman, J. R., et al. "A Randomized Trial of *Lactobacillus acidophilus* BG2FO4 to Treat Lactose Intolerance." *American Journal of Clinical Nutrition* 69 (1999): 140-146.

Shaukat, A., et al. "Systematic Review: Effective Management Strategies for Lactose Intolerance." *Annals of Internal Medicine* 152 (2010): 797-803.

See also: Calcium; Diarrhea; Food allergies and sensitivities; Gas, intestinal; Nondairy milk; Probiotics.

Lady's slipper orchid

RELATED TERM: *Cypripedium*
CATEGORY: Herbs and supplements
DEFINITION: Natural plant product used to treat specific health conditions.
PRINCIPAL PROPOSED USES: None
OTHER PROPOSED USES: Anxiety, insomnia, musculoskeletal pain

OVERVIEW

The common name "lady's slipper" refers to the distinctive shape of these beautiful orchids, members

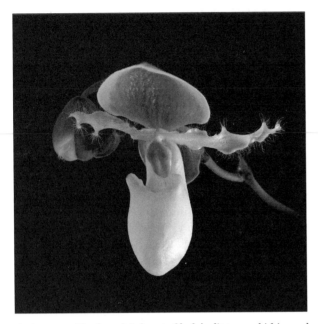

A tincture of fresh or dried root of lady's slipper orchid is used medicinally. (© Aetmeister/Dreamstime.com)

of the genus *Cypripedium* that are native to North America and Europe and of the *Paphiopedilum* species native to Southeast Asia. Other "slipper" orchid species are native to South America. Typically, the yellow lady's slipper *C. calceolus* var. *pubescens* (now called *C. parviflorum* var. *pubescens*) is used medicinally in Europe and North America. *C. montanum*, the rare mountain lady's-slipper that is native to North America, is also wildcrafted (collected in the wild).

Many of the *Cypripedium* lady's slipper species are endangered and have proven difficult to cultivate; even just collecting the flower may be enough to kill the plant, and transplantation from the wild is rarely successful. Alternatively, some herbalists recommend using the roots of another species called stream orchid or helleborine (*Epipactis helleborine*), which has the same purported effects, is more widespread, and is relatively easy to cultivate.

Traditionally, lady's slipper root was classified as a nervine, indicating its purported healing and calming effect on the nerves. The term "nervine," however, is no longer used in medicine.

THERAPEUTIC DOSAGES

The optimum oral dosage of lady's slipper is not known. A typical recommendation for *Cypripedium* species is 3 to 9 grams of root or 2 to 6 milliliters of a tincture of fresh or dried root. For muscle pain relief, a topical application of fresh or dried roots mashed into a poultice or plaster is sometimes used.

THERAPEUTIC USES

Despite a complete absence of scientific evidence that it is effective, lady's slipper is sometimes used either alone or as a component of formulas intended to treat anxiety or insomnia. Lady's slipper is also sometimes used topically as a poultice or plaster for the relief of muscular pain, but there is no evidence that it is effective.

SAFETY ISSUES

The safety of any medicinal application of these orchid species has not been established. Contact with the small hairs on some species can cause skin irritation.

Reviewed by EBSCO CAM Review Board

FURTHER READING

Moore, M. *Medicinal Plants of the Pacific West.* Santa Fe, N.M.: Red Crane Books, 1993.
Tierra, M. *The Way of Herbs.* New York: Pocket Books, 1998.

See also: Anxiety and panic attacks; Herbal medicine; Insomnia; Pain management.

Laetrile

CATEGORY: Herbs and supplements
RELATED TERMS: Amygdalin, apricot kernel, cyanide, vitamin B_{17}
DEFINITION: A potentially deadly, purported cancer cure dismissed as ineffective by the scientific community.

OVERVIEW

Laetrile is a pure form of the chemical amygdalin. This compound occurs naturally in many fruit pits and nuts. French chemists first identified it in 1830 and found that when amygdalin breaks down, it produces the poison cyanide.

Laetrile continues to attract the attention of health consumers and regulatory authorities. Cancer experts and health-fraud watchdogs are concerned about the risks of taking this substance and of patients being duped. There is little or no evidence in support of laetrile's proposed anticancer properties, and considerable evidence of its dangers. Even so, glowing testimonials fill supporters' Web sites.

"The primary risk of using any unproven treatment for cancer is the patient forgoes traditional treatment that could help them," says oncologist Clarence Brown, president of the M.D. Anderson Cancer Center in Orlando, Florida. "Secondly, they may be taking something that's harmful to them. It could interact with other medications. Or they could have a bad reaction. And they're spending, often times, big dollars to take a treatment that has absolutely no benefit."

Vitamin B_{17} and apricot kernels are other names for laetrile. It is not a vitamin. Some advocates believe cancer results from a vitamin deficiency that laetrile can presumably correct. Opponents think the term "laetrile" was coined to avoid federal drug safety and efficacy requirements.

THEORIES ON LAETRILE

During the nineteenth century, doctors tried using amygdalin to treat cancer. It proved too toxic. In the 1950s, a semisynthetic form, called laetrile, was produced and promoted as a cancer cure. Several theories exist about its anticancer action. In addition to the "vitamin" theory, some supporters believe an enzyme found primarily in cancer cells, but lacking in healthy cells, breaks down amygdalin. The amygdalin is broken down to cyanide, which then kills the cancer.

"Every cancer cell has a prodigious quantity of beta-glucosidase, or the unlocking enzyme," says G. Edward Griffin, who maintains that laetrile works and who published the supporting book *World Without Cancer: The Story of Vitamin B_{17}* (2001). None of these theories has held up well under scientific scrutiny.

SCIENTIFIC STUDIES

Laetrile gained notoriety in the 1970s, when doctors had fewer effective cancer treatments. Chemotherapy side effects were hard to control. Patients began looking for other options. More than seventy thousand Americans had tried laetrile by 1978. That year, the National Cancer Institute (NCI) reviewed cases submitted by doctors touting its benefits. Only two of sixty-seven patients had a complete response. Tumors got smaller in four others.

The NCI then sponsored research to evaluate laetrile. Two of the six persons in the first study died of cyanide poisoning after eating almonds. During the second study, patients received an infusion of amygdalin, followed by laetrile pills. Some participants reported feeling better while taking the drug, but cancer progressed in all 175 participants by the end of treatment. The agency decided not to investigate further. The American Cancer Society concluded laetrile had no role in cancer care.

CURRENT USE OF LAETRILE

The U.S. Food and Drug Administration (FDA) has not approved the use of laetrile and has taken action against companies in the United States to halt Web sales of laetrile. It is illegal to bring it into the United States for personal use. "This product has not been found to be safe and effective, so they're in violation of U.S. drug laws," says FDA spokesperson Susan Cruzan, of organizations that sell laetrile.

Mexican doctors, for example, still give laetrile to patients, despite the lack of scientific evidence. Oasis of Hope Hospital spokesperson Alex Phillips said that in several decades his Tijuana facility has treated 100,000 persons with laetrile. Patients initially receive laetrile through a vein. Then they take laetrile tablets, sometimes for the rest of their lives.

SAFETY ISSUES

Adverse reactions to laetrile are similar to those that occur with cyanide poisoning. Eating raw almonds or some fruits and vegetables when taking laetrile increases the risk of having an adverse reaction. Side effects tend to be more severe when laetrile is ingested, and some persons have died from laetrile treatment. Adverse effects of laetrile include nausea, vomiting, headache, dizziness, bluish skin color, droopy eyelids, trouble walking, fever, and confusion.

GENERAL ADVICE

Persons with cancer who want to try alternative therapies should consult a doctor if they are considering laetrile or other therapies. Also, consumers should know that herbal remedies can interfere with drugs ordered by a doctor.

Debra Wood, R.N.; reviewed by Brian Randall, M.D.

FURTHER READING

American Cancer Society. http://www.cancer.org.

SALEM HEALTH

Canadian Cancer Society. http://www.cancer.ca.

CancerNet. http://cancernet.nci.nih.gov.

Milazzo, Stefania, Edzard Ernst, et al. "Laetrile Treatment for Cancer." *Cochrane Database of Systematic Reviews* (2006): CD005476.

Milazzo, Stefania, Stephane Lejeune, et al. "Laetrile for Cancer: A Systematic Review of the Clinical Evidence." *Supportive Care in Cancer* 15, no. 6 (2007): 583-595.

U.S. Food and Drug Administration. http://www.fda.gov.

See also: Cancer risk reduction; Cancer treatment support; Pseudoscience; Science-based medicine; Vitamins and minerals.

Lapacho

RELATED TERMS: Isolapachone, lapachol, lapachone, Pau d'Arco, *Tabebuia avellanedae, T. impetiginosa*, taheebo

CATEGORY: Herbs and supplements

DEFINITION: Natural plant product used to treat specific health conditions.

PRINCIPAL PROPOSED USES: None

OTHER PROPOSED USES: Bladder infection, cancer, colds and influenza, diarrhea, pain, psoriasis, ulcers, vaginal infections, yeast hypersensitivity syndrome

OVERVIEW

The inner bark of the lapacho tree plays a central role in the herbal medicine of several South American indigenous cultures. The plant product is used to treat cancer and a variety of infectious diseases.

Little scientific investigation has been conducted of lapacho as a whole herb. However, an enormous amount of scientific interest has focused on three constituents of lapacho: lapachol, lapachone, and isolapachone. The relevance of these findings to the use of lapacho itself remains unclear.

THERAPEUTIC DOSAGES

Lapacho contains many components that do not dissolve in water, so making tea from the herb is not recommended. Instead, one should take powdered bark in capsule form; a typical dose is 300 to 500 milligrams three times daily. The inner bark of the lapacho tree is said to be the most effective part of the plant.

THERAPEUTIC USES

Based on its traditional uses, lapacho is sometimes recommended by herbalists as a treatment for cancer. However, there is no reliable scientific evidence that the herb is effective. Test-tube studies have found that lapachone can kill cancer cells by inhibiting an enzyme called topoisomerase, and there are hopes that effective anticancer drugs may eventually be produced through chemical modification of lapachone. Nonetheless, this does not indicate that lapacho is effective against cancer in humans; it would be difficult to take enough of the herb to provide active levels of lapachone.

Similarly, test-tube studies have found that constituents of lapacho (especially lapachone, isolapachone, and lapachol) may be able to kill various microorganisms, including various fungi and the parasites that cause schistosomiasis, malaria, and sleeping sickness. These findings have led to the widespread belief that lapacho is useful against the yeast *Candida albicans*, a common cause of vaginitis, and against the purported condition colloquially known as chronic candida; however, the supporting research remains far too preliminary to meaningfully show clinical benefits.

Similarly, these studies have been twisted to support claims that lapacho is useful for many infections, including colds and flu and bladder infections. However, there are at least two problems with this reasoning. First, lapacho has been tested primarily

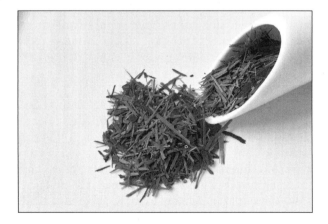

Lapacho bark. (© Darknightsky/Dreamstime.com)

against fungi and parasites; there is little evidence that it can kill viruses (the cause of colds) or bacteria (the cause of most bladder infections). Furthermore, even if lapacho can kill these microorganisms on direct contact, this does not imply that it would be effective if taken by mouth. Consider this analogy: Wine easily kills the cold virus on direct contact, but if one drinks wine when one has a cold, one is not likely to get well faster.

Similarly, hundreds of herbal products kill microorganisms in the test tube but fail to prove effective as systemic antibiotics. A substance taken by mouth has to survive the digestive tract and passage through the liver, and it has to reach sufficient concentrations in the bloodstream to produce a meaningful effect. Few substances can do this without simultaneously proving toxic to the body. Until lapacho's potential effects as an oral antibiotic are examined directly, it is not reasonable to assume that the herb is likely to help systemic infections.

Lapacho and its constituents have also been investigated for potential use in the treatment of pain, psoriasis, and ulcers. However, the evidence for benefit is too preliminary to rely upon.

SAFETY ISSUES

When taken in normal dosages, lapacho has not been found to cause any obvious side effects. However, full safety studies have not been performed. Furthermore, the anticancer actions of lapachone raise serious concerns about the safety of lapacho for pregnant women because, like cancer cells, cells of a developing fetus rapidly divide. Also, a study in animals found that lapachol caused fetal death. For all these reasons, pregnant or nursing women should not use lapacho. Safety in young children or those with severe liver or kidney disease also has not been established.

Reviewed by EBSCO CAM Review Board

FURTHER READING

Bailly, C. "Topoisomerase I Poisons and Suppressors as Anticancer Drugs." *Current Medicinal Chemistry* 7 (2000): 39-58.

Lima, N. M., et al. "Toxicity of Lapachol and Isolapachol and Their Potassium Salts Against *Biomphalaria glabrata, Schistosoma mansoni cercariae, Artemia salina,* and *Tilapia nilotica.*" *Acta Tropica* 83 (2002): 43-47.

Muller, K., et al. "Potential Antipsoriatic Agents: Lapacho Compounds as Potent Inhibitors of Hacat

Cell Growth." *Journal of Natural Products* 62 (1999): 1134-1136.

Portillo, A., et al. "Antifungal Activity of Paraguayan Plants Used in Traditional Medicine." *Journal of Ethnopharmacology* 76 (2001): 93-98.

Santos, A. F., et al. "Molluscicidal and Trypanocidal Activities of Lapachol Derivatives." *Planta Medica* 67 (2001): 92-93.

See also: Bladder infection; Cancer risk reduction; Candida/yeast hypersensitivity syndrome; Colds and flu; Folk medicine; Herbal medicine; Traditional healing; Vaginal infection.

Larch arabinogalactan

RELATED TERMS: Arabinogalactins, *Hypericum perforatum*, Western larch tree
CATEGORY: Herbs and supplements
DEFINITION: Natural plant product used to treat specific health conditions.
PRINCIPAL PROPOSED USE: Immune support
OTHER PROPOSED USES: Cancer treatment, ear infection

OVERVIEW

Arabinogalactins, substances found in many plants, are long molecules made of the sugars galactose and arabinose linked in a chain. Arabinogalactan extracted from the Western larch tree (*Larch arabinogalactan*, or LA) has been proposed as an immune stimulant.

THERAPEUTIC DOSAGES

A typical dose of powdered LA is 3 to 9 grams daily.

THERAPEUTIC USES

Test-tube and animal studies suggest that LA has several potentially positive effects on the immune system. It appears to activate a type of white blood cell called a natural killer or NK cell, and perhaps other white blood cells as well. LA also possibly alters levels of immune-related substances such as interleukins, interferon, and properdin.

On the basis of these findings, LA has been advocated as a supplement for general immune support. However, this recommendation is premature. It is a long way from basic science of this type to solid evidence that a treatment has real effective-ness.

Many plant substances appear to activate the immune system; this may be merely because the immune system regards them as "the enemy" and mobilizes to fight them. It takes double-blind, placebo-controlled trials to determine whether theoretical effects translate into real-life benefits, and only one such study has been performed on LA as an immune stimulant. This single meaningful trial was not designed to determine the actual medical benefits (if any) of LA. Rather, it primarily continued the theoretical investigation of LA's effects on components of the immune system.

In this trial, forty-eight healthy women were assigned to receive one of four treatments: LA, echinacea, LA plus echinacea, or placebo. Researchers evaluated various laboratory measurements of immune function. The results failed to show that LA by itself had any effect on immunity.

Other extremely preliminary research hints that LA might enhance the effectiveness of drugs used in cancer treatment, might help antibiotics fight ear infections and other infections, and might enhance the immune system in people with conditions such as chronic viral hepatitis, human immunodeficiency virus infection, and chronic fatigue syndrome. However, all these suggestions are highly speculative and lack reliable supporting evidence.

There is no doubt, however, that LA is a good dietary fiber source. Like less expensive forms of fiber, LA appears to have beneficial effects in the colon. A six-month study failed to find LA helpful for improving cholesterol profile.

SAFETY ISSUES

Based on animal studies and limited evidence in humans, LA appears to be essentially nontoxic. However, like other sources of dietary fiber, LA might lead to colonic problems like bloating and flatulence.

One additional set of potential risks derives from LA's supposed benefits: If LA does meaningfully stimulate the immune system, it might be dangerous. The immune system is highly balanced. An immune system that is too relaxed fails to defend the body against infections; an immune system that is too active attacks healthy tissues, causing autoimmune diseases. If LA truly boosts immunity, it might cause or worsen such conditions as lupus, Crohn's disease, asthma,

Graves' disease, Hashimoto's thyroiditis, multiple sclerosis, or rheumatoid arthritis. In addition, people who take immune suppressant drugs for organ transplants would be at risk of organ rejection. However, there is no actual evidence that LA causes problems.

Maximum safe doses in young children, pregnant or nursing women and people with severe liver or kidney disease have not been established. Persons taking an immunosuppressant drug such as cyclosporine, methotrexate, or corticosteroids should note that the use of LA could conceivably decrease the drug's effectiveness by stimulating the immune system.

Reviewed by EBSCO CAM Review Board

FURTHER READING

Currier, N. L., et al. "Effect over Time of In-Vivo Administration of the Polysaccharide Arabinogalactan on Immune and Hemopoietic Cell Lineages in Murine Spleen and Bone Marrow." *Phytomedicine* 10 (2003): 145-153.

Kim, L. S., et al. "Immunological Activity of *Larch arabinogalactan* and Echinacea." *Alternative Medicine Review* 7 (2002): 138-149.

Marett, R., and J. L. Slavin. "No Long-Term Benefits of Supplementation with Arabinogalactan on Serum Lipids and Glucose." *Journal of the American Dietetic Association* 104 (2004): 636-639.

Robinson, R. R., et al. "Effects of Dietary Arabinogalactan on Gastrointestinal and Blood Parameters in Healthy Human Subjects." *Journal of the American College of Nutrition* 20 (2001): 279-285.

See also: Cancer risk reduction; Ear infections; Echinacea; Immune support.

Lavender

RELATED TERMS: English lavender, essential oil of lavender, lavender oil, *Lavandula angustifolia*, *L. officinalis*

CATEGORY: Herbs and supplements

DEFINITION: Natural plant product used to treat specific health conditions.

PRINCIPAL PROPOSED USES: Insomnia, pregnancy support (pain after childbirth), wound healing

OVERVIEW

There are many plants in the lavender family, but the type most commonly used medicinally is English lavender. Traditionally, the essential oil of lavender was applied externally to treat joint pain, muscle aches, and a variety of skin conditions, including insect stings, acne, eczema, and burns. Lavender essential oil was also inhaled to relieve headaches, anxiety, and stress. Tincture of lavender was taken by mouth for joint pain, depression, migraines, indigestion, and anxiety. Lavender was additionally used as a hair rinse and as a fragrance in "dream pillows" and potpourri.

THERAPEUTIC DOSAGES

When used internally, lavender tincture is taken at a dose of 2 to 4 milliliters three times a day. Lavender essential oil is used externally or by inhalation only; it should not be used internally.

THERAPEUTIC USES

Lavender continues to be recommended for all its traditional uses. Only a few of these uses, however, have any supporting scientific evidence whatsoever, and for none of these is the evidence strong.

A few studies suggest that lavender oil, when taken by inhalation (aromatherapy) might reduce agitation in people with severe dementia. For example, in one well-designed but small study, a hospital ward was suffused with either lavender oil or water for two hours. An investigator who was unaware of the study's design and who wore a device to block inhalation of odors entered the ward and evaluated the behavior of the fifteen residents, all of whom had dementia. The results indicated that the use of lavender oil aromatherapy modestly decreased agitated behavior. A somewhat less rigorous study reported similar benefits. Rigor is essential in such studies, as it has been shown that merely creating expectations about the effects of aromas may be sufficient to cause these effects.

A preliminary controlled trial found some evidence that lavender, administered through an oxygen face mask, reduced the need for pain medications following gastric banding surgery. A small study performed in Iran reported that oral use of lavender tincture augmented the effectiveness of a pharmaceutical treatment for depression. However, this study suffered from numerous problems, both in design and reporting, and in the scientific reputation of the investigators involved.

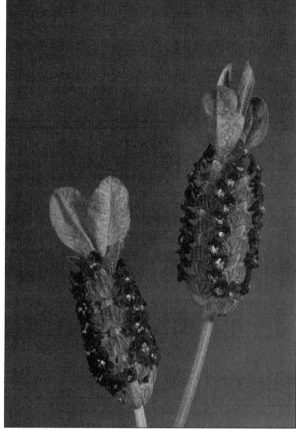

English lavender flowers. (Ray Coleman/Getty Images)

In a controlled trial with more than six hundred participants, lavender oil in bath water failed to improve perineal pain after childbirth. One poorly designed study found weak hints that lavender might be useful for insomnia. One animal study failed to find that lavender oil enhances wound healing. Lavender is also used in combination with other essential oils.

SAFETY ISSUES

No form of lavender has undergone comprehensive safety testing. Internal use of lavender essential oil is unsafe and should be avoided. Topical use is considered much safer. Allergic reactions are relatively common, as with all essential oils. In addition, one case suggests that a combination of lavender oil and tea tree oil applied topically caused gynecomastia (male breast enlargement) in three young boys.

A controlled study found that inhalation of lavender essential oil might impair some aspects of mental function. (Presumably, this was caused by the intended sedative effects of the treatment.) Oral use of tincture of lavender has not been associated with any severe adverse effects, but comprehensive safety testing has not been performed. Finally, the maximum safe doses of any form of lavender remain unknown for pregnant or nursing women, for young children, and for people with severe liver or kidney disease.

Reviewed by EBSCO CAM Review Board

FURTHER READING

Akhondzadeh, S., et al. "Comparison of *Lavandula angustifolia* Mill. Tincture and Imipramine in the Treatment of Mild to Moderate Depression." *Progress in Neuro-Psychopharmacology and Biological Psychiatry* 27 (2003): 123-127.

Henley, D. V., et al. "Prepubertal Gynecomastia Linked to Lavender and Tea Tree Oils." *New England Journal of Medicine* 356 (2007): 479-485.

Kim, J. T., et al. "Treatment with Lavender Aromatherapy in the Post-Anesthesia Care Unit Reduces Opioid Requirements of Morbidly Obese Patients Undergoing Laparoscopic Adjustable Gastric Banding." *Obesity Surgery* 17 (2007): 920-925.

Lewith, G. T., et al. "A Single-Blinded, Randomized Pilot Study Evaluating the Aroma of *Lavandula augustifolia* as a Treatment for Mild Insomnia." *Journal of Alternative and Complementary Medicine* 11 (2005): 631-637.

Lusby, P. E., et al. "A Comparison of Wound Healing Following Treatment with *Lavandula* x *allardii* Honey or Essential Oil." *Phytotherapy Research* 20, no. 9 (2006): 755-757.

Moss, M., et al. "Aromas of Rosemary and Lavender Essential Oils Differentially Affect Cognition and Mood in Healthy Adults." *International Journal of Neuroscience* 113 (2003): 15-38.

See also: Aromatherapy; Folk medicine; Pregnancy support; Tea tree; Wounds, minor.

Lecithin

RELATED TERMS: Egg lecithin, phosphatidylcholine in lecithin, soy lecithin

CATEGORY: Herbs and supplements
DEFINITION: Natural animal and plant substance used to treat specific health conditions.
PRINCIPAL PROPOSED USES: None
OTHER PROPOSED USES: Alzheimer's disease, bipolar disorder, high cholesterol, liver disease, Parkinson's disease, tardive dyskinesia, Tourette's syndrome, ulcerative colitis

OVERVIEW

For decades, lecithin has been a popular treatment for high cholesterol, although there is little evidence that it works. More recently, lecithin has been proposed as a remedy for various psychological and neurological diseases, such as Tourette's syndrome, Alzheimer's disease, and bipolar disorder (earlier known as manic depression).

Lecithin contains a substance called phosphatidylcholine that is presumed to be responsible for its medicinal effects. Phosphatidylcholine is a major part of the membranes surrounding human cells. However, when this substance is consumed, it is broken down into the nutrient choline rather than being carried directly to cell membranes. Choline acts like folate, trimethylglycine, and SAMe (S-adenosylmethionine) to promote methylation. It is also used to make acetylcholine, a nerve chemical essential for proper brain function.

REQUIREMENTS AND SOURCES

Neither lecithin nor its ingredient phosphatidylcholine is an essential nutrient; however, choline has recently been recognized as essential. For use as a supplement or a food additive, lecithin is often manufactured from soy.

THERAPEUTIC DOSAGES

Ordinary lecithin contains about 10 to 20 percent phosphatidylcholine. However, European research has tended to use products concentrated to contain 90 percent phosphatidylcholine in lecithin, and the following dosages are based on that type of product. For psychological and neurological conditions, doses as high as 5 to 10 grams (g) taken three times daily have been used in studies. For liver disease, a typical dose is 350 to 500 milligrams (mg) taken three times daily; for high cholesterol, 500 to 900 mg taken three times daily has been tried.

THERAPEUTIC USES

For some time, lecithin/phosphatidylcholine was one of the most commonly recommended natural treatments for high cholesterol. However, this idea appears to rest entirely on studies of unacceptably low quality. The best-designed studies have failed to find any evidence of benefit. In Europe, phosphatidylcholine is also used to treat liver diseases, such as alcoholic fatty liver, alcoholic hepatitis, liver cirrhosis, and viral hepatitis. However, research into these potential uses remains preliminary and has yielded contradictory results.

Researchers have recently become interested in the use of phosphatidylcholine as a supportive treatment in severe ulcerative colitis. There may be an insufficient quantity of phosphatidylcholine in the mucus lining the colon in persons with ulcerative colitis. Taking phosphatidylcholine may correct this deficiency.

In a small, double-blind, placebo-controlled study, sixty persons whose ulcerative colitis was poorly responsive to corticosteroids were randomized to receive either phosphatidylcholine (2 g per day) or placebo for twelve weeks. One-half of the participants taking phosphatidylcholine showed a significant improvement in symptoms versus only 10 percent taking placebo. Moreover, 80 percent taking phosphatidylcholine were able to discontinue their corticosteroids without disease flare-up, compared with 10 percent taking placebo.

Some evidence hints that phosphatidylcholine may reduce homocysteine levels, which in turn was thought likely to reduce heart disease risk. Because phosphatidylcholine plays a role in nerve function, it has also been suggested as a treatment for various psychological and neurological disorders, such as Alzheimer's disease, bipolar disorder, Parkinson's disease, Tourette's syndrome, and tardive dyskinesia (a late-developing side effect of drugs used for psychosis). However, the evidence that it works is limited to small studies with conflicting results.

SAFETY ISSUES

Lecithin is believed to be generally safe. However, some people taking high dosages (several grams daily) experience minor but annoying side effects, such as abdominal discomfort, diarrhea, and nausea. Maximum safe dosages for young children, pregnant or nursing women, and those with severe liver or kidney disease have not been determined.

Reviewed by EBSCO CAM Review Board

FURTHER READING

Olthof, M. R., et al. "Choline Supplemented as Phosphatidylcholine Decreases Fasting and Postmethionine-Loading Plasma Homocysteine Concentrations in Healthy Men." *American Journal of Clinical Nutrition* 82 (2005): 111-117.

Singh, N. K., and R. C. Prasad. "A Pilot Study of Polyunsaturated Phosphatidyl Choline in Fulminant and Subacute Hepatic Failure." *Journal of the Association of Physicians of India* 46 (1998): 530-532.

Stremmel, W., et al. "Phosphatidylcholine for Steroid-Refractory Chronic Ulcerative Colitis." *Annals of Internal Medicine* 147 (2007): 603-610.

See also: Alzheimer's disease and non-Alzheimer's dementia; Bipolar disorders; Cholesterol, high; Depression, mild to moderate; Food and Drug Administration; Liver disease; Mental health; Parkinson's disease; Soy; Tardive dyskinesia; Ulcerative colitis.

Lemon balm

RELATED TERMS: Essential oil of lemon balm, melissa, *Melissa officinalis*

CATEGORY: Herbs and supplements

DEFINITION: Natural plant product used to treat specific health conditions.

PRINCIPAL PROPOSED USES: Anxiety, insomnia, nervous stomach, oral and genital herpes, reducing agitation in dementia

OVERVIEW

Commonly called by its Latin first name, *Melissa*, lemon balm is a native of southern Europe, often planted in gardens to attract bees. Its leaves give off a delicate lemon odor when bruised.

Medical authorities of ancient Greece and Rome mentioned topical lemon balm as a treatment for wounds. The herb was later used orally as a treatment for influenza, insomnia, anxiety, depression, and nervous stomach.

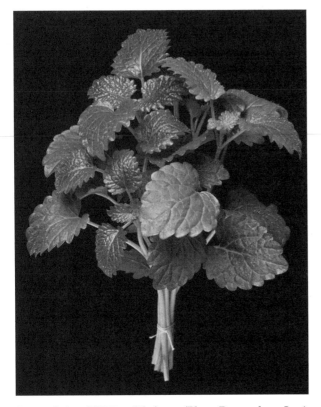

Lemon balm. (TH Foto-Werbung/Photo Researchers, Inc.)

THERAPEUTIC DOSAGES

For treatment of an active flare-up of herpes, the proper dosage is four thick applications daily of a standardized lemon balm (70:1) cream. The dosage may be reduced to twice daily for preventive purposes.

The best lemon balm extracts are standardized by their capacity to inhibit the growth of herpes virus in a petri dish. To make sure the extract has been properly prepared, manufacturers place cells in such a growing medium and then add herpes virus. Normally, the virus will gradually destroy all the cells. However, when little disks containing lemon balm are added, cells in the immediate vicinity are protected. Although manufacturers use this method as a form of quality control, it also provides evidence that lemon balm works.

When taken orally for its calming effect, the standard dosage of lemon balm is 1.5 to 4.5 grams of dried herb daily; extracts and tinctures should be taken according to label instructions.

THERAPEUTIC USES

Topical lemon balm is most popular today as a treatment for genital or oral herpes. It appears to make flare-ups less intense and to make them last for a shorter period of time, but it does not completely eliminate them. Regular use of lemon balm might help prevent flare-ups, but this potential use has not been properly studied.

Whereas conventional treatments can reduce infectivity and thereby help prevent the spread of herpes, there is no evidence that lemon balm offers this benefit. Common-sense methods of avoiding passing on herpes are not entirely effective: Many people are infectious even when they do not have obvious symptoms, and use of a condom does not entirely prevent the spread of the virus. Therefore, persons who are sexually active with a noninfected partner should use suppressive drug therapy.

There is some evidence that oral use of lemon balm has sedative effects, and it is currently used for insomnia, anxiety, and nervous stomach. Inhaled essential oil of lemon balm may also have calming effects.

SCIENTIFIC EVIDENCE

Herpes virus infection. Numerous test-tube studies have found that extracts of lemon balm possess antiviral properties. Experts do not know how it works, but the predominant theory is that the herb blocks viruses from attaching to cells.

One double-blind, placebo-controlled study followed sixty-six persons who were just starting to develop a cold sore (oral herpes). Treatment with melissa cream produced significant benefits on day two, reducing intensity of discomfort, number of blisters, and the size of the lesion. (The researchers specifically looked at day two because, according to them, that is when symptoms are most pronounced.)

Another double-blind study followed 116 persons with oral or genital herpes. Participants used either melissa cream or placebo cream for up to ten days. The results showed that the use of the herb resulted in a significantly better rate of recovery than for those persons given placebo. Relatively informal observations suggest that the regular use of lemon balm cream may help reduce the frequency of herpes flare-ups.

Sedative effect. Lemon balm extracts have been found to produce a sedative effect in mice. Based on this, human trials have been performed. In a four-month, double-blind, placebo-controlled study of forty-two people with Alzheimer's disease, the use of an oral lemon balm extract significantly decreased their tendency to become agitated.

In another study, lemon balm essential oil applied to the skin in the form of a cream also reduced agitation in seventy-one people with Alzheimer's disease. The researchers considered this a form of aromatherapy, a treatment in which the odor of a substance is said to produce the benefit. However, one of the first things to disappear in patients with Alzheimer's disease is the sense of smell; it is more likely, therefore, that the lemon balm worked by being absorbed through the skin.

Lemon balm also has shown sedative and anti-anxiety effects in two small studies of healthy people. In other studies, combination therapies containing lemon balm plus valerian have shown modest promise as sedatives for the treatment of insomnia.

SAFETY ISSUES

Topical lemon balm is not associated with any significant side effects, although allergic reactions are always possible. Oral lemon balm is on the GRAS (Generally Recognized As Safe) list of the U.S. Food and Drug Administration. However, according to one of the foregoing studies, lemon balm reduces alertness and impairs mental function; for this reason, persons engaging in activities that require alertness, such as operating a motor vehicle, should avoid using lemon balm beforehand.

In addition, one animal study suggests that if lemon balm is taken at the same time as standard sedative drugs, excessive sedation might occur. Persons taking sedative medications should note that the use of oral lemon balm might amplify the effect of the medications, potentially leading to excessive sedation.

Reviewed by EBSCO CAM Review Board

FURTHER READING

Akhondzadeh, S., et al. "*Melissa officinalis* Extract in the Treatment of Patients with Mild to Moderate Alzheimer's Disease." *Journal of Neurology, Neurosurgery, and Psychiatry* 74 (2003): 863-866.

Ballard, C. G., et al. "Aromatherapy as a Safe and Effective Treatment for the Management of Agitation in Severe Dementia: The Results of a Double-Blind, Placebo-Controlled Trial with *Melissa.*" *Journal of Clinical Psychiatry* 63 (2002): 553-558.

Kennedy, D. O., et al. "Attenuation of Laboratory-Induced Stress in Humans After Acute Administration of *Melissa officinalis* (Lemon Balm)." *Psychosomatic Medicine* 66 (2004): 607-613.

Snow, L. A., et al. "A Controlled Trial of Aromatherapy for Agitation in Nursing Home Patients with Dementia." *Journal of Alternative and Complementary Medicine* 10 (2004): 431-437.

See also: Alzheimer's disease and non-Alzheimer's dementia; Anxiety and panic attacks; Aromatherapy; Dyspepsia; Herbal medicine; Herpes.

Leukoplakia

CATEGORY: Condition
DEFINITION: Treatment of a disorder of the mucous membranes that manifests in areas such as the mouth, tongue, and female genitals.
PRINCIPAL PROPOSED NATURAL TREATMENT: Lycopene

INTRODUCTION

Leukoplakia is a disorder of the mucous membranes. Symptoms consist of white, grey, or red patches that form on the tongue, inside the mouth, or, more rarely, the female vulva. These patches are thick and slightly raised and often present a hardened surface. Areas of leukoplakia may be sensitive to touch, heat, or spicy foods.

The cause of leukoplakia is not clear, but it often develops in response to chronic irritation, such as rough surfaces on dentures, fillings, or crowns. One special type, known as hairy leukoplakia, involves a viral infection; it is found only in people who are infected with the human immunodeficiency virus.

Leukoplakia is associated also with an increased risk of cancer in the affected area. Removing an identifiable irritant may resolve the problem. In some cases, surgical treatment is advised.

PRINCIPAL PROPOSED NATURAL TREATMENTS

Vitamin A is known to play a role in the health of skin and mucous membranes. For this reason, vitamin A, used orally or topically, has been tried for leukoplakia. No clear benefits have been seen in scientific studies. However, the related substance lycopene might be helpful.

Lycopene is a carotenoid, a close chemical cousin of vitamin A. Found in high levels in tomato products, watermelon, and pink grapefruit, lycopene has shown promise in the treatment and prevention of prostate cancer and of macular degeneration (a disease of the eye). One study suggests that lycopene also might be useful for treating leukoplakia. In this double-blind, placebo-controlled study, fifty-eight persons with oral leukoplakia received either 8 milligrams (mg) or 4 mg oral lycopene daily or placebo capsules for three months. Participants were then followed by researchers for an additional two months. The results indicated that lycopene in either dose was more effective than placebo for reducing signs and symptoms of leukoplakia, and that 8 mg daily was more effective than 4 mg. Although one study cannot prove a treatment effective, these findings are definitely promising.

EBSCO CAM Review Board

FURTHER READING

Reamy, B. V., et al. "Common Tongue Conditions in Primary Care." *American Family Physician* 81 (2010): 627-634.

Singh, M., et al. "Efficacy of Oral Lycopene in the Treatment of Oral Leukoplakia." *Oral Oncology* 40 (2004): 591-596.

Zakrzewska, J. M. "Oral Lycopene: An Efficacious Treatment for Oral Leukoplakia?" *Evidence Based Dentistry* 6 (2005): 17-18.

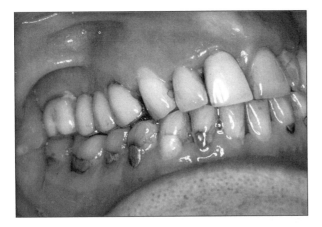

Leukoplakia in the mouth of a pipe smoker. (© Lester V. Bergman/Corbis)

See also: Burning mouth syndrome; Canker sores; Herpes; Lycopene; Vaginal infection; Vitamin A.

Levodopa/carbidopa

CATEGORY: Drug interactions

DEFINITION: Levodopa in combination with carbidopa is used in treating Parkinson's disease.

TRADE NAME: Sinemet

INTERACTIONS: Branched-chain amino acids, 5-HTP (5-hydroxytryptophan), iron, kava, policosanol, SAMe, traditional Chinese herbal medicine, vitamin B_6

5-HTP (5-HYDROXYTRYPTOPHAN)

Effect: Possible Harmful Interaction

The body uses the natural substance 5-HTP to manufacture serotonin, and supplemental forms of 5-HTP have been used for treating depression and migraine headaches. Since it is converted by the body to serotonin, 5-HTP might have antidepressant properties. For this reason, some people with Parkinson's-related depression have tried it.

However, the combination of 5-HTP and carbidopa might cause a scleroderma-like condition, in which the skin becomes hard and tight. Because of the risk of this side effect, persons taking levodopa/carbidopa for Parkinson's disease should avoid supplemental 5-HTP.

BRANCHED-CHAIN AMINO ACIDS (BCAAs)

Effect: Possible Harmful Interaction

Branched-chain amino acids (BCAAs) in supplement form have been used to improve appetite in cancer patients and to slow the progression of amyotrophic lateral sclerosis (ALS, or Lou Gehrig's disease). Dietary protein can decrease the effectiveness of levodopa in Parkinson's disease. Because it is the amino acids in proteins that affect levodopa, BCAAs might cause the same problem. Therefore, if one takes levodopa/carbidopa for Parkinson's, it may be advisable to avoid BCAAs and other amino acid supplements.

IRON

Effect: Take at a Different Time of Day

Iron appears to interfere with the absorption of both levodopa and carbidopa by binding to them.

Studies have found that blood levels of levodopa and carbidopa are reduced 30 to 51 percent and 75 percent, respectively, by iron supplementation, resulting in a worsening of symptoms of Parkinson's disease. Based on this finding, one should separate the times one takes iron and these drugs by as long as possible.

KAVA

Effect: Possible Harmful Interaction

The herb kava (*Piper methysticum*) has a sedative effect and is used for anxiety and insomnia. A few case reports suggest that kava might interfere with the action of dopamine in the body. This could at least partially neutralize the therapeutic effects of levodopa. In one individual, Parkinson's disease symptoms got worse following supplementation with kava extract of 150 milligrams (mg) twice daily for ten days. Based on these reports, it may be advisable to avoid kava during levodopa/carbidopa therapy.

TRADITIONAL CHINESE HERBAL MEDICINE

Effect: Possible Reduced Action of Drug

Certain herbal formulas used in traditional Chinese herbal medicine to treat upset stomach might reduce the effectiveness of levodopa.

VITAMIN B$_6$

Effect: Possible Reduced Action of Drug

If taking levodopa alone, one should not take more than 5 mg per day of vitamin B$_6$ or it might impair the effectiveness of the drug. However, if one uses levodopa/carbidopa combinations that provide a total daily dose of at least 75 mg of carbidopa, this issue is not a concern.

POLICOSANOL

Effect: Possible Benefits and Risks

Policosanol may increase both the effects and the side effects of levodopa.

SAME (S-ADENOSYLMETHIONINE)

Effect: Possible Benefits and Risks

SAMe is a naturally occurring compound derived from the amino acid methionine and the energy molecule adenosine triphosphate (ATP). SAMe is widely used as a supplement for treatment of osteoarthritis and depression. Preliminary evidence suggests that levodopa might deplete levels of SAMe in the body. This suggests (but definitely does not prove) that per-

sons taking levodopa/carbidopa might benefit from SAMe supplements.

One short-term (thirty-day) double-blind study suggests that such combination treatment is safe and might help depression related to Parkinson's disease. However, there are also concerns that SAMe could cause levodopa to be less effective over time. Persons taking levodopa/carbidopa should consult their physician about taking SAMe.

EBSCO CAM Review Board

FURTHER READING

Bottiglieri, T., K. Hyland, and E. H. Reynolds. "The Clinical Potential in Ademetionine (S-adenosylmethionine) in Neurological Disorders." *Drugs* 48 (1994): 137-152.

Liu, X., N. Lamango, and C. Charlton. "L-dopa Depletes S-adenosylmethionine and Increases S-adenosyl Homocysteine: Relationship to the Wearing Off Effects." *Social Neuroscience* 24 (1998): 1469.

Sunagane, N., et al. "Possibility of Interactions Between Prescription Drugs and OTC Drugs (2nd Report): Interaction Between Levodopa Preparation and OTC Kampo Medicines for Upset Stomach." *Yakugaku Zasshi* 126 (2006): 1191-1196.

See also: Branched-chain amino acids; 5-HTP (5-hydroxytryptophan); Food and Drug Administration; Iron; Kava; Policosanol; SAMe; Traditional Chinese herbal medicine; Supplements: Introduction; Vitamin B$_6$.

Licensing and certification of CAM practitioners

CATEGORY: Issues and overviews

RELATED TERMS: Acupuncture, chiropractic, homeopathy, hypnosis, massage therapy, midwifery, naturopathy, osteopathy

DEFINITION: The regulation of complementary and alternative medicine practice through licensing and certification.

REQUIREMENTS FOR PRACTICE

Licensure is a process in which the government reviews and verifies the credentials of a health care practitioner and then grants a license to practice within a given state. Certification is a credential issued by a professional organization that represents a complementary and alternative medicine (CAM) specialty. Persons seeking certification must pass a test of their knowledge of the specialty. Licensing is required to practice, but credentialing may not be.

In the United States, licensure for CAM practitioners is provided by the state in which the person seeks to practice. Licensure most often requires educational credentials and the passing of an examination that demonstrates the practitioner's knowledge. All licensed CAM practitioners are required to complete a specified number of hours of continuing education annually to maintain their licenses. Licensure and certification requirements for CAM practitioners vary with the CAM field. The CAM practices discussed here are chiropractic, acupuncture, homeopathy, osteopathy, naturopathy, midwifery, massage therapy, and hypnosis.

LICENSING

Chiropractors. Chiropractors are licensed by all fifty U.S. states and the District of Columbia. To be licensed, a chiropractor must complete four years of chiropractic education and then must pass the National Board of Chiropractic Examiners examination or a state-prepared examination.

Acupuncturists. Physician acupuncturists, as distinguished from nonphysician acupuncturists, can practice in any state and are, according to the American Academy of Medical Acupuncture, required to have medical training and two hundred hours of acupuncture training. Nonphysician acupuncturists receive different credentials depending on the type of acupuncture training program they attended. A nonphysician acupuncturist can be a certified acupuncturist, a licensed acupuncturist, a diplomate of acupuncture, or a master or doctor of Oriental medicine.

Training in acupuncture takes from two to four years and often includes clinical internships. Licensing of nonphysician acupuncturists varies from state to state. Many states license certified acupuncturists, but a few states have no regulations regarding acupuncture. Some states permit only physician acupuncturists to practice.

Homeopaths. Arizona, Connecticut, and Nevada are the only states that license homeopaths; homeopaths in these states are required to be medical doctors.

Rhode Island, California, and Minnesota permit homeopaths to practice without a license under the new health freedom laws. Homeopaths are not permitted to practice in the remaining states. General homeopathic education lasts four years, but it is shorter for already licensed medical doctors.

Naturopaths. The states of Alaska, Arizona, California, Connecticut, Florida, Hawaii, Idaho, Kansas, Maine, Montana, and New Hampshire, and the District of Columbia, license naturopaths. For licensure, the naturopath must complete four years of naturopathic medical college and pass the Naturopathic Physicians Licensing Examination. Several of these states also require that naturopaths be qualified to practice natural childbirth or acupuncture or to dispense natural substances. In Tennessee and South Carolina, practicing naturopathy is illegal. The remaining states do not license naturopaths and do not permit them to practice.

Osteopaths. Osteopaths are licensed as medical doctors in all U.S. states. Medical licensure requires graduation from an accredited medical or osteopathic school, an internship and residency, and, possibly, a fellowship in a specialty. In addition, they must pass either the U.S. Medical Licensing Exam or the Comprehensive Osteopathic Medical Licensing Exam.

Massage therapists. Massage therapists are licensed in thirty-seven U.S. states and the District of Columbia. The requirements for licensure vary from state to state, but many states require that massage therapists pass an examination and be certified.

Midwives. Midwives can be either nurse-midwives or non-nurse midwives. Most midwives in the United States are nurse-midwives. Non-nurse midwives are permitted to practice only in a few states (such as Arizona). Non-nurse midwives can attend a midwifery school and then serve as an apprentice to a licensed midwife. In Arizona, they must pass a state examination. Nurse-midwives must have a bachelor's degree in nursing and a master's degree in nursing with a concentration in midwifery. They must pass a nurse licensing examination and an advanced-practice nursing examination, then must work as an intern or apprentice for about two years in an emergency room, clinic, hospital, or obstetrician's office. To be licensed, nurse-midwives must pass the American Midwifery Certification Board exam.

Hypnotists. The states of Colorado, Connecticut, Indiana, and Washington require licensure for hypnotists. Each state has its own criteria for licensing. Indiana has an educational requirement for licensing, but the other three states do not. Some of the remaining states have regulations regarding the practice of hypnosis; others require that the hypnotist have other medical credentials; and others treat hypnotists as business persons and require no credentialing.

CERTIFICATION

No formal certification process exists for chiropractors. Nonphysician acupuncturists have to be certified to be licensed, but physician acupuncturists do not. To be certified, nonphysician acupuncturists must pass the National Certification Commission of Acupuncture and Oriental Medicine examination.

Medical doctors and osteopaths who become homeopaths can be certified by the American Board of Homeotherapeutics. They must be educated in homeopathy and must pass oral and written examinations. Nonphysician homeopaths can achieve certification by passing the examination of the Council for Homeopathic Certification. This credential is not required for state licensure.

Naturopaths do not have a certification process. Osteopaths can become board certified in their specialty, but it is not required for licensing. Massage therapists must be certified to practice. They can become certified by passing the Federation of State Massage Therapy Boards examination or by passing one of the National Certification Examination for Therapeutic Massage and Bodywork examinations.

A certification process exists for hypnotists, but it is not required for state licensure. The American Council of Hypnotist Examiners certifies hypnotists who pass its examination. Nurse-midwives must be certified to be licensed. Non-nurse midwives may become certified by the North American Registry of Midwives after completing their education.

Christine M. Carroll, R.N., M.B.A., B.S.N.

FURTHER READING

Arizona Department of Health Services. "Midwife Licensing Program: News and Updates." Available at http://www.azdhs.gov/als/midwife. A summary of Arizona law on the licensing of midwives.

Chiroweb. "Licensure and Legal Scope of Practice." Available at http://www.chirowweb.com/archives/ahcpr/chapter5.htm. Discusses the state licensing of chiropractors in the United States.

Tierney, Gillian. *Opportunities in Holistic Health Care Careers.* Rev. ed. New York: McGraw-Hill, 2007. This book addresses the job outlook, educational requirements, regulation, and salaries for many CAM practitioners.

See also: Education and training of CAM practitioners; History of alternative medicine; History of complementary medicine; Integrative medicine; Popular practitioners; Regulation of CAM; Scientific method.

Licorice

RELATED TERMS: Deglycyrrhizinated licorice, *Glycyrrhiza glabra*, licorice root
CATEGORY: Herbs and supplements
DEFINITION: Natural plant product used to treat specific health conditions.
PRINCIPAL PROPOSED USES: None
OTHER PROPOSED USES: Asthma, chronic fatigue syndrome, cough, eczema, heartburn, herpes, mouth sores, psoriasis, ulcers

OVERVIEW

A member of the pea family, licorice root has been used since ancient times both as a food and as a medicine. In Chinese herbology, licorice is an ingredient in nearly all herbal formulas for the traditional purpose of "harmonizing" the separate herbs involved.

The herb licorice contains a substance called glycyrrhizin. When taken in high enough amounts, glycyrrhizin produces effects similar to those of the natural hormone aldosterone, causing fluid retention, increased blood pressure, and loss of potassium. To prevent this, manufacturers have found a way to remove glycyrrhizin from licorice, producing the safer product deglycyrrhizinated licorice (DGL).

THERAPEUTIC DOSAGES

For supportive treatment of ulcer pain along with conventional medical care, the standard dose is two to four 380-milligram (mg) tablets of DGL taken before meals and at bedtime. The same tablets can be allowed to slowly dissolve in the mouth for possible relief from the pain of mouth sores.

A typical dose of whole licorice is 5 to 15 grams (g) daily. However, experts recommend against the use of doses this high for more than a few weeks. For long-term consumption, about 0.3 g of licorice root daily should be safe for most adults. Persons who wish to take a higher dose should do so only under the supervision of a physician. For the treatment of eczema, psoriasis, or herpes, 2 percent licorice gel or cream is applied twice daily to the affected area.

THERAPEUTIC USES

DGL has shown some promise for the treatment of ulcers. Weak evidence hints that it might also help prevent ulcers caused by anti-inflammatory drugs.

Licorice, in the form of a dissolving patch, is also sometimes recommended for relieving the discomfort of canker sores and other mouth sores.

Creams containing whole licorice (often combined with chamomile extract) are advocated for a variety of skin diseases, including eczema, psoriasis, and herpes, but there is supporting evidence for only the first of these uses. Whole licorice, not DGL, is used as an expectorant for respiratory problems such as coughs and asthma.

Licorice has been suggested as a treatment for chronic fatigue syndrome (CFS), based on the observation that people with CFS appear to suffer from low levels of certain adrenal hormones. The glycyrrhizin portion of licorice may relieve symptoms by mimicking the effects of these hormones. However, this is a dangerous approach to treatment that should be tried only under medical supervision. In addition, studies of drugs that even more closely imitate adrenal hormones have not found benefit.

Licorice extracts are used intravenously in Japan for treatment of viral hepatitis. However, there is no definite evidence that this treatment is effective; even if this were established, it would not imply that oral licorice would have a similar effect. Furthermore, the high dosages used for treatment of chronic hepatitis may cause an elevation of blood pressure and other serious medical problems. One should not inject preparations of licorice designed for oral use.

SCIENTIFIC EVIDENCE

Eczema. Creams containing whole licorice (often combined with extract of chamomile) are in wide use as "natural" hydrocortisone creams. However, only preliminary supporting evidence exists for this use. In one double-blind, placebo-controlled trial of thirty people, licorice gel at 2 percent was more effective

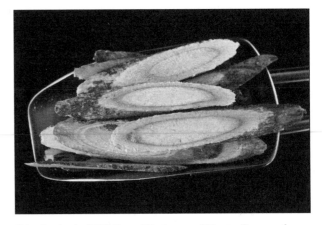

Licorice bark. (TH Foto-Werbung / Photo Researchers, Inc.)

than placebo or 1 percent gel for reducing symptoms of eczema.

Licorice has constituents that increase the activity of naturally occurring (or artificially supplied) corticosteroids, and this might explain some of the benefits seen. In addition, licorice contains licochalcone A, a substance hypothesized to have anti-inflammatory effects.

Ulcer treatment. Two controlled studies suggest that regular use of DGL in a combination product also containing antacids can heal ulcers as effectively as drugs in the Zantac family. These studies, however, do not prove that DGL was effective; antacids themselves can help heal ulcers, and in any case the studies were not double-blind.

Furthermore, if it does work, DGL would have to be taken continuously to avoid ulcer recurrence. In some cases, drug treatment can prevent the recurrence of ulcers permanently by eradicating the bacterium *Helicobacter pylori*, which is thought to cause some ulcers. There is no evidence that DGL can do the same.

Ulcer prevention. A preliminary study suggests that DGL might help prevent ulcers caused by aspirin and related medications, such as ibuprofen.

SAFETY ISSUES

The use of whole licorice has not been associated with significant adverse effects in the short term. However, two or more weeks of use may cause high blood pressure, fluid retention, and symptoms related to loss of potassium. Such effects are especially dangerous for people who take the drug digoxin or medications that deplete the body of potassium (such as thiazide and loop diuretics) or who have high blood pressure, heart disease, diabetes, or kidney disease.

Current evidence indicates that persons who wish to take whole licorice on a long-term basis without any risk of these side effects should not consume more than 0.2 mg of glycyrrhizin per kilogram of body weight daily. For a person who weighs 130 pounds, this works out to 12 mg of glycyrrhizin daily. Based on a typical 4 percent glycyrrhizin content, this is the equivalent of 0.3 grams of licorice root.

Whole licorice may have other side effects as well. For example, it appears to reduce testosterone levels in men. For this reason, men with impotence, infertility, or decreased libido may wish to avoid this herb. Licorice may also increase both the positive and negative effects of corticosteroids such as prednisone and hydrocortisone cream. In addition, some evidence suggests that licorice might affect the liver's ability to metabolize other medications, but the extent of this effect has not been fully determined.

Whole licorice possesses significant estrogenic activity, and some evidence indicates that licorice increases the risk of premature birth. For these reasons, it should not be taken by pregnant or nursing women or by women who have had breast cancer. Maximum safe doses for young children, nursing women, and those with severe liver or kidney disease have not been established.

It is believed, but not proven, that most or all of the major side effects of licorice are caused by glycyrrhizin. For this reason, DGL has been described as entirely safe. However, comprehensive safety studies on DGL have not been reported.

IMPORTANT INTERACTIONS

Persons taking digoxin should note that the long-term use of licorice can be dangerous. Persons taking thiazide or loop diuretics should note that the use of licorice might lead to excessive potassium loss. Persons undergoing corticosteroid treatment should note that licorice could increase both its negative and its positive effects. One should not take licorice internally if using corticosteroids.

Finally, persons taking aspirin or other anti-inflammatory drugs should note that the regular use of DGL might help lower the risk of ulcers.

Reviewed by EBSCO CAM Review Board

FURTHER READING

Lin, S. H., and T. Chau. "A Puzzling Cause of Hypokalaemia." *The Lancet* 360 (2002): 224.

Martin, M. D., et al. "A Controlled Trial of a Dissolving Oral Patch Concerning Glycyrrhiza (Licorice) Herbal Extract for the Treatment of Aphthous Ulcers." *General Dentistry* 56 (2008): 206-210.

Saeedi, M., et al. "The Treatment of Atopic Dermatitis with Licorice Gel." *Journal of Dermatological Treatment* 14 (2003): 153-157.

Somjen, D., et al. "Estrogen-Like Activity of Licorice Root Constituents, Glabridin and Glabrene, in Vascular Tissues In Vitro and In Vivo." *Journal of Steroid Biochemistry and Molecular Biology* 91 (2004): 147-155.

Strandberg, T. E., et al. "Preterm Birth and Licorice Consumption During Pregnancy." *American Journal of Epidemiology* 156 (2002): 803-805.

See also: Chronic fatigue syndrome; Cough; Eczema; Gastroesophageal reflux disease; Herbal medicine; Herpes; Psoriasis; Ulcers.

Life extension

CATEGORY: Therapies and techniques

RELATED TERMS: Antiaging medicine, biomedical gerontology, experimental gerontology

DEFINITION: Slowing the aging process and increasing the human lifespan through medicine, science, technology, and spirituality.

PRINCIPAL PROPOSED USES: Acquired immune deficiency syndrome, Alzheimer's disease, arthritis, cancer, cardiovascular disease, dementia, diabetes, fibromyalgia, leukemia, liver disease, lung disease, lupus, lymphoma, memory enhancement, multiple sclerosis, osteoporosis, Parkinson's disease, stroke

OTHER PROPOSED USES: Elderly revitalization, hearing enhancement, increased mobility, sexual potency, skin rejuvenation, sleep enhancement, vision enhancement

OVERVIEW

In 1980, when Saul Kent wrote a book entitled *The Life Extension Revolution* and established the nonprofit nutritional supplement organization the Life Extension Foundation, the term "life extension" came into worldwide prominence. Life extension primarily involves supporting the body's natural immune system, using various supplements and hormones that aid the body in delaying aging. Supplements are often combined with other forms of alternative medicine, such as meditation and yoga, to decrease stress, a major contributor in aging. Calorie-restricting plans, nanotechnology, cellular engineering, cryogenics, and cloning are more experimental versions of life extension.

MECHANISM OF ACTION

The primary benefit of life extension is to elevate the levels of vitamins or hormones that are already present in the human body by using supplements, because during aging, levels of vitamins and hormones drop sharply. Life expectancy today is eighty, up thirty years since 1900 (when life expectancy was fifty), so modern "seniors" seek to look, feel, and act younger longer. To achieve more youthful-appearing skin and sharper mental acuity, as well as greater sexual potency and more energy, many are using nutritional supplements to increase antioxidants in the body, which combat free radicals, agents of aging. Furthermore, the repletion of hormones to their younger levels helps turn back the clock.

USES AND APPLICATIONS

Numerous supplements and hormones are specifically used in life extension to combat aging: Pregnenolone hormone is used to bolster memory and mental clarity; dehydroepiandrosterone (DHEA) hormone is used to boost energy and vitality; testosterone hormone is used to increase sex drive in both males and females; estrogen and proestrogen hormones are used by women to increase sexuality and mental acuity and to counter the negative effects of menopause. The hormone melatonin is used to aid sleep, reduce fatigue, and help fight against degenerative diseases. In addition to hormones, various vitamin and nutrient supplements are also extremely important in life extension therapy: Lipoic acid and green tea extract are both powerful antioxidants that help protect the body from age and disease. Along with aspirin, vitamins B_6 and B_{12}, folic acid, and fish oil are all daily supplements recommended by life extension specialists for decreasing heart disease. Coenzyme Q_{10} and the amino acids carnosine and acetyl-L-carnitine, taken daily, boost energy.

SCIENTIFIC EVIDENCE

Since the 1930s, several hundred studies have shown that severe calorie restriction doubles the life span of mice, and many postulate that it lengthens the life span of humans as well, although there are no double-blind, placebo studies to prove that claim. Severe calorie restriction, without nutritional deficiency, does, however, drastically lower sugar and fat intake, resulting in less diabetes, stroke, and cardiovascular disease.

The most stunning scientific evidence to support life extension theory grew out of research for which American scientists were awarded the 2009 Nobel Prize in Physiology and Medicine. These studies proved that telomeres, the protective end caps for human chromosomes, may be healed and regenerated. Since aging is caused by chromosomal DNA material lost during repeated cell division (because of deteriorated telomere sheaths) being able to control telomeres makes it possible to control chromosomal deterioration and therefore aging. As a result, scientists in the laboratory can now take old, gray, sick mice that are unable to walk, genetically engineer their telomeres, and within only a few short weeks transform them into youthful, vibrant, running mice with sleek black fur. Scientists worldwide are hailing the discovery of telomeres and techniques used to genetically engineer them as the single greatest scientific advancement for expanding the human life span in history. Although current telomere experiments have been used in the laboratory only on mice, rabbits, frogs, and monkeys, scientists see no reason to believe that telomere research will not work equally well with humans. Hence, telomeres are being described in scientific circles as the newly discovered fountain of youth.

CHOOSING A PRACTITIONER

A licensed medical doctor, particularly a nutritionist who specializes in antiaging medicine, is the best choice for a life extension practitioner. The American Medical Association is the preeminent source for nutritional and antiaging physician referrals.

SAFETY ISSUES

Those taking prescription drugs should avoid taking any supplements unless approved by a licensed physician, to avoid adverse pharmaceutical effects or allergic reactions. Overdosing on supplements and hormones is also a great danger in life extension therapy.

For years, for example, it was thought that the more vitamin C consumed, the better, and many, particularly athletes, took massive doses of vitamin C daily. New scientific studies eventually demonstrated that huge doses of vitamin C taken daily, over a long time, actually decrease life span, resulting in a greater incidence of stroke. The key to taking life extension supplements and hormones is to consume them in moderation.

Mary E. Markland, M.A.

FURTHER READING

Fossel, M., et al. *The Immortality Edge: Realize the Secrets of Your Telomeres for a Longer, Healthier Life.* Hoboken, N.J.: John Wiley & Sons, 2011.

Ikeler, D. *Life Extension.* Seattle: Classic Day, 2008.

Maher, D., and Calvin Mercer. *Religion and the Implications of Radical Life Extension.* New York: Palgrave Macmillan, 2009.

Miller, Phillip, and Monica Reinagel. *The Life Extension Revolution: The New Science of Growing Older Without Aging.* New York: Bantam Books, 2006.

Tandy, Charles, Robin Hanson, and R. Michael Perry. *Doctor Tandy's First Guide to Life Extension and Transhumanity.* Palo Alto, Calif.: Ria University Press, 2001.

See also: Alzheimer's disease; Cancer risk reduction; Diabetes; Fibromyalgia: Homeopathic remedies; Liver disease; Lupus; Multiple sclerosis; Osteoporosis; Parkinson's disease; Strokes.

Lignans

CATEGORY: Functional foods
DEFINITION: Natural substance promoted as a dietary supplement for specific health benefits.
PRINCIPAL PROPOSED USES: None
OTHER PROPOSED USES: Cancer prevention, elevated cholesterol, kidney disease, menopausal symptoms

OVERVIEW

Lignans are naturally occurring chemicals widespread within the plant and animal kingdoms. Several lignans, with intimidating names such as secoisolariciresinol, are considered to be phytoestrogens, plant chemicals that mimic the hormone estrogen. Phytoestrogens are especially abundant in flaxseed and sesame seeds. Bacteria in the intestines convert the naturally occurring phytoestrogens from flaxseed into two other lignans, enterolactone and enterodiol, which also have estrogen-like effects. "Lignans" here refers to these two specific lignans and to the phytoestrogen kind, but not to the wide variety of other lignans.

Lignans are being studied for possible use in cancer prevention, particularly breast cancer. Like other phytoestrogens (such as soy isoflavones), they hook onto the same spots on cells where estrogen attaches. If there is little estrogen in the body (after menopause, for example), lignans may act like weak estrogen; but when natural estrogen is abundant in the body, lignans may instead reduce estrogen's effects by displacing it from cells. This displacement of the hormone may help prevent those cancers, such as breast cancer, that depend on estrogen to start and develop. In addition, at least one test-tube study suggests that lignans may help prevent cancer in ways that are unrelated to estrogen.

SOURCES

The richest source of lignans is flaxseed (sometimes called linseed), containing more than one hundred times the amount found in other foods. Flaxseed oil, however, does not contain appreciable amounts of lignans. Sesame seed is an equally rich source. Other food sources are pumpkin seeds, whole grains, cranberries, and black and green tea.

THERAPEUTIC DOSAGES

Effective dosages of purified lignans have not been determined. In studies of flaxseed as a source of lignans, flaxseed has been taken at a dose of 5 to 38 grams (g) daily. Cooking flaxseed apparently does not decrease the amount of lignans absorbed by the body.

THERAPEUTIC USES

A number of preliminary human and animal studies suggest that lignans may be helpful for cancer prevention, particularly of breast and colon cancer, and for the reduction of cholesterol. Other preliminary research suggests that flaxseed or lignans may decrease menopausal symptoms and improve kidney function in various types of kidney disease (specifically, lupus nephritis and polycystic kidney disease).

Flaxseed or other treatments for kidney disease should be taken only under a doctor's supervision because of the serious nature of these disorders. Despite positive preliminary results in animal studies, studies in humans have yielded mixed results for improving cholesterol levels.

Scientific Evidence

The most promising use for lignans is in cancer prevention. According to observational studies, people who eat more lignan-containing foods have a lower incidence of breast and perhaps colon cancer. This, however, does not prove that lignans are the cause of the benefit, for other factors in these foods, or in the characteristics of the people who consume these foods, may have been responsible. Double-blind, placebo-controlled studies are necessary to prove that a medical treatment provides benefits, and none have yet been reported for lignans. Nonetheless, animal studies offer additional support for a potential cancer-preventive or even cancer treatment effect.

Several studies showed that lignan-rich foods or lignans found in flax inhibited breast and colon cancer in animals and reduced metastases from melanoma (a type of skin cancer) in mice. Test-tube studies have found that flaxseed or one of its lignans inhibited the growth of human breast cancer cells and that the lignans enterolactone and enterodiol inhibited the growth of human colon tumor cells.

In many of these studies, it is not clear whether lignans are responsible for the benefit seen, because flaxseed contains many other substances. Animal and human studies have begun to examine specific lignans, and results seem to confirm that some of the positive effects probably come from the lignans themselves. Still, until more and better-designed trials are done, the precise effects of lignans on the human body, or the precise dose needed to prevent cancer, is not known.

Safety Issues

Women who are pregnant or breast-feeding should avoid high intake of flaxseed or purified lignans. One study found that pregnant rats who ate large amounts of flaxseed (5 or 10 percent of their diet), or a purified lignan present in flaxseed, gave birth to offspring with altered reproductive organs and functions, and that lignans were also transferred to the baby rats during nursing. In humans, eating 25 g of flaxseed per day amounts to about 5 percent of the diet.

High intake of lignans may not be safe for women with a history of estrogen-sensitive cancer, such as breast cancer or uterine cancer. A few test-tube studies suggest that certain cancer cells can be stimulated by lignans such as those present in flaxseed. Other studies found that lignans inhibit cancer cell growth. As with estrogen, lignans' positive or negative effects on cancer cells may depend on dose, type of cancer cell, and levels of hormones in the body. Persons with a history of cancer, particularly breast cancer, should consult a doctor before consuming large amounts of flaxseed.

EBSCO CAM Review Board

Further Reading

Coulman, K. D., et al. "Whole Sesame Seed Is as Rich a Source of Mammalian Lignan Precursors as Whole Flaxseed." *Nutrition and Cancer* 52 (2005): 156-165.

Hallund, J., et al. "A Lignan Complex Isolated from Flaxseed Does Not Affect Plasma Lipid Concentrations or Antioxidant Capacity in Healthy Postmenopausal Women." *Journal of Nutrition* 136 (2005): 112-116.

Hutchins, A. M., et al. "Flaxseed Consumption Influences Endogenous Hormone Concentrations in Postmenopausal Women." *Nutrition and Cancer* 39 (2001): 58-65.

Zhang, W., et al. "Dietary Flaxseed Lignan Extract Lowers Plasma Cholesterol and Glucose Concentrations in Hypercholesterolaemic Subjects." *British Journal of Nutrition* 99 (2008): 1301-1309.

See also: Cancer risk reduction; Cholesterol, high; Flaxseed; Functional foods: Introduction; Menopause.

Ligustrum

Related terms: Erzhi Wan, glossy privet tree, *Ligustrum lucidum*

Category: Herbs and supplements

Definition: Natural plant product used to treat specific health conditions.

Principal proposed use: Immune support

Other proposed uses: Cancer prevention, cancer treatment support, human immunodeficiency virus infection support, liver protection

Overview

The berries of the glossy privet tree *Ligustrum lucidum* have a long history of use in traditional Chinese herbal medicine as an herb that helps "tonify the yin." This expression cannot be fully explained without entering into the theoretical framework of traditional Chinese medicine, but it may be said loosely to indicate a strengthening effect on some of the functions of the body. As part of herbal combinations (traditional Chinese herbal medicine seldom uses single-herb preparations), ligustrum is used for such purposes as turning gray hair black, alleviating ringing in the ear, and treating vertigo.

One of the most famous combination therapies containing ligustrum is named Erzhi Wan, or "Two-Solstices Pill." It consists of ligustrum berries harvested at the winter solstice, combined with another herb (*Eclipta alba*) harvested at the summer solstice. The combined treatment is thought to provide a balance of two opposite "energies."

Therapeutic Dosages

A typical dose of ligustrum berries is 5 milligrams taken two or three times daily.

Therapeutic Uses

Ligustrum is marketed as a treatment for strengthening the immune system and, on this basis, is often recommended for use by people undergoing treatment for cancer or human immunodeficiency virus infection. However, there is no meaningful scientific

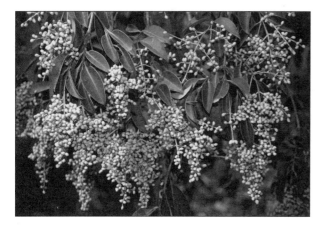

Berries on a ligustrum tree. (Pam Collins/Photo Researchers, Inc.)

evidence that ligustrum provides any benefit for these, or any other, conditions.

Weak evidence from test-tube and animal studies hints that ligustrum might have antiparasitic, antiviral, liver-protective, immunomodulatory (alters immune function), and cancer-preventive effects. However, this evidence is too preliminary to rely upon. Only double-blind, placebo-controlled studies can prove a treatment effective, and none have been performed on ligustrum.

Safety Issues

Although the use of ligustrum appears to be well tolerated in general, the herb has not undergone any meaningful safety evaluation at the level of modern scientific standards. Safety in young children, pregnant or nursing women, and people with severe liver or kidney disease is definitely not established.

Reviewed by EBSCO CAM Review Board

Further Reading

Baronikova, S., et al. "Changes in Immunomodulatory Activity of Human Mononuclear Cells After Cultivation with Leaf Decoctions from the Genus *Ligustrum* L." *Phytotherapy Research* 13 (1999): 692-695.

Lirussi, D., et al. "Inhibition of *Trypanosoma cruzi* by Plant Extracts Used in Chinese Medicine." *Fitoterapia* 75 (2004): 718-723.

Ma, S. C., et al. "In Vitro Evaluation of Secoiridoid Glucosides from the Fruits of *Ligustrum lucidum* as Antiviral Agents." *Chemical and Pharmaceutical Bulletin* 49 (2001): 1471-1473.

See also: Cancer treatment support; Herbal medicine; HIV/AIDS support; Immune support; Liver disease; Traditional Chinese herbal medicine.

Linden

Related terms: Lime flower, linden flower, *Tilia cordata, T. platyphyllos*

Category: Herbs and supplements

Definition: Natural plant product used to treat specific health conditions.

Principal proposed use: Common cold

OTHER PROPOSED USES: Anxiety, dyspepsia, insomnia, liver protection, viral hepatitis

OVERVIEW

Linden flowers have a pleasant, tangy taste, and for this reason the tree is sometimes called lime flower. Besides use in beverages and liqueurs, linden flower has a long history of medicinal use for such conditions as colds and flu, digestive distress, anxiety, migraine headaches, and insomnia. The wood of the linden tree has been used for liver problems, kidney stones, and gout.

THERAPEUTIC DOSAGES

Linden flower is usually taken at a dose of 2 to 4 grams (g) daily, often as tea. A daily dose of linden wood is prepared by boiling 15 to 40 g in water for several hours.

THERAPEUTIC USES

Linden flower has been approved by Germany's Commission E for the treatment of cold symptoms. However, there is no meaningful evidence that it is helpful for this purpose. Linden is said to promote sweating, and this in turn has long been presumed to be helpful for people with colds; however, there is no meaningful evidence that sweating helps colds or that linden promotes sweating.

Other proposed uses of linden also lack scientific support. Two preliminary studies that evaluated linden flower for potential sedative or antianxiety effects returned contradictory results. Weak evidence hints that linden flower might help reduce symptoms of digestive upset and protect the liver from toxins. One preliminary study found possible anti-inflammatory and pain-relieving effects with linden leaf. However, none of this research approaches the level of meaningful evidence. Only double-blind, placebo-controlled studies can show a treatment effective, and none have been performed on linden.

Other proposed benefits of linden that lack any meaningful supporting evidence include the claims that linden flower reduces blood pressure, prevents blood clots, and decreases risk of stroke or heart attack, and that linden bark can treat viral hepatitis.

SAFETY ISSUES

Linden is widely believed to be a safe herb, but it has not undergone comprehensive safety testing. Numerous texts state that when taken in high doses, linden can be toxic to the heart, but this appears to have been a case of authors quoting one another for decades in succession; the original source of this concern is unclear. Safety in young children, pregnant or nursing women, and people with severe liver or kidney disease has not been established.

Reviewed by EBSCO CAM Review Board

FURTHER READING

Coleta, M., et al. "Comparative Evaluation of *Melissa officinalis* L., *Tilia europaea* L., *Passiflora edulis* Sims., and *Hypericum perforatum* L. in the Elevated plus Maze Anxiety Test." *Pharmacopsychiatry* 34 (2001): S20-S21.

Matsuda, H., et al. "Hepatoprotective Principles from the Flowers of *Tilia argentea* (Linden): Structure Requirements of Tiliroside and Mechanisms of Action." *Bioorganic and Medicinal Chemistry* 10 (2002): 707-712.

Toker, G., et al. "Flavonoids with Antinociceptive and Anti-inflammatory Activities from the Leaves of *Tilia argentea* (Silver Linden)." *Journal of Ethnopharmacology* 95 (2004): 393-397.

See also: Colds and flu; Common cold: Homeopathic remedies; Herbal medicine.

Lipoic acid

CATEGORY: Herbs and supplements
RELATED TERMS: Alpha-lipoic acid, thioctic acid
DEFINITION: Essential natural substance used as a dietary supplement for specific health benefits.
PRINCIPAL PROPOSED USE: Diabetic neuropathy (peripheral neuropathy and cardiac autonomic neuropathy)
OTHER PROPOSED USES: Burning mouth syndrome, cancer prevention, cataract prevention, diabetes (blood sugar control), glaucoma, heart disease prevention, liver disease, migraine headaches, sun-damaged skin

OVERVIEW

Lipoic acid, also known as alpha-lipoic acid, is a sulfur-containing fatty acid. It is found inside every cell of the body, where it helps generate the energy

Lipoic Acid for Diabetic Neuropathies

Proponents of the use of lipoic acid believe that this natural substance can help prevent nerve cell damage in persons with diabetic neuropathies. Diabetic neuropathies are peripheral nerve disorders caused by diabetes or poor blood sugar control.

The most common types of diabetic neuropathy result in problems with sensation in the feet, a condition that can develop early in the disease or slowly after many years of diabetes. The symptoms include numbness, pain, or tingling in the feet or lower legs. The pain can be intense and require treatment to relieve the discomfort. The loss of sensation in the feet may also increase the possibility that foot injuries will go unnoticed and develop into ulcers or lesions that become infected. In some cases, diabetic neuropathy can be associated with difficulty walking and some weakness in the foot muscles.

Other types of diabetic-related neuropathies affect specific parts of the body. For example, diabetic amyotrophy causes pain, weakness and wasting of the thigh muscles, or cranial nerve infarcts that may result in double vision, a drooping eyelid, or dizziness. Diabetes can also affect the autonomic nerves that control blood pressure, the digestive tract, bladder function, and sexual organs. Problems with the autonomic nerves may cause lightheadedness, indigestion, diarrhea or constipation, difficulty with bladder control, and impotence.

that keeps humans alive and functioning. Lipoic acid is a key part of the metabolic machinery that turns glucose (blood sugar) into energy for the body's needs.

Lipoic acid is an antioxidant, which means that it neutralizes naturally occurring but harmful chemicals known as free radicals. Unlike other antioxidants, which work only in water or fatty tissues, lipoic acid is unusual in that it functions in both water and fat. By comparison, vitamin E works only in fat, and vitamin C works only in water. This gives lipoic acid an unusually broad spectrum of antioxidant action.

Lipoic acid also may help regenerate other antioxidants that have been used up. In addition, lipoic acid may be able to do the work of other antioxidants when the body is deficient in them.

It is thought that certain nerve diseases are at least partially caused by damaging free radicals. Because

of its combined fat and water solubility, lipoic acid can get into all the parts of a nerve cell and potentially protect it against such damage. This is the rationale for studies on the potential benefits of lipoic acid for diabetic neuropathy.

SOURCES

A healthy body makes enough lipoic acid to supply its requirements; external sources are not necessary. However, several medical conditions appear to be accompanied by low levels of lipoic acid (specifically diabetes, liver cirrhosis, and atherosclerosis), which suggests (but does not prove) that supplementation would be helpful. Liver and yeast contain some lipoic acid. Nonetheless, supplements are necessary to obtain therapeutic dosages.

THERAPEUTIC DOSAGES

The typical dosage of oral lipoic acid for treating complications of diabetes is 100 to 200 milligrams (mg) three times daily. In studies that found benefits, several weeks of treatment were often necessary for full effects to develop.

For use as a general antioxidant, a lower dosage of 20 to 50 mg daily is commonly recommended, although there is no evidence that taking lipoic acid in this way offers any health benefit.

THERAPEUTIC USES

Lipoic acid has been widely used for decades in Germany to treat diabetic peripheral neuropathy. This is a condition caused by diabetes in which nerves leading to the arms and legs become damaged, resulting in numbness, pain, and other symptoms. Free radicals are hypothesized to play a role in neuropathy, and on this basis, lipoic acid has been tried as a treatment. However, the evidence for benefit is largely limited to studies that used the intravenous form of this supplement.

Another set of nerves also may become damaged in diabetes: the autonomic nerves that control internal organs. When this occurs in the heart (cardiac autonomic neuropathy), it leads to irregularities of heart rhythm. There is some evidence that lipoic acid supplements may be helpful for this condition.

Preliminary and sometimes contradictory evidence suggests that lipoic acid may improve other aspects of diabetes, including blood sugar control and the development of long-term complications, such as diseases of the heart, kidneys, and small blood vessels.

Mixed evidence exists for the benefits of lipoic acid in the treatment of burning mouth syndrome, a condition characterized by unexplained scalding sensations in the mouth. Weak evidence hints that use of lipoic acid might help prevent migraine headaches. A cream containing 5 percent lipoic acid has shown promise for the treatment of sun-damaged skin.

One animal study suggests that lipoic acid might help prevent age-related hearing loss. Similarly weak evidence hints that lipoic acid might be helpful for glaucoma and for reducing the side effects (specifically, cardiac toxicity) of the cancer chemotherapy drug doxorubicin. Other uses for which lipoic acid has been proposed include preventing cancer and heart disease and treating or preventing cataracts.

SCIENTIFIC EVIDENCE

Diabetic peripheral neuropathy. There is some evidence that intravenous lipoic acid can reduce symptoms of diabetic peripheral neuropathy, at least in the short term. However, the evidence for oral lipoic acid remains weak and contradictory.

For example, a double-blind, placebo-controlled study of five hundred people with diabetic neuropathy found that intravenous lipoic acid helped reduce symptoms over a three-week period; however, long-term oral supplementation did not prove effective.

Benefits were seen with oral lipoic acid in a study published in 2006. In this double-blind, placebo-controlled trial, 181 people with diabetic peripheral neuropathy were given either placebo or one of three doses of lipoic acid: 600, 1,200, or 1,800 mg daily. Over the five-week study period, benefits were seen in all three lipoic acid groups compared with the placebo group.

While this outcome may sound promising, one feature of the results tends to reduce the faith one can put in them: the absence of a dose-related effect. Ordinarily, when a treatment is effective, higher doses produce relatively better results. When such a spectrum of outcomes is not observed, the study becomes questionable. Other than this one study, the positive evidence for oral lipoic acid in diabetic peripheral neuropathy is limited to open studies of minimal to no validity and double-blind trials too small to be relied upon. There is some preliminary evidence that lipoic acid could be more effective if it were combined with gamma-linolenic acid, another supplement used for diabetic peripheral neuropathy.

Diabetic autonomic neuropathy. There is better evidence for oral lipoic acid in a form of diabetic neuropathy affecting the nerves that supply the heart: autonomic neuropathy. Not only does diabetes damage the nerves in the arms and legs; it can also affect deep nerves that control organs such as the heart and digestive tract.

The Deutsche Kardiale Autonome Neuropathie study followed seventy-three people with diabetes who had symptoms caused by nerve damage affecting the heart. Treatment with 800 mg daily of oral lipoic acid showed statistically significant improvement compared with placebo and caused no significant side effects.

Burning mouth syndrome. Persons with burning mouth syndrome (BMS) feel chronic scalding pain in the mouth, as if they had consumed an excessively hot drink. Although the cause of BMS is not known, the symptoms resemble those of neuropathy, and for that reason, researchers have investigated the potential benefits of lipoic acid.

In a two-month, double-blind trial involving sixty people with BMS, the use of lipoic acid significantly reduced symptoms, compared with placebo. However, three small double-blind trials failed to find any benefit for lipoic acid.

SAFETY ISSUES

Lipoic acid appears to have no significant side effects at dosages up to 1,800 mg daily. Safety for young children, women who are pregnant or nursing, and those with severe liver or kidney disease has not been established.

EBSCO CAM Review Board

FURTHER READING
Carbone, M., et al. "Lack of Efficacy of Alpha-Lipoic Acid in Burning Mouth Syndrome." *European Journal of Pain* 13, no. 5 (2009): 492-496.
Cavalcanti, D. R., and F. R. da Silveira. "Alpha Lipoic Acid in Burning Mouth Syndrome." *Journal of Oral Pathology and Medicine* 38 (2009): 254-261.
Magis, D., et al. "A Randomized, Double-Blind, Placebo-Controlled Trial of Thioctic Acid in Migraine Prophylaxis." *Headache* 47 (2007): 52-57.
Ziegler, D., et al. "Oral Treatment with Alpha-Lipoic Acid Improves Symptomatic Diabetic Polyneuropathy." *Diabetes Care* 29 (2006): 2365-2370.

See also: Antioxidants; Burning mouth syndrome; Diabetes; Pain management; Supplements: Introduction.

Lithium

CATEGORY: Drug interactions
DEFINITION: Medication used to treat bipolar disorder.
INTERACTIONS: Citrate, herbal diuretic, inositol
TRADE NAMES: Eskalith, Eskalith CR, Lithane, Lithobid, Lithonate, Lithotabs

INOSITOL

Effect: Possible Helpful Interaction

Lithium may cause or exacerbate symptoms of psoriasis. One small, double-blind study found that the use of supplemental inositol may help alleviate this problem.

HERBAL DIURETIC

Effect: Possible Harmful Interaction

The use of lithium as a therapy requires careful attention to lithium levels in the blood. If there is too little lithium, the treatment will not work; if lithium levels get too high, toxicity may result.

One cause of excessively high lithium levels is dehydration. When the amount of water in the blood decreases, lithium levels proportionally rise. For this reason, persons taking lithium are warned that they must be sure to drink sufficient liquids when they are exposed to heat. Diuretic drugs (water pills) can also cause problems, by causing the body to excrete water.

One case report suggests that herbal diuretics can also lead to increased lithium levels. Certain herbs are thought to act as diuretics, including buchu, celery seed, cleavers, corn silk, couch grass, dandelion, goldenrod, gravel root, horsetail, juniper, parsley, rosemary, and wild carrot.

This report noted the case of a twenty-six-year-old woman who had been taking a constant dose of lithium for five months without any problems. When she suddenly developed drowsiness, tremor, unsteadiness in walking, and rapid involuntary movements of the eyes, doctors conducted a laboratory examination and found that her lithium level had skyrocketed. It turned out that a few weeks before this episode she had started taking an herbal weight-loss formula that included numerous herbal diuretics.

Manufacturers frequently add herbal diuretics to weight-loss formulas to cause short-term loss of water weight. This has no value for long-term weight loss, but it does give some immediate sense of success. However, in this case, the herbal diuretics also caused lithium levels to rise.

CITRATE

Effect: Possible Harmful Interaction

Potassium citrate, sodium citrate, and potassium-magnesium citrate are sometimes used to prevent kidney stones. These supplements reduce urinary acidity and can therefore lead to decreased blood levels and effectiveness of lithium.

EBSCO CAM Review Board

FURTHER READING

Allan, S. J., et al. "The Effect of Inositol Supplements on the Psoriasis of Patients Taking Lithium." *British Journal of Dermatology* 150 (2004): 966-969.

Pyevich, D., and M. P. Bogenschutz. "Herbal Diuretics and Lithium Toxicity." *American Journal of Psychiatry* 158 (2001): 1329.

See also: Antidepressants; Depression, mild to moderate; Food and Drug Administration; Inositol; Mental health; SSRIs.

Liver disease

CATEGORY: Condition
RELATED TERMS: Cholestasis, Gilbert's syndrome, liver support, liver-toxic herbs
DEFINITION: Treatment of diseases of the liver.
PRINCIPAL PROPOSED NATURAL TREATMENTS: Milk thistle, S-adenosylmethionine
OTHER PROPOSED NATURAL TREATMENTS: Andrographis, artichoke leaf, beet leaf, betaine (trimethylglycine), choline, dandelion, inositol, lecithin, licorice, lipoic acid, liver extracts, noni, phyllanthus, *Picrorhiza kurroa*, schisandra, sweet potato, taurine, thymus extract, turmeric
HERBS AND SUPPLEMENTS TO BE USED WITH CAUTION: Beta-carotene, blue-green algae, chaparral, coltsfoot, comfrey, germander, germanium, green tea extracts, greater celandine, kava, kombucha, mistletoe, pennyroyal, pokeroot, sassafras, skullcap,

spirulina, traditional Chinese herbal medicine, vitamin A, vitamin B_3

INTRODUCTION

The liver is a sophisticated chemical laboratory, capable of carrying out thousands of chemical transformations on which the body depends. The liver produces important chemicals from scratch, modifies others to allow the body to use them better, and neutralizes an enormous range of toxins. However, this last function of the liver, neutralizing toxins, is also the organ's Achilles' heel. The process of rendering toxins harmless to the body at large may bring harm to the liver itself.

Alcohol is the most common chemical responsible for toxic damage to the liver, causing fatty liver, alcoholic hepatitis, and, potentially, cirrhosis of the liver. Exposure to industrial chemicals may harm the liver. Many prescription medications may damage the liver too, including cholesterol-lowering drugs in the statin family and high-dose niacin (also used to reduce cholesterol levels.) The over-the-counter drug acetaminophen (Tylenol) is highly toxic to the liver when taken to excess. Finally, numerous natural herbs and supplements contain chemicals that may cause or accelerate harm to the liver.

Chemicals are not the only source of harm to the liver. Viruses may infect it, causing viral hepatitis; hepatitis C, in particular, may become chronic and gradually destroy the liver. In addition, during pregnancy, the liver may become backed up with bile, a condition called cholestasis of pregnancy.

Conventional treatment of liver disease depends on the source of the problem. People who abuse alcohol will at the very least avoid further liver damage by stopping alcohol use, and, in cases short of liver cirrhosis, full liver recovery may be expected. When drugs are at fault, it may be possible to switch to a different drug.

Conventional treatment of liver injury caused by chronic viral hepatitis involves sophisticated immune-regulating therapies, which have become fairly successful. In extreme cases of liver injury, a liver transplant may be necessary.

PRINCIPAL PROPOSED NATURAL TREATMENTS

This article examines the herbs and supplements that may harm the liver and that, therefore, should not be taken by people who already have liver disease.

Milk thistle. The herb milk thistle has shown promise for a variety of liver conditions, and for this reason it is often said to have general liver-protective properties. Some evidence suggests benefit for viral hepatitis (especially chronic hepatitis), cirrhosis of the liver, alcoholic hepatitis, and liver toxicity caused by industrial chemicals, mushroom poisons, and medications. However, the evidence that milk thistle works remains incomplete and contradictory.

For example, a double-blind, placebo-controlled study performed in 1981 followed 106 Finnish soldiers with alcoholic liver disease for four weeks. The treated group showed a significant decrease in elevated liver enzymes and improvement in liver histology (appearance of cells under a microscope), as evaluated by biopsy in twenty-nine persons.

Two similar studies provided essentially equivalent results. However, a three-month, randomized, double-blind study of 116 people showed little to no additional benefit, perhaps because most participants reduced their alcohol consumption and almost one-half stopped drinking entirely. Another study found no benefit in seventy-two persons followed for fifteen months.

Study results similarly conflict on whether milk thistle is helpful in liver cirrhosis.

In a double-blind, placebo-controlled study of 170 people with alcoholic or nonalcoholic cirrhosis, researchers found that the four-year survival rate was 58 percent in the group treated with milk thistle, compared to only 38 percent in the placebo group. This difference was statistically significant.

A double-blind, placebo-controlled trial that enrolled 172 people with cirrhosis for four years also found reductions in mortality, but they just missed the conventional cutoff for statistical significance. Another study, a two-year, double-blind, placebo-controlled trial of two hundred people with alcoholic cirrhosis, found no reduction in mortality attributable to the use of milk thistle.

A 2007 review of published and unpublished studies on milk thistle as a treatment for liver disease concluded that benefits were seen only in low-quality trials, and even in those studies, milk thistle did not show more than a slight benefit.

Milk thistle is also used in a vague condition known as minor hepatic insufficiency, or "sluggish liver." This term is mostly used by European physicians and American naturopathic practitioners (conventional

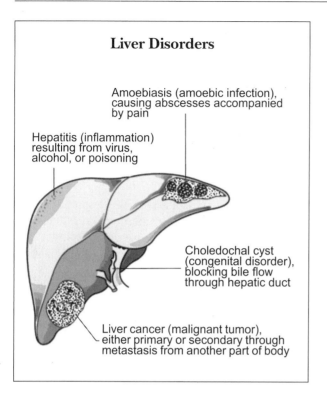

Liver Disorders

Amoebiasis (amoebic infection), causing abscesses accompanied by pain

Hepatitis (inflammation) resulting from virus, alcohol, or poisoning

Choledochal cyst (congenital disorder), blocking bile flow through hepatic duct

Liver cancer (malignant tumor), either primary or secondary through metastasis from another part of body

physicians in the United States do not recognize it). Symptoms reportedly include aching under the ribs, fatigue, unhealthy skin appearance, general malaise, constipation, premenstrual syndrome, chemical sensitivities, and allergies.

S-adenosylmethionine. The body manufactures S-adenosylmethionine (SAMe) for use in converting certain chemicals to other chemicals (specifically, through the processes of transmethylation and trans-sulfuration). Some evidence suggests that SAMe taken as an oral supplement may have value in the treatment of various liver diseases, including chronic viral hepatitis, liver cirrhosis, jaundice of pregnancy, and liver toxicity caused by drugs or chemicals.

Perhaps the best evidence regards cholestasis (backup of bile in the liver) caused by serious liver disease. In a two-week double-blind study of 220 people with cholestasis, the use of SAMe (1,600 milligrams daily) significantly improved liver-related symptoms compared with placebo. Most participants in this study had chronic viral hepatitis.

Another large study evaluated the potential benefits of SAMe for the treatment of people with alcoholic liver cirrhosis. This two-year, double-blind, placebo-controlled study of 117 people failed to find

SAMe helpful for the group as a whole. However, in a subgroup of those with less advanced disease, treatment with SAMe appeared to reduce the number of people who needed a liver transplant, or who died.

Gilbert's syndrome is an unexplained but harmless condition in which levels of bilirubin rise in the body, causing an alarming yellowing of the skin (jaundice). Weak evidence hints that SAMe may help reduce bilirubin levels in this condition.

OTHER PROPOSED NATURAL TREATMENTS

One double-blind study found evidence that a beverage made from sweet potato could improve measures of liver function in people with mild hepatitis of unspecified cause. Preliminary evidence suggests that the supplement betaine (trimethylglycine, not to be confused with betaine hydrochloride) may be helpful for treating fatty liver caused by alcohol and other causes, and also for protecting the liver from toxins in general.

Despite early promise, the herb phyllanthus does not appear to be helpful for viral hepatitis. Green tea has long been considered to play a protective role against liver disease. However, the evidence is unconvincing.

Numerous other herbs and supplements have shown some promise in test-tube studies for protecting the liver. These herbs and supplements include andrographis, artichoke leaf, beet leaf, choline, dandelion, inositol, lecithin, licorice, lipoic acid, liver extracts, *Picrorhiza kurroa*, schisandra, taurine, thymus extract, and turmeric.

Hundreds of other herbs and supplements could be included on this list. However, it is a long way from test-tube studies to effects in people, and none of these treatments should be regarded as having proven or even probable liver-protective properties.

HERBS AND SUPPLEMENTS TO USE WITH CAUTION

Many natural products have the capacity to harm the liver. Furthermore, because of the generally inadequate regulation of dietary supplements, there are real risks that herbal products may contain liver-toxic contaminants even if the actual herbs listed on the label are safe. For this reason, it is recommended that people with liver disease not use medicinal herbs except under the supervision of a physician.

High doses of the supplements beta-carotene and vitamin A are thought to accelerate the progression of alcoholic liver disease in people who abuse alcohol. (Nutritional supplementation at the standard daily requirement level should not cause a problem.) All forms of vitamin B_3, including niacin, niacinamide (nicotinamide), and inositol hexaniacinate, may damage the liver when taken in high doses. (Again, nutritional supplementation at the standard daily requirement level should not cause a problem.)

A great many herbs and supplements have known or suspected liver-toxic properties, including chaparral, coltsfoot, corydalis, comfrey, germander, germanium (a mineral), greater celandine, green tea extract (despite its proposed benefits), kava, kombucha, mistletoe, noni, pennyroyal, pokeroot, sassafras, and various herbs and minerals used in traditional Chinese herbal medicine.

In addition, herbs that are not toxic to the liver in themselves are sometimes adulterated with other herbs of similar appearance that are accidentally harvested in a misapprehension of their identity (for example, germander found in skullcap products). Furthermore, blue-green algae species such as spirulina may at times be contaminated with liver-toxic substances called microcystins, for which no highest safe level is known.

Some articles claim that the herb echinacea is potentially toxic to the liver, but this concern appears to have been based on a misunderstanding of its constituents. Echinacea contains substances in the pyrrolizidine alkaloid family. However, while many pyrrolizidine alkaloids are toxic to the liver, those found in echinacea are not believed to have that property.

Whole valerian contains liver-toxic substances called valepotriates; however, valepotriates are thought to be absent from most commercial valerian products. Case reports suggest that even very high doses of valerian do not harm the liver.

EBSCO CAM Review Board

FURTHER READING

Abdelmalek, M. F., et al. "Betaine, a Promising New Agent for Patients with Nonalcoholic Steatohepatitis." *American Journal of Gastroenterology* 96 (2001): 2711-2717.

Charlton, M. "Branched-Chain Amino Acid Enriched Supplements as Therapy for Liver Disease." *Journal of Nutrition* 136 (2005): 295S-298S.

Jin, X., R. H. Zheng, and Y. M. Li. "Green Tea Consumption and Liver Disease." *Liver International* 28 (2008): 990-996.

Rambaldi, A., and C. Gluud. "S-adenosyl-l-methionine for Alcoholic Liver Diseases." *Cochrane Database of Systematic Reviews* (2001): CD002235. Available through *EBSCO DynaMed Systematic Literature Surveillance* at http://www.ebscohost.com/dynamed.

Rambaldi, A., B. Jacobs, and C. Gluud. "Milk Thistle for Alcoholic and/or Hepatitis B or C Virus Liver Diseases." *Cochrane Database of Systematic Reviews* (2007): CD003620. Available through *EBSCO DynaMed Systematic Literature Surveillance* at http://www.ebscohost.com/dynamed.

Suda, I., et al. "Intake of Purple Sweet Potato Beverage Effects on Serum Hepatic Biomarker Levels of Healthy Adult Men with Borderline Hepatitis." *European Journal of Clinical Nutrition* 62 (2008): 60-67.

See also: Bile acid sequestrant drugs; Cholesterol, high; Cirrhosis; Gallstones; Gastrointestinal health; Hepatitis, alcoholic; Hepatitis, viral; Kidney stones; Milk thistle; SAMe.

Lobelia

RELATED TERM: *Lobelia inflata*

CATEGORY: Herbs and supplements

DEFINITION: Natural plant product used to treat specific health conditions.

PRINCIPAL PROPOSED USE: Cigarette addiction

OTHER PROPOSED USES: Asthma, chemical dependency, depression, enhancing memory, insomnia, pain reduction

OVERVIEW

The herb *Lobelia inflata* was originally used by Native Americans in the New England region of the United States. It was subsequently popularized by Samuel Thomson, the founder of an idiosyncratic form of medicine that came to be called Thomsonianism. The enduring popularity of lobelia is one of the legacies of this nineteenth-century enthusiasm. (Goldenseal is another herb popularized by Thomson.)

The traditional names of the herb capture its traditional uses: wild tobacco, asthma weed, gagroot, and pukeweed. Dried lobelia tastes and smells somewhat like tobacco, and for this reason it was sold as a tobacco substitute. Lobelia was also used to treat asthma and to stimulate vomiting.

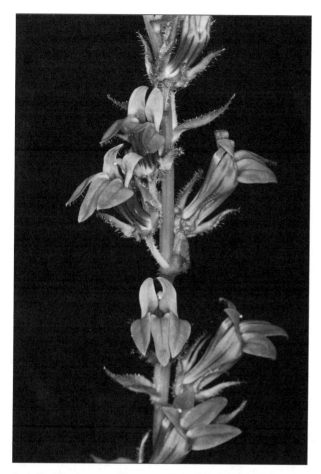

Lobelia plant was used as a medicinal herb by Native Americans. (© Jochenschneider/Dreamstime.com)

The Thomsonians additionally claimed that lobelia could relax muscles and nerves. On this basis, they used it for anxiety, epilepsy, kidney stones, insomnia, menstrual cramps, muscle spasms, spastic colon, and tetanus.

THERAPEUTIC DOSAGES

Lobelia is generally sold in the form of a vinegar tincture. The typical dose of this tincture is 20 to 60 drops taken three times daily.

THERAPEUTIC USES

The major active ingredient of lobelia is a substance called lobeline. It is widely stated that lobeline is chemically similar to nicotine, and on this basis it has been marketed as a smoking cessation treatment.

However, this belief appears to be a type of urban legend, because lobeline is not chemically similar to nicotine.

Chemists investigating the lobeline-nicotine myth found that lobeline may diminish certain effects of nicotine in the body, specifically nicotine-induced release of the substance dopamine. Because dopamine is believed to play a significant role in drug addiction, these findings can be taken as hinting that lobeline might be useful for treating drug addiction. Potential benefits have been found for addiction to amphetamines.

Dopamine also plays a role in cigarette addiction. For this reason, despite lobeline's lack of similarity to nicotine, it is possible that lobelia could be helpful for people who wish to stop smoking. However, despite the widespread marketing of lobelia for this purpose, there is no meaningful evidence that it works.

Other proposed uses of lobelia also lack supporting evidence. For example, although studies in horses have found that injected lobeline causes the animals to breathe more deeply, it is a long way from a finding like this to the widespread claims that lobelia is helpful for asthma in humans. Similarly, animal studies hint that lobeline might enhance memory and reduce pain, and, in addition, that beta-amyrin palmitate, another constituent of lobelia, might have antidepressant and sedative properties. However, no human studies on these potential benefits of the herb have been conducted.

SAFETY ISSUES

It is widely stated that lobelia is a dangerously toxic herb. However, herbalist Paul Bergner reviewed published literature on the subject and discovered that each author who described lobelia as toxic was merely quoting another author, going back nearly to the early nineteenth century. The original published reference on which this sequence of hearsay reporting appears to have been based is a note in the *American New Dispensatory* of 1810, in which an "eminent physician" is quoted as stating that if a person consumes lobelia and does not vomit, death will follow. The ultimate origin of this warning may have been the claims made by the prosecution in a widely publicized trial of Samuel Thomson in which he was accused of committing murder through the use of lobelia.

There have been no reported cases of death caused by *Lobelia inflata* in animals or humans. Considering

On Lobelia

Samuel Thompson, an early and controversial proponent of the herb Lobelia inflata *for medicinal uses, here discusses the herb's emetic (vomit-inducing) functions in preventing and curing illness.*

The emetic herb [*Lobelia inflata*] is of great value in preventing sickness, as well as curing it. By taking a dose when first attacked by any complaint, it will throw it off, and frequently prevent long sickness. It not only acts [as] an emetic, and throws off from the stomach everything that nature does not require to support the system, but extends its effects to every part of the body. It is searching, enlivening, quickening, and has great power in removing obstructions; but it soon exhausts itself, and if not followed by some other medicine to hold the vital heat till nature is able to support itself by digesting the food, it will not be sufficient to remove a disease that has become seated.

how widely lobelia was used under the Thomsonians and subsequently, the concern that it causes death appears to be a significant overstatement. Lobelia may present health risks, but if it does, these risks have not been documented.

Short-term side effects that have been reported in association with lobelia include stomach pain, heartburn, nausea, vomiting, and dizziness. Lobeline also appears to trigger coughing and a sense of choking, for reasons that are unclear.

That lobeline restricts dopamine release suggests that lobelia might worsen symptoms of Parkinson's disease (in which dopamine levels are low) and could possibly interfere with the action of drugs used for schizophrenia or attention deficit disorder (which also act on dopamine). These concerns are, however, purely theoretical. Also, safety in young children, pregnant or nursing women, or people with severe liver or kidney disease has not been established.

Reviewed by EBSCO CAM Review Board

FURTHER READING

Butler, J. E., et al. "Changes in Respiratory Sensations Induced by Lobeline After Human Bilateral Lung Transplantation." *Journal of Physiology* 534 (2001): 583-593.

Miller, D. K., et al. "Lobeline Inhibits the Neurochemical and Behavioral Effects of Amphetamine." *Journal of Pharmacology and Experimental Therapeutics* 296 (2001): 1023-1034.

Raj, H., et al. "How Does Lobeline Injected Intravenously Produce a Cough?" *Respiratory Physiology and Neurobiology* 145 (2005): 79-90.

See also: Addiction; Folk medicine; Herbal medicine; Smoking addiction; Thomson, Samuel.

Lomatium

RELATED TERM: *Lomatium dissectum*
CATEGORY: Herbs and supplements
DEFINITION: Natural plant product used to treat specific health conditions.
PRINCIPAL PROPOSED USE: Antiviral
OTHER PROPOSED USES: Acute bronchitis, colds and influenza, herpes, human immunodeficiency virus infection support, sinusitis, viral hepatitis

OVERVIEW

An herb of bright yellow, umbrella-shaped flowers, lomatium was widely used among indigenous peoples of North America as a treatment for a variety of infections, especially those involving the lungs. Reportedly, the use of this herb protected the Washoe tribe of Nevada from suffering any deaths during the 1917/1918 worldwide pandemic of influenza. It was also said to be useful for pneumonia and tuberculosis.

THERAPEUTIC DOSAGES

Lomatium is typically used in the form of a resin-free extract, taken at a dose of 1 to 3 milliliters daily.

THERAPEUTIC USES

Lomatium is now regarded by some herbalists as an effective treatment for many types of viral infection, including human immunodeficiency virus (HIV) infection, viral hepatitis, colds and flu, acute bronchitis, sinusitis, and herpes. However, there is no meaningful scientific evidence that lomatium is helpful for these conditions, or that it has any antiviral effects at all. Its alleged effects in the great influenza pandemic of 1917/1918 cannot be taken as meaningful evidence of benefit; like all other great plagues, the influenza pandemic gave rise to innumerable rumors of cures, none of which have held up to scientific testing.

At most, there is exceedingly weak evidence from a small number of test-tube studies hinting that *Lomatium* species might have antiviral properties. However, tens or hundreds of thousands of substances have shown antiviral effects in the test tube; the benefits hypothesized from preliminary test-tube studies rarely hold up when human studies are performed. Only double-blind, placebo-controlled studies can show a treatment effective, and no studies of this type have been performed on lomatium.

SAFETY ISSUES

Lomatium has not undergone any modern safety testing. Reportedly, lomatium resin frequently causes allergic reactions leading to a whole-body rash; this is why resin-free products are sold. In addition, lomatium may cause digestive distress. Safety in young children, pregnant or nursing women, and persons with severe liver or kidney disease has not been evaluated.

Reviewed by EBSCO CAM Review Board

FURTHER READING

Lee, T. T., et al. "Suksdorfin: An Anti-HIV Principle from *Lomatium suksdorfii*, Its Structure-Activity Correlation with Related Coumarins, and Synergistic Effects with Anti-AIDS Nucleosides." *Bioorganic and Medicinal Chemistry* 2 (1995): 1051-1056.

McCutcheon, A. R., et al. "Antiviral Screening of British Columbian Medicinal Plants." *Journal of Ethnopharmacology* 49 (1996): 101-110.

See also: Bronchitis; Colds and flu; Hepititis, viral; Herbal medicine; Herpes; HIV/AIDS support.

Loop diuretics

CATEGORY: Drug interactions
DEFINITION: Used to reduce fluid accumulation in the body.
INTERACTIONS: Dong quai, licorice, magnesium, potassium, St. John's wort, vitamin B_1
DRUGS IN THIS FAMILY: Bumetanide (Bumex), ethacrynic acid (Edecrin), furosemide (Lasix), torsemide (Demadex)

POTASSIUM
Effect: Probable Need for Supplementation
Loop diuretics cause a constant and significant loss of potassium. The classic treatment for this is to eat bananas and drink orange juice. Potassium supplements are also frequently prescribed.

MAGNESIUM
Effect: Probable Need for Supplementation
Long-term use (more than six months) of loop diuretics might lead to magnesium deficiency. In turn, magnesium depletion can increase loss of potassium.

Since magnesium deficiency is common anyway, taking a magnesium supplement at the standard U.S. Dietary Reference Intake (formerly known as the Recommended Dietary Allowance) levels might make sense.

VITAMIN B_1
Effect: Probable Need for Supplementation
Evidence suggests that loop diuretics interfere with the body's metabolism of vitamin B_1 (thiamin). This effect may cause adverse consequences in one group of persons who commonly take loop diuretics: people with heart failure. The heart depends on B_1 for proper function; therefore, this finding suggests that taking a B_1 supplement may be advisable. In fact, preliminary evidence suggests that thiamin supplementation does indeed improve heart function in persons with congestive heart failure (CHF).

LICORICE
Effect: Possible Dangerous Interaction
Licorice, too, affects potassium, and the combination of licorice and loop diuretics might cause unexpectedly rapid potassium loss. However, the special form of licorice known as DGL (deglycyrrhizinated licorice) should not affect potassium levels.

DONG QUAI, ST. JOHN'S WORT
Effect: Possible Harmful Interaction
Loop diuretics have been reported to cause increased sensitivity to the sun, amplifying the risk of sunburn or skin rash. Because St. John's wort and dong quai may also cause this problem, taking these herbal supplements during treatment with loop diuretics might add to this risk. It may be a good idea to wear a sunscreen or protective clothing during sun

exposure if one takes one of these herbs while using a loop diuretic.

EBSCO CAM Review Board

FURTHER READING

Brady, J. A., C. L. Rock, and M. R. Horneffer. "Thiamin Status, Diuretic Medications, and the Management of Congestive Heart Failure." *Journal of the American Dietetic Association* 95 (1995): 541-544.

Hardig, L., et al. "Reduced Thiamine Phosphate, but Not Thiamine Diphosphate, in Erythrocytes in Elderly Patients with Congestive Heart Failure Treated with Furosemide." *Journal of Internal Medicine* 247 (2000): 597-600.

Sole, M. J., and K. N. Jeejeebhoy. "Conditioned Nutritional Requirements: Therapeutic Relevance to Heart Failure." *Deutsches Herzzentrum München* 27 (2002): 174-178.

Yue, Q. Y., et al. "No Difference in Blood Thiamine Diphosphate Levels Between Swedish Caucasian Patients with Congestive Heart Failure Treated with Furosemide and Patients Without Heart Failure." *Journal of Internal Medicine* 242 (1997): 491-495.

See also: Dong quai; Food and Drug Administration; Licorice; Magnesium; Potassium; St. John's wort; Supplements: Introduction; Vitamin B_1.

Low-carbohydrate diet

CATEGORY: Therapies and techniques
RELATED TERMS: Atkins diet, high-protein diet, low-carbohydrate diet, Zone diet
DEFINITION: Weight loss and maintenance through diets that are low in carbohydrates.

OVERVIEW

Mainstream groups such as the American Heart Association and the American Dietetic Association endorse a unified set of dietary guidelines for people who wish to lose weight: Eat a low-fat diet and cut calories. However, many popular weight-loss and diet books take a very different approach. The Atkins diet, the Zone diet, Protein Power, and numerous other dietary approaches reject the low-fat guideline. Instead, these methods recommend cutting down on carbohydrates. According to proponents of these theories, when a person reduces the carbohydrates in his or

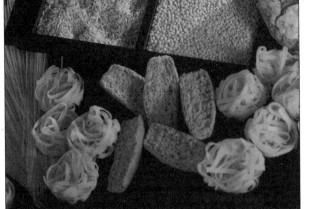

Assorted carbohydrates. (Garo/Phanie/Photo Researchers, Inc.)

her diet (and, correspondingly, increases protein or fat, or both), that person will find it much easier to reduce calorie intake and may even lose weight without cutting calories.

The controversy over these contradictions has been heated. Proponents of the low-fat diet claim that low-carbohydrate (low-carb) diets are ineffective and even dangerous, while low-carb proponents say much the same about the low-fat approach. However, an article published in the *Journal of the American Medical Association* suggests that neither side has a strong case. Researchers concluded, essentially, that a calorie is a calorie, regardless of whether it comes from a low-carb or a low-fat diet. They did not find any consistent evidence that the low-carb diet makes it easier to lose weight than the low-fat diet, but neither did they find any consistent evidence for the reverse. Furthermore, the authors of the review did not find any compelling reason to conclude that low-carb diets are unsafe, although they did point out that the long-term safety of such diets remains unknown.

Subsequent studies confirmed these findings for a variety of low-carb diets. In some studies, one particular diet method may do better than others, but in other studies a different diet will stand out. Researchers reviewing thirteen studies comparing low-carb with low-fat/low-calorie diets in overweight participants for a minimum of six months concluded that the low-carb diets tended to perform better at reducing weight and cardiovascular disease factors for up to one year. Nevertheless, a consensus has yet to emerge among nutrition scientists as to what diet performs better overall. Many of the foregoing studies suggest that if a diet causes weight loss, cholesterol will improve regardless of the diet used to achieve that weight loss. However, the manner of change in a person's cholesterol profile differs between the two approaches. Low-fat diets tend to improve total and LDL (low-density lipoprotein, or bad) cholesterol levels, but they tend to worsen HDL (high-density lipoprotein, or good) cholesterol and triglyceride levels; low-carb, high-fat diets have the opposite effect.

The Mediterranean diet, which is relatively high in fiber and monounsaturated fats (such as olive oil) has also attracted the attention of nutrition researchers. There is good evidence that it is as effective as low-carb diets for weight reduction and probably more effective than low-fat diets. It also seems to have the added advantage of benefiting persons with diabetes more than the other two diets.

However, if one undertakes a low-carb (or low-fat) diet that does not cause weight loss, that person's cholesterol profile will probably not improve significantly. In addition, there is little to no evidence that the low-carb approach improves blood sugar control except insofar as it leads to weight loss. However, there is some evidence that a low-carb diet that is high in mono-unsaturated fats reduces blood pressure to a slightly greater extent than does a high-carb, low-fat diet. Contrary to claims by some low-carb proponents, low-fat, high-carb diets do not seem to backfire metabolically and promote weight gain.

Based on this information, it seems that the most sensible course to take to lose weight is to experiment with different diets and determine which one cuts the most calories (and keeps them cut). If the low-carb diet approach works, one should continue with it. However, if it does not help one lose weight, it should not be continued indefinitely.

Any form of extreme dieting can cause serious side effects or even death. All people who intend to adopt an unconventional diet should first seek medical advice. Furthermore, people with kidney failure should not use low-carb, high-protein diets, as high protein intake can easily overstress failing kidneys. (High-protein diets are probably not harmful for people with healthy kidneys.)

In addition, people who take the blood thinner warfarin (Coumadin) may need to have their blood coagulation tested after beginning a high-protein, low-carb diet. Two case reports suggest that such diets may decrease the effectiveness of warfarin, requiring a higher dose. Conversely, a person who is already on warfarin and a high-protein, low-carb diet and then goes off the diet, may need to reduce his or her warfarin dose.

EBSCO CAM Review Board

FURTHER READING

Berglund, L., et al. "Comparison of Monounsaturated Fat with Carbohydrates as a Replacement for Saturated Fat in Subjects with a High Metabolic Risk Profile: Studies in the Fasting and Postprandial States." *American Journal of Clinical Nutrition* 86 (2007): 1611-1620.

Dansinger, M. L., et al. "Comparison of the Atkins, Ornish, Weight Watchers, and Zone Diets for Weight Loss and Heart Disease Risk Reduction." *Journal of the American Medical Association* 293 (2005): 43-53.

Ebbeling, C. B., et al. "Effects of a Low-Glycemic Load vs Low-Fat Diet in Obese Young Adults." *Journal of the American Medical Association* 297 (2007): 2092-2102.

Gardner, C. D., et al. "Comparison of the Atkins, Zone, Ornish, and LEARN Diets for Change in Weight and Related Risk Factors Among Overweight Premenopausal Women: The A to Z Weight Loss Study." *Journal of the American Medical Association* 297 (2007): 969-977.

Hession, M., et al. "Systematic Review of Randomized Controlled Trials of Low-Carbohydrate vs. Low-Fat/Low-Calorie Diets in the Management of Obesity and Its Comorbidities." *Obesity Reviews* 10 (2009): 36-50.

Howard, B. V., J. E. Manson, et al. "Low-Fat Dietary Pattern and Weight Change over Seven Years: The Women's Health Initiative Dietary Modification Trial." *Journal of the American Medical Association* 295 (2006): 39-49.

Howard, B. V., L. Van Horn, et al. "Low-Fat Dietary Pattern and Risk of Cardiovascular Disease: The Women's Health Initiative Randomized Controlled Dietary Modification Trial." *Journal of the American Medical Association* 295 (2006): 655-666.

Luscombe-Marsh, N. D., et al. "Carbohydrate-Restricted Diets High in Either Monounsaturated Fat or Protein Are Equally Effective at Promoting Fat Loss and Improving Blood Lipids." *American Journal of Clinical Nutrition* 81 (2005): 762-772.

Nordmann, A. J., et al. "Effects of Low-Carbohydrate vs Low-Fat Diets on Weight Loss and Cardiovascular Risk Factors: A Meta-analysis of Randomized Controlled Trials." *Archives of Internal Medicine* 166 (2006): 285-293.

Shai, I., et al. "Weight Loss with a Low-Carbohydrate, Mediterranean, or Low-Fat Diet." *New England Journal of Medicine* 359 (2008): 229-241.

Tay, J., et al. "Metabolic Effects of Weight Loss on a Very-Low-Carbohydrate Diet Compared with an Isocaloric High-Carbohydrate Diet in Abdominally Obese Subjects." *Journal of the American College of Cardiology* 51 (2008): 59-67.

Wal, J. S., et al. "Moderate-Carbohydrate Low-Fat Versus Low-Carbohydrate High-Fat Meal Replacements for Weight Loss." *International Journal of Food Sciences and Nutrition* 58 (2007): 321-329.

See also: Anti-inflammatory diet; Diet-based therapies; Low-glycemic index diet; Macrobiotic diet; Obesity and excess weight; Raw foods diet; Vegan diet; Vegetarian diet.

Low-glycemic-index diet

CATEGORY: Therapies and techniques

RELATED TERMS: GI diet, GL diet, low-glycemic-load diet

DEFINITION: Nutritional approach based on the consumption of low-fat foods and foods that have particular kinds of carbohydrates.

OVERVIEW

Mainstream organizations, such as the American Heart Association and the American Dietetic Association, endorse a unified set of guidelines for the optimum diet. According to these organizations, the majority of calories in the daily diet should come from carbohydrates (55 to 60 percent), fat should provide no more than 30 percent of total calories, and protein should be kept to 10 to 15 percent.

However, many popular diet books turn the standard diet upside down. The Atkins diet, the Zone diet, Protein Power, and other alternative dietary approaches reject carbohydrates and advocate increased consumption of fat or protein, or both. According to theory, the low-carbohydrate (carb) approach aids in weight loss (and provides a variety of other health benefits) by reducing the body's production of insulin.

The low-glycemic-index (low-GI) diet splits the difference between the low-carb and low-fat approaches. It maintains the low-carb diet's focus on insulin, but it suggests choosing certain carbohydrates over others rather than restricting carbohydrate intake.

Evidence suggests that carbohydrates are not created equal. Some carbohydrates, such as pure glucose, are absorbed quickly and create a rapid, strong rise in both blood sugar and insulin. However, other carbohydrates (such as brown rice) are absorbed much more slowly and produce only a modest blood sugar and insulin response. According to proponents of the low-GI diet, eating foods in the latter category will enhance weight loss and improve health. However, despite some promising theory, there is no solid evidence that low-GI diets enhance weight loss.

Besides weight loss, preliminary evidence suggests that the low-GI approach (or, even better, a related method called low-glycemic load, which is discussed later in this article) may help prevent heart disease. The low-GI approach has also shown promise for treating and possibly preventing diabetes.

WHAT IS THE GLYCEMIC INDEX?

The precise measurement of the glucose-stimulating effect of a food is called its glycemic index. The lower a food's GI, the less potent its effects on blood sugar (and, therefore, on insulin).

The GI of glucose is arbitrarily set at 100. The ratings of other foods are determined as follows. First, researchers calculate a portion size for the food to supply 50 grams (g) of carbohydrates. Next, they give that amount of the food to a minimum of eight to ten people and measure the blood sugar response. (By using a group of people rather than one person, researchers can ensure that the idiosyncrasies of one person do not skew the results.) On another occasion, researchers also give each participant an equivalent amount of glucose and perform the same measurements. The GI of a food is then determined by comparing the two outcomes. For example, if a food causes one-half of the blood sugar rise of glucose, it is assigned a GI of 50; if it causes one-quarter of the rise, it is assigned a GI of 25. The lower the GI, the better.

When scientists first began to determine the GI of foods, some of the results drew skepticism. It did not surprise anyone when jellybeans turned out to have a high GI of 80 (after all, jellybeans are mostly sugar). Also, it was not unexpected that kidney beans have a low GI of 27 because they are notoriously difficult to digest. However, when baked potatoes showed an index of 93, researchers were stunned. This rating is higher than that of almost all other foods, including ice cream (61), sweet potatoes (54), and white bread (70). Based on this finding, low-GI diets recommend that people avoid potatoes.

There are other surprises hidden in the GI tables. For example, fructose (the sweetener in honey) has an extraordinarily low GI of 23, lower than brown rice and almost three times lower than white sugar. Candy bars also tend to have a relatively good (low) GI, presumably because their fat content makes them digest slowly.

Dietary Changes and Type 2 Diabetes

More than any other disease, type 2 diabetes is related to lifestyle. It is often the case that people prefer having an injection or taking a pill to improve their quality of life rather than changing their diet and level of physical activity. Attention to diet and exercise results in a dramatic decrease in the need for drug therapy in nine of ten persons with diabetes. In some cases, the loss of only a small percentage of body weight results in an increased sensitivity to insulin. Permanent weight reduction and exercise also help to prevent long-term complications and permit a healthier and more active lifestyle.

It is difficult to predict the GI of a food without specifically testing it, but there are some general factors that can be recognized. Fiber content tends to reduce the GI of a food, presumably by slowing down digestion. For this reason, whole grains usually have a lower GI score than refined, processed grains. Fat content also reduces GI score. Simple carbohydrates (such as sugar) often have a higher GI score than complex carbohydrates (such as brown rice).

However, there are numerous exceptions to these rules. Factors such as the acid content of food, the size of the food particles, and the precise mixture of fats, proteins, and carbohydrates can substantially change the GI measurement. For a measurement like the GI to be meaningful, it has to be generally reproducible among people. In other words, if a potato has a GI of 93 in one person, it should have nearly the same GI when given to another person. Science suggests that the GI passes this test. The GI of individual foods is fairly constant among people, and even mixed meals have a fairly predictable effect according to most studies.

Thus, the GI of a food really does indicate its propensity to raise insulin levels. Whether a diet based on the index will aid in weight loss, however, is a different issue.

FOLLOWING A LOW-GLYCEMIC-INDEX DIET

Following a low-GI diet is fairly easy. Basically, one should follow the typical diet endorsed by authorities such as the American Dietetic Association, but in doing so, one should choose carbohydrates that fall toward the lower end of the GI scale. Popular books such as *The Glucose Revolution* (1999) give a great deal of information on how to make these choices.

DO LOW-GLYCEMIC-INDEX DIETS AID IN WEIGHT LOSS?

There are two primary theoretical reasons given why low-GI diets should help reduce weight. The most prominent reason given in books on the low-GI approach involves insulin levels. Basically, these books show that low-GI diets reduce insulin release, and then take almost for granted the idea that reduced insulin levels should aid in weight loss. However, there is little justification for the second part of this argument. Excess weight is known to lead to elevated insulin levels, but there is little meaningful evidence for the reverse: that reducing insulin levels will help remove excess weight.

Books on the low-GI diet give another reason for using their approach. They state that low-GI foods fill a person up more quickly than do high-GI foods and that they also keep one feeling full for longer. However, there is more evidence against this belief than for it.

The satiety index. A measurement called the satiety index assigns a numerical quantity to the filling quality of a food. These numbers are determined by feeding people fixed caloric amounts of those foods and then determining how soon they get hungry again and how much they eat at subsequent meals. The process is similar to the methods used to establish the GI index.

The results of these measurements do not corroborate the expectations of low-GI diet proponents. As it happens, foods with the worst (highest) GI index are often the most satiating, exactly the reverse of what low-GI-theory proponents would say. For example, the satiety index claims that potatoes are among the most satiating of foods. However, the GI analysis gave potatoes a bad rating. According to the low-GI theory, one should feel hunger pangs shortly after eating a big baked potato. In real life, this does not happen.

There are numerous other contradictions between research findings and the low-GI/high-satiety theory. For example, one study found no difference in satiety between fructose (fruit sugar) and glucose when taken as part of a mixed meal, even though fructose has a GI more than four times lower than glucose.

Some studies do seem to suggest that certain low-GI foods are more filling than high-GI foods. However, in these studies the bulkiness and lack of palatability of the low-GI foods chosen may have played a more important role than the foods' GI. Thus, the satiety argument for low-GI diets does not appear to hold up to scrutiny.

IS THE GLYCEMIC INDEX THE RIGHT MEASUREMENT?

There is another problem with the low-GI approach: It is probably the wrong way to assess the insulin-related effects of food. The GI measures blood sugar response per gram of carbohydrate contained in a food, not per gram of the food. This leads to some odd numbers. For example, a parsnip has a GI of 98, almost as high as pure sugar. If taken at face value, this figure suggests that dieters should avoid parsnips. However, parsnips are mostly indigestible fiber, and a person would have to eat a few bushels to trigger a major glucose and insulin response.

The reason for the high number is that the GI rates the effects per gram of carbohydrate rather than per gram of total parsnip, and the sugar present in minute amounts in a parsnip itself is highly absorbable. The high GI rating of parsnips is thus extremely misleading. Books such as *The Glucose Revolution* address issues like this on a case-by-case basis by arguing, for example, that one can consider most vegetables "free foods" regardless of their GI. In fact, the same considerations apply to all foods and distort the meaningfulness of the scale as a whole.

A different measurement, the glycemic load (GL), takes this into account. The GL is derived by multiplying the GI by the percent carbohydrate content of a food. In other words, it measures the glucose/insulin response per gram of food rather than per gram of carbohydrate in that food. Using this system, the GL of a parsnip is 10, while glucose has a relative load of 100. Also, the GL of a typical serving of potato is only 27.

SCIENTIFIC EVIDENCE

Theory is one thing and practice is another. It is certainly possible that making sure to focus on low-GI or low-GL foods will help a person lose weight, even if the theoretical justification for the idea is weak. However, there is only preliminary positive evidence to support this possibility, and the largest and longest-term trial failed to find benefit.

In one of the positive studies, 107 overweight adolescents were divided into two groups: a low-GI group and a low-fat group. The low-GI group was counseled to follow a diet consisting of 45 to 50 percent carbohydrates (preferably low-GI carbohydrates), 20 to 25 percent protein, and 30 to 35 percent fat. Calorie restriction was not emphasized. The low-fat group received instructions for a standard low-fat, low-calorie diet divided into 55 to 60 percent carbohydrates, 15 to 20 percent protein, and 25 to 30 percent fat. In about four months, participants on the low-GI diet lost about 4.5 pounds, while those on the standard diet lost just under 3 pounds.

This study does not say as much about the low-GI approach as it might seem. Perhaps the most obvious problem is that the low-GI diet used here was also a high-protein diet. It is possible that high-protein diets might help weight loss regardless of the GI of the foods consumed. (In fact, this is precisely what proponents of high-protein diets claim.)

Another problem is that participants were not assigned to the two groups randomly. Rather, researchers consciously picked what group each participant should join. This is a major flaw because it introduces the possibility of intentional or unintentional bias. It is quite possible, for example, that researchers placed adolescents with greater self-motivation into the low-GI group, based on an unconscious desire to see results from the study. This is not an academic problem, and modern medical studies always use randomization to circumvent it.

Finally, researchers made no effort to determine how well participants followed their diets. It might be that those in the low-fat diet group simply did not follow the rules as well as those in the low-GI diet group because the rules were more challenging. Despite these many flaws, the study results are still promising. Losing weight without deliberately cutting calories is potentially a great thing.

In another study, thirty overweight women with excessively high insulin levels were put on either a normal low-calorie diet or one that supplied the same amount of calories but used low-GI foods. The results during twelve weeks showed that women following the low-GI diet lost several pounds more than those following the normal diet.

In yet another small study, this one involving overweight adolescents, a conventional reduced-calorie diet was compared with a low-GL diet that did not have any calorie restrictions. The results showed that simply by consuming low-GI foods, without regard for calories, the participants on the low-GI diet were able to lose as much or more weight as those on the low-calorie diet.

However, in a large and long-term study, an eighteen-month trial of 203 Brazilian women, the use of a low-GI diet failed to prove more effective than a high-GI diet. Additionally, a smaller study failed to find a low-GI diet more effective for weight loss than a low-fat diet except in people with high levels of circulating insulin.

POSSIBLE HEALTH BENEFITS

There is some evidence that a low-GI diet (or, even better, a low-GL diet) might help prevent cancer and heart disease. The low-GI approach has also shown promise for preventing or treating diabetes.

Heart disease prevention. One large observational study evaluated the diets of more than 75,000 women

and found that those women whose diets provided a lower GL had a lower incidence of heart disease. In this study, 75,521 women age thirty-eight to sixty-three years were followed for ten years. Each filled out detailed questionnaires regarding her diet. Using this data, researchers calculated the average GL of each participant. The results showed that women who consumed a diet with a high GL were more likely to experience heart disease than those who consumed a diet of low GL.

Other observational studies suggest that the consumption of foods with lower GL may improve cholesterol profile: specifically, reduced triglyceride levels and higher HDL (good cholesterol) levels. These effects, in turn, might lead to decreased risk of heart disease. However, other observational studies have found little or no relationship between heart disease and GI or GL.

These contradictory results are not surprising, but even if the observational study results were entirely consistent, it would not prove the case for a low-GI approach. Conclusions based on observational studies are notoriously unreliable because of the possible presence of unidentified confounding factors. For example, because there is an approximate correlation between fiber in the diet and GL, it is possible that benefits, when seen, are from fiber intake instead. Factors such as this one may easily obscure the effects of the factor under study, leading to contradictory or misleading results.

Intervention trials (studies in which researchers actually intervene in participants' lives) are more reliable, and some have been conducted to evaluate the low-GI diet. For example, in the foregoing large weight-loss trial, the low-GI diet failed to prove more effective than a high-GI diet in terms of weight loss. The results did suggest, though, that a low-GI diet can improve cholesterol profile. However, this study was not primarily designed to look at effects on cholesterol.

A study that primarily focused on this outcome followed thirty people with high lipid levels for three months. During the second month, low-GI foods were substituted for high-GI foods, while other nutrients were kept similar. Improvements were seen in total cholesterol, LDL (bad) cholesterol, and triglycerides, but not in HDL. A close analysis of the results showed that only participants who had high triglycerides at the beginning of the study showed benefit. Another controlled trial found that a high carb, low-GL diet optimized lipid profile compared with several other diets. However, another study found that low-fat and low-GI diets were about equally effective in terms of profile.

Another approach to the issue involves analysis of effects on insulin resistance. Evidence suggests that increased resistance of the body to its own insulin raises the risk of heart disease. One study found that the use of a low-GI diet versus a high-GI diet improved the body's sensitivity to insulin in women at risk for heart disease. Similar results were seen in a group of people with severe heart disease and in healthy people. While these results are preliminary, taken together they do suggest that consumption of low-GI foods might have a beneficial effect on heart disease risk.

Low-GL diet and diabetes. Two large observational studies, one involving men and the other involving women, found that diets with lower GLs were associated with a lower rate of diabetes. For example, one trial followed 65,173 women for six years. Women whose diets had a high GL had a 47 percent increased risk of developing diabetes compared with those whose diets had the lowest GL. Fiber content of diet also makes a difference. People who consumed a diet that was both low in fiber and high in GL had a 250 percent increased incidence of diabetes.

However, as always, the results of these observational studies have to be taken with caution. It is quite possible that unrecognized factors are responsible for the results seen. For example, magnesium deficiency is widespread and may contribute to the development of diabetes; whole grains contain magnesium and are also low-GI foods. Therefore, it could be that the benefits seen in these studies are actually caused by increased magnesium intake in the low-GI group, rather than by effects on blood sugar and insulin.

Furthermore, one observational study found no connection between the glycemic values of foods and the incidence of diabetes. Another observational study did find a correlation between carbohydrate intake (especially pastries) and the onset of diabetes, but no consistent relationship with GI. Other studies have found no relationship between sugar consumption (a high-GI food) and diabetes onset.

Thus, reducing dietary GL may help prevent diabetes, but this is not known for sure. Whether or not low-GI diets can prevent diabetes, going on a low-GI diet might improve blood sugar control for people who already have diabetes. However, the benefits seem to be small at most.

OTHER USES AND APPLICATIONS

Weak evidence hints that a low-GI diet might help prevent macular degeneration. Although there are theoretical reasons to believe that the use of white sugar and other high-GI foods might promote colon cancer, a large observational study failed to find any association between colon cancer rates and diets high in sugar, carbohydrates, or GL.

It has been proposed that low-GI foods may enhance sports performance. One study involving a simulated sixty-four-kilometer bicycle race found no performance differences between the use of honey (low GI) and the use of dextrose (high GI) as a carbohydrate source. However, another study did find benefit with the consumption of a low-GI snack before endurance exercise. Finally, one study compared a low-GL diet with a high-carb diet in people with acne and found evidence that the low-GL diet reduced acne symptoms.

CONCLUSION

The evidence that a low-GI diet will help one lose weight is not impressive. Its theoretical foundation is weak, and it appears to be using the wrong method of ranking foods regarding their effects on insulin. Conversely, however, there is no reason to believe a low-GI diet causes harm.

While the most popular low-GI-diet books, such as *The Glucose Revolution* and *Sugar Busters* (1995), recommend a diet that is generally reasonable and should be safe, it is easy to design some fairly extreme low-GI diets. For example, a diet consisting of nothing but lard would be a very, very low-GI diet, because the GI of lard is 0. Although it no longer seems that saturated fat is as harmful as it was once thought to be, a pure lard diet is probably not a good idea. Any diet book or other source that recommends achieving a low GI by consuming an extreme diet should be approached with caution.

EBSCO CAM Review Board

FURTHER READING

Chiu, C. J., et al. "Dietary Glycemic Index and Carbohydrate in Relation to Early Age-Related Macular Degeneration." *American Journal of Clinical Nutrition* 83 (2006): 880-886.

Clapp, J. F., and B. Lopez. "Low- Versus High-Glycemic Index Diets in Women: Effects on Caloric Requirement, Substrate Utilization, and Insulin Sensitivity." *Metabolic Syndrome and Related Disorders* 5 (2007): 231-242.

Ebbeling, C. B., et al. "Effects of a Low-Glycemic Load vs Low-Fat Diet in Obese Young Adults." *Journal of the American Medical Association* 297 (2007): 2092-2102.

Noakes, M., et al. "The Effect of a Low Glycaemic Index (GI) Ingredient Substituted for a High GI Ingredient in Two Complete Meals on Blood Glucose and Insulin Levels, Satiety, and Energy Intake in Healthy Lean Women." *Asia Pacific Journal of Clinical Nutrition* 14, suppl. (2005): S45.

Pittas, A. G., et al. "The Effects of the Dietary Glycemic Load on Type 2 Diabetes Risk Factors During Weight Loss." *Obesity* 14 (2006): 2200-2209.

Smith, R. N., et al. "A Low-Glycemic-Load Diet Improves Symptoms in Acne Vulgaris Patients." *American Journal of Clinical Nutrition* 86 (2007): 107-115.

Tavani, A., et al. "Carbohydrates, Dietary Glycaemic Load, and Glycaemic Index, and Risk of Acute Myocardial Infarction." *Heart* 89 (2003): 722-726.

Wu, C. L., and C. Williams. "A Low Glycemic Index Meal Before Exercise Improves Endurance Running Capacity in Men." *International Journal of Sport Nutrition and Exercise Metabolism* 16 (2006): 510-527.

See also: Diet-based therapies; Low-carbohydrate diet.

Lupus

RELATED TERMS: SLE, systemic lupus erythematosus

CATEGORY: Condition

DEFINITION: Treatment of an autoimmune disease in which antibodies develop to fight foreign substances in the body.

PRINCIPAL PROPOSED NATURAL TREATMENT: Dehydroepiandrosterone

OTHER PROPOSED NATURAL TREATMENTS: Beta-carotene, *Cordyceps*, fish oil, flaxseed, food allergen identification and avoidance, magnesium, pantothenic acid, selenium, vitamin B_3, vitamin B_{12}, vitamin E

NATURAL PRODUCT TO AVOID: Alfalfa

INTRODUCTION

Systemic lupus erythematosus (also known as lupus or SLE) is an autoimmune disease that primarily affects young and middle-aged women. Its cause is unknown but is believed to involve both genetic inheritance and factors in the environment. Whatever the cause, people with lupus develop antibodies against substances in their own bodies, including deoxyribonucleic acid (DNA). These antibodies cause widespread damage and are believed to be primarily responsible for the many symptoms of this disease.

Lupus may begin with such symptoms as fatigue, weight loss, fever, malaise, and loss of appetite. Other common early symptoms include muscle pain, joint pain, and a facial rash. As lupus progresses, symptoms may develop in virtually every part of the body. Kidney damage is one of the most devastating effects of lupus, but many other serious problems may develop, including seizures, mental impairment, anemia, and inflammation of the heart, blood vessels, eyes, and digestive tract.

Conventional treatment for lupus centers on a variety of anti-inflammatory drugs. In mild cases, taking nonsteroidal anti-inflammatory drugs (NSAIDs) may help; more severe forms of lupus require long-term use of corticosteroid anti-inflammatory drugs such as prednisone. The side effects of these medications can be quite serious themselves. Cytotoxic agents (azathioprine, cyclophosphamide, and chlorambucil) might also be helpful, but they too have many side effects. Close physician supervision is always required with lupus because of the risk of complications in so many organs.

PRINCIPAL PROPOSED NATURAL TREATMENTS

A meaningful body of evidence indicates that the hormone dehydroepiandrosterone (DHEA) may be helpful for the treatment of lupus when used as part of a comprehensive, physician-directed treatment approach. DHEA is the most abundant steroid hormone found in the bloodstream. The body uses DHEA as the starting material for making the sex hormones testosterone and estrogen. DHEA has been tried as a treatment for a variety of medical conditions, including osteoporosis, but it is showing its greatest promise in the treatment of lupus.

A twelve-month, double-blind, placebo-controlled trial of 381 women with mild or moderate lupus

Treating Lupus

Because of the nature and cost of the medications used to treat lupus and because of the potential for serious side effects, many persons seek other ways of treating the disease. Some alternative approaches include special diets, nutritional supplements, fish oils, ointments and creams, chiropractic treatment, and homeopathy. Although these methods may not be harmful in and of themselves and may be associated with symptomatic or psychosocial benefit, no research to date shows that they affect the disease process or prevent organ damage.

Some alternative or complementary approaches may help the patient cope or reduce some of the stress associated with living with a chronic illness. If the doctor feels the approach has value and will not be harmful, it can be incorporated into the patient's treatment plan. However, it is important not to neglect regular health care or treatment of serious symptoms. An open dialogue between patient and doctor about the relative values of complementary and alternative therapies enables the patient to make an informed choice about treatment options.

evaluated the effects of DHEA at a dose of 200 milligrams (mg) daily. Although many participants in both groups improved (the power of placebo is often amazing), DHEA was more effective than placebo, reducing many symptoms of the disease.

Similarly, in a double-blind, placebo-controlled study of 120 women with lupus, the use of DHEA at a dose of 200 mg daily significantly decreased symptoms and reduced the frequency of disease flare-ups. A smaller study found equivocal evidence that a lower dose of DHEA (30 mg daily for women older than age forty-five years and 20 mg daily for women aged forty-five years) might also work.

A 2007 review of all published studies concluded that the use of DHEA may meaningfully improve quality of life in the short term for people with lupus, but that it probably does not alter the long-term course of the disease.

OTHER PROPOSED NATURAL TREATMENTS

Flaxseed contains lignans and alpha-linolenic acid, substances with a wide variety of effects in the body. In particular, flaxseed may antagonize the activity of a substance called platelet-activating factor (PAF) that plays a role in lupus kidney disease (lupus nephritis). Preliminary evidence suggests that flaxseed might help prevent or treat lupus nephritis.

Fish oil contains omega-3 fatty acids, which have some anti-inflammatory effects. Fish oil has been found useful in rheumatoid arthritis, a disease related to lupus. The results of two small double-blind studies suggest that fish oil might also be useful for lupus. However, evidence suggests that fish oil is not effective for lupus nephritis.

Other treatments sometimes recommended for lupus include beta-carotene, *Cordyceps*, magnesium, selenium, vitamin B_3, vitamin B_{12}, vitamin E, pantothenic acid, and food allergen identification and avoidance. However, there is no meaningful evidence that these treatments work for lupus. Another study failed to find copper supplements helpful for lupus symptoms.

HERBS AND SUPPLEMENTS TO AVOID

The herb alfalfa contains a substance called L-canavanine, which can worsen lupus or bring it out of remission. People with lupus should avoid alfalfa entirely. Also, various herbs and supplements may interact adversely with drugs used to treat lupus.

EBSCO CAM Review Board

FURTHER READING

Chang, D. M., et al. "Dehydroepiandrosterone Treatment of Women with Mild-to-Moderate Systemic Lupus Erythematosus." *Arthritis and Rheumatism* 46 (2002): 2924-2927.

Crosbie, D., et al. "Dehydroepiandrosterone for Systemic Lupus Erythematosus." *Cochrane Database of Systematic Reviews* (2007): CD005114. Available through *EBSCO DynaMed Systematic Literature Surveillance* at http://www.ebscohost.com/dynamed.

Duffy, E. M., et al. "The Clinical Effect of Dietary Supplementation with Omega-3 Fish Oils and/or Copper in Systemic Lupus Erythematosus." *Journal of Rheumatology* 31 (2004): 1551.

Nordmark, G., et al. "Effects of Dehydroepiandrosterone Supplement on Health-Related Quality of Life in Glucocorticoid Treated Female Patients with Systemic Lupus Erythematosus." *Autoimmunity* 38 (2005): 531-540.

See also: Corticosteroids; Dehydroepiandrosterone (DHEA); Fatigue; Fibromyalgia: Homeopathic remedies;

Nonsteroidal anti-inflammatory drugs (NSAIDs); Weight loss, undesired; Women's health.

Lust, Benedict

CATEGORY: Biography
IDENTIFICATION: German cofounder of naturopathic medicine
BORN: February 3, 1872; Michelbach, Germany
DIED: September 5, 1945; Butler, New Jersey

OVERVIEW

German natural medicine proponent Benedict Lust cofounded naturopathic medicine, which focuses on using natural remedies and the body's natural ability to heal and maintain itself. Lust has been referred to as the founder of naturopathy in the United States.

Lust worked as a professional waiter for many years in several countries (including Germany, Switzerland, and the United States) until he became sick with what he self-diagnosed as tuberculosis. Upon being struck ill, he decided to return to Germany to be treated by a religious leader—Father Sebastian Kneipp—who also was one of the founders of the naturopathic medicine movement. After being treated for some time, Lust claimed that his health had improved dramatically. The recovery turned him into a strong believer and proponent of natural medicine.

Kneipp advised Lust to return to the United States to spread the ideas of the homeopathic movement. Upon returning to the United States, Lust opened a health food store and eventually began publishing multiple magazines that advocated practices associated with natural medicine. Later, he formally studied the principles of homeopathy, and in 1901, he obtained a degree from the New York Homeopathic Medical College. The following year, he obtained a degree in osteopathy from the Universal College of Osteopathy in New York.

Upon completing his formal education, Lust decided to purchase the rights to the term "naturopathy" from John Scheel, a German physician and homeopath who first coined the term around 1895. Lust subsequently opened the first medical school in the world devoted to naturopathy, which he named the American School of Naturopathy. Some years later he also established the American Naturopathic Association, which reportedly was the first professional organization for naturopathic practitioners in the United States. Lust continued to publish several works on naturopathy, including a magazine called *Nature's Path* and the collection *Universal Naturopathic Encyclopedia* (1918), which outlined drugless forms of therapy.

Lust was scrutinized for his beliefs by many of his colleagues during his formal education, and well into his career. He was arrested more than one dozen times for his approach to natural healing, which often involved spa treatments (such as massage and sunbathing) in the nude at his established health spas.

Brandy Weidow, M.S.

FURTHER READING

Kirchfeld, Friedhelm, and Wade Boyle. *Nature Doctors: Pioneers in Naturopathic Medicine.* 2d ed. Portland, Ore.: NCNM Press, 2005.
Lust, Benedict. *Collected Works of Dr. Benedict Lust: Containing the Works "Yungborn," "The Life and Times of Dr. Benedict Lust," and "Pilgrimages to the Great Masters."* East Wenatchee, Wash.: Healing Mountain, 2006.
Lust, Benedict, and Jared Zeff. *Collected Works of Benedict Lust ND, Founder of Naturopathic Medicine.* Edited by Anita Boyd and Eric Yarnell. East Wenatchee, Wash.: Healing Mountain, 2006.

See also: Biologically based therapies; Naturopathy; Osteopathic manipulation; Thomson, Samuel.

Lutein

CATEGORY: Functional foods
DEFINITION: Natural substance promoted as a dietary supplement for specific health benefits.
PRINCIPAL PROPOSED USES: None
OTHER PROPOSED USES: Atherosclerosis, cataracts, macular degeneration, retinitis pigmentosa

OVERVIEW

Lutein, a chemical found in green vegetables, is a member of a family of substances known as carotenoids. Beta-carotene is the best-known nutrient in this class. Like beta-carotene, lutein is an antioxidant that protects cells against damage caused by dangerous, naturally occurring chemicals known as free radicals.

Evidence has shown that lutein may play an important role in protecting eyes and eyesight. It may work in two ways: by acting directly as a kind of natural sunblock and also by neutralizing free radicals that can damage the eye.

SOURCES

Lutein is not an essential nutrient. However, it is possible that it may be useful for optimal health. Green vegetables are the best source of lutein, especially spinach, kale, collard greens, romaine lettuce, leeks, and peas. Unlike beta-carotene, lutein is not found in high concentrations in yellow and orange vegetables such as carrots.

THERAPEUTIC DOSAGES

It is not known how much lutein is necessary for a therapeutic effect, but estimates range from 5 to 30 milligrams (mg) daily.

THERAPEUTIC USES

According to theoretical findings and two preliminary double-blind studies, it appears that the use of lutein supplements might help prevent or slow the development of age-related macular degeneration and possibly cataracts, the two most common causes of vision loss in the elderly. Lutein has also shown some promise for the treatment of retinitis pigmentosa, an inherited form of eye disease that causes progressive vision loss. Weak evidence hints that lutein might help prevent atherosclerosis.

SCIENTIFIC EVIDENCE

Most observational studies suggest that people who eat foods containing lutein are less likely to develop cataracts and perhaps macular degeneration, the two most common causes of vision loss in adults. Furthermore, there are good theoretical reasons to believe that lutein may play an important role in protecting the eyes.

Lutein is the main pigment (coloring chemical) in the center of the retina, the region of maximum visual sensitivity known as the macula. Macular degeneration consists of injury to the macula and leads to a severe loss in vision. One of the main causes of macular degeneration appears to be sun damage to the sensitive tissue. Lutein appears to act as a natural eyeshade, protecting the retina against too much light. It is also an antioxidant, meaning that it fights free radicals. Free radicals may play a role in macular degeneration.

Based on this information, researchers conducted a double-blind, placebo-controlled trial of lutein. The study enrolled ninety people with dry-type macular degeneration and followed them for twelve months. The participants received either lutein (10 mg), lutein plus other antioxidants and a multivitamin-multimineral supplement, or placebo. At the end of the study period, participants who had taken lutein alone or lutein plus the other nutrients showed improvements in vision, while no change in vision was seen in the placebo group.

A subsequent study failed to find benefit with lutein, but it used a lower dose (6 mg daily) and involved fewer people. Ultimately, further study is needed to establish whether lutein is actually helpful for macular degeneration.

Besides protecting the macula, lutein might also shield the lens of the eye from light damage, slowing the development of cataracts. One small, two-year, double-blind, placebo-controlled trial found some evidence that lutein may improve vision in people who already have cataracts. A trial involving 225 adults with retinitis pigmentosa found that four years of daily supplementation with lutein and vitamin A slowed the rate of visual loss in the mid-peripheral field.

SAFETY ISSUES

Although lutein is a normal part of the diet, there has not been much evaluation of lutein's safety when taken as a concentrated supplement. One study found evidence that lutein is safe in doses up to the highest tested dose of 10 mg daily. A review of other evidence concluded that long-term use of lutein should be safe when taken at a dose of up to 20 mg per day. A 2009 study following 77,126 adults (older than age fifty years), however, suggests that there may be some harm in long-term supplementation with lutein. This study found that long-term use of beta-carotene, lutein, or retinol supplements may increase lung cancer risk. Long-term supplement use was determined by participants' memory of the previous ten years, so the results of this large study should be interpreted with some caution. Finally, maximum safe dosages for young children, pregnant or nursing women, and those with severe liver or kidney disease have not been established.

EBSCO CAM Review Board

FURTHER READING

Olmedilla, B., et al. "Lutein, but Not Alpha-Tocopherol, Supplementation Improves Visual Function in Patients with Age-Related Cataracts." *Nutrition* 19 (2003): 21-24.

Shao, A., and J. N. Hathcock. "Risk Assessment for the Carotenoids Lutein and Lycopene." *Regulatory Toxicology and Pharmacology* 45 (2006): 289-298.

Rosenthal, J. M., et al. "Dose-Ranging Study of Lutein Supplementation in Persons Aged Sixty Years or Older." *Investigative Ophthalmology and Visual Science* 47 (2006): 5227-5233.

Satia, J. A., et al. "Long-Term Use of Beta-Carotene, Retinol, Lycopene, and Lutein Supplements and Lung Cancer Risk." *American Journal of Epidemiology* 169 (2009): 815-828.

Berson, E. L., et al. "Clinical Trial of Lutein in Patients with Retinitis Pigmentosa Receiving Vitamin A." *Archives of Ophthalmology* 128 (2010): 403-411.

See also: Atherosclerosis and heart disease prevention; Beta-carotene; Cataracts; Macular degeneration; Retinitis pigmentosa.

Lycopene

CATEGORY: Functional foods

DEFINITION: Natural substance promoted as a dietary supplement for specific health benefits.

PRINCIPAL PROPOSED USES: None

OTHER PROPOSED USES: Cancer prevention and treatment, cataracts, exercise-induced asthma, gingivitis, heart disease, high blood pressure, intrauterine growth retardation, leukoplakia, macular degeneration, male infertility, oral submucous fibrosis, preeclampsia

OVERVIEW

Lycopene is a powerful antioxidant found in tomatoes and pink grapefruit. Like the better-known supplement beta-carotene, lycopene belongs to the family of chemicals known as carotenoids. As an antioxidant, it is about twice as powerful as beta-carotene.

SOURCES

Lycopene is not a necessary nutrient. However, like other substances found in fruits and vegetables, it may be important for optimal health.

Tomatoes are the best source of lycopene. Cooking does not destroy lycopene, so pizza sauce is just as good as a fresh tomato. Some studies indicate that cooking tomatoes in oil may provide lycopene in a way that is better used by the body, although not all studies agree. Lycopene is also found in watermelon, guava, and pink grapefruit. Synthetic lycopene is also available and appears to be as well absorbed as natural-source lycopene.

THERAPEUTIC DOSAGES

The optimum dosage for lycopene has not been established, but the amount found helpful in studies generally fell in the range of 4 to 8 milligrams (mg) daily. It has been suggested the lycopene is better absorbed when it is taken with fats such as olive oil, but one study failed to find any meaningful change in absorption.

THERAPEUTIC USES

Some observational studies suggest that foods containing lycopene may help prevent macular degeneration, cataracts, cardiovascular disease, and cancer. However, observational studies are highly unreliable means of determining the effectiveness of medical treatments; only double-blind studies can do so, and few have been performed that relate to these potential uses of lycopene.

The best study of lycopene evaluated its possible benefits for pregnant women. Participants in this double-blind study of 251 women received either placebo or 2 mg of lycopene twice daily. For reasons that are not clear, the use of lycopene appeared to reduce the risk of preeclampsia, a dangerous complication of pregnancy. In addition, the use of lycopene appeared to help prevent inadequate growth of the fetus. However, despite these promising results, researchers are cautious about drawing conclusions: Several other nutritional substances have shown promise for preventing preeclampsia in preliminary trials, only to fail when larger and more definitive studies were done.

Lycopene has also shown promise for leukoplakia, a precancerous condition of the mouth and other mucous membranes. In a double-blind, placebo-controlled study, fifty-eight people with oral leukoplakia received either 8 mg oral lycopene daily, 4 mg daily, or placebo capsules for three months. Participants were then followed for an additional two months.

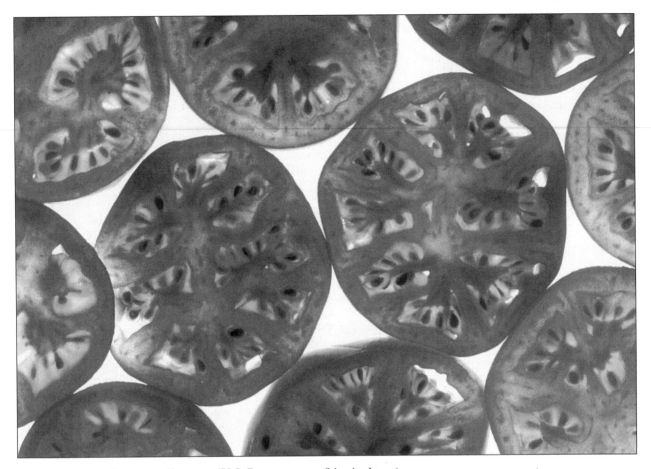

Tomatoes are a major source of lycopene. (U.S. Department of Agriculture)

The results indicated that lycopene in either dose was more effective than placebo for reducing signs and symptoms of leukoplakia, and that 8 mg daily was more effective than 4 mg.

Lycopene (taken at a dose of 16 grams daily) has shown promise for oral submucous fibrosis, a severe condition of the mouth primarily associated with excessive chewing of betel nuts. Regarding yet another mouth condition, gingivitis (periodontal disease), the results of a small double-blind trial suggest that lycopene can offers benefits when taken on its own or when used to augment the effectiveness of standard care.

Much weaker evidence (far too weak to rely upon) hints that lycopene or a standardized tomato extract containing lycopene might be helpful for treating a number of conditions, including prostate cancer, hypertension, breast cancer, and male infertility, and for preventing heart disease, sunburn, and testicular damage caused by the cancer chemotherapy drug adriamycin. Weak evidence hints that lycopene might help protect against side effects, specifically damage to the heart and to developing sperm cells, caused by the drug doxorubicin.

Results of studies have been inconsistent regarding the effects of lycopene and exercise-induced asthma. Finally, one observational study failed to find that high consumption of lycopene reduced the risk of developing diabetes.

SAFETY ISSUES

Lycopene is believed to be a safe supplement, as evidenced by researchers feeling comfortable giving it to pregnant women. One evaluation of the literature concluded that the long-term use of lycopene should be generally safe in doses up to 75 mg per day. Pregnant women should consult with a physician before taking any herbs or supplements. Maximum safe dosages for young children, pregnant or nursing women, and those with severe liver or kidney disease have not been established.

EBSCO CAM Review Board

FURTHER READING

Barber, N. J., et al. "Lycopene Inhibits DNA Synthesis in Primary Prostate Epithelial Cells In Vitro and Its Administration Is Associated with a Reduced Prostate-Specific Antigen Velocity in a Phase II Clinical Study." *Prostate Cancer and Prostatic Diseases* 9 (2006): 407-413.

Chandra, R. V., et al. "Efficacy of Lycopene in the Treatment of Gingivitis." *Oral Health and Preventive Dentistry* 5 (2007): 327-336.

Engelhard, Y. N., et al. "Natural Antioxidants from Tomato Extract Reduce Blood Pressure in Patients with Grade-1 Hypertension." *American Heart Journal* 151 (2006): 100.

Falk, B., et al. "Effect of Lycopene Supplementation on Lung Function After Exercise in Young Athletes Who Complain of Exercise-Induced Bronchoconstriction Symptoms." *Annals of Allergy, Asthma, and Immunology* 94 (2005): 480-485.

Sesso, H. D., J. E. Buring, et al. "Plasma Lycopene, Other Carotenoids, and Retinol and the Risk of Cardiovascular Disease in Men." *American Journal of Clinical Nutrition* 81 (2005): 990-997.

Sesso, H. D., S. Liu, et al. "Dietary Lycopene, Tomato-Based Food Products, and Cardiovascular Disease in Women." *Journal of Nutrition* 133 (2003): 2336-2341.

Shao, A., and J. N. Hathcock. "Risk Assessment for the Carotenoids Lutein and Lycopene." *Regulatory Toxicology and Pharmacology* 45 (2006): 289-298.

Singh, M., et al. "Efficacy of Oral Lycopene in the Treatment of Oral Leukoplakia." *Oral Oncology* 40 (2004): 591-596.

Wang, L., et al. "The Consumption of Lycopene and Tomato-Based Food Products Is Not Associated with the Risk of Type 2 Diabetes in Women." *Journal of Nutrition* 136 (2006): 620-625.

See also: Atherosclerosis and heart disease prevention; Cancer risk reduction; Cancer treatment support; Cataracts; Heart attack; Macular degeneration.

Lysine

CATEGORY: Herbs and supplements
RELATED TERMS: L-lysine, lysine hydrochloride
DEFINITION: Natural substance of the human body used as a supplement to treat specific health conditions.
PRINCIPAL PROPOSED USE: Herpes simplex prevention (cold sores, genital herpes)

OVERVIEW

Lysine is an essential amino acid that is obtained from food. Some evidence suggests that supplemental lysine may be able to help prevent herpes infections such as cold sores and genital herpes.

REQUIREMENTS AND SOURCES

Most people need about 1 gram (g) of lysine per day. The requirement may be greater for athletes and people recovering from major injuries, especially burns. The richest sources of lysine are animal proteins such as meat and poultry, but it is also found in dairy products, eggs, and beans.

THERAPEUTIC DOSAGES

A typical therapeutic dosage of lysine for herpes infections is 1 g three times daily. Lysine can be taken as a regular part of the diet in hopes of preventing herpes flare-ups, or, perhaps, at the first sign of an attack. Although the evidence is not strong, there may be some advantage to restricting the intake of foods that contain a lot of arginine, such as chocolate, peanuts, other nuts and seeds, and, to a lesser extent, wheat.

THERAPEUTIC USES

Some small studies suggest that regular use of lysine supplements can help prevent flare-ups of cold sores and genital herpes, although other studies have not found any benefit. Lysine has also been proposed as a treatment to take at the onset of a flare-up, but at least one study failed to find it effective for this purpose.

Both cold sores and genital herpes are caused by a virus called herpes simplex. After a person is first infected, this virus hides in certain nerve cells and re-emerges during times of stress. Test-tube research suggests that lysine fights this virus by blocking arginine, an amino acid the virus needs to replicate. For this reason, lysine might be most effective when used in conjunction with a low-arginine diet. However, this widely stated claim has not been proven. (Note that if this were true, people who have herpes would need to avoid taking arginine supplements.)

SCIENTIFIC EVIDENCE

It appears that regular use of lysine supplements, when taken in sufficient doses, might be able to reduce the number and intensity of herpes flare-ups. One double-blind, placebo-controlled study followed fifty-two participants with a history of herpes flare-ups. While receiving 3 g of L-lysine every day for six months, the treatment group experienced an average of 2.4 fewer herpes flare-ups than the placebo group, a significant difference. The lysine group's flare-ups were also significantly less severe and healed faster.

Another double-blind, placebo-controlled crossover study on forty-one subjects also found improvements in the frequency of attacks. This study found that 1,250 milligrams (mg) of lysine daily worked, but 624 mg did not. Other studies, including one that followed sixty-five individuals, found no benefit, but they used lower dosages of lysine.

Although some of these studies are promising, none of them was large enough to give conclusive answers. At this point, more evidence is needed to determine whether lysine is effective for preventing herpes simplex.

Many people use lysine in a different way: They take it at the onset of a herpes attack. However, a double-blind, placebo-controlled study evaluating this method found no benefit. One should consider using the herb lemon balm instead.

SAFETY ISSUES

Although lysine is an essential part of the diet, the safety of concentrated lysine supplements has not been well studied. In animal studies, high dosages have caused gallstones and elevated cholesterol levels, so those persons with either of these problems may want to use caution when using lysine. Maximum safe dosages for young children, pregnant or nursing women, and those with severe liver or kidney disease have not been established. In persons taking lysine to treat herpes, arginine might counteract the potential benefit.

EBSCO CAM Review Board

FURTHER READING

Flodin, N. W. "The Metabolic Roles, Pharmacology, and Toxicology of Lysine." *Journal of the American College of Nutrition* 16 (1997): 7-21.

See also: Herbal medicine; Herpes; Lemon balm.

M

Maca

CATEGORY: Herbs and supplements
RELATED TERM: *Lepidium meyenii*
DEFINITION: Natural plant product used to treat specific health conditions.
PRINCIPAL PROPOSED USE: Male sexual dysfunction
OTHER PROPOSED USES: Adaptogen, benign prostate enlargement, diabetes, fatigue, female infertility, female sexual dysfunction, hypertension, male infertility, osteoarthritis

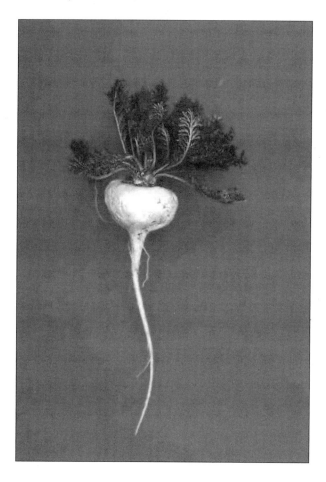

Peruvian maca root. (PR Newswire)

OVERVIEW

Maca is a Peruvian root vegetable used as both food and medicine. It is sometimes called Peruvian ginseng, not because the plants have any botanical relationship, but because their traditional uses are somewhat similar. Traditionally, maca has been said to increase energy and stamina and to enhance both fertility and sex drive in men and women.

THERAPEUTIC DOSAGES

The usual dose of maca is 500 to 1,000 milligrams (mg) three times a day.

THERAPEUTIC USES

Maca is widely marketed for improving male sexual function, female sexual function, and both male fertility and female fertility. However, at present there is no reliable evidence that it actually provides any benefits. Much of the evidence for maca comes from animal studies. In one study in rats, use of maca enhanced male sexual function. Animal studies have had mixed results regarding male and female fertility.

There are two published human trials on maca, performed by a single research group. In one small twelve-week, double-blind, placebo-controlled study, use of maca at 1,500 mg or 3,000 mg increased male libido. While this was an interesting finding, the study did not report benefits in male sexual function, just in desire. Since loss of sexual function (for example, impotence) is a more common problem in men than loss of sexual desire, these results do not justify the widespread claim that maca has been shown to act like a kind of herbal Viagra.

Another small study found that four months of maca use increased sperm count and sperm function. This study failed to use a control group, and for this reason, its results are essentially meaningless. There have been no human trials on maca for female fertility or female sexual function. Contrary to widespread reports, maca does not appear to increase testosterone levels or, in fact, to affect any male hormones.

Other animal studies hint that maca might offer benefits for prostate enlargement, stress, diabetes, and high blood pressure. However, this evidence is too weak to justify any claims regarding maca and these conditions. One human trial evaluated a combination of maca and cat's claw for osteoarthritis, but because it failed to include a placebo group, its results mean little.

SAFETY ISSUES

In the two reported human clinical trials, use of maca has not led to any serious adverse effects. However, this herb has not undergone comprehensive safety testing. Safety in young children, pregnant or nursing women, and people with severe liver or kidney disease has not been established.

EBSCO CAM Review Board

FURTHER READING

Gonzales, G. F., et al. "Effect of *Lepidium meyenii* (Maca), a Root with Aphrodisiac and Fertility-Enhancing Properties, on Serum Reproductive Hormone Levels in Adult Healthy Men." *Journal of Endocrinology* 176 (2003): 163-168.

_____. "Effect of *Lepidium meyenii* (Maca) on Sexual Desire and Its Absent Relationship with Serum Testosterone Levels in Adult Healthy Men." *Andrologia* 34 (2002): 367.

_____. "*Lepidium meyenii* (Maca) Improved Semen Parameters in Adult Men." *Asian Journal of Andrology* 3 (2002): 301-303.

Lopez-Fando, A., et al. "*Lepidium peruvianum chacon* Restores Homeostasis Impaired by Restraint Stress." *Phytotherapy Research* 18 (2004): 471-474.

Mehta, K., et al. "Comparison of Glucosamine Sulfate and a Polyherbal Supplement for the Relief of Osteoarthritis of the Knee." *BMC Complementary and Alternative Medicine* 7 (2007): 34.

See also: Ginseng; Herbal medicine; Sexual dysfunction in men.

Macrobiotic diet

CATEGORY: Therapies and techniques
RELATED TERM: Macrobiotics
DEFINITION: A philosophy of living based on the need for balance and harmony in which a person's diet consists primarily of whole grains and fresh vegetables and is low in fat and protein.
PRINCIPAL PROPOSED USES: Acquired immunodeficiency syndrome, cancer, general health and well-being
OTHER PROPOSED USE: Heart disease risk

OVERVIEW

Japanese philosopher George Ohsawa developed the macrobiotic lifestyle, which includes the macrobiotic diet, meditation, exercise, and stress reduction. The lifestyle also involves limiting exposure to pesticides. Ohsawa also believed that eating healthy food is part of a process that promotes world peace and harmony.

The macrobiotic diet is based on the traditional Japanese diet. Food choices for the diet are based on the principle of yin and yang, opposing forces that are viewed as needing to balance each other. In the 1960s, Ohsawa's student Michael Kushi, of the Kushi Institute, popularized the macrobiotic diet in the United States. The original diet proposed by Ohsawa is now viewed by macrobiotic diet teachers to be too restrictive; the current macrobiotic diet has been modified to prevent problems such as scurvy, other forms of malnutrition, and death, which were reported in some followers of the original diet.

Organic foods that are minimally processed are recommended for the macrobiotic diet. Up to 60 percent of the diet's components are whole grains and up to 30 percent are vegetables, with the remainder of the diet being made up of beans and seaweed. The diet does not include meat, animal fats, dairy, eggs, refined sugar, or artificial sweeteners. Warm drinks are to be avoided too.

The diet also recommends specific approaches to food preparation. For example, only gas stoves are to be used, and cooking vessels or utensils containing copper, aluminum, or Teflon are to be avoided.

MECHANISM OF ACTION

As a means of restoring the balance of yin and yang, teachers of macrobiotics attempt to adjust the individual person's diet based on the areas affected by illness.

USES AND APPLICATIONS

Proponents of the macrobiotic diet state that it can have curative properties for cancer and acquired immunodeficiency syndrome (AIDS), can prevent heart disease, and can contribute to an overall sense of well-being.

SCIENTIFIC EVIDENCE

No randomized-controlled clinical trials of the macrobiotic diet exist. Reports of macrobiotic dieters who have recovered from cancer are anecdotal.

SAFETY ISSUES

The macrobiotic dieter may become deficient in vitamins B_{12} or D, fluid, calcium, iron, and riboflavin. Experts recommend that pregnant or nursing women and children on the macrobiotic diet may need to consume eggs, dairy products, or other forms of supplementation to prevent nutritional deficiencies that can lead to rickets, retarded growth, or slow motor or mental development in the fetus.

Katherine Hauswirth, R.N., M.S.N.

FURTHER READING

American Cancer Society. "Macrobiotic Diet." Available at http://www.cancer.org/treatment.

Kushi Institute. "What Is Macrobiotics?" Available at http://www.kushiinstitute.org/html/what_is_macro.html.

MD Anderson Cancer Center, University of Texas. "Macrobiotics: Detailed Scientific Review." Available at http://www.mdanderson.org/education-and-research.

See also: Diet-based therapies; Low-carbohydrate diet; Low-glycemic index diet; Raw foods diet; Vegan diet; Vegetarian diet.

Macular degeneration

CATEGORY: Condition

RELATED TERMS: Dry macular degeneration, maculopathy, wet macular degeneration

DEFINITION: Treatment of the gradual deterioration of the macula, an area of the retina.

PRINCIPAL PROPOSED NATURAL TREATMENTS: Carotenoids (such as lutein and zeaxanthin), zinc with or without antioxidants

OTHER PROPOSED NATURAL TREATMENTS: Beta-carotene, bilberry, ginkgo, low-glycemic-index diet, oligomeric proanthocyanidins, vitamin E

INTRODUCTION

The lens of the eye focuses an image on a portion of the retina called the macula, the area of finest visual perception. Gradual deterioration of the macula is called macular degeneration. After cataracts, damage to the macula is the second most common cause of visual impairment in persons older than age sixty-five years. Smoking, high blood pressure, and atherosclerosis are associated with progressive damage to the macula. Ultraviolet light may also play a role by creating harmful free radicals in the eye.

In the most common form of macular degeneration (dry macular degeneration), a substance known as lipofuscin accumulates in the lining of the retina. A much less common form of macular degeneration involves the abnormal growth of blood vessels (wet macular degeneration). This can be treated successfully if attended to soon enough, but it may lead to irreversible blindness if left untreated. For this reason, medical consultation in all cases of macular degeneration (or any other type of vision loss) is essential.

PRINCIPAL PROPOSED NATURAL TREATMENTS

The treatments described in this section are intended as support to standard ophthalmological care, not as a substitute for it. In addition, all studies refer primarily to the more common type of macular degeneration, dry macular degeneration.

Zinc and antioxidants. A single, solid study suggests that zinc, or a mixture of zinc and antioxidants, can prevent or slow the progression of early macular degeneration. However, it is not clear whether the antioxidant portion of this mixture added any additional benefit. This double-blind, placebo-controlled trial evaluated the effects of zinc with or without antioxidants on macular degeneration in 3,640 persons in the early stage of the disease. Participants were randomly assigned to receive one of the following treatments: antioxidants (vitamin C at 500 milligrams [mg], vitamin E at 400 international units, and beta-carotene at 15 mg), zinc (80 mg) and copper (2 mg), antioxidants plus zinc, or placebo. The results indicate that zinc alone or zinc plus antioxidants significantly slowed the progression of the disease. It is not clear how much the antioxidants in the mixture contributed to the benefits.

Zinc at doses of 80 mg and higher daily can be harmful. One of the problems is that high-dose zinc supplementation impairs copper absorption. This is why extra copper was provided in the foregoing study. However, there may be other risks too, so physician supervision is advised.

There is no convincing evidence that antioxidants alone are effective for preventing or delaying the onset of macular degeneration. A four-year, double-blind, placebo-controlled trial of 1,193 people with macular degeneration failed to find vitamin E alone helpful for preventing or treating macular degeneration. An even larger and longer study, following more than twenty thousand people for more than ten years, failed to find that beta-carotene alone reduced the incidence of macular degeneration. A mixture of beta-carotene, vitamin E, and vitamin C has also failed to prove beneficial. A review of three randomized controlled trials involving a total of 23,099 subjects found no evidence of benefit for vitamin E and beta-carotene.

Lutein and other carotenoids. Carotenoids are a group of substances that are found in many fruits and vegetables, especially those that are yellow-orange and dark green. (Beta-carotene is the best known carotenoid.) Observational studies suggest that the higher intake of dietary carotenoids is associated with a lower incidence of macular degeneration.

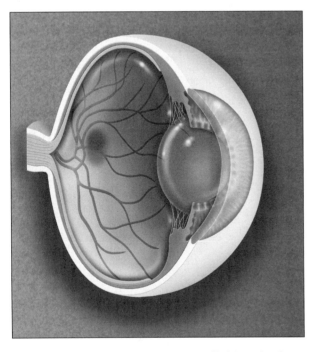

Gradual deterioration of the macula is called macular degeneration. (BSIP/Photo Researchers, Inc.)

However, observational studies prove little about cause and effect. To determine whether carotenoids can actually prevent or treat macular degeneration, double-blind, placebo-controlled studies are necessary.

In the large study mentioned, beta-carotene failed to prove effective for preventing macular degeneration. However, the less well-known carotenoids lutein and zeaxanthin might be more promising. These carotenoids, principally found in corn and dark-green leafy vegetables, are found in high concentrations in the eye. It has been suggested that they may protect the macula from light-induced damage by dyeing it yellow, thereby acting as a kind of natural pair of sunglasses. They also act in the usual antioxidant fashion by neutralizing free radicals.

These hopes received support from a double-blind, placebo-controlled trial that enrolled ninety people with dry macular degeneration and followed them for twelve months. The participants received either lutein (10 mg), lutein plus antioxidants and a multivitamin-multimineral supplement, or placebo. At the end of the study period, participants who had taken lutein alone or lutein plus the other nutrients showed improvements in vision, while no change in vision was seen in the placebo group. A subsequent study failed to find benefit with lutein, but it used a lower dose (6 mg daily) and involved fewer people. Ultimately, further study will be needed to establish whether lutein is actually helpful for macular degeneration.

OTHER PROPOSED NATURAL TREATMENTS

Like carotenoids, flavonoids are found in many plants and may offer a variety of beneficial effects. Weak but interesting evidence suggests that bilberry and oligomeric proanthocyanidins, both rich in flavonoids, may prevent or treat macular degeneration.

The herb *Ginkgo biloba* also contains many flavonoids and is also thought to increase circulation. In a six-month, double-blind, placebo-controlled study of twenty people with macular degeneration, the use of ginkgo at a dose of 160 mg daily resulted in improved visual acuity. Furthermore, positive results were seen in a twenty-four-week double-blind study of ninety-nine people with macular degeneration that compared ginkgo extract at a dose of 240 mg per day with ginkgo at a dose of 60 mg per day. Vision improved in both groups, but to a greater extent with the higher dose. This study would have been more meaningful if it had included a placebo group, but nonetheless, "dose-related" effects of this type hint that a treatment may really work. It has been suggested that ginkgo aids vision by increasing blood flow to the optic nerve, but one study designed to evaluate this possible mechanism of action failed to document such an effect.

Weak evidence hints that moderate wine consumption might help prevent macular degeneration. Similarly weak evidence suggests possible benefit with a low-glycemic-index diet.

In observational studies, people who happen to consume a diet rich in omega-3 fatty acids (fish oil) seem to lower their risk of macular degeneration. However, in the absence of randomized-controlled trials, it is not possible to say whether or not it is the omega-3 that produces this benefit. One controlled study that failed to use a placebo group appeared to find benefit with a combination of acetyl-L-carnitine, fish oil, and coenzyme Q_{10}.

EBSCO CAM Review Board

FURTHER READING

Bartlett, H. E., and F. Eperjesi. "Effect of Lutein and Antioxidant Dietary Supplementation on Contrast Sensitivity in Age-Related Macular Disease." *European Journal of Clinical Nutrition* 61 (2007): 1121-1127.

Chiu, C. J., et al. "Dietary Glycemic Index and Carbohydrate in Relation to Early Age-Related Macular Degeneration." *American Journal of Clinical Nutrition* 83 (2006): 880-886.

Chong, E. W., et al. "Dietary Omega-3 Fatty Acid and Fish Intake in the Primary Prevention of Age-Related Macular Degeneration." *Archives of Ophthalmology* 126 (2008): 826-833.

Christen, W. G., et al. "Beta-Carotene Supplementation and Age-Related Maculopathy in a Randomized Trial of U.S. Physicians." *Archives of Ophthalmology* 125 (2007): 333-339.

Evans, J., and K. Henshaw. "Antioxidant Vitamin and Mineral Supplements for Preventing Age-Related Macular Degeneration." *Cochrane Database of Systematic Reviews* (2008): CD000253. Available through *EBSCO DynaMed Systematic Literature Surveillance* at http://www.ebscohost.com/dynamed.

Feher, J., et al. "Improvement of Visual Functions and Fundus Alterations in Early Age-Related Macular Degeneration Treated with a Combination of Acetyl-L-Carnitine, N-3 Fatty Acids, and Coenzyme Q10." *Ophthalmologica* 219 (2005): 154-166.

Preventing Macular Degeneration

The following recommendations for a healthful lifestyle apply to those with age-related macular degeneration (AMD) and to those who are at risk of developing the disease:

- *Healthy eating.* Although scientific evidence is inconclusive, a diet rich in nutrients may lower one's risk of AMD. To ingest a high level of antioxidants, one should eat a minimum of five servings per day of varied fruits and vegetables. Green leafy vegetables such as spinach, kale, and collard greens are particularly recommended. Eating fish and other foods that contain omega-3 fatty acid may also reduce one's risk of AMD. Also, moderate wine consumption may help decrease the risk of developing AMD.

- *Exercise.* Cardiovascular exercise improves the body's overall health and helps maintain a healthy circulatory system. One should always wear a hat or cap when outdoors and should also wear sunglasses or protective lenses all year.

- *Doctor visits.* One should consult a doctor to treat hypertension, high cholesterol, or other heart-related conditions; to get regular eye examinations (once every other year before age fifty years, and every year after that); and before taking any type of antioxidant supplement.

Reviewed by Brian Randall, M.D.

Taylor, H. R., et al. "Vitamin E Supplementation and Macular Degeneration." *British Medical Journal* 325 (2002): 11.

Wimpissinger, B., et al. "Influence of *Ginkgo biloba* on Ocular Blood Flow." *Acta Ophthalmologica Scandinavica* 85 (2007): 445-449.

See also: Aging; Blepharitis; Carotenoids; Cataracts; Elder health; Glaucoma; Lutein; Night vision, impaired; Retinitis pigmentosa; Uvietis; Zinc.

Magnesium

CATEGORY: Herbs and supplements
RELATED TERMS: Magnesium chloride, magnesium citrate, magnesium fumarate, magnesium gluconate,

magnesium malate, magnesium orotate, magnesium oxide, magnesium sulfate

DEFINITION: Natural substance of the human body used as a supplement to treat specific health conditions.

PRINCIPAL PROPOSED USES: Diabetes, hypertension, kidney stones, migraine headaches, noise-related hearing loss

OTHER PROPOSED USES: Angina, asthma, atherosclerosis, autism, cholesterol, congestive heart failure, coronary artery disease, dysmenorrhea, fatigue, fibromyalgia, glaucoma, mitral valve prolapse, osteoporosis, preeclampsia, pregnancy-induced leg cramps, premenstrual syndrome, restless legs syndrome, stroke

OVERVIEW

Magnesium is an essential nutrient, meaning that the body needs it for healthy functioning. It is found in significant quantities throughout the body and used for numerous purposes, including muscle relaxation, blood clotting, and the manufacture of ATP (adenosine triphosphate, the body's main energy molecule).

Magnesium has been called nature's calcium channel blocker because of its ability to block calcium from entering muscle and heart cells. A group of prescription heart medications work in a similar way, although much more powerfully. This may be the basis for some of magnesium's effects when it is taken as a supplement in fairly high doses.

REQUIREMENTS AND SOURCES

Requirements for magnesium increase as people grow and age. The official U.S. and Canadian recommendations for daily intake are as follows: 30 milligrams (mg) for infants up to six months old, 75 mg for infants seven to twelve months old, 80 mg for children one to three years old, 130 mg for children four to eight years old, and 240 mg for persons nine to thirteen years old. For those fourteen to eighteen years old, the recommendations are 410 mg for males and 360 mg for females; for those nineteen to thirty years old, 400 mg for males and 310 for females; and for those aged thirty-one and over, 420 mg for males and 320 mg for women. The recommendations for pregnant women are 400 mg for those eighteen and younger, 350 mg for those nineteen to thirty years old, and 360 mg for those thirty-one to fifty years old; for nursing women, they are 360 mg for those aged eigh-

teen and younger, 310 mg for those nineteen to thirty, and 320 mg for those thirty-one to fifty years old.

These recommendations refer to total intake from food plus supplements. The average diet provides a daily intake of magnesium very close to these amounts. In the United States, the average dietary intake of magnesium is lower than the recommended daily allowance; however, it is unclear whether this truly indicates deficiency, or if the recommended allowance is too high. Alcohol abuse, surgery, diabetes, zinc supplements, certain types of diuretics (thiazide and loop diuretics, but not potassium-sparing diuretics), estrogen and oral contraceptives, and the medications cisplatin and cyclosporin have been reported to reduce the body's level of magnesium or increase magnesium requirements. Those taking potassium supplements may receive greater benefit from them if they take extra magnesium as well. While it is sometimes said that calcium interferes with magnesium absorption, this effect is apparently too small to have a significant effect on overall magnesium status.

Kelp is very high in magnesium, as are wheat bran, wheat germ, almonds, and cashews. Other good sources include blackstrap molasses, brewer's yeast (not to be confused with nutritional yeast), buckwheat, nuts, and whole grains. One can also get appreciable amounts of magnesium from collard greens, dandelion greens, avocado, sweet corn, cheddar cheese, sunflower seeds, shrimp, dried fruit (figs, apricots, and prunes), and from many other common fruits and vegetables.

THERAPEUTIC DOSAGES

A typical supplemental dosage of magnesium ranges from the nutritional needs described above to as high as 600 mg daily. For premenstrual syndrome (PMS) and dysmenorrhea (painful menstruation), an alternative approach is to start taking 500 to 1,000 mg daily, beginning on day fifteen of the menstrual cycle and continuing until menstruation begins. Magnesium citrate may be slightly more absorbable than other forms of magnesium.

THERAPEUTIC USES

Preliminary double-blind studies suggest that regular use of magnesium supplements may help prevent migraine headaches, hearing loss caused by exposure to loud noises, and kidney stones and may help treat high blood pressure, angina, dysmenorrhea (menstrual cramps), pregnancy-induced leg cramps, and premenstrual syndrome (including menstrual migraines).

People with diabetes are often deficient in magnesium, and according to some (but not all) studies, magnesium supplementation may enhance blood sugar control and insulin sensitivity in people with diabetes or prediabetic conditions. Magnesium may also help control blood pressure in people with both hypertension and diabetes.

One study found that magnesium supplements might be helpful for people with mitral valve prolapse who also have low levels of magnesium in the blood. There is some evidence that magnesium may decrease the atherosclerosis risk caused by hydrogenated oils, the margarine-like fats found in many junk foods.

Magnesium supplements do not appear to be helpful for preventing preeclampsia. (Magnesium, taken by injection rather than orally, however, is probably helpful for treating preeclampsia that already exists.)

Magnesium is sometimes said to decrease symptoms of restless legs syndrome, but the evidence that it works consists solely of open trials without a placebo group, and such studies are not trustworthy. Weak evidence hints at possible benefits for insomnia.

It is often said that magnesium supplements are essential for preventing or treating osteoporosis, but there is only minimal supporting evidence for this claim. Studies on magnesium supplements for improving sports performance have returned contradictory results.

Magnesium has also been suggested as a treatment for Alzheimer's disease, attention deficit disorder, fatigue, fibromyalgia, low high-density lipoproteins (HDL, or good cholesterol), periodontal disease, rheumatoid arthritis, and stroke. However, there is virtually no evidence that it is helpful for any of these conditions. Despite some early enthusiasm, combination therapy with vitamin B_6 and magnesium has not been found helpful in autism. One double-blind, placebo-controlled study failed to find magnesium helpful in glaucoma.

Magnesium is sometimes advocated for stabilizing the heart after a heart attack, but one study actually found that use of magnesium slightly increased risk of sudden death, repeat heart attack, or need for bypass surgery in the year following the initial heart attack. However, magnesium may be helpful in congestive heart failure. In a well-designed trial involving seventy-nine patients with severe congestive heart failure,

magnesium (as magnesium orotate) significantly improved survival and clinical symptoms after one year compared with a placebo.

Alternative medical literature frequently mentions magnesium as a treatment for asthma. However, this idea seems to be based primarily on the use of intravenous magnesium as an emergency treatment for asthma. Taking something by mouth is very different from having it injected into the veins. Studies of oral magnesium for asthma have shown more negative than positive results. Inhaled, aerosolized magnesium, however, has shown some promise.

Although magnesium is sometimes mentioned as a treatment to help keep the heart beating normally, a six-month double-blind trial of 170 people did not find it effective for preventing a particular heart rhythm abnormality called atrial fibrillation. However, a small double-blind, placebo-controlled trial found that magnesium supplements reduced episodes of arrhythmia in individuals with congestive heart failure (CHF). One possible explanation: People with congestive heart failure often take drugs (loop diuretics) that deplete magnesium. The combination of magnesium deficiency with digoxin (another drug given for CHF) may cause arrhythmias. Thus, it is possible that the benefits seen here were caused by correction of that depletion.

Magnesium and Diabetes

Magnesium plays an important role in carbohydrate metabolism. It may influence the release and activity of insulin, the hormone that helps control blood glucose (sugar) levels. Low blood levels of magnesium (called hypomagnesemia) are frequently seen in persons with type 2 diabetes. Hypomagnesemia may worsen insulin resistance, a condition that often precedes diabetes, or may be a consequence of insulin resistance.

Persons with insulin resistance do not use insulin efficiently and require greater amounts of insulin to maintain blood sugar within normal levels. The kidneys possibly lose their ability to retain magnesium during periods of severe hyperglycemia (significantly elevated blood glucose). The increased loss of magnesium in urine may then result in lower blood levels of magnesium. In older adults, correcting magnesium depletion may improve insulin response and action.

SCIENTIFIC EVIDENCE

Migraine headaches. A double-blind study found that regular use of magnesium helps prevent migraine headaches. In this twelve-week trial, eighty-one people with recurrent migraines were given either 600 mg of magnesium daily or a placebo. By the last three weeks of the study, the treated group's migraines had been reduced by 41.6 percent, compared with a reduction of 15.8 percent in the placebo group. The only side effects observed were diarrhea (in about one-fifth of the participants) and, less often, digestive irritation.

Similar results have been seen in other, smaller double-blind studies. One study found no benefit, but it has been criticized on many significant points, including using an excessively strict definition of what constituted benefit.

Noise-related hearing loss. One double-blind, placebo-controlled study on three hundred military recruits suggests that 167 mg of magnesium daily can prevent hearing loss due to exposure to high-volume noise.

Kidney stones. Magnesium inhibits the growth of calcium oxalate stones in the test tube and decreases stone formation in rats. However, human studies have had mixed results. In one two-year open study, 56 people taking magnesium hydroxide had fewer recurrences of kidney stones than 34 people not given magnesium. In contrast, a double-blind (and, hence, more reliable) study of 124 people found that magnesium hydroxide was essentially no more effective than a placebo.

Hypertension. Magnesium works with calcium and potassium to regulate blood pressure. Several studies suggest that magnesium supplements can reduce blood pressure in people with hypertension, although some studies have not shown this.

In one study, eighty-two people (ages forty to seventy-five years) with diabetes, high blood pressure, and low levels of magnesium were randomized to receive 2.5 g of magnesium chloride or a placebo for four months. Those in the treatment group had lower blood pressure readings compared with those in the control group.

Angina. In a double-blind, placebo-controlled trial of 187 people with angina, six months of treatment with magnesium at a dose of 730 mg daily improved exercise tolerance and enhanced overall quality of life. Benefits were also seen in a similar, smaller double-blind trial.

After a heart attack. In a one-year double-blind, placebo-controlled trial of 468 individuals who had just experienced a heart attack, use of a magnesium supplement at a dose of 360 mg daily failed to prevent heart-related events (defined as heart attack, sudden cardiac death, or need for cardiac bypass) and actually may have increased the risk slightly.

Dysmenorrhea. A six-month double-blind, placebo-controlled study of fifty women with menstrual pain found that treatment with magnesium significantly improved symptoms. The researchers reported evidence of reduced levels of prostaglandin F 2 alpha, a hormone-like substance involved in pain and inflammation. Similarly positive results were seen in a double-blind, placebo-controlled study of twenty-one women.

Premenstrual syndrome (PMS). A double-blind, placebo-controlled study of thirty-two women found that magnesium taken from day fifteen of the menstrual cycle to the onset of menstrual flow could significantly improve PMS symptoms, specifically mood changes.

Another small, double-blind preliminary study found that regular use of magnesium could reduce symptoms of PMS-related fluid retention. In this study, thirty-eight women were given magnesium or placebo for two months. The results showed no effect after one cycle, but by the end of two cycles, magnesium significantly reduced weight gain, swelling of extremities, breast tenderness, and abdominal bloating. In addition, one small double-blind study (twenty participants) found that magnesium supplementation can help prevent menstrual migraines. Preliminary evidence suggests that the combination of magnesium and vitamin B_6 might be more effective than either treatment alone.

Pregnancy-induced leg cramps. Pregnant women frequently experience painful leg cramping. One double-blind trial of seventy-three pregnant women found that three weeks of magnesium supplements significantly reduced leg cramps compared with a placebo.

SAFETY ISSUES

The U.S. government has set the following upper limits for use of magnesium supplements: 65 mg for children aged one to three, 110 mg for children four to eight, 350 mg for adults, and 350 mg for pregnant or nursing women. In general, magnesium appears to be quite safe when taken at or below recommended dosages. The most common complaint is loose stools. However, people with severe kidney or heart disease should not take magnesium (or any other supplement) except on the advice of a physician. Maximum safe dosages have not been established for children of all ages. There has been one case of death caused by excessive use of magnesium supplements in a developmentally and physically disabled child. Pregnant or nursing women should not exceed the nutritional dosages presented in the Requirements and Sources section.

If taken at the same time, magnesium can interfere with the absorption of antibiotics in the tetracycline family and, possibly of the drug nitrofurantoin. Also, when combined with oral diabetes drugs in the sulfonylurea family, magnesium may cause blood sugar levels to fall more than expected.

IMPORTANT INTERACTIONS

Persons taking potassium supplements, manganese, loop and thiazide diuretics, oral contraceptives, estrogen replacement therapy, cisplatin, digoxin, or medications that reduce stomach acid may need extra magnesium. Persons taking antibiotics in the tetracycline family or nitrofurantoin (Macrodantin) should separate their magnesium dose from doses of these medications by at least two hours to avoid absorption problems. Those taking oral diabetes medications in the sulfonylurea family (Tolinase, Micronase, Orinase, Glucotrol, Diabinese, DiaBeta) should work closely with their physicians when taking magnesium to avoid hypoglycemia. Those taking amiloride should not take magnesium supplements except on medical advice.

EBSCO CAM Review Board

FURTHER READING

Guerrero-Romero, F., and M. Rodríguez-Morán. "The Effect of Lowering Blood Pressure by Magnesium Supplementation in Diabetic Hypertensive Adults with Low Serum Magnesium Levels." *Journal of Human Hypertension* 23, no. 4 (2009): 245-251.

Hatzistavri, L. S., et al. "Oral Magnesium Supplementation Reduces Ambulatory Blood Pressure in Patients with Mild Hypertension." *American Journal of Hypertension* 22, no. 10 (2009): 1070-1075.

Kazaks, A. G., et al. "Effect of Oral Magnesium Supplementation on Measures of Airway Resistance and Subjective Assessment of Asthma Control and Quality of Life in Men and Women with Mild to Moderate Asthma." *Journal of Asthma* 47, no. 1 (2010): 83-92.

Stepura, O. B., and A. I. Martynow. "Magnesium Orotate in Severe Congestive Heart Failure (MACH)." *International Journal of Cardiology* 134, no. 1 (2009): 145-147.

See also: Diabetes; Hearing loss; Herbal medicine; Hypertension; Kelp; Kidney stones.

Magnet therapy

CATEGORY: Therapies and techniques
RELATED TERMS: Electromagnetic therapy, magnetic stimulation, pulsed electromagnetic field therapy, repetitive transcranial magnet therapy, static magnets, transcranial magnetic stimulation
DEFINITION: Technique using magnets and magnetic fields on or near the body.
PRINCIPAL PROPOSED USES:

- *Static magnets:* Diabetic peripheral neuropathy and other forms of peripheral neuropathy, fibromyalgia, low back pain and other forms of chronic musculoskeletal pain, post-polio syndrome, rheumatoid arthritis, wound healing after plastic surgery
- *Pulsed electromagnetic field therapy:* Migraines, non-healing bone fractures, osteoarthritis, postoperative pain, stress incontinence and bed-wetting
- *Repetitive transcranial magnet therapy:* Depression

OTHER PROPOSED USES

- *Static magnets:* Carpal tunnel syndrome, chronic pelvic pain in women, edema, fatigue, insomnia, menstrual pain, osteoarthritis, rheumatoid arthritis, scar tissue, sports and fitness support, surgery support, tinnitus
- *Pulsed electromagnetic field therapy:* Erectile dysfunction, multiple sclerosis
- *Repetitive transcranial magnet therapy:* Epilepsy, myofascial pain syndrome, obsessive-compulsive disorder, Parkinson's disease, post-traumatic stress disorder, schizophrenia

OVERVIEW

Long popular in Japan, magnet therapy has entered public awareness in the United States, stimulated by golfers and tennis players extolling the virtues of magnets in the treatment of sports-related injuries. Magnetic knee, shoulder, and ankle pads, and insoles and mattress pads, are widely available and are thought to provide myriad healing benefits.

Despite this enthusiasm, there is little scientific evidence to support the use of magnets for any medical condition. However, some small studies suggest that various forms of magnet therapy might have a therapeutic effect in certain conditions.

History of magnet therapy. Magnet therapy has a long history in traditional folk medicine. Reliable documentation indicates that Chinese doctors have believed in the therapeutic value of magnets for two thousand years or more. In sixteenth-century Europe, Paracelsus used magnets to treat a variety of ailments. Two centuries later, Franz Mesmer became famous for treating various disorders with magnets.

In the middle decades of the twentieth century, scientists in various parts of the world began performing studies on the therapeutic use of magnets. From the 1940s on, magnets became increasingly popular in Japan. Yoshio Manaka, one of the influential Japanese acupuncturists of the twentieth century, used magnets in conjunction with acupuncture. Magnet therapy also became a commonly used technique of self-administered medicine in Japan. For example, a type of plaster containing a small magnet became popular for treating aches and pains, especially among the elderly. Magnetic mattress pads, bracelets, and necklaces also became popular, mainly among the elderly. During the 1970s, both magnets and electromagnetic machines became popular among athletes in many countries for treating sports-related injuries.

These developments led to a rapidly growing industry creating magnetic products for a variety of conditions. However, the development of this industry preceded any reliable scientific evidence that static magnets actually work for the purposes intended. In the United States, it was only in 1997 that properly designed clinical trials of magnets began to be reported. Subsequently, results of several preliminary studies suggested that both static magnets and electromagnetic therapy may indeed offer therapeutic benefits for several disorders. These findings have escalated research interest in magnet therapy.

Types of magnet therapy and their uses. The term "magnet therapy" usually refers to the use of static magnets placed directly on the body, generally over regions of pain. Static magnets are either attached to the body by tape or encapsulated in specially designed

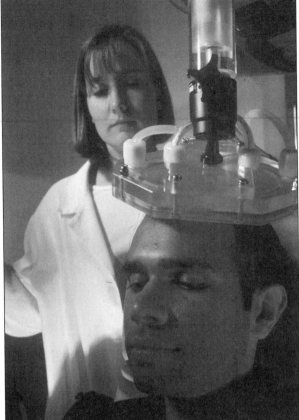

A patient receiving an experimental treatment for depression using repetitive transcranial magnetic stimulation. (Richard T. Nowitz/Photo Researchers, Inc.)

products such as belts, wraps, or mattress pads. Static magnets are also sometimes known as permanent magnets.

Static magnets come in various strengths. The units of measuring magnet strength are gauss (G) and tesla (T); 1 tesla equals 10,000 G. A refrigerator magnet, for example, is around 200 G. Therapeutic magnets measure anywhere from 200 to 10,000 G, but the most commonly used measure from 400 to 800 G.

Therapeutic magnets come in two different types of polarity arrangements: unipolar magnets and alternating-pole devices. Magnets that have north on one side and south on the other are known, rather confusingly, as unipolar magnets. Bipolar or alternating-pole magnets are made from a sheet of magnetic material with north and south magnets arranged in an alternating pattern, so that both north and south face the skin. This type of magnet exerts a weaker magnetic field because the alternating magnets tend to oppose each other. Each type of magnet has its own recommended uses and enthusiasts. (There are many heated opinions, with no supporting evidence, on this matter.)

More complex magnetic devices have also been studied, not for home use, but for use in physicians' offices and hospitals. A special form of electromagnetic therapy, repetitive transcranial magnetic stimulation (rTMS), is undergoing particularly close study. rTMS is designed specifically to treat the brain with low-frequency magnetic pulses. A large body of small studies suggest that rTMS might be beneficial for depression. It is also being studied for the treatment of amyotrophic lateral sclerosis (ALS), Parkinson's disease, epilepsy, schizophrenia, and obsessive-compulsive disorder.

MECHANISM OF ACTION

Many commercial magnets have such a weak field that it is hard to believe they could affect the body at all. Some, however, are quite powerful and could conceivably cause effects at some depth. Nonetheless, biophysicists are skeptical that static magnets could significantly affect the body. (The moving magnetic fields of rTMS and pulsed electromagnetic therapy, or PEMF, act differently, and there is little doubt that they can affect nerve tissue and possibly other parts of the body.)

A commonly held misconception is that magnets attract the iron in blood cells, thus moving the blood and stimulating circulation. However, the iron in the blood is not in a magnetic form. Static magnets could affect charged particles in the blood, nerves, and cell membranes or subtly alter biochemical reactions, although whether the effect is strong enough to make a difference remains to be shown. Some research results suggest that static magnets affect local blood circulation, but a rigorously designed double-blind trial found that commercially available static magnets have no effect on blood flow. Another well-designed trial also failed to find effects on blood circulation. However, there is some weak evidence that static magnets may affect muscle metabolism. Further research will be necessary to sort out these possibilities.

SCIENTIFIC EVIDENCE

Static magnets. In double-blind, placebo-controlled trials, static magnets have shown promise for a number of conditions, but in no case is the evidence strong enough to be relied upon. In a 2007 review of all studies of static magnets as a treatment for pain, researchers concluded that there is no meaningful evidence that they are effective; they further concluded that current evidence suggests that, for some pain-related conditions, static magnets are not effective (a much stronger statement than the first).

Some magnet proponents claim that it is impossible to carry out a truly double-blinded study on magnets because participants can simply use a metal pin or a similar object to discover whether they have a real magnet or not. Some researchers have gotten around this by using a weak magnet as the placebo treatment. Other researchers have designed more complicated placebo devices that participants have been found unable to identify as fake treatments.

Rheumatoid arthritis. A double-blind, controlled trial of sixty-four people with rheumatoid arthritis of the knee compared the effects of strong alternating polarity magnets with the effects of a deliberately weak unipolar magnet. Researchers used the weakened magnet as a control group so that participants would not find it easy to break the blind by testing the magnetism of their treatment.

After one week of therapy, 68 percent of the participants using the strong magnets (the treatment group) reported relief, compared with 27 percent

---

How Magnet Therapy Might Work

No scientific theory or manufacturer claim about how magnet therapy might work has been proven. Although some preliminary research has been conducted in animals and in small clinical trials, the mechanisms by which magnets might affect the human body are not yet known. Scientific researchers and magnet manufacturers have proposed that magnets might work by:

- Changing how nerve cells function and by blocking pain signals to the brain
- Restoring the balance between cell death and growth
- Increasing the flow of blood and the delivery of oxygen and nutrients to tissues
- Increasing the temperature of the area of the body being treated

in the control group. This difference was statistically significant. Two of four other subjective measurements of disease severity also showed statistically significant improvements. However, no significant improvements were seen in objective evaluations of the condition, such as blood tests for inflammation severity or physician's assessment of joint tenderness, swelling, or range of motion. This study suggests that magnet therapy may reduce the pain of rheumatoid arthritis without altering actual inflammation. However, the mixture of statistically significant and insignificant results indicates that a larger trial is necessary to factor out "statistical noise."

Post-polio syndrome. A double-blind, placebo-controlled study of fifty people with post-polio syndrome found evidence that magnets are effective for relieving pain. The magnets or placebo magnets were placed on previously determined trigger points (one per person) for forty-five minutes. (Trigger points are sore areas within muscle that, when pressed, cause relief in other areas of the muscle and conversely, when inflamed, cause pain in other parts of the muscle.) In the treatment group, 76 percent of the participants reported improvement, compared with 19 percent in the placebo group.

Fibromyalgia. A six-month, double-blind, placebo-controlled trial of 119 people with fibromyalgia compared two commercially available magnetic mattress pads with sham treatment and no treatment. Group 1 used a mattress pad designed to create a uniform magnetic field of negative polarity. Group 2 used a mattress pad that varied in polarity. In both groups, manufacturer's instructions were followed. Groups 3 and 4 used sham treatments designed to match in appearance the magnets used in groups 1 and 2. Group 5 received no treatment.

On average, participants in all groups showed improvement in the six months of the study. Participants in the treatment groups, especially group 1, showed a trend toward greater improvement; however, the differences between real treatment and sham or no treatment failed to reach statistical significance in most measures. This outcome suggests that magnetic mattress pads might be helpful for fibromyalgia, but a larger study would be necessary to identify benefits.

An earlier double-blind, placebo-controlled study of thirty women with fibromyalgia did find significant improvement with magnets compared with placebo. The women slept on magnetic mattress pads (or sham pads for the control group) every night for four months. Of the twenty-five women who completed the trial, participants sleeping on the experimental mattress pads experienced a significant decrease in pain and fatigue compared with the placebo group, along with significant improvement in sleep and physical functioning.

A single-blind study of somewhat convoluted design provides weak evidence that a gown made from a special "electromagnetic shielding fabric" can reduce fibromyalgia symptoms. The rationale for using this fabric is, however, somewhat scientifically implausible.

Peripheral neuropathy. A four-month, double-blind, placebo-controlled, crossover study of nineteen people with peripheral neuropathy found a significant reduction in symptoms compared with placebo. Participants wore magnetic foot insoles during the day throughout the trial period. Reduction in the symptoms of burning, numbness, and tingling were especially marked in those cases of neuropathy associated with diabetes.

Based on these results, a far larger randomized, placebo-controlled, follow-up study was performed by the same researchers. This trial enrolled 375 people with peripheral neuropathy caused by diabetes and tested the effectiveness of four months of treatment with magnetic insoles. The results indicated that the insoles produced benefits beyond that of the placebo effect, reducing such symptoms as burning pain, numbness, tingling, and exercise-induced pain.

Surgery support. A double-blind, placebo-controlled study looked at the effect of magnets on healing after plastic surgery. The study examined the use of magnets on twenty persons who had suction lipectomy (liposuction). Magnets contained in patches were placed over the operative region immediately after surgery and left in place for fourteen days. The treatment group experienced statistically significant reduction of pain and swelling on postoperative days one through four, and of discoloration on days one through three, compared with the control group. Another study of 165 people, however, failed to find that the use of static magnets over the surgical incision reduced post-surgical pain. Furthermore, the positioning of static magnets at the acupuncture/acupressure point P6 in persons undergoing ear, nose, and throat or gynecological surgeries reduced nausea and vomiting no better than placebo in a randomized trial.

Low back pain and other forms of chronic musculoskeletal pain. A double-blind, placebo-controlled, crossover trial of fifty-four people with knee or back pain compared a complex static magnet array with a sham magnet array. Participants used either the real or the sham device for twenty-four hours; then, after a seven-day rest period, they used the opposite therapy for another twenty-four hours. Evaluations showed that the use of the real magnet was associated with greater improvements than the sham treatment.

Benefits were also seen in a double-blind, placebo-controlled trial of forty-three people with chronic knee pain who used fairly high-power but otherwise ordinary static magnets continuously for two weeks. In another placebo-controlled trial, the use of a magnetic knee wrap for twelve weeks was associated with a significant increase in quadriceps (thigh muscle) strength in persons with knee osteoarthritis.

A double-blind, placebo-controlled, crossover study of twenty people who had chronic low back pain for a minimum of six months failed to find any evidence of benefit. However, the alternating-pole magnet used in this study produced a very weak magnetic field. Another study found some benefit that failed to reach statistical significance.

In a double-blind study of 101 people with chronic neck and shoulder pain, the use of a magnetic necklace failed to prove more effective than placebo treatment. Another study failed to find magnetic insoles helpful for heel pain.

Osteoarthritis. A widely publicized twelve-week study of 194 people reportedly found that the use of magnetic bracelets reduced osteoarthritis pain in the hip and knee. However, the study actually found statistically similar benefits among participants given a placebo treatment. The researchers suggest that this failure to show superior effects may have been caused, in part, by an error: The study utilized weak magnets as the placebo treatments, but thirty-four persons in the placebo group accidentally received strong magnets instead. This would tend to decrease the difference in outcome seen between the treatment and the placebo group and could therefore hide a real treatment benefit. Nonetheless, this study does not provide evidence that magnetic bracelets offer any benefit for osteoarthritis beyond that of the placebo effect.

A much smaller study also failed to find statistically significant benefit, but it was too small to be able to produce statistically meaningful results. Rather, it was designed to evaluate a special placebo magnet device. After the study, researchers polled the participants to see if they could correctly identify whether they had been given the real treatment or the placebo: They could not.

Pelvic pain. A double-blind, placebo-controlled study of 14 women with chronic pelvic pain (from endometriosis or other causes) found no significant benefit when magnets were applied to abdominal trigger points for two weeks. However, statistical analysis showed that it would have been necessary to enroll a larger number of participants to detect an effect. A larger study did find some evidence of benefit after four weeks of treatment, but a high dropout rate and other design problems compromise the meaningfulness of the results. Another small study found possible evidence of benefit in menstrual pain.

Carpal tunnel syndrome. A double-blind, placebo-controlled study of thirty people with carpal tunnel syndrome found that a single treatment with a static magnet produced dramatic and long-lasting benefits. However, identical dramatic benefits were seen in the placebo group. In two more small, randomized trials, researchers again found that there were no differences between the treatment and the placebo groups. Both groups experienced similar improvements in symptoms.

In a small study involving thirty-one people with long-standing carpal tunnel syndrome, a combination of static magnet and pulsed electromagnetic field therapy modestly improved deep pain but had no significant effect on overall pain in a two-month period.

Sports performance. People who undergo intense exercise often experience muscle soreness afterwards. One study tested magnet therapy for reducing this symptom. However, while the use of magnets did reduce muscle soreness, so did placebo treatment, and there was no significant difference between the effectiveness of magnets and placebo. Another study, of more complex design, also failed to find benefit.

Magnetic insoles have been advocated for increasing sports performance. However, a study of fourteen college athletes failed to find that magnetic insoles improved vertical jump, bench squat, forty-yard dash, or performance of a soccer-specific fitness test.

Pulsed electromagnetic field therapy. Pulsed electromagnetic field therapy (PEMF) is quite distinct from magnet therapy itself. (The term "electromagnetic field" does not, in this case, refer to magnetism in the ordinary sense.) Nonetheless, for historical reasons, PEMF is often classified with true magnetic therapies.

Bone has a remarkable capacity to heal from injury. In some cases, though, the broken ends do not join, leading to what is called nonunion fractures. PEMF therapy has been used to stimulate bone repair in nonunion and other fractures since the 1970s; this is a relatively accepted use. More controversially, PEMF has shown promise for osteoarthritis, stress incontinence, and possibly other conditions.

Osteoarthritis. Three double-blind, placebo-controlled studies enrolling more than 350 people suggest that PEMF therapy can improve symptoms of osteoarthritis. For example, a double-blind, placebo-controlled study tested PEMF in eighty-six people with osteoarthritis of the knee and eighty-one people with osteoarthritis of the cervical spine. Participants received eighteen half-hour sessions with either a PEMF machine or a sham device. The treated participants showed significantly greater improvements in disease severity than those given placebo. For both osteoarthritis conditions, benefits lasted for a minimum of one month after treatment was stopped.

A later double-blind trial evaluated low-power, extremely low-frequency PEMF for the treatment of knee osteoarthritis. A total of 176 people received eight sessions of either sham or real treatment for two weeks. The results showed significantly greater pain reduction in the treated group.

Urinary incontinence. Many women experience stress incontinence, the leakage of urine following any action that puts pressure on the bladder. Laughter, physical exercise, and coughing can all trigger this unpleasant occurrence. A recent study suggests that PEMF treatment might be helpful. In this placebo-controlled study, researchers applied high-intensity pulsating magnetic fields to sixty-two women with stress incontinence. The intention was to stimulate the nerves that control the pelvic muscles.

The results showed that one session of magnetic stimulation significantly reduced episodes of urinary leakage over the following week, compared with placebo. In the treated group, 74 percent experienced significant improvement, compared with only 32 percent in the placebo group. Presumably, the high-intensity magnetic field used in this treatment created electrical currents in the pelvic muscles and nerves. This was confirmed by objective examination of thirteen participants, which found that magnetic stimulation was increasing the strength of closure at the exit from the bladder. However, there was one serious flaw in this study: It does not appear to have been double-blind. Researchers apparently knew which participants were getting real treatment and which were not and, therefore, might have unconsciously biased their observations to conform to their expectations. Thus, the promise of electromagnetic therapy for stress incontinence still needs to be validated in properly designed trials.

Similarly, magnetic stimulation has been studied for the treatment of bed-wetting (nocturnal enuresis). In a small preliminary study, the use of PEMF day and night for two months was helpful in girls.

Multiple sclerosis. A two-month, double-blind, placebo-controlled study of thirty people with multiple sclerosis was conducted using a PEMF device. Participants were instructed to tape the device to one of three different acupuncture points on the shoulder, back, or hip. The study found statistically significant improvements in the treatment group, most notably in bladder control, hand function, and muscle spasticity. Benefits were seen in another small study too.

Erectile dysfunction. In a three-week, double-blind, placebo-controlled trial, twenty men with erectile dys-

Paracelsus on Magnets and Disease

Physician-botanist-alchemist Paracelsus (1493-1541), an early proponent of what is now called magnet therapy, discusses the use of magnets in treating disease in humans. Two perspectives are presented here.

Fortified by experience which is the mistress of all things, and by mature theory, based on experience, I affirm that the Magnet is a stone which not only undeniably attracts steel and iron, but has also the same power over the matter of all diseases in the whole body of man.

By the attractive power of a magnet acting upon the diseased aura of the blood in an affected part, that aura may be made to return into the center from which it originated, and be absorbed therein, and thereby we may destroy the herd of the virus and cure the patient, and we need not wait idly to see what Nature will do. The magnet is therefore useful in all inflammations, in fluxes and ulcerations, in diseases of the bowels and uterus, in internal as well as in external disease.

function received PEMF therapy or placebo. The magnetic therapy was administered by means of a small box worn near the genital area and kept in place as continuously as possible during the study period; neither participants nor observers knew whether the device was activated or not. The results showed that the use of PEMF significantly improved sexual function compared with placebo.

Migraines. In a double-blind trial, forty-two people with migraine headaches were given treatment with real or placebo PEMF therapy to the inner thighs for one hour, five times per week for two weeks. The results showed benefits in headache frequency and severity. However, the study design was rather convoluted and nonstandard, so the results are difficult to interpret.

Postoperative pain. In a small, randomized trial, eighty women undergoing breast augmentation surgery were divided into three groups. The first group received PEMF therapy for seven days after surgery to both breasts, the second group received fake PEMF therapy to both breasts as a control, and the third group received real and fake PEMF therapy to either breast. Compared to the control, women receiving PEMF therapy reported significantly less discomfort and used less pain medications by the third postoperative day.

Electromagnetic therapy. Unlike PEMF, repetitive transcranial magnetic stimulation (rTMS) involves magnetic fields and is, therefore, more closely related to standard magnet therapy. rTMS, which involves applying low-frequency magnetic pulses to the brain, has been investigated for treating emotional illnesses and other conditions that originate in the brain. The results of preliminary studies have been generally promising.

Depression. About twenty small studies have evaluated rTMS for the treatment of depression, including severe depression that does not respond to standard treatment and the depressive phase of bipolar illness, and most found it effective. In one of these studies, seventy people with major depression were given rTMS or sham rTMS in a double-blind setting of two weeks. The results showed that participants who had received actual treatment experienced significantly greater improvement than did those receiving sham treatment. In a far larger study involving 301 depressed persons, none of whom were being treated with antidepressant medications, real rTMS was sig-

nificantly more effective than fake rTMS after four to six weeks of treatment.

In another trial involving ninety-two elderly persons whose depression had been linked to poor blood flow to the brain (vascular depression), actual rTMS was significantly more effective than sham rTMS. Benefits were more notable in younger participants. In a particularly persuasive piece of evidence, researchers pooled the results of thirty double-blind trials involving 1,164 depressed persons and determined that real rTMS was significantly more effective than sham rTMS.

Two separate studies suggest that rTMS may be an effective additional treatment for the 20 to 30 percent of depressed people for whom conventional drug therapy is not successful. Another group of researchers pooled the results of twenty-four studies involving 1,092 persons and found rTMS to be more effective than sham for treatment-resistant depression. Electroconvulsive therapy (shock treatment) is often used for people in this category, but rTMS may be an equally effective alternative.

Epilepsy. In a double-blind, placebo-controlled trial, twenty-four people with epilepsy (technically, partial complex seizures or secondarily generalized seizures) not fully responsive to drug treatment were given treatment with rTMS or sham rTMS twice daily for one week. The results showed a mild reduction in seizures among the people given real rTMS. However, the benefits rapidly disappeared when treatment was stopped. Similarly short-lived effects were seen in an open trial.

Schizophrenia. A double-blind, placebo-controlled, crossover trial looked at the use of low-frequency rTMS in twelve people diagnosed with schizophrenia and manifesting frequent and treatment-resistant auditory hallucinations (hearing voices). Participants received rTMS for four days, with the length of treatment building from four minutes on the first day to sixteen minutes on the fourth day. Active stimulation significantly reduced the incidence of auditory hallucinations compared with sham stimulation. The extent of the benefit varied widely, lasting from one day in one participant to two months in another. Possible benefits were seen in other small studies. Researchers pooling the results of six controlled trials, which involved 232 persons with schizophrenia resistant to conventional treatment, found that real, low-frequency rTMS was significantly better at reducing auditory hallucinations than sham rTMS.

Parkinson's disease. In a double-blind, placebo-controlled trial of ninety-nine people with Parkinson's disease, real rTMS was more effective than sham rTMS delivered in eight weekly treatments. Similar benefits were seen in three other small studies. Even more encouraging, the combined results of ten randomized trials in persons with Parkinson's indicated significant benefit for rTMS (using higher frequencies).

Chronic pain syndromes. rTMS technology has also been applied to areas other than the brain. Myofascial pain syndrome is a condition similar to fibromyalgia but is more localized. Whereas fibromyalgia involves tender trigger points all over the body, myofascial pain syndrome involves trigger points clustered in one portion of the body only. One controlled trial found indications that a form of repetitive magnetic stimulation applied to the painful area may be effective for myofascial pain syndrome of the trapezius muscle.

In a placebo-controlled trial involving sixty-one people with long-standing diabetes, low-frequency repetitive magnetic stimulation failed to diminish the pain associated with diabetic peripheral neuropathy. However, in another study involving twenty-eight people with peripheral neuropathy, high-frequency rTMS applied to the brain was more effective at reducing pain and improving quality of life than was fake rTMS.

Tinnitus. One preliminary study found indications that rTMS may be helpful for tinnitus (ringing in the ear).

Post-traumatic stress disorder. A small, double-blind, placebo-controlled study found that the use of rTMS may be able to reduce symptoms of post-traumatic stress disorder.

Cigarette addiction. A small, double-blind, placebo-controlled study found evidence that rTMS may reduce the craving for cigarettes in people attempting to quit smoking.

Obsessive-compulsive disorder. A double-blind, placebo-controlled study of eighteen people with obsessive-compulsive disorder found no evidence of benefit with rTMS.

Amyotrophic lateral sclerosis. Amyotrophic lateral sclerosis, also called Lou Gehrig's disease, is a nerve disorder that causes progressive muscle weakness. A small pilot study hinted that rTMS may be beneficial at least temporarily.

HOW TO USE MAGNET THERAPY

The following is a brief description of the use of magnet therapy. However, one should keep in mind that the ways that magnets are used have not been fully evaluated by long-term clinical testing. A full medical evaluation is advisable before using magnets. One should not treat a painful back with magnets if the underlying cause of pain is a fracture or a tumor.

Types of magnets. There are a number of theories on the best size and type of magnets to use and where to apply them, based on the type of condition being treated and other factors. Because unipolar magnets have greater depth of magnetic field penetration, some researchers consider these more effective in treating deeper tissues. Conversely, it is considered that alternating-pole magnet devices might be more effective at stimulating surface tissue. Thus, it might be appropriate to use a unipolar high-gauss magnet for low back pain that originates deep in the tissue and an alternating-pole configuration for an injury closer to the surface, such as a wrist sprain. However, there is no meaningful scientific evidence to support these distinctions.

In addition, some practitioners hold that the north side of the magnet calms and the south side excites, and that using the correct side of the magnet is crucial. However, from a scientific perspective, it is difficult to see how there could be any difference between the two poles of the magnet in terms of the effect upon body tissue.

There is general consensus that the magnet should be placed as close to the affected part of the body as possible. This can be done by taping the magnet to the skin, slipping the magnet inside a bandage over the affected area, or using a wrap device that has embedded magnets.

Taping magnets to the body might irritate the skin; in addition, some research scientists and practitioners suspect that the body may accommodate to the magnetic field over time, thus reducing the therapeutic effect. To prevent both the irritation and the accommodation, practitioners usually recommend intermittent use, such as five days on, two days off or twelve hours on, twelve hours off.

Magnetic devices available. Manufacturers make a wide range of magnetic devices. For treating large areas of the body, wraps and belts containing magnets are available. Wraps are specifically designed for the wrist, elbow, knee, ankle, neck, shoulder, and back, and are often made from thermal material to have the added effect of warming the area. These wraps are often recommended in cases of injury and arthritis, where heat feels better. Proponents of magnet therapy often recommend the use of magnetic mattress pads and mattresses for people with problems affecting several areas of the body, such as fibromyalgia or arthritis; they also recommend magnetic mattress pads for insomnia and fatigue.

Proponents of magnet therapy recommend magnetic foot insoles for people with diabetic peripheral neuropathy, leg aches and pains, circulatory problems of the lower extremities, or foot injuries and problems, and for people who stand all day. Magnetic necklaces are said to be useful for neck and shoulder pain and for generalized aches and pains, and magnetic bracelets are advocated for wrist pain and general problems.

SAFETY ISSUES

In general, magnets appear to be safe; the biggest risk appears to be skin irritation from any tape that is used to hold them in place. Magnetic resonance imaging (MRI) machines, for example, expose the body to gigantic magnetic fields, and extensive investigation has found no evidence of harm. However, during the MRI, a person is subjected to a high level of magnetism for a short period of time, whereas people who use static magnets daily or sleep on them every night are subjected to a low level of magnetism over a long period of time. It is not known whether this type of exposure has any deleterious effects. Nonetheless, one study, in which participants slept on a magnetic mattress pad every night for four months, found no side effects. In addition, a safety study of rTMS found no evidence of harm. In a large study in which rTMS was administered to numerous people with depression, totaling more than ten thousand cumulative treatment sessions, no significant adverse effects were reported. Transient headache and scalp discomfort were the most frequent problems reported. There were no seizures or changes in hearing or cognition.

It was previously thought that persons with an implantable cardioverter-defibrillator (ICD) or a pacemaker should not use magnetic devices at all, but this recommendation has been adjusted. One study found that with the exception of magnetic mattresses and mattress pads, most magnets sold for therapeutic purposes do not interfere with the magnetically activated switches present in most pacemakers. Magnetic mattress pads can deactivate and alter the function of ICDs and pacemakers, but other therapeutic magnets are safe if kept six inches or farther from these devices.

There are theoretical concerns that magnets might be risky for people with epilepsy. Similarly, until the physiological effects of magnet treatments are better understood, pregnant women should avoid them.

EBSCO CAM Review Board

FURTHER READING

Andre-Obadia, N., et al. "Pain Relief by rTMS: Differential Effect of Current Flow but No Specific Action on Pain Subtypes." *Neurology* 71 (2008): 833-840.

Bretlau, L. G., et al. "Repetitive Transcranial Magnetic Stimulation (rTMS) in Combination with Escitalopram in Patients with Treatment-Resistant Major Depression." *Pharmacopsychiatry* 41 (2008): 41-47.

Cepeda, M. S., et al. "Static Magnetic Therapy Does Not Decrease Pain or Opioid Requirements." *Anesthesia and Analgesia* 104 (2007): 290-294.

Chen, C. Y., et al. "Effect of Magnetic Knee Wrap on Quadriceps Strength in Patients with Symptomatic Knee Osteoarthritis." *Archives of Physical Medicine and Rehabilitation* 89 (2008): 2258-2264.

Colbert, A. P., et al. "Static Magnetic Field Therapy for Carpal Tunnel Syndrome." *Archives of Physical Medicine and Rehabilitation* 91 (2010): 1098-1104.

Heden, P., and A. A. Pilla. "Effects of Pulsed Electromagnetic Fields on Postoperative Pain: A Double-Blind Randomized Pilot Study in Breast Augmentation Patients." *Aesthetic Plastic Surgery* 32 (2008): 660-666.

Klaiman, P., et al. "Magnetic Acupressure for Management of Postoperative Nausea and Vomiting." *Minerva Anestesiologica* 74 (2008): 635-642.

Pittler, M. H., E. M. Brown, and E. Ernst. "Static Magnets for Reducing Pain." *CMAJ: Canadian Medical Association Journal* 177 (2007): 736-742.

Wrobel, M. P., et al. "Impact of Low Frequency Pulsed Magnetic Fields on Pain Intensity, Quality of Life, and Sleep Disturbances in Patients with Painful Diabetic Polyneuropathy." *Diabetes and Metabolism* 34 (2008): 349-354.

See also: Electromagnetic hypersensitivity; Pain management.

Mahesh Yogi, Maharishi

ALSO KNOWN AS: Maharishi (honorific); Mahesh Prasad Varma (given name)

CATEGORY: Biography

IDENTIFICATION: Indian philosopher and teacher who developed and promoted Transcendental Meditation

BORN: October 18, c. 1911; Jabalpur, Madhya Pradesh, India

DIED: February 5, 2008; Vlodrop, the Netherlands

OVERVIEW

Maharishi Mahesh Yogi was an Indian philosopher and teacher born in India. He developed Transcendental Meditation, which combines mantra meditation and spiritual techniques. The Maharishi has been called the guru of this technique, which has more recently been termed a spiritual movement.

The Maharishi earned a degree in physics from Allahabad University in 1942. Around this same time, he became a disciple and helper to Swami Brahmananda Saraswati, a notable spiritual leader in India and the Maharishi's inspiration. Around 1955, the Maharishi began to promote Transcendental Meditation and related techniques that are aimed at holistic well-being.

The Maharishi gained particular popularity in the 1960s and 1970s both because of his worldwide tours to promote his teachings and because of his association with various celebrities, including members of the band The Beatles. He later detailed his travel experiences in the book *Thirty Years Around the World* (1986). He founded the International Meditation Society in 1959, the same year his movement was renamed Transcendental Meditation, and in 1966 he founded the Students' International Meditation Society. He soon began promoting regular yoga in combination with meditation, practices that are in line with the modern teachings that stemmed from his original approach.

The Maharishi later mentored Deepak Chopra, a popular Indian American physician, writer, and public speaker, during the early 1990s. The two parted ways around 1994, when Chopra left the movement, reportedly because of a disagreement about Chopra's decision to expand his own teaching and writing career.

An estimated several million people have studied the Maharishi's techniques, and his work has been recognized by many academic and clinical institutions,

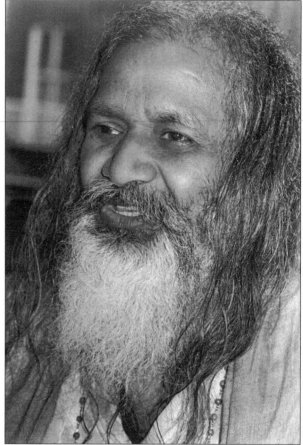

Maharishi Mahesh Yogi. (Hulton Archive/Getty Images)

including universities and holistic practices. According to various media sources (including *Time* and *Newsweek*), the Maharishi has been criticized by other Indian scholars and sages for presenting an overly simplified program that supposedly contradicts traditional Hindu beliefs and practices. Furthermore, others criticized the Maharishi and his affiliates for lavish spending and for gaining popularity for his business acumen, rather than for his spiritual and holistic teachings. The Maharishi stepped down from his active leadership and administrative roles in 2008, and he observed a period of spiritual silence (*mauna*), until his death a few weeks later.

Brandy Weidow, M.S.

FURTHER READING

Humes, Cynthia A. "Maharishi Mahesh Yogi: Beyond the T. M. Technique." In *Gurus in America*, edited by Thomas A. Forsthoefel and Cynthia A. Humes. *Gurus in America*. Albany: State University of New York Press, 2005.

Mason, Paul. *The Maharishi: The Biography of the Man Who Gave Transcendental Meditation to the World*. Shaftsbury, Dorset, England: Element Books, 1994.

See also: Charaka; Chopra, Deepak; Mind/body medicine; Popular practitioners; Spirituality; Transcendental Meditation.

Maitake

CATEGORY: Herbs and supplements
RELATED TERM: *Grifola frondosa*
DEFINITION: Natural plant product used to treat specific health conditions.
PRINCIPAL PROPOSED USES: Adaptogen, strengthen immunity
OTHER PROPOSED USES: Diabetes, cancer treatment, human immunodeficiency virus infection support, high cholesterol, hypertension

OVERVIEW

Maitake is a medicinal mushroom used in Japan as a general promoter of robust health. As with *Coriolus versicolor*, shiitake, and reishi (all fungi), innumerable healing powers have been attributed to maitake, ranging from curing cancer to preventing heart disease. There has not been enough reliable research to determine whether any of these ancient beliefs are really true.

THERAPEUTIC DOSAGES

Maitake is an edible mushroom that can be eaten as food or made into tea. A typical dosage of dried maitake in capsule or tablet form is 3 to 7 grams daily.

THERAPEUTIC USES

Contemporary herbalists classify maitake as an adaptogen, a substance said to help the body adapt to stress and resist infection. However, there is no definitive scientific evidence to show that maitake (or any other purported adaptogen) really functions in this way.

Most investigation has focused on the polysaccharide constituents of maitake. This family of substances is known to affect the human immune system in complex ways, and one substance in particular, beta-D-glucan, has been studied for its potential benefit in treating cancer and human immunodeficiency virus infection. Highly preliminary studies also suggest that maitake may be useful in treating diabetes, hypertension (high blood pressure), and high cholesterol. However, there is no real evidence that maitake is effective for these or any other illnesses.

SAFETY ISSUES

Maitake is widely believed to be safe, although formal safety studies have not been performed. Safety in young children, pregnant or nursing women, and those with severe liver or kidney disease has not been established.

EBSCO CAM Review Board

FURTHER READING

Konno, S. "Maitake SX-fraction: Possible Hypoglycemic Effect on Diabetes Mellitus." *Alternative and Complementary Therapy* 7 (2001): 366-370.

Kubo, K., H. Aoki, and H. Nanba. "Anti-diabetic Activity Present in the Fruit Body of *Grifola frondosa* (Maitake)." *International Biological and Pharmaceutical Bulletin* 17 (1994): 1106-1110.

Kubo, K., and H. Nanba. "Anti-hyperliposis Effect of Maitake Fruit Body (*Grifola frondosa*)." *International Biological and Pharmaceutical Bulletin* 20 (1997): 781-785.

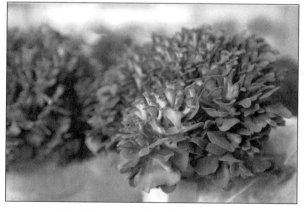

Innumerable healing powers have been attributed to maitake, ranging from curing cancer to preventing heart disease. There has not been enough reliable research to determine whether any of these ancient beliefs are really true. (AP Photo)

Yamada, Y., H. Nanba, and H. Kuroda. "Antitumor Effect of Orally Administered Extracts from Fruit Body of *Grifola frondosa* (Maitake)." *Chemotherapy* 38 (1990): 790-796.

See also: Coriolus versicolor; Ginseng; Herbal medicine; Immune support; Reishi; Shiitake.

Malic acid

CATEGORY: Herbs and supplements
RELATED TERM: Apple acid
DEFINITION: Natural substance of the human body used as a supplement to treat specific health conditions.
PRINCIPAL PROPOSED USES: None
OTHER PROPOSED USE: Fibromyalgia

OVERVIEW

The body synthesizes malic acid during the process of converting carbohydrates to energy. Extremely preliminary evidence suggests that individuals with the disease fibromyalgia (a disorder that involves fatigue and chronic pain in the muscles) might have difficulty creating or utilizing malic acid. Such a deficiency could interfere with normal muscle function.

Based on this supposition, products containing malic acid and other nutrients were widely offered for sale to people with fibromyalgia. However, there is no evidence that these products are in fact helpful.

REQUIREMENTS AND SOURCES

The body produces its own malic acid. Many fruits and vegetables also supply malic acid, most notably apples.

THERAPEUTIC DOSAGES

In studies and commercial products, the usual dose of malic acid for fibromyalgia is 1,200 to 2,800 milligrams (mg) per day, generally combined with magnesium and other nutrients.

THERAPEUTIC USES

Malic acid is a major ingredient in combination treatments used for fibromyalgia. However, there is no meaningful evidence that it works.

SCIENTIFIC EVIDENCE

In a double-blind, placebo-controlled trial, twenty-four individuals with fibromyalgia were given either a placebo or malic acid (1,200 mg per day) combined with magnesium (300 mg daily). After four weeks of treatment, there was no significant difference between the placebo and malic acid groups.

The researchers then gave all participants the malic acid combination and increased the dose over a six-month period. A significant improvement in fibromyalgia symptoms was found after the dose reached about 1,600 mg of malic acid with 400 mg of magnesium. However, because this part of the trial was not blind or controlled, the results may be entirely due to the placebo effect. Only a properly designed double-blind, placebo-controlled trial of the higher malic acid dose could demonstrate that it really works, and no such trial has been reported.

SAFETY ISSUES

Malic acid appears to be safe at recommended dosages. A few people reported loose stools at the higher doses in the above studies, possibly because of the magnesium in the combination. Safety in pregnant or nursing women, children, and individuals with severe liver or kidney disease has not been established.

EBSCO CAM Review Board

FURTHER READING

Abraham, G. E., and J. D. Flechas. "Management of Fibromyalgia: Rationale for the Use of Magnesium and Malic Acid." *Journal of Nutrition and Medicine* 3 (1992): 49-59.

Russell, I. J., et al. "Treatment of Fibromyalgia Syndrome with Super Malic." *Journal of Rheumatology* 22 (1995): 953-958.

See also: Chronic fatigue syndrome; Fibromyalgia: Homeopathic remedies; Herbal medicine; Magnesium; Pain management.

Manganese

CATEGORY: Herbs and supplements
RELATED TERMS: Manganese chloride, manganese gluconate, manganese picolinate, manganese sulfate

DEFINITION: Natural substance of the human body used as a supplement to treat specific health conditions.

PRINCIPAL PROPOSED USES: Dysmenorrhea, osteoporosis

OTHER PROPOSED USES: Diabetes, epilepsy, muscle sprains and strains, rheumatoid arthritis, tardive dyskinesia

OVERVIEW

The human body contains only a very small amount of manganese, but this metal is important as a constituent of many key enzymes. The chemical structure of these enzymes is interesting: Large protein molecules cluster around a tiny atom of metal.

Manganese plays a particularly important role as part of the natural antioxidant enzyme superoxide dismutase (SOD), which helps fight damaging free radicals. It also helps energy metabolism, thyroid function, blood sugar control, and normal skeletal growth.

REQUIREMENTS AND SOURCES

The official U.S. recommendations for daily manganese intake are as follows: 0.003 mg for infants up to six months of age, 0.6 mg for infants seven to twelve months old, 1.2 mg for children one to three years old, 1.5 mg for children four to eight years old, 1.9 mg for males nine to thirteen years old, 2.2 mg for males fourteen to eighteen years old, 1.6 mg for females nine to eighteen years old, 2.3 mg for males nineteen years of age and older, and 1.8 mg for females nineteen years of age and older. The recommendation for pregnant women is 2 mg and for nursing women 2.6 mg. The absorption of manganese may be impaired by simultaneous intake of antacids or calcium or iron supplements.

The best sources of dietary manganese are whole grains, legumes, avocados, grape juice, chocolate, seaweed, egg yolks, nuts, seeds, boysenberries, blueberries, pineapples, spinach, collard greens, peas, and green vegetables.

THERAPEUTIC DOSAGES

A typical dosage used in studies on manganese is 3 to 6 mg daily. It is sometimes recommended at a much higher dose of 50 to 200 mg daily for two weeks following a muscle sprain or strain, but this dosage exceeds recommended safe intake levels.

THERAPEUTIC USES

Because manganese plays a role in bone metabolism, it has been suggested as a treatment for osteoporosis, a condition in which bone mass deteriorates with age. However, there is no direct evidence that manganese is helpful, except perhaps in combination with other minerals. Manganese has also been suggested for the treatment of muscle strains and sprains, rheumatoid arthritis, and tardive dyskinesia, but there is no reliable evidence to indicate that it actually helps.

One small but rigorous study suggests that making sure to get enough manganese may help control symptoms of dysmenorrhea (menstrual pain). People with epilepsy or diabetes have lower-than-normal levels of manganese in their blood. This suggests (but definitely does not prove) that manganese supplements might be useful for these conditions. However, studies that could prove or disprove this idea have not been performed.

SCIENTIFIC EVIDENCE

Osteoporosis. Although manganese is known to play a role in bone metabolism, there is no direct evidence that manganese supplements can help prevent osteoporosis. However, one double-blind, placebo-controlled study suggests that a combination of minerals including manganese may be helpful. Fifty-nine women took either a placebo, calcium (1,000 mg daily), or calcium plus a daily mineral supplement consisting of 5 mg of manganese, 15 mg of zinc, and 2.5 mg of copper. After two years, the group receiving calcium plus minerals showed better bone density than the group receiving calcium alone. But this study does not reveal whether it was the manganese or the other minerals that made the difference.

Dysmenorrhea. One very small but well-designed and carefully conducted double-blind study suggested that 5.6 mg of manganese daily might ease menstrual discomfort. In the same study, a lower dosage of 1 mg daily was not effective.

SAFETY ISSUES

Manganese is thought to be safe when taken by adults at a dose of 11 mg daily or less. The maximum safe dosage of manganese for pregnant or nursing women has also been established as 11 mg daily, or 9 mg if the woman is eighteen years old or younger.

Very high exposure to manganese (due either to environmental pollution or manganese mining) has resulted in a serious psychiatric disorder known as manganese madness.

IMPORTANT INTERACTIONS

Persons taking iron, copper, zinc, magnesium, or calcium may need extra manganese; those taking manganese may need extra iron, copper, zinc, magnesium, and calcium. Those taking antacids may also need extra manganese.

EBSCO CAM Review Board

FURTHER READING

Freeland-Graves, J. H., and P. H. Lin. "Plasma Uptake of Manganese as Affected by Oral Loads of Manganese, Calcium, Milk, Phosphorous, Copper, and Zinc." *Journal of the American College of Nutrition* 10 (1991): 38-43.

Penland, J. G., and P. E. Johnson. "Dietary Calcium and Manganese Effects on Menstrual Cycle Symptoms." *American Journal of Obstetrics and Gynecology* 168 (1993): 1417-1423.

Strause, L., et al. "Spinal Bone Loss in Postmenopausal Women Supplemented with Calcium and Trace Minerals." *Journal of Nutrition* 124 (1994): 1060-1064.

See also: Dysmenorrhea; Herbal medicine; Osteoporosis; Women's health.

Manipulative and body-based practices

CATEGORY: Therapies and techniques
RELATED TERMS: Acupressure, acupuncture, Bowen therapy, chiropractic, massage, physical therapy, reflexology, shiatsu
DEFINITION: Manual techniques that release muscle tension and increase circulation to stimulate the body's natural healing abilities.
PRINCIPAL PROPOSED USES: Flexibility, pain relief, physical symptom relief, relaxation
OTHER PROPOSED USES: Anxiety, autism, burns, depression, fatigue, fibromyalgia, headaches, hypertension, insomnia, migraines, nightmares, stress

OVERVIEW

Manipulative and body-based therapies use manual pressure to effect changes in a body's physical state. Some techniques release muscle tension, some stimulate nerve pathways, and some aim to balance a body's vital energy. All of these practices are intended to restore the body to a natural state of balance and to encourage its innate healing abilities.

MECHANISM OF ACTION

Acupressure is the technique of applying pressure with the fingertips to specific trigger points on the body to discharge muscle tension and release the body's obstructed energy. Acupuncture is the insertion of needles into these trigger points and along energy meridians to disrupt neurological signals and relieve pain.

The Bowen technique is a method of gently rolling muscles and tissues with the fingers and thumbs. These moves produce energy surges that stimulate the body to reset and heal itself. Bowen therapy also incorporates periods of rest during the treatment to allow the body to find balance.

Chiropractic is a method of practicing medicine that heals without the use of surgery or pharmaceuticals. One element of chiropractic is manipulation of the spine to restore posture, balance, and freedom from pain. Other elements of chiropractic include electrical muscle stimulation, traction, and therapeutic ultrasound.

Massage therapy is the kneading of the superficial muscles to bring more oxygen to tissues and clear waste products to reduce pain and stiffness throughout the body. It creates relaxation and enhances immune function.

Physical therapy is a treatment plan of body manipulations and exercises designed to maximize mobility and limb function impaired by injury, disease, or birth defect or disorder. Progress can be measured as increased strength, range of motion, and time of unsupported balance.

Reflexology is a technique of applying manual pressure to specific sites on the hands and feet that trigger physical changes in related parts of the body. This technique targets pressure sensors in the hands and feet to disrupt reflexive stress signals and allow the body to return to a natural state.

Shiatsu is similar to acupressure in that pressure is applied with the fingertips to specific targets to clear

Body-Based Therapies for Back Pain

When back pain becomes chronic or when medications and other conventional therapies do not provide relief, many people try complementary and alternative (CAM) treatments. Although such therapies will not cure diseases or heal the injuries that cause pain, some people find CAM useful for managing or relieving pain. Following are some of the most commonly used complementary therapies for back pain.

Manipulation. Spinal manipulation refers to procedures in which professionals use their hands to mobilize, adjust, massage, or stimulate the spine or surrounding tissues. This type of therapy is often performed by osteopathic doctors and chiropractors. It tends to be most effective in people with uncomplicated pain and when used with other therapies. Spinal manipulation is not appropriate for persons with medical problems such as osteoporosis, spinal cord compression, or inflammatory arthritis (such as rheumatoid arthritis) or for persons taking blood-thinning medications such as warfarin (Coumadin) or heparin (Calciparine, Liquaemin).

Acupuncture. This ancient Chinese practice has been increasingly gaining acceptance and popularity in the United States. Acupuncture is based on the theory that a life force called qi flows through the body along certain channels, which if blocked can cause illness. According to the theory, the insertion of thin needles at precise locations along these channels by practitioners can unblock the flow of qi, relieving pain and restoring health. Practitioners believe that inserting needles, and then providing stimulation by twisting or passing a low-voltage electrical current through them, may foster the production of the body's natural pain-numbing chemicals, such as endorphins, serotonin, and acetylcholine.

Acupressure. As with acupuncture, the theory behind acupressure is that it unblocks the flow of qi. The difference between acupuncture and acupressure is that no needles are used in acupressure. Instead, a therapist applies pressure to points along the channels with his or her hands, elbows, or even feet. (In some cases, patients are taught to do their own acupressure.) Acupressure has not been well studied for back pain.

Rolfing. A type of massage, Rolfing involves using strong pressure on deep tissues in the back to relieve tightness of the fascia, a sheath of tissue that covers the muscles, which can cause or contribute to back pain. The theory behind Rolfing is that releasing muscles and tissues from the fascia enables the back to align itself properly. The effectiveness of Rolfing for back pain has not been scientifically proven.

obstructions in the body's vital energy. This energy travels along pathways called meridians. Shiatsu differs from acupressure in that a continuous meridian, rather than a discrete trigger point, is the target.

USES AND APPLICATIONS

Acupressure involves gradually increasing finger pressure on a specific point on the body, typically applied for three minutes. The amount of pressure, the duration of pressure, and the choice of points depend upon the present condition of the body. Acupressure has been shown to bring effective pain relief in cases of migraines, cluster headaches, neuralgias, and childbirth.

The Bowen technique involves a gentle rolling of muscles and connective tissues, yet it targets the nervous and bioenergy systems to boost the body's natural ability to heal and balance itself. Bowen therapy has been shown to bring effective pain relief in cases of fibromyalgia, sciatica, migraine, and frozen shoulder. It is also used to manage aspects of anxiety and panic attacks, Parkinson's disease, and cerebral palsy.

Chiropractic treatment often involves the realignment of the spinal column to ease any irritation to the spinal nerves that may be causing pain or malfunction. It brings effective pain relief in cases of headaches, neck pain, lower back strain, and sciatica.

Massage therapy manipulates muscles to increase the circulation of blood and lymph. Additional benefits include increased muscle relaxation, the release of endorphins and serotonin, and improved sleep. Massage therapy may be practiced to promote muscle recovery in athletes; to prevent the formation of scar tissue in persons recovering from surgery, trauma, or burns; and to ease depression.

Physical therapy works to improve a person's mobility to promote independence and enhance the quality of life. Each treatment plan is tailored to the patient's present condition and the underlying cause of the impairment. Physical therapy is commonly prescribed following joint replacement and limb amputation.

Reflexology is based on a connection between sites on the hands and feet and the corresponding internal organs. Thus, it is often sought as a noninvasive, non-pharmacological treatment for hormonal imbalances, infertility, sleep disorders, and adverse stress effects.

Like other manipulative body techniques Shiatsu promotes: relaxation, increased flexibility, and enhanced stamina. It also affects the digestive and endocrine systems, may be used to treat constipation, insomnia, and metabolic disorders.

Scientific Evidence

Double-blind studies are difficult to apply to manipulative and body-based therapies because the subjects know what therapy they are receiving. The effectiveness of such therapies may be demonstrated, however, by measuring specific parameters before and after treatment and determining the statistical significance of any difference in a population of subjects. Such parameters include quantitative range of motion and grip strength; blood levels of serotonin, dopamine, epinephrine, and cortisol; and qualitative scales of pain, depression, and disability. Effectiveness may also be compared among therapies and compared with self-care or pharmacological treatment alone.

Choosing a Practitioner

Qualified practitioners are typically required to hold a current state license; the names of licensed practitioners are available from each state's licensing board. Many practitioners are members of professional associations; membership information by geographical area may be available to potential clients.

Safety Issues

Trained, licensed professionals often hold certificates in first aid and cardiopulmonary resuscitation to address unexpected reactions to therapy. Because each person's body is different, the reaction to therapy may vary. Injuries may be exacerbated, bruising and swelling may occur, and pain may persist after treatment from nerve inflammation and muscle ache.

Bethany Thivierge, M.P.H.

Further Reading

American Chiropractic Association. http://www.acatoday.org. The largest professional association for chiropractic doctors.

American Massage Therapy Association. http://www.amtamassage.org. A professional association for massage therapists.

Association of Reflexologists. http://www.aor.org.uk. A nonprofit organization for professional practitioners of reflexology.

Baker, Julian. *The Bowen Technique*. Champaign, Ill.: Human Kinetics, 2002. A paperback textbook with photographs illustrating proper hand placement.

Gach, Michael Reed, and Beth Ann Henning. *Acupressure for Emotional Healing: A Self-Care Guide for Trauma, Stress, and Common Emotional Imbalances*. New York: Bantam Books, 2004. A clearly written guide to practicing self-care with acupressure.

See also: Acupressure; Acupuncture; Alexander technique; Aston-Patterning; Biodynamic massage; Craniosacral therapy; Dance movement therapy; Energy medicine; Feldenkrais method; Massage therapy; Meridians; Metamorphic technique; Mind/body medicine; Osteopathic manipulation; Pain management; Progressive muscle relaxation; Qigong; Reflexology; Relaxation therapies; Rolfing; Shiatsu; Soft tissue pain; Tai Chi; Therapeutic touch.

Mann, Felix

Category: Biography
Identification: German-born British acupuncturist and writer credited with developing scientific acupuncture
Born: April 10, 1931; Frankfurt, Germany

Overview

Felix Mann, a British acupuncturist especially noted for his written contributions to the study of acupuncture, is a critic of the idea of the existence of acupuncture points and meridians, concepts associated with traditional acupuncture. In contrast, Mann came to develop what is called scientific acupuncture, which is grounded in quite different principles.

In his book *Reinventing Acupuncture: A New Concept of Ancient Medicine* (1992), Mann argues that traditional acupuncture practices must be updated to reflect modern advances in medicine. Mann originally studied the traditional acupuncture system under a number of different teachers. He even studied Chinese language and writing so that he could read traditional texts that had not been translated into English or other languages. Upon completing many years of study of traditional acupuncture approaches, and after reportedly directly observing patients gain little benefit from such methods, he concluded that the traditional methods of acupuncture involving placement of needles into particular points of the body were ineffective.

Mann introduced new ideas into the field of acupuncture, including the idea that certain persons are "strong reactors"; that is, they are particularly sensitive to the effects of the treatment. In addition, he is known for using a novel technique termed "micro-acupuncture," which involves the insertion of a single needle into one side of a person's body. After only a few seconds, the needle is withdrawn without excessive movement or stimulation. It is estimated that Mann used this particular technique in the majority of his patients.

Mann was the founder and president of the Medical Acupuncture Society (1959 to 1980), was the first president of the British Medical Acupuncture Society (1980), and has published several books on acupuncture, including *The Treatment of Disease by Acupuncture* (1963), *Atlas of Acupuncture* (1966), and the first English-language textbook in the field, *Acupuncture: The Ancient Chinese Art of Healing* (1962). Of note, some of his early publications were based on traditional acupuncture beliefs, as they were written before he changed his opinions of the field. He has lectured on acupuncture in more than one dozen countries and has taught physicians from about forty-five countries. He won a German Pain Prize in 1995.

Brandy Weidow, M.S.

FURTHER READING

Baldry, P. "The Integration of Acupuncture Within Medicine in the UK: The British Medical Acupuncture Society's Twenty-Fifth Anniversary." *Acupuncture in Medicine* 23, no. 1 (2005): 2-12.

Bauer, Matthew. "The Final Days of Traditional Beliefs? Part One." *Chinese Medical Times* 1, issue 4 (August, 2006). Available at http://www.chinesemedicinetimes.com/section.php?xsec=122.

Mann, Felix. *Reinventing Acupuncture: A New Concept of Ancient Medicine.* 2d ed. Boston: Butterworth-Heinemann, 2000.

_____. *Scientific Aspects of Acupuncture.* 2d ed. Maryland Heights, Mo.: Butterworth-Heinemann, 1983.

See also: Acupuncture; Meridians; Traditional healing.

Mannose

CATEGORY: Herbs and supplements
RELATED TERM: D-mannose
DEFINITION: Natural substance of the human body used as a supplement to treat specific health conditions.
PRINCIPAL PROPOSED USE: Urinary tract infection

OVERVIEW

Mannose is a six-carbon-sugar, as are the better-known and closely related substances glucose and fructose. Relying on evidence that is both exceedingly preliminary and highly inconsistent, some alternative medicine practitioners have popularized mannose as a treatment for urinary tract infections.

REQUIREMENTS AND SOURCES

Mannose plays an important role in human physiology. However, there is no nutritional need for this substance, as the body can easily produce it from glucose. Nonetheless, significant quantities of it can be found in many fruits and vegetables, including peaches, apples, blueberries, green beans, cabbage, and tomatoes.

THERAPEUTIC DOSAGES

A typical recommended dose of mannose for the treatment or prevention of bladder infections is 1.5 grams (g) daily, often divided into three doses of 500 milligrams (mg) each.

THERAPEUTIC USES

The idea that mannose supplements can help prevent or treat bladder infections derives from a property of the *Escherichia coli* bacterium. *E. coli* is one of the common causes of bladder infections. Many strains of *E. coli* have the ability to attach to the mannose present in the wall of the bladder by means of threadlike structures called pili. This process of attachment allows them to initiate the process of infection.

Reasoning from this fact of basic science, medical researchers in the 1980s hypothesized that consumption of mannose as a supplement would increase levels of mannose in the urine to such an extent that this free mannose would saturate the *E. coli*'s mannose-binding pili and thereby make the bacteria unable to grapple onto the cells of the bladder wall.

It is essentially this reasoning that is restated by proponents of mannose for bladder infections. However, the argument has at least four problems. First, one of the main ways that the body's white blood cells recognize and kill *E. coli* is via these mannose-sensitive pili. When these pili are saturated by mannose, white blood cells (specifically, macrophages) are less able to consume the *E. coli* bacteria. Second, many species of *E. coli*, including some of the most dangerous, do not have mannose-sensitive pili. Third, there are numerous other bacteria that cause bladder infections, and these are not known or suspected to have mannose-sensitive pili.

Perhaps the most important point is that the use of mannose for preventing or treating bladder infections has never undergone any meaningful scientific study in human beings. There is a bit of evidence from animal studies performed in the 1980s, but it is a long way from animal studies to efficacy in humans. Proponents of mannose also cite numerous testimonials, but the placebo effect and related confounding factors are quite sufficient to produce numerous testimonials for any treatment. Only double-blind, placebo-controlled studies can actually prove a treatment effective, and none have been performed on mannose. There is no meaningful scientific reason to believe that mannose is useful for the prevention or treatment of bladder infections.

SAFETY ISSUES

As a sugar widely present in foods, mannose is assumed to be safe. However, the maximum safe dosage has been established neither in healthy adults nor in pregnant or nursing women or young children. Very weak evidence from test-tube studies hints that consumption of gigantic amounts of mannose by pregnant women could conceivably increase risk of birth defects in their offspring.

EBSCO CAM Review Board

FURTHER READING

Felipe, I., et al. "Inhibition of Macrophage Phagocytosis of *Escherichia coli* by Mannose and Mannan." *Brazilian Journal of Medicine and Biology Research* 24 (1991): 919-924.

See also: Bladder infection; Herbal medicine.

Marshmallow

CATEGORY: Herbs and supplements
RELATED TERM: *Althaea officinalis*
DEFINITION: Natural plant product used as a dietary supplement for specific health benefits.
PRINCIPAL PROPOSED USES: Asthma, colds, cough, Crohn's disease, skin inflammation, sore throat, ulcers

OVERVIEW

The similarity in name between the herb marshmallow and the sweet treat is more than a coincidence, although the modern sugar-puff ball no longer bears much relationship to the old-fashioned candy flavored with marshmallow herb.

Besides inspiring makers of campfire food, the marshmallow has also been used medicinally since the time of ancient Greece. Hippocrates spoke of it as a treatment for bruises and blood loss, and subsequent Roman physicians recommended marshmallow for toothaches, insect bites, chilblains, and irritated skin. In medieval Europe, herbalists used marshmallow to soothe toothaches, coughs, sore throats, chapped skin, indigestion, and diarrhea.

THERAPEUTIC DOSAGES

Marshmallow can be made into a soothing tea by steeping roots overnight in water and diluting to taste. This tea can be drunk as desired for symptomatic relief. Alternatively, one can take marshmallow in capsules (5 to 6 grams daily) or in tincture according to label directions. Marshmallow ointments can be applied directly to soothe inflamed or irritated skin.

THERAPEUTIC USES

Marshmallow contains large sugar molecules called mucilage, which are thought to exert a soothing effect on mucous membranes; this is the basis of most proposed uses of the herb. However, only double-blind, placebo-controlled studies can prove a treatment effective, and no such studies of marshmallow have been reported.

On the basis of its supposed soothing properties, tea or lozenges containing marshmallow tea are often recommended for asthma, cough, colds, and sore throat. Marshmallow taken as tea or in capsules is sometimes

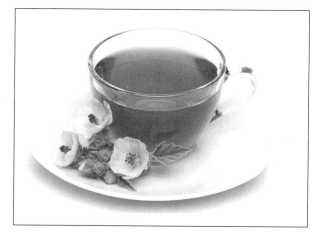

The flowers of the marshmallow plant, along with the herbal tea prepared from it. (Bildagentur-online/TH Foto-Werbung/Photo Researchers, Inc.)

recommended for Crohn's disease or ulcers, on the theory that mucilage might sooth the lining of the digestive tract. Finally, marshmallow ointment is sometimes recommended for irritated skin.

SAFETY ISSUES

Marshmallow is believed to be entirely safe. It is approved for use in foods, and its chemical makeup does not suggest any but benign effects. However, detailed safety studies have not been performed. One study suggests that marshmallow can slightly lower blood sugar levels. For this reason, people with diabetes should use caution when taking marshmallow. Safety in young children, pregnant or nursing women, and those with severe liver or kidney disease has not been established.

EBSCO CAM Review Board

FURTHER READING

"*Althaea officinalis*, Marshmallow." In *The Western Herbal Tradition*, by Graeme Tobyn, Alison Denham, and Margaret Whitelegg. New York: Churchill Livingstone/Elsevier, 2011.

Tomoda, M., et al. "Hypoglycemic Activity of Twenty Plant Mucilages and Three Modified Products." *Planta Medica* 53 (1987): 8-12.

See also: Asthma; Colds and flu; Ulcers.

Massage therapy

CATEGORY: Therapies and techniques

RELATED TERMS: Acupressure, deep-tissue massage, effleurage massage, neuromuscular massage, reflexology, Rolfing structural integration, St. John method, shiatsu, structural integration, Swedish massage, touch-based therapy

DEFINITION: A touch-based therapy involving manipulation of the muscles.

PRINCIPAL PROPOSED USES: General stress reduction, low back pain and other forms of muscular pain

OTHER PROPOSED USES: Anorexia, anxiety, asthma, attention deficit disorder, autism, bulimia, cancer treatment support, cystic fibrosis, depression, diabetes, eczema, fibromyalgia, human immunodeficiency virus infection support, iliotibial band pain, juvenile rheumatoid arthritis, migraine headaches, neck pain, neonatal sepsis, premenstrual syndrome, pregnancy support, recovery from severe burns, smoking cessation, spinal cord injury

OVERVIEW

Along with herbal treatment, touch-based therapy is one of the most ancient forms of medical care. Humans stroke and rub areas of the body that hurt; massage therapy develops this human impulse into a professional treatment. There is no doubt that massage relieves pain and induces relaxation temporarily. Whether it offers any lasting benefits, however, remains unclear.

Forms of massage. There are many schools of massage. In most cases, massage therapists combine several techniques, although there are also purists who use one method only. The most common technique is Swedish massage, which combines long strokes and gentle kneading movements that primarily affect surface muscle tissues. Deep-tissue massage utilizes greater pressure to reach deeper levels of muscles. This may be called the "hurts-good-and-feels-great-after" approach. Shiatsu or acupressure massage also uses deep pressure but does so according to the principles of acupuncture theory. Neuromuscular massage (such as the St. John method of neuromuscular therapy) applies strong pressure to tender spots, technically known as trigger points.

Several other techniques are best described as relatives of massage. Rolfing structural integration aims to affect not muscles, but the connective tissue (fascia) surrounding muscles and everything else in the body. This highly organized technique aims to permanently improve the body's structure. Reflexology is a form of foot massage based on the theory that the whole body is reflected in the foot.

MECHANISM OF ACTION

There are many theories about how massage might work, but none have been proved true. Little doubt exists that massage temporarily increases blood circulation in the massaged area, but it is not clear that this makes any lasting difference. Some massage therapists and massage therapy schools promote the notion that massage breaks up calcium deposits in the muscle, but there is no objective substantiation for this claim. A completely different explanation is that massage promotes healing in a more general way, by reducing stress and inducing relaxation. Massage also satisfies the basic human need to be touched.

Some forms of massage (such as Rolfing, acupressure, and reflexology) have elaborate theories behind them. However, there is little to no scientific evidence for these theories; moreover, there is some evidence that the theory behind reflexology is incorrect.

USES AND APPLICATIONS

Massage is most commonly used to relieve muscular tension and to promote relaxation. Massage is also said to be helpful as an aid to the treatment of various conditions, including attention deficit disorder (ADD), asthma, autism, bedsores, bulimia, cystic fibrosis, diabetes, eczema, fibromyalgia, human immunodeficiency virus infection, iliotibial band pain, juvenile rheumatoid arthritis, low back pain, lymphedema, neck pain, premenstrual syndrome (PMS), pregnancy, severe burns, and spinal cord injury.

SCIENTIFIC EVIDENCE

Although there is some evidence that massage may be helpful for various medical purposes, in general the evidence is not strong. There are several reasons for this, but one is most fundamental: Even with the best of intentions, it is difficult to properly ascertain the effectiveness of a hands-on therapy like massage.

Only one form of study can truly prove that a treatment is effective: the double-blind, placebo-controlled trial. However, it is not possible to fit massage into a study design of this type. What could researchers use for placebo massage, and how could they make sure that both participants and practitioners did not know who was receiving real massage and who was receiving fake massage?

Because of these problems, all studies of massage fall short of optimum design. Many have compared massage to no treatment. However, studies of this type cannot provide reliable evidence about the efficacy of a treatment. If a benefit is seen, there is no way to determine whether it was caused by massage specifically, or just by attention generally. (Attention alone will almost always produce some reported benefit.)

More meaningful trials used some sort of fake treatment for the control group, such as phony laser acupuncture. However, using a placebo treatment that is very different in form from the treatment under study is less than ideal. One study compared

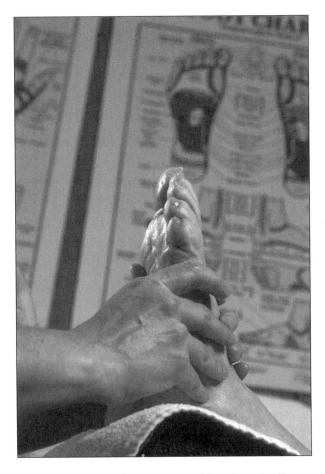

Pressure points on a foot are massaged by a therapist. (Larry Mulvehill/Photo Researchers, Inc.)

real reflexology with fake reflexology. However, it is quite likely that the reflexologists unconsciously conveyed more enthusiasm and optimism when performing the real therapy than when performing the fake therapy; this, too, could affect the outcome. It has been suggested that the only way to avoid this last problem would be to compare the effectiveness of trained practitioners with actors trained only enough to provide a simulation of treatment; however, such studies have not been reported.

Still other studies have simply involved giving people massages and seeing whether they improved. These trials are particularly meaningless; it has been long since proven that both participants and examining physicians will, at minimum, think that they observe improvement in people given a treatment, whether or not the treatment does anything on its own.

Finally, other trials have compared massage to competing therapies, such as acupuncture or relaxation therapy. When one compares unproven therapies to each other, the results cannot possibly prove that any of the tested treatments are effective. Given these caveats, the following is a summary of what science knows about the effects of massage.

Low back pain. Although the evidence is far from complete, it does appear that massage may offer benefits for low back pain. However, these benefits may last for only a short time. One study compared massage with fake laser therapy in 107 people with low back pain. The results indicate that massage is more effective than fake laser therapy for relieving low back pain, and that massage therapy with exercise and posture training is even more effective.

Another study compared acupuncture, massage, and self-care education in 262 people with persistent back pain. By the end of the ten-week treatment period, massage had shown itself more effective than self-care (or acupuncture). However, at a one-year follow-up, no difference was seen in symptoms between the massage group and the self-care group. In another study, acupressure-style massage was more effective than Swedish massage for the treatment of low back pain.

In a review of thirteen randomized trials, researchers concluded that massage may be effective for nonspecific low back pain, and that the beneficial effects can last for up to one year in persons with chronic pain. Researchers also noted that exercise and education appear to enhance the effectiveness of massage.

Cancer. Massage therapy has been studied for its benefits in managing the symptoms associated with cancer and its treatment. In a randomized study investigating the effects of massage on 348 persons with advanced cancer who had moderate to severe pain, the researchers found that, compared with simple touch, massage was significantly more effective at reducing pain and improving mood immediately following treatment; the effect, however, was not sustained. The authors of a review of ten massage therapy studies could not draw firm conclusions about its benefits for a wide range of symptoms in persons undergoing treatment for cancer.

Massage without aromatherapy has shown promise for reducing nausea caused by chemotherapy. However, a small randomized trial found that effleurage massage, a common massage technique, had no significant effect on anxiety, depression, or quality of life among twenty-two women undergoing radiation therapy for breast cancer.

Other conditions. Preliminary controlled trials of varying quality suggest that massage may provide benefit in a number of conditions, including the following: ADD, anorexia nervosa, asthma in children, autism, bulimia, cystic fibrosis, anxiety, diabetes, eczema, fibromyalgia, iliotibial band pain (a form of tendonitis that can cause knee or hip pain), juvenile rheumatoid arthritis, migraine headaches, pregnancy and childbirth, quitting smoking, burn recovery, and spinal cord injury. One study found that massaging premature infants three times daily for ten days at acupressure locations resulted in greater weight compared with similar infants receiving routine care.

One study commonly cited as evidence that ordinary massage therapy is helpful for PMS was flawed by the absence of a control group. However, a better-designed trial compared reflexology with fake reflexology in thirty-eight women with PMS symptoms and found evidence that real reflexology was more effective.

Several studies indicate that massage with aromatherapy may be helpful for relieving anxiety. One study evaluated this combination therapy for treating anxiety or depression (or both) in people undergoing treatment for cancer. The treatment did appear to provide some short-term benefits. A 2008 review could find no convincing evidence for the effectiveness of massage therapy against depression in general.

Study results are mixed on whether massage can improve measures of immune function in people with human immunodeficiency virus infection. For chronic neck pain, one study found that massage is less effective than acupuncture. In fact, in this trial, massage was no more effective than fake acupuncture. Finally, a review of the literature published in 1997 suggests that massage is not helpful for preventing pressure sores (bedsores).

CHOOSING A PRACTITIONER

As with all medical therapies, it is best to choose a licensed practitioner. Where licensure is not available, persons should seek a referral from a qualified and knowledgeable medical practitioner. However, most states in the United States license massage therapists.

Note that massage, like other hands-on therapies, involves personal talents that go beyond specific training, certification, or licensure: Some people are simply gifted with their hands. Furthermore, what works for one person may not work for another. For these reasons, some trial and error is often necessary to find the best massage therapist.

SAFETY ISSUES

Massage is generally safe. However, it can sometimes exacerbate pain temporarily, even when properly performed. In addition, massage that is performed too forcefully on fragile people could cause bone fractures and other internal injuries. However, licensed massage therapists have been trained in ways to avoid causing these problems. Finally, machines designed to perform elements of massage may be less safe than standard massage.

EBSCO CAM Review Board

FURTHER READING

Billhult, A., I. Bergbom, and E. Stener-Victorin. "Massage Relieves Nausea in Women with Breast Cancer Who Are Undergoing Chemotherapy." *Journal of Alternative and Complementary Medicine* 13 (2007): 53-58.
Coelho, H. F., K. Boddy, and E. Ernst. "Massage Therapy for the Treatment of Depression." *International Journal of Clinical Practice* 62 (2008): 325-333.
Ernst, E. "The Safety of Massage Therapy." *Rheumatology* 42 (2003): 1101-1106.
Furlan A. D., et al. "Massage for Low-Back Pain." *Cochrane Database of Systematic Reviews* (2008): CD001929. Available through *EBSCO DynaMed Systematic Literature Surveillance* at http://www.ebscohost.com/dynamed.
Kutner, J. S., et al. "Massage Therapy Versus Simple Touch to Improve Pain and Mood in Patients with Advanced Cancer." *Annals of Internal Medicine* 149 (2008): 369-379.
Lawler, S. P., and L. D. Cameron. "A Randomized, Controlled Trial of Massage Therapy as a Treatment for Migraine." *Annals of Behavioral Medicine* 32 (2006): 50-59.
Sherman, K. J., et al. "Effectiveness of Therapeutic Massage for Generalized Anxiety Disorder." *Depression and Anxiety* 27 (2010): 441-450.
Wang, M. Y., et al. "The Efficacy of Reflexology." *Journal of Advanced Nursing* 62 (2008): 512-520.
Wilkinson, S., K. Barnes, and L. Storey. "Massage for Symptom Relief in Patients with Cancer." *Journal of Advanced Nursing* 63 (2008): 430-439.
Wilkinson, S., et al. "Effectiveness of Aromatherapy Massage in the Management of Anxiety and Depression in Patients with Cancer." *Journal of Clinical Oncology* 25 (2007): 532-539.

See also: Aston-Patterning; Craniosacral therapy; Fibromyalgia: Homeopathic remedies; Hellerwork; Manipulative and body-based practices; Pain management; Reflexology; Relaxation therapies; Rolfing; Shiatsu.

Maté

CATEGORY: Herbs and supplements
RELATED TERMS: *Ilex paraguariensis, Yerba mate*
DEFINITION: Natural plant product used to treat specific health conditions.
PRINCIPAL PROPOSED USES: Enhancing mental function (with caffeine content), enhancing sports performance (with caffeine content)
OTHER PROPOSED USES: Cancer prevention, weight loss

OVERVIEW

Maté is an evergreen tree native to Argentina, Brazil, Paraguay, and Uruguay. The leaves and small stems of the tree are used to make a tealike caffeinated beverage. Maté has traditionally been used to enhance alertness and mental function and also to treat digestive problems.

THERAPEUTIC DOSAGES

A typical dose of maté is 3 to 10 grams (g) of dried herb per cup. Concentrated extracts are also available. These should be taken according to label instructions.

THERAPEUTIC USES

Maté is widely advertised as a healthful beverage, said to provide all the presumed benefits of green tea, such as preventing cancer and heart disease. However, the basis for this claim is largely theoretical. Maté does contain antioxidant polyphenols similar to those in tea, but this by itself does not demonstrate that maté is health-promoting; numerous substances with strong antioxidant properties have failed to prove beneficial in double-blind, placebo-controlled studies. Even green tea itself has not been proven to offer any health benefits.

In the test tube, maté has shown effects that suggest possible value for reducing cancer risk. However, these findings are far too preliminary to rely upon; in fact, there is stronger evidence that maté could under certain circumstances increase the risk of cancer.

Other proposed benefits of maté also largely lack foundation. One study found that an extract of mate could help slow glycation, a metabolic side effect of diabetes. These findings have been used to claim that maté is healthful for people with diabetes. However, this study did not involve people with diabetes; it involved chemicals in a test tube. Tens of thousands of substances show benefits in the test tube that fail to translate into real life; it is greatly premature to claim that maté is helpful for people with diabetes based on these exceedingly preliminary findings.

Similarly weak evidence hints that maté might increase fat metabolism, and on this basis maté has been proposed as a weight-loss agent. However, there are no published human studies of maté that show any weight-loss benefit. One small double-blind, placebo-controlled study evaluated an herbal preparation containing maté combined with guarana and damiana. The herbal mixture appeared to cause participants to feel full more quickly during a meal, and to continue to feel full for longer after the meal; this led to modest, short-term weight loss. However, it is not clear to what extent the maté in this product played a role. Another study found that maté might increase bile flow and speed the action of the intestines; these reported effects, even if real, do not indicate any particular health benefit.

Although some maté proponents attempted for many years to maintain that maté does not contain caffeine (supposedly it contained a chemical called mateine, which, in fact, does not exist), maté does in fact contain caffeine. Depending on how it is brewed, maté tea contains somewhat more caffeine than black tea and slightly less caffeine than coffee. Based on this caffeine content, maté would be expected to enhance mental function and improve sports performance.

SAFETY ISSUES

As a widely consumed beverage, maté is generally assumed to be entirely safe. However, this may be an incorrect assumption. Numerous studies have found associations between high consumption of maté in South America and increased rates of cancer of the esophagus, mouth, throat, and larynx. It is widely stated that this increased risk is entirely due to the practice of drinking maté at very high temperatures. However, the underlying evidence is not so clear-cut. The data actually suggest that at least some of this increased risk is because of the maté itself, rather than the temperature at which it is consumed. In addition, maté consumption has also been associated with increased risk of kidney and lung cancer, which would not be expected to be influenced by beverage temperature. Finally, there is some direct evidence that mate has carcinogenic effects. Putting all this information together, it does appear that maté is at the very least slightly carcinogenic. However, so is charred hamburger; moderate use of maté is not likely to significantly increase one's cancer risk.

Other potential problems with maté relate to its caffeine content. Potential side effects of caffeine include heartburn, gastritis, insomnia, anxiety, and heart arrythmias (benign palpitations or more serious disturbances of heart rhythm.) All drug interactions that can occur with caffeine would be expected to occur with maté as well.

Maximum safe doses have not been established in pregnant or nursing women, young children, or people with severe liver or kidney disease.

IMPORTANT INTERACTIONS

In persons taking MAO inhibitors, the caffeine in maté could cause dangerous drug interactions. Those taking stimulant drugs such as Ritalin may find the stimulant effects of maté to be amplified. Also, the caffeine in maté may interfere with the action of drugs to prevent heart arrythmias or treat insomnia, heartburn, ulcers, or anxiety.

EBSCO CAM Review Board

FURTHER READING

Chandra, S., and E. De Mejia Gonzalez. "Polyphenolic Compounds, Antioxidant Capacity, and Quinone Reductase Activity of an Aqueous Extract of *Ardisia compressa* in Comparison to Maté (*Ilex paraguariensis*) and Green (*Camelliasinensis*) Teas." *Journal of Agricultural and Food Chemistry* 52 (2004): 3583-3589.

Goldenberg, D., et al. "The Beverage Maté: A Risk Factor for Cancer of the Head and Neck." *Head and Neck* 25 (2003): 595-601.

_____. "Habitual Risk Factors for Head and Neck Cancer." *Otolaryngology and Head and Neck Surgery* 131 (2004): 986-993.

Gonzalez de Mejia, E., et al. "Effect of Yerba Maté (*Ilex paraguariensis*) Tea on Topoisomerase Inhibition and Oral Carcinoma Cell Proliferation." *Journal of Agricultural and Food Chemistry* 53 (2005): 1966-1973.

Lunceford, N., and A. Gugliucci. "*Ilex paraguariensis* Extracts Inhibit AGE Formation More Efficiently than Green Tea." *Fitoterapia* 76, no. 5 (2005): 419-427.

Ramirez-Mares, M. V., et al. "In Vitro Chemopreventive Activity of *Camellia sinensis, Ilexparaguariensis,* and *Ardisia compressa* Tea Extracts and Selected Polyphenols." *Mutatation Research* 554 (2004): 53-65.

Sewram, V., et al. "Maté Consumption and the Risk of Squamous Cell Esophageal Cancer in Uruguay." *Cancer Epidemiology, Biomarkers, and Prevention* 12 (2003): 508-513.

See also: Damiana; Green tea; Guarana; Herbal medicine.

Meditation

CATEGORY: Therapies and techniques

RELATED TERMS: Mindfulness meditation, relaxation, Transcendental Meditation, Zen meditation

DEFINITION: An awake, relaxed state characterized by decreased metabolic activity in the body.

PRINCIPAL PROPOSED USES: Anxiety, depression, insomnia, stress-related illness

OTHER PROPOSED USES: Alcohol or tobacco abuse, attention deficit disorder, chronic fatigue syndrome, chronic pain, fibromyalgia, hypertension, peripheral neuropathy

OVERVIEW

Meditation has been practiced around the world for thousands of years. Physiologically, it occupies a position between wakefulness and sleep. In a large survey conducted in the United States in 2007, 9.4 percent of the adult population reported using meditation for health purposes in the past year, an increase of almost 2 percent from similar data collected in 2002.

Several styles of meditation are practiced, all within a continuum of two classes: concentrative and nonconcentrative. Techniques for concentrative meditation encourage the practitioner to focus on a specific stimulus (the breath or repetition of a word such as "om"), which limits incoming stimuli. Examples of this type of meditation include yogic meditation and Buddhist *samatha* meditation, both of which focus on the breath.

Nonconcentrative meditative techniques increase stimuli, encouraging the practitioner to pay attention to the thoughts, feelings, and sensations experienced, but in a nonjudgmental way. Examples of this type of meditation include Zen and mindfulness. Techniques that involve meditating while actively moving include mindful yoga, Tai Chi, and qigong. Another type of meditation, compassionate, involves meditating while feeling complete love and harmony with others.

Transcendental Meditation (TM), created by Maharishi Mahesh Yogi, encourages focusing on a specific mantra depending on the expertise level of the practitioner. The objective is to repeat the mantra without concentrative effort and to develop awareness without thought. Therefore, this type of meditation falls between the concentrative and the nonconcentrative types. Brain activity, measured by cerebral blood flow and functional magnetic resonance imaging, has been found to have varying patterns within the same person, depending on the type of meditation being practiced.

MECHANISM OF ACTION

Meditation affects so many systems of the body it is difficult to pinpoint a mechanism of action; indeed, there would be multiple mechanisms involved with so many effects. Meditation results in lower oxygen consumption, respiration rate, and heart rate, and it

How to Meditate

There are many different types of meditation, but there is no "right" technique for every person. Most types of meditation include the following basic elements: position, focus, attitude, and breathing.

Position. Before engaging your mind, you should follow these guidelines to make your body comfortable: Sit in a comfortable position on the floor or in a chair. If you choose a chair, keep your knees comfortably apart and rest your hands in your lap. If you sit on the floor, choose one of these poses: tailor fashion (cross-legged), with a cushion under your buttocks; Japanese fashion (on your knees, with your big toes touching and your buttocks resting on the soles of your feet), with a cushion between your feet and buttocks; the yoga full lotus position (not recommended for beginners), in which you keep your spine straight and vertical, but not rigid, and then briefly rock from side to side and from front to back until you feel comfortable and balanced on your hips.

Focus. To direct your thoughts, close your eyes (unless the focus of attention is an object). Focus attention on a silent thought, word, or prayer, or on a mental image. Focus on the sensation of each breath during inhaling and exhaling, or on an object such as a candle flame, flower, painting, or bare wall.

Attitude. It is important to maintain a gentle and non-judgmental attitude while you meditate. This will help you to relax. Do not be concerned about your goals or whether or not you are meditating correctly. As a beginner, it is natural for your attention to wander frequently. When your attention wanders, gently redirect it back. Do not try to force attention. Meditation should not be stressful.

Breathing. Proper breathing can enhance your experience. Breathe through your nose, if possible. Place your tongue on the ridge behind your upper teeth. Focus your attention on your stomach and diaphragm rather than your nostrils and chest. Place your hand on your stomach and feel the sensations as you inhale and exhale. Your stomach should rise when you inhale and should fall when you exhale. Be attentive to your breathing, but stay relaxed and breathe naturally.

Progress. Meditation should become easier with regular practice. You should experiment to find out what technique works best for you, and you should consider taking a meditation class. Many different techniques are taught. Some have a spiritual focus and others are more focused on stress reduction.

Amy Scholten, M.P.H.; reviewed by Brian Randall, M.D.

---

impacts brain activity. These effects vary depending on the amount of time one spends meditating and the type of meditation being done.

Meditation was once thought to be a sort of hibernation or to be similar to sleep, but physiologic testing shows that neither is the case. Regular practice lowers cortisol levels, increases serotonin availability, and better-controls homeostasis.

Uses and Applications

Meditation is used by persons worldwide. It is also prescribed by health care practitioners for specific conditions. Meditation has shown efficacy in treating anxiety, depression, drug addiction, fibromyalgia, and insomnia, and it is used for pain management. A randomized clinical trial of mindfulness-based stress reduction versus medication for insomnia showed comparable changes in sleep duration and quality in the two groups studied.

Meditation is useful for the elderly to assist in pain management, improve sleep quality and quantity, and decrease the need for pharmaceutical agents. In children, various types of meditation (including mindfulness, Tai Chi, and TM) have led to improvements in cognitive tasks and to decreased anxiety and distractibility. Tai Chi was associated with mood and quality of life improvements in a studied group of high school girls. TM training also has been shown to decrease blood pressure in teenagers who had high blood pressure before the training.

Scientific Evidence

It is impossible to conduct double-blind studies on meditation because participants must know they are meditating; therefore, they would not be blinded. There are some compelling studies with relatively good designs comparing physiologic measures pre- and post-meditation training. Research on persons who had magnetic resonance imaging scans before and after undergoing an eight-week mindfulness-based stress reduction course has shown that their brains are actually different. Studies show that participants have more dense gray matter in specific areas of the brain after the course. Other research has found that the specific type of meditation practiced leads to different patterns of brain activity.

Other researchers have looked at the impact of long-term meditation practice on modifying electro-encephalogram (EEG) results, brain activity, and even structure of the brain, providing evidence for neural plasticity related to meditation practice. EEG alpha waves and theta waves are often found to be increased during meditation, compared with control conditions.

Comparison of the brains of long-time meditators (Western meditation practitioners) with nonpractitioners showed an increase in cortical thickness in the prefrontal cortex and right anterior insula of the brain. Scientists have studied Buddhist monks who have practiced meditation for an average of 19,000 hours in comparison with novices and found increased brain activation as measured by functional magnetic resonance imaging; those who had practiced 44,000 hours on average had lower brain activation than study controls. The researchers used distracter sounds and found that the "expert meditators" had decreased brain activity response related to the sounds, compared with study controls.

Additional research on expert Buddhist meditators versus study controls (during the meditation exercise and at rest) involved measuring brain activity during compassion meditation, when they were asked to generate an unconditional state of loving kindness. Areas of the limbic system were activated in both groups, but the response was stronger in expert meditators. When meditation was compared with rest, activation occurred in the amygdala, temporo-parietal junction, and right posterior superior temporal sulcus.

TM seems to reduce the response to pain while allowing the sensory experience of pain to remain fully activated. Research on the effect of meditating on a regular basis on the experience of pain found that meditators reported the same level of pain as those who did not meditate. However, this study was not conducted during meditation. The brains of meditators showed 40 to 50 percent decreased responsiveness by fMRI. The nonmeditators also were trained, and five months later, both groups showed the 40 to 50 percent responsiveness rate, indicating that the TM training they received had affected the brain's reaction to pain.

CHOOSING A PRACTITIONER

Meditation can be self-taught. However, if one wants to select a teacher to learn meditation, it is important to feel comfortable with the teacher and to be aware of the various types of meditation, because one style may be better suited than another. Some types of meditation, such as TM, require specific classes taught by an approved teacher.

For persons seeking help with stress or anxiety, a program called mindfulness-based stress reduction has been shown to be effective; TM has been found to be helpful for decreasing blood pressure.

SAFETY ISSUES

Meditation is generally safe for almost everyone. There have been some case reports of people with psychological illnesses such as psychosis and severe depression experiencing exacerbation of the condition in connection with meditation. Some healthy people experience repressed memories or emotions in association with meditation. Some persons may find they cannot meditate for more than a few minutes at a time, as it is too taxing for them. They can start with shorter time periods and work their way up to longer sessions gradually. For some persons who take antidepressants or thyroid medications, the dosage may actually need to be reduced after meditation becomes a regular daily practice.

Dawn M. Bielawski, Ph.D.

FURTHER READING

Barinaga, Marcia. "Studying the Well-Trained Mind." *Science* 302 (2003): 44-46. Discusses collaboration among scientists and Buddhist monks in a study measuring the effects of meditation on the brain.

Cormody, James, and Ruth A. Baer. "Relationships Between Mindfulness Practice and Levels of Mindfulness, Medical and Psychological Symptoms, and Well-Being in a Mindfulness-Based Stress Reduction Program." *Journal of Behavioral Medicine* 31 (2008): 23-33. The researchers conducted pre- and postintervention surveys of 174 adults who participated in this mindfulness program.

Gross, Cynthia R., et al. "Mindfulness-Based Stress Reduction Versus Pharmacotherapy for Chronic Primary Insomnia." *Explore* 7 (2011): 76-87. The researchers studied thirty adults with diagnosed insomnia and randomized them to either mindfulness-based stress reduction training or pharmacotherapy, comparing various indices of sleep quality and quantity between the two treatments.

Sibinga, Erica M. S., and Kathi J. Kemper. "Complementary, Holistic, and Integrative Medicine: Meditation Practices for Pediatric Health." *Pediatrics in Review* 31 (2010): 91-103. Directed to pediatric clinicians, this article describes cases for which meditative practices may be helpful, then provides summary tables of data from studies of various types of pediatric-focused meditation.

Wang, D., et al. "Cerebral Blood Flow Changes Associated with Different Meditation Practices and Perceived Depth of Meditation." *Psychiatry Research: Neuroimaging* 191 (2011): 60-67. This study involved comparing two types of meditation (focus-based and breath-based) within subjects and looked at functional MRI and cerebral blood flow in relation to the subjects' reported experiences.

See also: Autogenic training; Biofeedback; Guided imagery; Humor and healing; Hypnotherapy; Maharishi Mahesh Yogi; Mental health; Mind/body medicine; Relaxation therapies; Traditional healing; Transcendental Meditation; Walking, mind/body.

Medium-chain triglycerides

CATEGORY: Herbs and supplements

DEFINITION: Natural substance of the human body used as a supplement to treat specific health conditions.

PRINCIPAL PROPOSED USE: Undesired weight loss (especially from acquired immunodeficiency syndrome)

OTHER PROPOSED USES: Diabetes, performance enhancement, weight loss

OVERVIEW

Medium-chain triglycerides (MCTs) are fats with an unusual chemical structure that allows the body to digest them easily. Most fats are broken down in the intestine and remade into a special form that can be transported in the blood. However, MCTs are absorbed intact and taken to the liver, where they are used directly for energy. In this sense, they are processed very similarly to carbohydrates.

MCTs are different enough from other fats that they can be used as fat substitutes by people (especially those with AIDS) who need calories but are unable to absorb or metabolize normal fats. MCTs have also shown a bit of promise for improving body composition and enhancing athletic performance.

REQUIREMENTS AND SOURCES

There is no dietary requirement for MCTs. Coconut oil, palm oil, and butter contain up to 15 percent MCTs (plus a lot of other fats). MCTs can be purchased as purified supplements.

THERAPEUTIC DOSAGES

MCTs can be eaten as salad oil or used in cooking. When taken as an athletic supplement, dosages around 85 milligrams (mg) daily are common.

THERAPEUTIC USES

Preliminary evidence suggests that MCTs are a useful fat substitute for those who have difficulty digesting fat. This makes MCTs potentially helpful for people with AIDS, who need to find a way to gain weight but cannot digest fat easily. MCTs might theoretically be helpful for those who have trouble digesting fatty foods because they lack the proper enzymes (pancreatic insufficiency), but taking digestive enzymes appears to be more effective.

Although this may sound paradoxical given the above, some evidence suggests that MCT consumption might also enhance the body's natural tendency to burn fat. On this basis, the supplement has been proposed as a weight-loss aid. The results of studies have generally failed to find any weight-loss benefits. Some studies have, however, found that use of MCTs might produce improvements in body composition (ratio of fat to lean tissue). A related supplement called structured medium- and long-chain triacylglycerols (SMLCT) has been created to provide the same potential benefits as MCTs, but in a form that can be used as cooking oil. In a preliminary double-blind trial, SMLCT has also shown some promise for enhancing body composition. One placebo-controlled study found hints that use of MCTs by people with type 2 diabetes might improve insulin sensitivity and aid weight loss.

Athletes often sip carbohydrate-loaded drinks during exercise. MCTs may provide an alternative. Like other fats, they provide more energy per ounce than carbohydrates; but unlike normal fats, this energy can be released rapidly. A number of double-blind trials using MCTs for improving high-intensity or endurance exercise performance have been conducted, but the results have been thoroughly inconsistent. This is not surprising, as none of these studies enrolled enough participants to provide trustworthy results. Larger studies are necessary to discover whether MCTs are really as useful for athletes as the supplement's proponents claim.

SCIENTIFIC EVIDENCE

Fat malabsorption. A double-blind, placebo-controlled study on twenty-four men and women with AIDS suggests that MCTs can help improve AIDS-related fat malabsorption. In this disorder, fat is not digested; it passes unchanged through the intestines, and the body is deprived of calories as well as of fat-soluble vitamins.

The study participants were split into two groups: One received a liquid diet containing normal fats, whereas the other group received mostly MCTs. After twelve days, the participants on the MCT formula showed significantly less fat in their stool and better fat absorption than the other group. Another double-blind study found similar results in twenty-four men with AIDS-related fat malabsorption.

The body depends on enzymes from the pancreas to digest fat. In one study, individuals with inadequate pancreatic function due to chronic pancreatitis appeared to be better able to absorb MCTs than ordinary fatty acids. However, this did not turn out to mean much on a practical basis, because without taking extra digestive enzymes, they could only just barely absorb the MCTs, whereas, if they took digestive enzymes, they absorbed ordinary fats as well as MCTs without difficulty.

SAFETY ISSUES

Studies in animals and humans reveal that MCTs are quite safe when consumed at a level of up to 50 percent of total dietary fat. However, some people who consume MCTs, especially on an empty stomach, experience annoying (but not severe) abdominal cramps and bloating. The maximum safe dosage of MCTs in young children, pregnant or nursing women, and people with serious kidney or liver disease has not been established.

EBSCO CAM Review Board

FURTHER READING

Beermann, C., et al. "Short Term Effects of Dietary Medium-Chain Fatty Acids and n-3 Long-Chain Polyunsaturated Fatty Acids on the Fat Metabolism of Healthy Volunteers." *Lipids in Health and Disease* 2 (2003): 10.

Han, J. R., et al. "Effects of Dietary Medium-Chain Triglyceride on Weight Loss and Insulin Sensitivity in a Group of Moderately Overweight Free-Living Type 2 Diabetic Chinese Subjects." *Metabolism* 56 (2007): 985-991.

Matsuo, T., et al. "Effects of a Liquid Diet Supplement Containing Structured Medium- and Long-Chain Triacylglycerols on Body Fat Accumulation in Healthy Young Subjects." *Asia Pacific Journal of Clinical Nutrition* 10 (2001): 46-50.

Nosaka, N., et al. "Effects of Dietary Medium-Chain Triacylglycerols on Serum Lipoproteins and Biochemical Parameters in Healthy Men." *Bioscience, Biotechnology, and Biochemistry* 66 (2002): 1713-1718.

St-Onge, M. P., et al. "Medium-Chain Triglycerides Increase Energy Expenditure and Decrease Adiposity in Overweight Men." *Obesity Research* 11 (2003): 395-402.

_____. "Medium- Versus Long-Chain Triglycerides for Twenty-seven Days Increases Fat Oxidation and Energy Expenditure Without Resulting in Changes in Body Composition in Overweight Women." *International Journal of Obesity Related Metabolic Disorders* 27 (2003): 95-102.

Tsuji, H., et al. "Dietary Medium-Chain Triacylglycerols Suppress Accumulation of Body Fat in a Double-Blind, Controlled Trial in Healthy Men and Women." *Journal of Nutrition* 131 (2001): 2853-2859.

See also: Herbal medicine; Weight loss, undesired.

Melatonin

CATEGORY: Herbs and supplements

DEFINITION: Natural substance of the human body used as a supplement to treat specific health conditions.

PRINCIPAL PROPOSED USES: Insomnia, jet lag, other sleep disorders

OTHER PROPOSED USES

- *Oral:* Aging in general, Alzheimer's disease and non-Alzheimer's dementia, attention deficit disorder, cancer (as an addition to conventional therapy), cluster headaches, epilepsy in children, fibromyalgia, functional dyspepsia (chronic indigestion of no known cause), immune support, irritable bowel syndrome, migraine, preventing heart disease, reducing anxiety before surgery, seasonal affective disorder, smoking cessation, tardive dyskinesia
- *Topical:* Thinning hair in women

OVERVIEW

Melatonin is a natural hormone that regulates sleep. During daylight, the pineal gland in the brain produces an important neurotransmitter called serotonin. (A neurotransmitter is a chemical that relays messages between nerve cells.) However, at night, the pineal gland stops producing serotonin and instead makes melatonin. This melatonin release helps trigger sleep. The production of melatonin varies according to the amount of light to which a person is exposed; for example, people produce more melatonin in a completely dark room than in a dimly lit one.

Melatonin supplements appear to be helpful for people whose natural sleep cycle has been disturbed, such as travelers suffering from jet lag. The hormone may also be helpful in various other sleep disorders.

Based on early reports that melatonin levels decline with age, the hormone was briefly marketed as a kind of fountain of youth. However, newer evidence suggests that melatonin levels do not decline with age after all. Other potential benefits of melatonin remain largely speculative. Very weak evidence hints that melatonin might be helpful for functional dyspepsia (chronic indigestion of unknown cause).

REQUIREMENTS AND SOURCES

Melatonin is not a nutrient. However, travelers and workers on rotating or late shifts can experience sleep disturbances that seem to be caused by changing melatonin levels. A person can boost melatonin production naturally by getting thicker blinds for the bedroom windows or wearing a night mask. One can also take melatonin tablets.

THERAPEUTIC DOSAGES

Melatonin is typically taken half an hour before bedtime for the first four days after traveling. For ordinary insomnia, melatonin is usually taken about 30 minutes to 1 hour before bedtime. To fall asleep on Sunday night after staying up late Friday and Saturday, one study suggests using melatonin 5.5 hours before the desired bedtime. The optimum dose of melatonin is not clear, but it is probably in the range of 1 to 5 milligrams (mg).

Melatonin is available in two forms: immediate-release (just plain melatonin, also called quick-release) and slow-release (a special preparation, also called controlled-release, designed to spread melatonin absorption over many hours). It seems reasonable to suppose that quick-release melatonin helps in falling asleep, while slow-release melatonin helps in staying asleep, but study results are inconsistent on this issue.

THERAPEUTIC USES

Reasonably good evidence reveals that melatonin can help people with jet lag adjust to a new schedule. Although it probably works in part by resetting the biological clock, it also appears to decrease or block wakefulness-promoting circuits in the nervous system and may have other direct sedative effects. Based on this, melatonin has been tried for insomnia of various types, but results have been inconsistent.

Three small double-blind studies suggest that use of melatonin might reduce symptoms of irritable bowel syndrome. It has been suggested that melatonin might work through effects on the nervous system in the digestive tract.

Four double-blind studies performed by Saudi researchers reported that melatonin was useful for reducing anxiety prior to surgery, presumably because of its sedative effects. However, other researchers have been unable to confirm these results.

Three small, double-blind, and placebo-controlled studies found evidence that melatonin may slightly reduce nighttime blood pressure. Two preliminary double-blind trials hint that use of melatonin at a dose of 10 mg per day may reduce symptoms of tardive dyskinesia.

A preliminary double-blind study suggests that melatonin may improve quality of life in children with epilepsy, perhaps by improving sleep and reducing medication side effects. One surprising double-blind study suggests that topical application of melatonin may increase hair growth in women with thinning hair, for reasons that are entirely unclear.

Oral melatonin has shown some potential for treating seasonal affective disorder, cluster headaches, and irritable bowel syndrome.

Highly preliminary studies, including nonblind controlled trials, suggest that melatonin may enhance the effectiveness of standard therapy for breast cancer, prostate cancer, brain glioblastomas, non-small-cell lung cancer, and other forms of cancer. Melatonin has also shown some promise in animal studies for reducing side effects (specifically, cardiac toxicity) of the chemotherapy drug doxorubicin; however, the only human trials supporting this use fall considerably below modern scientific standards.

Weak evidence supports a role for melatonin in reducing nicotine withdrawal symptoms. On the basis of one uncontrolled trial, melatonin has been promoted as a treatment for fibromyalgia.

Based on theoretical reasoning and scant evidence, it has been suggested that melatonin can boost the immune system, prevent heart disease, and fight aging in general. Evidence to date suggests that melatonin is not helpful for menopausal symptoms, chronic fatigue syndrome, or migraines.

SCIENTIFIC EVIDENCE

Sleep disorders. Melatonin appears to produce sedation comparable to that of conventional pharmaceuticals used for inducing sleep without impairing mental function. Melatonin has shown promise as a treatment for a variety of sleep disorders, of which the best studied is jet lag.

Jet lag. There is good evidence that melatonin can help people fall asleep when their bedtime rhythms have been disturbed by travel (jet lag). For example, one double-blind, placebo-controlled study enrolled 320 people and followed them for four days after a long plane trip. The participants were divided into four groups and given a daily dose of 5 mg of standard melatonin, 5 mg of slow-release melatonin, 0.5 mg of standard melatonin, or a placebo. The group that received 5 mg of standard melatonin slept better, took less time to fall asleep, and felt more energetic and awake during the day than the other three groups.

Another small double-blind trial found that airplane crews experienced improved rest when using melatonin (10 mg) compared with placebo, and equivalent benefits when compared with the drug zopiclone. Neither group experienced any impairment in mental function the following morning.

According to one review of the literature, melatonin treatment for jet lag is most effective for those who have crossed a significant number of time zones, perhaps eight.

Shift work. Studies of melatonin for the treatment of insomnia related to shift work have yielded mixed results. Researchers have been surprised by these findings but suggest that perhaps working at night upsets the biological rhythm even more profoundly than traveling over many time zones, too profoundly for melatonin to help.

Sleep in the elderly. Mixed results have been seen with the use of melatonin for treating insomnia in the elderly. Not only have many studies failed to find melatonin helpful, but those studies with positive results found widely varying benefits; for example, some studies found a decreased time to falling asleep, but no change in sleep throughout the night, while others found the reverse. These differences have not followed dose or type of melatonin in any obvious way, making them somewhat suspect.

General insomnia. One small study failed to find benefit for general insomnia in healthy people.

Sleep problems in children. A four-week double-blind trial evaluated the benefits of melatonin for children with difficulty falling asleep. A total of forty children who had experienced this type of sleep problem for at least one year were given either a placebo or melatonin at a dose of 5 mg. The results showed that use of melatonin helped participants fall asleep significantly more easily. Similar results were seen in a double-blind, placebo-controlled study of sixty-two children and in a study of twenty developmentally disabled children with sleep problems.

Delayed weekend sleep pattern (Monday morning fatigue). Many individuals stay up late on Friday and Saturday nights and then find it difficult to get to sleep at a reasonable hour on Sunday. A small double-blind, placebo-controlled study found evidence that taking melatonin 5.5 hours before the desired Sunday bedtime improved the ability of participants to fall asleep.

Sleep in hospitalized persons. Benefits were seen in a small, double-blind trial of patients in a pulmonary intensive care unit (ICU). It is famously difficult to sleep in an ICU, and the resulting sleep deprivation is not helpful for those recovering from disease or surgery. In this study of eight hospitalized individuals, 3 mg of controlled-release melatonin dramatically improved sleep quality and duration.

Other sleep problems. Small double-blind trials have found benefits for improving sleep in people with diabetes, asthma, head injury, schizophrenia, Alzheimer's disease, and Parkinson's disease. Melatonin has also shown benefit for improving sleep in people with attention deficit disorder; it has failed, however, to show benefit for the symptoms of ADD per se.

Blind people often have trouble sleeping on any particular schedule, because there are no light cues available to help them get tired at night. A small double-blind, placebo-controlled, crossover trial found that the use of melatonin at a dose of 10 mg per day was able to resynchronize participants' sleep schedules.

Some individuals find it impossible to fall asleep until early morning, a condition called delayed sleep phase syndrome (DSPS). Melatonin may be beneficial for this syndrome.

Individuals trying to stop using sleeping pills in the benzodiazepine family may find melatonin helpful. A double-blind, placebo-controlled study of thirty-four individuals who regularly used such medications found that melatonin at a dose of 2 mg nightly (controlled-release formulation) could help them discontinue the use of the drugs. Interestingly, another study failed to find melatonin helpful for reducing benzodiazepine use among people taking drugs in that family for anxiety. There can be risks in discontinuing benzodiazepine drugs; those who plan to discontinue their use should do so with their physician's advice.

Cancer treatment. Melatonin has been used with conventional anticancer therapy in more than a dozen clinical studies. Results have been surprisingly good, although this research must be considered preliminary. For example, a double-blind study on thirity people with advanced brain tumors suggested that melatonin might prolong life and also improve the quality of life. Participants received standard radiation treatment with or without 20 mg daily of melatonin. After one year, six of fourteen individuals in the melatonin group were still alive, compared with just one of sixteen from the control group. The melatonin group also had fewer side effects from the radiation treatment–a notable improvement in their quality of life.

Improvements in symptoms and a possible reduction of mortality were also seen in other studies. Melatonin appears to work by increasing levels of the body's own tumor-fighting proteins, known as cytokines.

Headaches. Some evidence suggests that individuals with cluster headaches have lower than average levels of the hormone melatonin. In a double-blind, placebo-controlled study of twenty individuals with cluster headaches, use of melatonin (10 mg daily) for fourteen days appeared to reduce headache severity or frequency (or both) in about one-half the participants. Overall, the use of melatonin produced better effects than placebo.

In a small randomized, crossover study, forty-eight men and women who suffered from migraines took melatonin (2 mg) every night for eight weeks. The supplement did not decrease the number of migraine attacks.

Seasonal affective disorder. One study found that people with seasonal affective disorder (SAD) have higher levels of melatonin than those without the condition. On this basis, it would seem that supplemental melatonin should worsen SAD symptoms. However, the evidence for such an effect is inconsistent. Some researchers have proposed that interaction between SAD and melatonin might be more complex than merely high or low levels and that, when taken at certain times of day, melatonin might help the condition. A very small study found that

Melatonin for Irritable Bowel Syndrome

While melatonin is best known as a sleep aid, it is also hypothesized to play a role in the neurological regulation of the intestinal tract. Some evidence suggests that it can influence pain sensation and muscular contraction.

In three small, double-blind, placebo-controlled studies enrolling a total of more than one hundred persons with irritable bowel syndrome (IBS), the use of melatonin appeared to improve IBS symptoms independent of its effects on sleep. The most recent of these studies was performed by Indian researchers and published in the *Journal of Clinical Gastroenterology* in 2007. In this trial, eighteen people with IBS were given either placebo or 3 mg of melatonin before bed for eight weeks. The results showed that compared with placebo, melatonin markedly improved IBS symptoms as measured by total symptom scores.

Steven Bratman, M.D.

when melatonin was given in the afternoon, it produced some benefit for people with SAD. However, a study of melatonin used in the early morning or the late evening failed to find any benefit.

Melatonin has shown equivocal effects for two conditions related to SAD: subsyndromal seasonal affective disorder (S-SAD) and weather-associated syndrome (WAS). According to the one reported study, use of melatonin improved some symptoms but worsened others.

Dementia. In a sizable Danish trial, researchers investigated the effects of melatonin on mood, sleep, and cognitive decline in elderly patients, most of whom suffered from dementia. They found that melatonin (2.5 mg) given nightly for an average of fifteen months slightly improved sleep but worsened mood. The latter effect was reversed by adding light therapy during the day. Melatonin apparently had no significant effect on cognition. In a systematic review of five randomized trials including 323 people with dementia, researchers failed to find evidence that melatonin is helpful in enhancing memory and other cognitive abilities. In two of the trials, however, melatonin was associated with short-term improvement in mood and behavior.

SAFETY ISSUES

A safety study found that melatonin at a dose of 10 mg daily produced no toxic effects when given to forty healthy males for a period of twenty-eight days. However, this does not prove that melatonin is safe when taken on a regular basis over the long term. Melatonin is not truly a food supplement but a hormone. As with other hormones used in medicine, such as estrogen and cortisone, harmful effects can take years to appear. Hormones are powerful substances that have many subtle effects in the body, and these effects are far from fully understood. While in one small study, use of melatonin over an eight-day period by healthy men did not affect natural release of melatonin or levels of pituitary or sex hormones, another study found effects on testosterone and estrogen metabolism in men and possible impairment of sperm function. Also, a small study in women found possible effects on the important female hormone luteinizing hormone (LH).

Melatonin appears to cause drowsiness and decreased mental attention for about two to six hours after its use and may also impair balance. For this reason, people should not drive or operate machinery for several hours after taking melatonin. In a study of healthy middle-aged and older adults, however, an extended-release version of melatonin, which is said to more closely mimic natural fluctuations of the hormone in the body, did not impair mental ability or driving skills one to four hours later compared with a placebo. In either case, melatonin does not appear to have any lingering effects the following day.

Based on theoretical ideas of how melatonin works, some authorities specifically recommend against using it in people with depression, schizophrenia, autoimmune diseases, and other serious illnesses. One study in postmenopausal women found evidence that melatonin might impair insulin action and glucose tolerance, suggesting that people with diabetes should not use it. However, another study found melatonin safe and effective for people with diabetes. Because of these contradictions, individuals with diabetes should seek a physician's supervision before using melatonin.

Two exceedingly preliminary studies reported by one research group have led to publicized concerns that use of the supplement melatonin might increase nighttime asthma. However, one double-blind study of melatonin in people with asthma found evidence of improved sleep without worsening of symptoms. Again, at the current state of knowledge, caution must be advised for people with nighttime asthma who wish to try melatonin.

There is some evidence that melatonin may interfere with the ability of blood to clot normally, at least in healthy volunteers, though the clinical significance of this finding is unknown. Maximum safe dosages for young children, pregnant or nursing women, or those with serious liver or kidney disease have not been established.

EBSCO CAM Review Board

FURTHER READING
Alstadhaug, K. B., et al. "Prophylaxis of Migraine with Melatonin." *Neurology* 75 (2010): 1527-1532.

Jansen, S., et al. "Melatonin for the Treatment of Dementia." *Cochrane Database of Systemic Reviews* 1 (2011): CD003802.

Klupinska, G., et al. "Therapeutic Effect of Melatonin in Patients with Functional Dyspepsia." *Journal of Clinical Gastroenterology* 42 (2007): 270-274.

Otmani, S., et al. "Effects of Prolonged-Release Melatonin, Zolpidem, and Their Combination on Psychomotor Functions, Memory Recall, and Driving Skills in Healthy Middle-Aged and Elderly Volunteers." *Human Psychopharmacology* 23, no. 8 (2008): 693-705.

Riemersma-van der Lek, R. F., et al. "Effect of Bright Light and Melatonin on Cognitive and Noncognitive Function in Elderly Residents of Group Care Facilities." *Journal of the American Medical Association* 299 (2008): 2642-2655.

Saha, L., et al. "A Preliminary Study of Melatonin in Irritable Bowel Syndrome." *Journal of Clinical Gastroenterology* 41 (2007): 29-32.

Van der Heijden, K. B., et al. "Effect of Melatonin on Sleep, Behavior, and Cognition in ADHD and Chronic Sleep-Onset Insomnia." *Journal of the American Academy of Child and Adolescent Psychiatry* 46 (2007): 233-241.

Wirtz, P. H., et al. "Oral Melatonin Reduces Blood Coagulation Activity: A Placebo-Controlled Study in Healthy Young Men." *Journal of Pineal Research* 44 (2008): 127-133.

See also: Benzodiazepines; Herbal medicine; Insomnia.

Memory and mental function impairment

CATEGORY: Condition

RELATED TERMS: Age-associated memory impairment, age-related cognitive decline, brain boosters, cognitive impairment

DEFINITION: Treatment of impaired memory and cognitive function.

PRINCIPAL PROPOSED NATURAL TREATMENTS: *Bacopa monniera* (brahmi), ginkgo, ginseng, phosphatidylserine

OTHER PROPOSED NATURAL TREATMENTS: Carnitine, cranberry, creatine, dehydroepiandrosterone, folate, guarana, huperzine A, isoflavones, lobelia, muira puama, multivitamin-multimineral supplements, neuropeptides, *Rhodiola rosea*, ribose, rosemary, saffron, Spanish sage, tyrosine, vinpocetine, whey protein, vitamin B_1, vitamin B_{12}, vitamin E, zinc

INTRODUCTION

Mental function often declines particularly under conditions of stress or fatigue. In addition, most people age forty and older experience some memory loss, technically known as age-related cognitive decline or age-associated memory impairment. It is not known what causes this normal experience, and there is no conventional treatment available for it. A few natural treatments might be helpful.

PRINCIPAL PROPOSED NATURAL TREATMENTS

Statistically speaking, it is easier to demonstrate a big improvement than a small one, and for that reason, it is more difficult to prove the effectiveness of a treatment in a mild condition than in a severe one. Because of this, there is far more evidence supporting the use of natural supplements for treating Alzheimer's disease than for improving mental function in healthy people. Nonetheless, there is some evidence for the latter.

Ginkgo biloba. An extract made from the herb *Ginkgo biloba* is a well-established herbal treatment for Alzheimer's disease. Ginkgo may also be helpful for improving normal age-related memory loss and even for enhancing mental function in younger people.

Age-related mental decline. In six of nine double-blind studies, the use of *Ginkgo biloba* extract significantly improved age-related mental decline compared with placebo. For example, in a double-blind, placebo-controlled trial, 241 elderly people complaining of mildly impaired memory were given either placebo or ginkgo for twenty-four weeks. The results showed that ginkgo produced modest improvements in certain types of memory.

Another double-blind, placebo-controlled trial examined the effects of ginkgo extract in forty men and women (age fifty-five to eighty-six years) who were not mentally impaired. In a six-week period, the results showed improvements in measurements of mental function. Benefits were seen in four other trials too, involving about 135 participants.

Set against these positive findings is a large (214 people) twenty-four-week study that found no benefit in ordinary age-related memory loss. It has been suggested that flaws in the trial's design led to this negative outcome. However, three other studies enrolling about four hundred elderly persons also failed to find significant benefit with daily use of ginkgo. Another double-blind, placebo-controlled study used a one-time dose of ginkgo and found no benefits. Also, a small, double-blind, placebo-controlled study looking for immediate mind-stimulating effects did not find them.

Besides these negative trials, there is another weakness in the evidence. There are numerous measurable aspects of memory and mental function, and studies of ginkgo for improving memory and mental function have examined a great many of these. The exact areas of benefits seen vary widely. For example, in one positive study, ginkgo may speed up the ability to memorize letters but not expand the number of letters that can be retained, while in another positive study, the reverse may be true. This type of inconsistency tends to decrease the confidence one can place in these apparently positive studies, because if ginkgo were really working, one would expect its effects to be more reproducible. Ginkgo may help normal age-related memory loss, but more research is necessary to determine whether this is the case.

Improving memory and mental function in younger people. Several studies enrolling about 250 people

What Is Alzheimer's Disease?

Alzheimer's disease (AD), a serious form of memory and mental function impairment, is also the most common form of dementia among older people. Dementia is a brain disorder that seriously affects a person's ability to carry out daily activities.

AD begins slowly. It first involves the parts of the brain that control thought, memory, and language. People with AD may have trouble remembering things that happened recently or have trouble remembering the names of people they know. A related problem, mild cognitive impairment (MCI), causes more memory problems than normal for older adults. Many, but not all, people with MCI will develop AD.

In AD, symptoms progressively get worse. People may not recognize family members or may have trouble speaking, reading, or writing. They may forget how to brush their teeth or comb their hair. Later on, they may become anxious or aggressive or may wander from home. Eventually, they need total care. This can cause great stress for family members who must care for them.

AD usually begins after age sixty. The risk goes up as a person gets older. One's risk is also higher if a family member has had the disease. No treatment can stop the disease, but some drugs and some alternative therapies may help keep symptoms from getting worse for a limited time.

have examined the effects of ginkgo on memory and mental function in younger people. However, the benefits seen in the positive trials were inconsistent, and the largest study failed to find any effect. One study hints that benefits may occur initially and then decline after several weeks.

Besides ginkgo alone, several double-blind, placebo-controlled studies evaluated combined treatment with ginseng and ginkgo, or vinpocetine and ginkgo, for enhancing mental function in young people, and most found some evidence of benefit. Weak evidence suggests that combining phosphatidylserine with ginkgo might increase its efficacy. However, in two studies, ginkgo combined with the Ayurvedic herb brahmi failed to improve mental function.

Phosphatidylserine. Like ginkgo, the supplement phosphatidylserine (PS) is widely used in Europe to treat various forms of dementia. There is some evidence that PS can also help people with ordinary age-related memory loss.

In one double-blind study that enrolled 149 people with memory loss (but not dementia), PS provided significant benefits compared with placebo. Persons with the most severe memory loss showed the most improvement.

Another double-blind trial of 120 older people with memory complaints (but not dementia) found no benefits. This discrepancy may have to do with the type of PS used (the second trial used the more modern soy-derived form of the supplement). Phosphatidylserine might enhance the effectiveness of ginkgo.

Ginseng. Several studies have found indications that the herb ginseng might enhance mental function. However, the specific benefits seen have varied considerably from trial to trial, tending to make the actual cognitive effects of ginseng (if there are any) difficult to discern.

For example, in a two-month, double-blind, placebo-controlled study of 112 healthy, middle-aged adults given either ginseng or placebo, results showed that ginseng improved abstract thinking ability. However, there was no significant change in reaction time, memory, concentration, or overall subjective experience between the two groups.

Another double-blind, placebo-controlled study of fifty men found that eight-week treatment with a ginseng extract improved ability to complete a detail-oriented editing task. A double-blind trial of sixteen healthy males found favorable changes in the ability to perform mental arithmetic in those given ginseng for twelve weeks.

More comprehensive benefits were seen in a double-blind, placebo-controlled trial of sixty elderly persons given fifty or one hundred days of treatment. The results showed that *Panax ginseng* produced improvements in numerous measures of mental function, including memory, attention, concentration, and ability to cope. Benefits were still evident at the fifty-day follow-up. However, virtually no improvement was seen in the placebo group, a result that is highly unusual and raises doubts about the accuracy of the study. Finally, four double-blind, placebo-controlled studies evaluated combined treatment with ginseng and ginkgo and found inconsistent evidence of improved mental function.

Bacopa monniera (brahmi). The Ayurvedic herb *Bacopa monniera* (brahmi) has a traditional reputation for improving memory. However, a twelve-week, double-blind, placebo-controlled trial of seventy-six persons that tested the potential memory-enhancing benefits of brahmi generally failed to find much evidence of benefit. The only significant improvement seen among all the many measures used was one that evaluated retention of new information. A randomized trial involving forty-eight healthy elderly persons found some memory-enhancing effects of *B. monniera* compared with placebo, but the outcomes measured were too numerous to be convincing.

In another double-blind, placebo-controlled study of thirty-eight persons, short-term use of brahmi failed to produce any measurable improvements in memory, while in a third double-blind, placebo-controlled study, the use of brahmi over a two-week period did produce some benefits, but in quite a different pattern. Finally, a study found that one-time combined treatment with ginkgo (120 milligrams [mg]) and brahmi (300 mg) failed to improve mental function.

Slightly more promising results have been seen in studies of a proprietary Ayurvedic mixture containing brahmi and about thirty other ingredients. However, these studies were generally not up to modern scientific standards.

OTHER PROPOSED NATURAL TREATMENTS
On the basis of one small double-blind study, a proprietary mixture of substances called neuropep-

tides has been extensively marketed for improving mental function. Radio, television, and Web advertisements state that this product has been shown to bring about "a reversal of ten years of short-term memory decline." However, this claim is not founded in reliable evidence. Another single study suggests that the supplement nicotinamide adenine dinucleotide might help improve temporary mental impairment caused by jet lag.

Evidence conflicts on whether multivitamin-multimineral tablets may improve cognitive function in people of various age groups. In general, the best-designed studies have failed to find benefit. However, it is quite possible that multivitamin-multimineral supplements are helpful for people with marked vitamin or mineral malnutrition. Studies of isoflavone-rich soy or red clover for enhancing mental function in women have found little to no beneficial effects at best.

Huperzine A is a potent chemical derived from a particular type of club moss (*Huperzia serrata*). This substance is really more a drug than an herb, but it is sold over the counter as a dietary supplement for memory loss and mental impairment. Some evidence indicates that it may be helpful for Alzheimer's disease and related conditions; very weak evidence suggests benefit for healthy people. Much the same can be said about the substance vinpocetine.

Creatine, best known for its use as a sports-performance enhancer, may improve mental function in sleep-deprived, but not necessarily well-rested, young persons. Sage and vitamin B_{17} have slight supporting evidence from preliminary double-blind trials.

Mild vitamin B_{12} deficiency may impair mental function. Because such deficiency is relatively common in the elderly, it has been suggested that vitamin B_{12} supplements may be appropriate in this age group. However, in the two studies that tried it, no benefits were seen.

The elderly are also commonly deficient in vitamin B_6, but a review of the literature failed to find meaningful evidence that vitamin B_6 offers any benefits. One study failed to find folate helpful either; however, in another study, folate supplementation improved mental function in older persons with high levels of homocysteine. Combinations of B vitamins, including B_{12}, B_6, and folate, have proved ineffective.

One study failed to find any benefit with zinc. Other preliminary double-blind trials suggest that the amino acid tyrosine may improve memory and mental function under conditions of sleep deprivation or other forms of stress. Other double-blind trials suggest that a proprietary extract of the herb *Rhodiola rosacea* may offer a similar benefit.

Whey protein contains alpha-lactalbumin, a protein that in turn contains high levels of the amino acid tryptophan. Tryptophan is the body's precursor for serotonin and is thought to affect mental function. In a small double-blind study, the use of alpha-lactalbumin in the evening improved morning alertness, perhaps by enhancing sleep quality. Another small double-blind study found weak evidence that alpha-lactalbumin improved mental function in people sensitive to stress. A third study failed to find that alpha-lactalbumin significantly improved memory in women experiencing premenstrual symptoms.

Herbs that contain caffeine would be expected to enhance mental function in healthy people, at least temporarily. These herbs include green tea, black tea, maté, and guarana. For example, in a double-blind, placebo-controlled study of 129 healthy young adults, the one-time use of guarana plus vitamins and minerals improved mental function and reduced mental fatigue among those undergoing a battery of cognitive tests. In another double-blind, placebo-controlled study, the use of guarana alone or guarana plus ginseng appeared to improve mental function. However, these studies had some design problems. In two other studies, no benefits were seen.

Some reports suggested that declining levels of the hormone dehydroepiandrosterone (DHEA) cause impaired mental function in the elderly. On this basis, DHEA has been promoted as a brain-boosting supplement. However, large studies have failed to find any correlation between DHEA levels and mental function, and there is no direct evidence that DHEA supplements provide any benefit in the elderly. One study did find potential benefits in younger people.

Weak evidence culled from a large, double-blind, placebo-controlled study hints that the use of beta-carotene over many years might enhance mental function. However, long-term use of beta-carotene might present safety risks.

Other herbs and supplements that have been proposed for enhancing memory and mental function, but that lack meaningful supporting evidence, include gotu kola, rosemary, saffron, muira puama, sage, and lobelia. In one small double-blind study, the supplement ribose failed to prove effective for enhancing mental function. However, the researchers suggested that the dose they used (2 grams daily) may have been insufficient.

A large study failed to find that the use of vitamin E helped maintain healthy mental function in women older than age sixty-five years. Also, women who are marginally deficient in iron may experience improved mental function when they correct this deficiency. Carnitine has shown some benefit for reducing mental fatigue and enhancing cognitive function in centenarians.

EBSCO CAM Review Board

FURTHER READING

Ataka, S., et al. "Effects of Oral Administration of Caffeine and D-Ribose on Mental Fatigue." *Nutrition* 24 (2008): 233-238.

Balk, E. M., et al. "Vitamin B6, B12, and Folic Acid Supplementation and Cognitive Function." *Archives of Internal Medicine* 167 (2007): 21-30.

Calabrese, C., et al. "Effects of a Standardized *Bacopa monnieri* Extract on Cognitive Performance, Anxiety, and Depression in the Elderly." *Journal of Alternative and Complementary Medicine* 14 (2008): 707-713.

Crews, W. D., et al. "A Double-Blinded, Placebo-Controlled, Randomized Trial of the Neuropsychologic Efficacy of Cranberry Juice in a Sample of Cognitively Intact Older Adults." *Journal of Alternative and Complementary Medicine* 11 (2005): 305-309.

Durga, J., et al. "Effect of Three-Year Folic Acid Supplementation on Cognitive Function in Older Adults in the FACIT Trial." *The Lancet* 369 (2007): 208-216.

Fournier, L. R., et al. "The Effects of Soy Milk and Isoflavone Supplements on Cognitive Performance in Healthy, Postmenopausal Women." *Journal of Nutrition, Health, and Aging* 11 (2007): 155-164.

Grodstein, F., et al. "A Randomized Trial of Beta Carotene Supplementation and Cognitive Function in Men: The Physicians' Health Study II." *Archives of Internal Medicine* 167 (2007): 2184-2190.

Hvas, A. M., et al. "No Effect of Vitamin B-12 Treatment on Cognitive Function and Depression." *Journal of Affective Disorders* 81 (2004): 269-273.

Kang, J. H., et al. "A Randomized Trial of Vitamin E Supplementation and Cognitive Function in Women." *Archives of Internal Medicine* 166 (2006): 2462-2468.

Kennedy, D. O., C. F. Haskell, et al. "Improved Cognitive Performance and Mental Fatigue Following a Multivitamin and Mineral Supplement with Added Guarana (*Paullinia cupana*)." *Appetite* 50 (2008): 506-513.

Kennedy, D. O., P. A. Jackson, et al. "Modulation of Cognitive Performance Following Single Doses of 120 mg *Ginkgo biloba* Extract Administered to Healthy Young Volunteers." *Human Psychopharmacology* 22 (2007): 559-566.

Kennedy, D. O., S. Pace, et al. "Effects of Cholinesterase Inhibiting Sage (*Salvia officinalis*) on Mood, Anxiety, and Performance on a Psychological Stressor Battery." *Neuropsychopharmacology* 31 (2006): 845-852.

Kritz-Silverstein, D., et al. "Effects of Dehydroepiandrosterone Supplementation on Cognitive Function and Quality of Life." *Journal of the American Geriatrics Society* 56 (2008): 1292-1298.

McNeill, G., et al. "Effect of Multivitamin and Multimineral Supplementation on Cognitive Function in Men and Women Aged Sixty-Five Years and Over." *Nutrition Journal* 6 (2007): 10.

Malaguarnera, M., et al. "L-carnitine Treatment Reduces Severity of Physical and Mental Fatigue and Increases Cognitive Functions in Centenarians." *American Journal of Clinical Nutrition* 86 (2007): 1738-1744.

Markus, C. R., et al. "Evening Intake of Alpha-lactalbumin Increases Plasma Tryptophan Availability and Improves Morning Alertness and Brain Measures of Attention." *American Journal of Clinical Nutrition* 81 (2005): 1026-1033.

Maylor, E. A., et al. "Effects of Zinc Supplementation on Cognitive Function in Healthy Middle-aged and Older Adults." *British Journal of Nutrition* 96 (2006): 752-760.

Murray-Kolb, L. E., and J. L. Beard. "Iron Treatment Normalizes Cognitive Functioning in Young Women." *American Journal of Clinical Nutrition* 85 (2007): 778-787.

The NEMO Study Group. "Effect of a Twelve-mo Micronutrient Intervention on Learning and Memory in Well-Nourished and Marginally Nourished School-Aged Children." *American Journal of Clinical Nutrition* 86 (2007): 1082-1093.

Rawson, E. S., et al. "Creatine Supplementation Does Not Improve Cognitive Function in Young Adults." *Physiology and Behavior* 95 (2008): 130-134.

Van Uffelen, J. G., et al. "Walking or Vitamin B for Cognition in Older Adults with Mild Cognitive Impairment?" *British Journal of Sports Medicine* 42 (2008): 344-351.

See also: Alzheimer's disease; Beta-carotene; Brahmi; Ginkgo; Ginseng; Mental health; Phosphatidylserine.

Menopause

CATEGORY: Condition
RELATED TERM: Hot flashes/flushes
DEFINITION: Treatment of symptoms related to the cessation of a woman's menstrual cycle.
PRINCIPAL PROPOSED NATURAL TREATMENTS: Black cohosh, isoflavones, soy
OTHER PROPOSED NATURAL TREATMENTS: Acupuncture, alfalfa, chasteberry, dehydroepiandrosterone, dong quai, estriol, evening primrose oil, flaxseed, gamma oryzanol, grass pollen, licorice, lignans, oligomeric proanthocyanidins, *Pueraria mirifica*, progesterone cream, red clover, rhubarb, royal jelly, St. John's wort, suma, traditional Chinese herbal medicine, vitamin C, vitamin E, yoga

INTRODUCTION

The hormonal changes of menopause can produce a variety of symptoms, ranging from hot flashes and vaginal dryness to anxiety, depression, and insomnia. Many of these symptoms are undoubtedly caused by the natural decrease in estrogen production that occurs at menopause; however, the human body is so complex that other hormonal factors undoubtedly also play a role.

Menopause is not a disease. It is clearly a natural process, but one that many women prefer not to experience. No longer do women accept as merely part of life the decrease in libido, pain during intercourse, years of hot flashes, and other uncomfortable problems that may accompany menopause. One of the most valued ideals of alternative medicine is the desire to trust nature, but not without exception. For example, in a state of nature, both infant and maternal mortality are high. This survival of the fittest helps humanity as a species to be stronger, but it is not something that a compassionate society can tolerate. Thus, no matter what their ideals, humans frequently find themselves tampering with nature. The treatment of menopause is simply one example among many.

Estrogen-replacement therapy can alleviate many of the problems associated with menopause. However, it creates counterbalancing risks. The most frightening issue is the increased risk of breast cancer that appears to be associated with replacement estrogen. In addition, estrogen therapy can cause blood clots in the legs, and it appears to raise the risk of heart disease rather than lower it (as previously thought). The decision whether to use estrogen-replacement therapy for menopausal symptoms should involve a careful examination of the risks and benefits in consultation with a physician.

PRINCIPAL PROPOSED NATURAL TREATMENTS

Several natural treatments, compared with placebo, may reduce menopausal symptoms. (The comparison is essential, as placebo itself is dramatically effective for menopause, generally reducing the rate of hot flashes by 50 percent.) It is not known if any of these treatments reduces the risk of osteoporosis.

Soy and soy (or other source) isoflavones. Both soy and red clover contain phytoestrogens (naturally occurring substances with estrogen-like actions) called isoflavones. It is thought that the isoflavones in these herbs may offer some benefits of estrogen with less risk. However, the evidence base for this hypothesis is conflicting.

Improvements in hot flashes and other symptoms, such as vaginal dryness and mood, have been seen in many studies of soy, mixed soy isoflavones, aglycone isoflavones, and the isoflavone genistein alone. However, about as many studies of soy or concentrated isoflavones have failed to find significant benefit compared with placebo.

For example, a double-blind study of 247 women with menopausal hot flashes compared the effects of placebo and genistein over a period of one year. Genistein was taken at a dose of 54 milligrams (mg) per day. The results indicated that the use of genistein significantly reduced hot flashes compared with placebo. In addition, isoflavones from red clover have shown inconsistent results in studies, with the best and largest study finding no benefit.

What can one make of this mixed evidence? One problem here is that placebo treatment has a strong effect on menopausal symptoms. In such circumstances, statistical "noise" can easily drown out the real benefits of a treatment under study. Unlike estrogen, which has such a powerful effect on hot flashes and other menopausal symptoms that its benefits are almost always clear in studies, soy and concentrated isoflavones likely have a modest effect, one that does not always show itself above the background noise of statistical variation. It has also been suggested that the placebo used in many of these studies, polyunsaturated fatty acids, may have efficacy of its own; this would tend to hide actual benefits.

Another explanation may be that certain women benefit from soy isoflavones more than others. In about one-third of people, isoflavones are converted by intestinal bacteria into a substance called equol. A minimum of two studies suggests that these equol producers may experience greater reduction in their menopausal symptoms than non-equol producers.

Evidence regarding whether soy or soy isoflavones are helpful for osteoporosis remains conflicting. On balance, it is probably fair to summarize evidence as indicating that isoflavones (either as soy, genistein, mixed isoflavones, or tofu extract) have a modestly beneficial effect on bone density. One small but long-term study suggests that progesterone cream (another treatment proposed for use in preventing or treating osteoporosis) may decrease the bone-sparing effect of soy isoflavones.

Black cohosh. The herb black cohosh is widely used for treatment of menopause, but the evidence that it works remains incomplete and inconsistent. The best

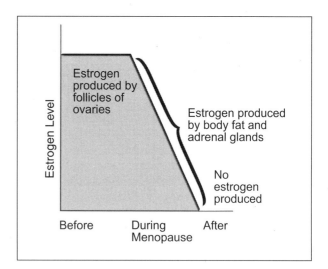

During menopause, which may last for several years, estrogen production diminishes; after menopause, estrogen is no longer produced by the body.

study was a twelve-week, double-blind, placebo-controlled trial of 304 women with menopausal symptoms. This study appeared to find that black cohosh was more effective than placebo. The best evidence was for a reduction in hot flashes. However, the statistical procedures used in the study were somewhat unusual and open to question.

Promising results were also seen in a three-month double-blind study of 120 menopausal women. Participants were given either black cohosh or fluoxetine (Prozac). Over the course of the trial, black cohosh proved more effective than fluoxetine for hot flashes, but fluoxetine was more effective than black cohosh for menopause-related mood changes.

Earlier, smaller studies have found improvements not only in hot flashes but also in other symptoms of menopause. For example, in a double-blind, placebo-controlled study, ninety-seven menopausal women received black cohosh, estrogen, or placebo for three months. The results indicated that the herb reduced overall menopausal symptoms (including hot flashes) to the same extent as the drug. In addition, microscopic analysis showed that black cohosh had an estrogen-like effect on the cells of the vagina. This is a positive result because it suggests that black cohosh might reduce vaginal thinning. However, black cohosh did not affect the cells of the uterus in an estrogen-like manner; this too is a positive result, as estrogen's effects on the uterus are potentially harmful. Finally, the study found hints that black cohosh might help protect bone. However, a great many of the study participants dropped out, making the results less than reliable.

One study, too small to have reliable results from a statistical point of view, found black cohosh just as effective as 0.6 mg daily of conjugated estrogens. A study reported in 2006 found that black cohosh has weak estrogen-like effects on vaginal cells and possible positive effects on bone (specifically, stimulating new bone formation).

A substantial (244-participant) double-blind study published in 2007 compared black cohosh with the synthetic hormone tibolone and found them equally effective for treating menopausal symptoms. Though not approved as a drug in the United States, tibolone does appear to be effective for menopausal symptoms, and, therefore, these results are somewhat promising. However, this study lacked a placebo group, and because the placebo effect is powerful for

menopausal symptoms, this omission significantly reduces the meaningfulness of the results.

One double-blind study evaluated a combination therapy containing black cohosh and St. John's wort in 301 women with general menopausal symptoms and depression. The results showed that the use of the combination treatment was significantly more effective than placebo for both problems. A smaller study using a combination of the same two herbs found improvements in overall menopausal symptoms and in cholesterol profile.

In contrast, there have been several studies that failed to find benefit. For example, in a twelve-month, double-blind, placebo-controlled study of 350 women, participants were given either black cohosh, a supplement containing ten herbs, the multibotanical plus soy, standard hormone replacement therapy, or placebo. The results showed significant benefits compared with placebo for hormone replacement therapy, but only slight, nonsignificant benefits with the other treatments. In addition, a double-blind study of 122 women failed to find statistically significant benefits with black cohosh compared with placebo, as did another study enrolling 132 women and one double-blind, placebo-controlled study that involved 124 women given a black cohosh-soy isoflavone combination. These negative outcomes were quite possibly caused by the relatively small sizes of the black cohosh groups. In a condition such as menopausal symptoms, where the placebo effect is strong and treatment is relatively weak, large numbers of participants are necessary to show benefit above and beyond the placebo effect. Nonetheless, this is an impressive number of negative studies, and some question must remain about the efficacy of this herb. Black cohosh may be modestly effective, however, for reducing hot flashes and other symptoms of menopause, but doubts remain.

Some information has developed regarding how black cohosh might work. In the past, the herb was described as a phytoestrogen. However, subsequent evidence indicates that black cohosh is not a general phytoestrogen, but that it may act like estrogen in only a few parts of the body: the brain (reducing hot flashes), bone (potentially helping to prevent or treat osteoporosis), and possibly the vagina (alleviating dryness and thinning). It does not appear to act like estrogen in the breast or the uterus, which is good news, as estrogen is carcinogenic in those tissues. If this theory is true, black cohosh is a selective-estrogen receptor modifier, somewhat like the drug raloxifen (Evista). However, more evidence is needed.

OTHER PROPOSED NATURAL TREATMENTS

Rhubarb contains the phytoestrogenic substance lindleyin. On this basis, extracts of rhubarb have been tried for control of menopausal symptoms. In a twelve-week, double-blind, placebo-controlled trial of 109 women with menopause-related problems, the use of a special rhubarb extract significantly improved symptoms compared with placebo. (Raw rhubarb is toxic when taken in excessive quantities.) The special standardized extract used in these trials was processed so as to remove toxic components.

Grass pollen extracts have shown promise for treatment of benign prostate enlargement. Their benefits in that condition may result from a hormonal effect. On this basis, grass pollens have been proposed for treatment of menopausal symptoms. One double-blind, placebo-controlled study followed fifty-four women with menopausal symptoms and found benefits with a supplement containing grass pollen extract.

The herb *Pueraria mirifica*, which contains numerous phytoestrogens, is promoted as an effective treatment for menopausal symptoms. In one double-blind study, the herb showed promise for improving vaginal dryness. In another trial comparing *P. mirifica* to standard estrogen treatment (0.625 mg conjugated equine estrogen), researchers found the herb to be equally effective at relieving a range of menopausal symptoms. In addition, another double-blind study found benefit with a combination product containing standardized extracts of black cohosh, dong quai, milk thistle, red clover, American ginseng, and chasteberry.

For many years, the hormone progesterone ("natural progesterone," as distinguished from the synthetic progestins used in birth control pills and hormone replacement therapy) was aggressively promoted by some alternative medicine practitioners as the true cure for osteoporosis. However, at that time there was no meaningful evidence that progesterone helps prevent osteoporosis (these claims were based largely on anecdotes, plausible reasoning, and "studies" that did not come close to modern scientific standards). When the subject was finally studied properly, the first results indicated that progesterone does not work for osteoporosis after all. However, it may

work for other menopausal symptoms. A one-year, double-blind, placebo-controlled study of 102 women found that cream containing 20 mg of the hormone progesterone may be effective against hot flashes, though it did not appear to protect bone from breakdown. However, another double-blind trial failed to find 32 mg daily effective for osteoporosis or any other menopause-related symptoms.

The hormone dehydroepiandrosterone (DHEA) has been tested as a treatment for menopausal symptoms, with some promising results in a small, preliminary trial. Because it is a naturally occurring hormone, there has been some concern regarding the safety of supplemental DHEA. However, a placebo-controlled trial with ninety-three postmenopausal women found DHEA supplementation for one year was not associated with increased adverse endometrial effects or changes in blood lipids or insulin sensitivity. Another, double-blind study found benefit with a mixture of isoflavones, lignans and black cohosh.

A small double-blind study conducted in Iran reported that vitamin E (400 international units daily) was more effective than placebo for treating menopausal hot flashes. However, a larger study in the United States failed to find vitamin E significantly helpful for hot flashes associated with breast cancer treatment.

An extract (HPE) made from human placenta is used in South Korea and other areas of East Asia as a treatment for numerous conditions. One study compared HPE with normal saline solution for treating menopause. In this eight-week trial, participants were given either normal saline or HPE as a subcutaneous injection through the skin of the abdomen. The results appear to indicate that HPE might improve some symptoms of menopause.

Evidence that is far too weak to be relied upon has been quoted in support of flaxseed, gamma oryzanol, multivitamin-multimineral combinations, and St. John's wort. Other proposed treatments that lack meaningful supporting evidence include bioflavonoids, chasteberry, licorice, suma, and vitamin C. In one trial, a combination of St. John's wort and chasteberry for sixteen weeks failed to produce any significant benefit compared with placebo in one hundred women with hot flashes.

Evidence regarding whether acupuncture might improve menopausal symptoms remains unconvincing. For example, one study that appears on the

Traditional Use of Black Cohosh

Black cohosh (known as both *Actaea racemosa* and *Cimicifuga racemosa*), a member of the buttercup family, is a perennial plant native to North America. Other common names include black snakeroot, bugbane, bugwort, rattleroot, rattletop, rattleweed, and macrotys. Insects avoid it, which accounts for some of these common names.

Black cohosh was used in North American Indian medicine for gynecological disorders, malaise, kidney disorders, malaria, rheumatism, and sore throat. It was also used for colds, cough, constipation, hives, and backache, and to induce lactation. In nineteenth-century America, black cohosh was a home remedy used for rheumatism and fever, as a diuretic, and to bring on menstruation. It was extremely popular among a group of alternative practitioners who called black cohosh macrotys and prescribed it for rheumatism, lung conditions, neurological conditions, and conditions that affected women's reproductive organs (including menstrual problems, inflammation of the uterus or ovaries, infertility, threatened miscarriage, and relief of labor pains).

surface to be well designed found no benefit in the placebo group. This is so unusual as to cast significant doubt on the results. Another pilot study found no significant difference between the sham (fake) acupuncture and real acupuncture for hot flashes. A small, placebo-controlled study among women with breast cancer who also had hot flashes because of their treatments did suggest some benefit for acupuncture, though the results were inconclusive. Two studies involving 462 postmenopausal women each concluded that acupuncture, when added to usual self-care, effectively reduces the frequency of hot flashes for a minimum of two months. This effect may only be short-term, however. In one of these studies, researches reevaluating participants at six and twelve months found the acupuncture group was no better than the group who received only self-care.

A double-blind, placebo-controlled study of questionable validity reported benefits in "all menopausal symptoms" through the use of oligomeric proanthocyanidins from pine bark. Also, it has been suggested that royal jelly is beneficial for menopausal symptoms, but there is no evidence to support this claim. The same is true regarding traditional Chinese herbal medicine for menopause. One study has been widely reported as proving the effectiveness of a particular Chinese herbal formula, but it lacked a placebo group. Another study failed to find the Chinese herb *Pueraria lobata* helpful for menopausal symptoms. Some evidence suggests that evening primrose oil, dong quai, and ginseng are not effective for menopausal symptoms. The herb alfalfa contains strong phytoestrogens. This might make it helpful for menopause, but no studies have been reported.

One double-blind, placebo-controlled study failed to find melatonin more helpful than placebo for menopausal symptoms. (Actually, placebo did a little better than melatonin in this study.) Another study failed to find that ginkgo improved mood, general energy level, or mental function in menopausal women.

Heavy exercise causes increased calcium loss through sweat, and the body does not compensate for this by reducing calcium loss in the urine. The result can be a net calcium loss so great that it presents health concerns for menopausal women. One study found that the use of an inexpensive calcium supplement (calcium carbonate), taken at a dose of 400 mg twice daily, is sufficient to offset this loss.

In a randomized, controlled trial, eight weeks of daily supervised yoga was modestly more effective than a similar amount of supervised physical exercise in relieving menopausal symptoms (such as hot flashes), decreasing psychological stress, and improving cognitive abilities among 120 women. Another study failed to find exercise helpful for reducing menopausal symptoms.

ESTRIOL: A SAFER FORM OF ESTROGEN?

Some alternative medicine practitioners have popularized the use of a special form of estrogen called estriol, claiming that, unlike standard estrogen, it does not increase the risk of cancer. However, this claim is unfounded.

There is no real doubt that estriol is effective. Controlled and double-blind trials have found oral or vaginal estriol effective for reducing hot flashes, night sweats, insomnia, vaginal dryness, recurrent urinary tract infections, and osteoporosis.

Estriol might cause less vaginal bleeding as a side effect than other forms of estrogen, but this has not been proven. However, like other forms of estrogen, oral estriol stimulates the growth of uterine tissue.

This leads to a risk of uterine cancer. In a placebo-controlled study of 1,110 women, uterine tissue stimulation was seen among women given estriol orally (1 to 2 mg daily) compared to those given placebo. Another large study found that oral estriol increased the risk of uterine cancer. In another study of forty-eight women given estriol 1 mg twice daily, uterine tissue stimulation was seen in the majority of cases.

In contrast, a twelve-month double-blind trial of oral estriol (2 mg daily) in sixty-eight Japanese women found no effect on the uterus. It may be that the high levels of soy in the Japanese diet altered the results.

Additionally, test-tube studies suggest that estriol is just as likely to cause breast cancer as any other form of estrogen. Women who are considering using estriol should think of it as equivalent to any other form of estrogen.

EBSCO CAM Review Board

FURTHER READING

Borrelli, F., and E. Ernst. "Black Cohosh (*Cimicifuga racemosa*) for Menopausal Symptoms." *Pharmacological Research* 58 (2008): 8-14.

Borud, E. K., et al. "The Acupuncture on Hot Flashes Among Menopausal Women Study." *Menopause* 17 (2010): 262-268.

Chattha, R., et al. "Effect of Yoga on Cognitive Functions in Climacteric Syndrome." *BJOG: An International Journal of Obstetrics and Gynaecology* 115 (2008): 991-1000.

Elavsky, S., and E. McAuley. "Physical Activity and Mental Health Outcomes During Menopause." *Annals of Behavioral Medicine* 33 (2007): 132-142.

Jou, H. J., et al. "Effect of Intestinal Production of Equol on Menopausal Symptoms in Women Treated with Soy Isoflavones." *International Journal of Gynaecology and Obstetrics* 102 (2008): 44-49.

Kim, K. H., et al. "Effects of Acupuncture on Hot Flashes in Perimenopausal and Postmenopausal Women." *Menopause* 17 (2010): 269-280.

Martin, B. R., et al. "Exercise and Calcium Supplementation: Effects on Calcium Homeostasis in Sportswomen." *Medicine and Science in Sports and Exercise* 39 (2007): 1481-1486.

Panjari, M., et al. "The Safety of Fifty-Two Weeks of Oral DHEA Therapy for Postmenopausal Women." *Maturitas* 63 (2009): 240.

Pruthi, S., et al. "Pilot Evaluation of Flaxseed for the Management of Hot Flashes." *Journal of the Society for Integrative Oncology* 5 (2007): 106-112.

Reed, S. D., et al. "Vaginal, Endometrial, and Reproductive Hormone Findings: Randomized, Placebo-Controlled Trial of Black Cohosh, Multibotanical Herbs, and Dietary Soy for Vasomotor Symptoms." *Menopause* 15 (2008): 51-58.

Rotem, C., and B. Kaplan. "Phyto-Female Complex for the Relief of Hot Flushes, Night Sweats, and Quality of Sleep." *Gynecological Endocrinology* 23 (2007): 117-122.

Sammartino, A., et al. "Short-Term Effects of a Combination of Isoflavones, Lignans, and *Cimicifuga racemosa* on Climacteric-related Symptoms in Postmenopausal Women." *Gynecological Endocrinology* 22 (2006): 646-650.

Ziaei, S., A. Kazemnejad, and M. Zareai. "The Effect of Vitamin E on Hot Flashes in Menopausal Women." *Gynecologic and Obstetric Investigation* 64 (2007): 204-207.

See also: Aging; Black cohosh; Dehydroepiandrosterone (DHEA); Estrogen; Isoflavones; Osteoporosis; Pain management; Premenstrual syndrome (PMS); Progesterone; Soy; Women's health.

Men's health

CATEGORY: Issues and overviews
DEFINITION: The use of nutrients, dietary supplements, herbal extracts, and alternative therapies for preventing and treating health conditions specific to men, such as prostate disorders and erectile dysfunction.

OVERVIEW

The use of complementary and alternative medicine (CAM) for managing men's health is increasing worldwide. A survey released in December of 2008 by the National Institutes of Health found that 33.5 percent of men use some form of complementary or alternative medicine. In North America, about 30 percent of men diagnosed with prostate disease use some form of CAM therapy.

Many dietary, phytotherapeutic, supplemental, and herbal agents have been used to prevent or treat prostate cancer, benign prostate hyperplasia, erectile dysfunction, and male infertility, but the role of CAM in managing men's health conditions continues to be debated. If CAM is evaluated by criteria of evidence-based medicine, available data have not clearly established the efficacy of many alternative agents. Different extraction procedures, variations in the quality of raw products, and the lack of knowledge regarding mechanisms of action of active ingredients make comparisons between various products virtually impossible and lead to conflicting results in clinical trials. Nonetheless, many health care professionals believe that when used properly, CAM can be beneficial in improving men's health.

Prostate Cancer

Prostate cancer is the most common cancer diagnosed in men and the second leading cause of cancer-related deaths in men in the United States. No complementary or alternative treatments will cure prostate cancer, but several CAM alternatives may be helpful in preventing the disease. CAM therapies present valuable opportunities for prostate cancer, particularly in the watchful waiting population. A June 2010, survey revealed that more than one-third of recently diagnosed persons with prostate cancer utilize some form of CAM therapy.

Foods that protect against prostate cancer. Several types of foods have shown potential for preventing prostate cancer. Of special interest are soy and soy products. Epidemiological data show a ten- to one-hundred-times lower incidence of prostate cancer in Asia, compared with Western countries. Soy products are a traditional staple in the diets of Eastern countries, suggesting that nutrition plays an important role in prostate cancer prevention. Legumes such as soybeans are rich in a variety of phytochemicals and are rich in isoflavones such as genistein and several other anticarcinogens that inhibit the growth of prostate cancer cells.

Lycopene, a carotenoid found mainly in tomatoes and tomato-derived products, has been shown in a number of clinical studies to have protective effects against the development of prostate cancer. Lycopene is an acyclic isomer of beta-carotene, and its most important anticancer property may be its strong antioxidant activity.

Cruciferous vegetables such as cabbage, Brussels sprouts, and broccoli have been shown to possess

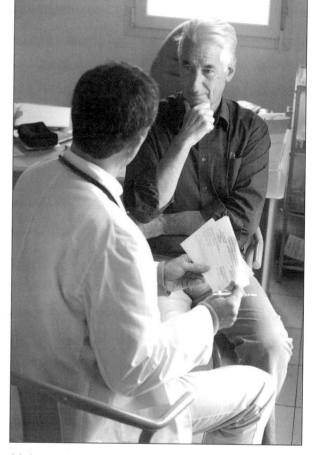

Male patient talking with his doctor. (Phanie/Photo Researchers, Inc.)

anticancer activities, possibly because of the substances they contain, such as indole-3-carbinol, glucaric acid, and sulforaphane, and because of their high concentration of the carotenoids lutein and zeaxantin.

The role of dietary supplements. The effectiveness of selenium in preventing prostate cancer has been the subject of numerous clinical trials, and different trials have yielded conflicting results concerning this trace element's protective efficacy. It is thought that selenium's antioxidant properties may help repair deoxyribonucleic acid (DNA), prevent cell invasion, and stimulate the signaling of transforming growth factor beta.

The Nutritional Prevention of Cancer Trial, which studied 1,312 men with low selenium levels, found a 63 percent reduction in prostate cancer incidence in men supplemented with selenium, compared with placebo. The men showed a 49 percent lower risk of prostate cancer through a seven-plus-year follow-up period. Reaching opposite conclusions, the Selenium and Vitamin E Cancer Prevention Trial of 35,000 men concluded that selenium and vitamin E, taken alone or together, do not prevent prostate cancer.

The Alpha-Tocopherol, Beta-Carotene Cancer Prevention Trial studied the protective effects of vitamin E and beta-carotene in 29,133 male smokers age fifty to sixty-nine. In this trial, vitamin E supplementation led to a 32 percent reduction in prostate cancer incidence and a 41 percent decrease in prostate cancer deaths.

Herbal therapy. Interest has been growing in the use of herbs in preventing prostate cancer. Among these agents, the catechins in green tea have shown encouraging results. In a one-year trial, men with precancerous changes in the prostate received green tea extract providing 600 milligrams of catechins per day, or a placebo. Prostate cancer developed in 3.3 percent of the men receiving green tea extract and in 30 percent of those given a placebo.

Benign Prostatic Hyperplasia

CAM therapies have also been useful in treating benign prostatic hyperplasia (BPH), an affliction that eventually affects at least 80 percent of men after age fifty. BPH is not related to cancer and is more bothersome than dangerous. The cause is thought to be related to variations in levels of hormones such as dihydrotestosterone or estrogen (or both), causing enlargement of the prostate, which partially blocks the urethra and hinders urinary voiding.

Some nutraceuticals have produced results equal to or better than pharmaceuticals prescribed to treat BPH. Several meta-analyses suggest clinical efficacy and good tolerability for extracts from *Serenoa repens* (saw palmetto), *Pygeum africanum* (from the bark of the African plum tree), stinging nettle, and pumpkin seeds.

Saw palmetto extract, derived from the fruit of *S. repens*, the American dwarf palm, is the botanical best studied and most used to treat symptoms of BPH. It appears to contain substances that have activity similar to (but weaker than) 5-alpha-reductase inhibitors, which prevent conversion of testosterone to dihydrotestosterone. Some studies have found that the efficacy of *S. repens* extract is comparable to that of finasteride and alpha-blockers.

Extract of the bark of the African plum tree *P. africanum* moderately improves urinary symptoms associated with BPH. Numerous studies report that pygeum significantly reduces urinary hesitancy, frequency, nocturia, and pain with urination in men with mild to moderate symptoms.

Clinical studies have shown that pumpkin seed oil (*Cucurbita pepo*), in combination with saw palmetto, effectively reduces symptoms of BPH. Researchers have suggested that the zinc, free fatty acid, or plant sterol content of pumpkin seeds may account for their efficacy.

Stinging nettle root (*Urtica dioica*), in combination with other herbs (especially saw palmetto), is effective in relieving symptoms of BPH. Clinical studies have shown stinging nettle to be comparable to finasteride in slowing the growth of certain prostate cells. Unlike finasteride, however, the herb does not decrease prostate size.

Erectile Dysfunction

The inability of men to achieve or maintain an erection sufficient for satisfactory sexual function can have considerable impact on interpersonal relationships and quality of life. According to Douglas MacKay, writing in *Alternative Medicine Review*, erectile dysfunction (ED) affects 50 percent of men forty to seventy years of age in the United States; by extrapolation, about thirty million men in the United States are affected. While prescription drugs have proven valuable in managing ED, they are not without limitations.

Over the centuries, many products have been touted as enhancing male vigor and libido. While the effectiveness of many of these substances cannot be adequately confirmed, arginine, yohimbine, *Panax ginseng*, and *Ginkgo biloba* all provide some degree of evidence that they are helpful for treating ED.

Nitric oxide (NO) is intimately related to penile erections. When a man becomes aroused, NO secretion begins in the blood vessels that lead into the penis, allowing the vessels to relax and widen to allow an increased flow of blood to enter the penis and harden it. NO levels decline as men age, resulting in ED. L-arginine, an amino acid found in muscle and cell tissues, is the biological precursor of NO. The formation of NO depends on sufficient levels of L-arginine in the body. L-arginine supplementation is particularly effective for treating men with abnormal NO metabolism, and most clinical trials have shown positive treatment results, often doubling levels of vascular NO.

Derived from the bark of an African evergreen tree (*Corynanthe yohimbe* or *Pausinystalia yohimbe*), yohimbine (also known as yohimbe) is regulated as a drug in some countries, where it is pharmacologically classified as an alpha-2-adrenergic receptor

Study: Prostate Genes Altered by Intensive Diet and Lifestyle Changes

A 2008 pilot study, conducted by researchers at the University of California, San Francisco, suggests that intensive lifestyle and diet changes, forms of complementary and alternative medicine, may alter gene expression (the way a gene acts) in the prostate—possibly affecting the progression of prostate cancer. Although the study's findings suggest directions for future research, such lifestyle and diet changes are not a substitute for proven prostate cancer therapies.

This study, known as Gene Expression Modulation by Intervention with Nutrition and Lifestyle, included a group of thirty-one men with low-risk prostate cancer. These men declined immediate surgery, hormonal therapy, or radiation and participated in an intensive three-month nutritional and lifestyle intervention while researchers monitored their tumor progression. The men stuck to a low-fat, plant-based diet and took dietary supplements including fish oil, selenium, and vitamins C and E. They also participated in stress management activities such as yoga-based stretching, breathing, meditation, imagery, and progressive relaxation; did moderate aerobic exercise; and attended group support sessions.

The researchers created "gene expression profiles" and took samples of the men's ribonucleic acid (RNA) before and after the intervention. They found that there were changes in the men's RNA following the lifestyle and diet modifications. Certain RNA transcripts that play a critical role in tumor formation had "up-regulated" (increased), and others had "down-regulated" (decreased).

The researchers concluded that intensive nutrition and lifestyle changes may alter gene expression in the prostate. They believe that understanding how these changes affect the prostate may lead to more effective prevention and treatment for prostate cancer, and they recommend larger, randomized-controlled trials to confirm the results of this pilot study.

antagonist. As such, it blocks brain receptors involved in releasing norepinephrine in the genitals. Norepinephrine is the principal neurotransmitter involved in the vascular smooth muscle contraction that reduces penile blood flow, ending an erection. Therefore, blocking norepinephrine receptors helps prolong tumescence. Yohimbine increases the amount of blood that is allowed to flow into the penis and prevents it from flowing out.

For more than two millennia, *P. ginseng* has been used by Chinese healers for its restorative properties. Modern scientists have identified active constituents, including triterpene saponin glycosides known as ginsenosides, which may be responsible for some of ginseng's antioxidant and health-preserving properties. Ginsenosides have been shown to increase the release of NO, and preliminary studies suggest that this is ginseng's primary mechanism of action, resulting in improved penile hemodynamics.

The herb *Ginkgo biloba* also has vasodilating properties. It is used in many alternative herbal supplements to help increase blood flow to the genitals. Recent evidence supports indications that *Ginkgo biloba* extract is effective in the treatment of ED caused by the lack of blood flow to the genitals. It enhances blood circulation and appears to help ED by increasing blood flow to the penis. It can also relax the muscles and assist with penis blood flow.

INFERTILITY

Reports show that about 6 percent of adult males are believed to be infertile. Male infertility is usually associated with a decrease in the number, quality, or motility (power of movement) of sperm. Taken together, low sperm count in the semen, decreased sperm motility, and abnormal shape of the sperm are responsible for infertility in about 40 percent of men.

Excessive reactive free radicals can be very damaging to sperm. Elements in the sperm cell membrane are highly susceptible to oxidative damage. Several antioxidant supplements that regulate the effects of oxidative stress, such as vitamin C, vitamin E, glutathione, selenium, and coenzyme Q_{10} (CoQ_{10}), have proven to be effective in treating this cause of male infertility.

The effects of oxidative DNA damage and the role of dietary ascorbic acid (vitamin C) in preventing this damage have encouraged examination of these factors in relation to human sperm DNA. One study showed that dietary ascorbic acid protects human sperm from oxidative DNA damage that could affect sperm quality and increase the risk of genetic defects. Another study found that daily supplementation with 200 to 1,000 milligrams of vitamin C increased the fertility of men with a condition called agglutination, in which sperm stick together.

Vitamin E supplementation has been shown to enhance fertility in men, most probably by decreasing free-radical damage to sperm cells. In another study, men with low fertilization rates were given 200 IU (international units) of vitamin E daily. After one month of supplementation, fertilization rates increased significantly, and the amount of oxidative stress on sperm cells decreased.

Glutathione and selenium are vital to the antioxidant defenses of sperm and have shown positive effects on sperm motility. Deficiencies in either of these substances can lead to defective sperm motility. In a clinical study of twenty infertile men, glutathione demonstrated a statistically significant improvement in sperm motility. Another study reported that fertile males had significantly higher selenium levels in their seminal fluid than infertile men.

Zinc deficiency is associated with decreased testosterone levels and reduced sperm count. An adequate amount of zinc ensures proper sperm production and motility. Several studies have found supplemental zinc to be helpful in treating cases of low sperm count or of decreased testosterone levels.

The amino acid L-arginine is a biochemical precursor of substances that are thought to be essential to sperm production and motility. L-arginine is also essential for the production of testosterone, the predominant hormone necessary for healthy sperm production. In one study, 74 percent of men with low sperm count experienced significant improvement in sperm count and motility after taking 4 grams of L-arginine per day for three months.

Carnitine, derived from an amino acid, contributes directly to sperm motility and may be involved in the successful maturation of sperm. This is especially important because sperm tend to accumulate carnitine while in the epididymis. Low levels of carnitine lead to potential alterations in sperm motility. One study found a direct correlation between semen carnitine content and sperm motility.

CoQ_{10} is concentrated in the mitochondria of sperm cells, where it is involved in energy production. It also functions as an antioxidant, preventing lipid peroxidation of sperm membranes. In one study, 10 milligrams per day of an analog of CoQ_{10} was given to infertile men, resulting in increases in sperm count and motility.

Gerald W. Keister, M.S.

FURTHER READING

National Cancer Institute. Complementary and Alternative Medicine. http://www.cancer.gov/cancertopics/cam.

National Center for Complementary and Alternative Medicine. http://nccam.nih.gov.

Trivieri, Larry, Jr., and John W. Anderson. eds. *Alternative Medicine: The Definitive Guide.* 2d ed. Berkeley, Calif.: InnoVision Health Media, 2002.

See also: Benign prostatic hyperplasia; Cancer risk reduction; Cancer treatment support; Heart attack; Infertility, male; Prostatitis; Sexual dysfunction in men.

Mental health

CATEGORY: Issues and overviews
RELATED TERMS: Emotional health, psychological health
DEFINITION: Treatment of psychological and other mental health disorders.

OVERVIEW

People with psychological problems, including mood, anxiety, eating, sleep, and sexual disorders, seek complementary and alternative medicine (CAM) treatments. In some cases, they rely on these treatments in lieu of extant therapies; in other cases, they use CAM treatments along with traditional therapies.

CAM treatments for mental illness are remarkably diverse in scope. One 2002 review listed more than twenty widely used CAM techniques for mental health. These techniques include aromatherapy, acupuncture, herbal remedies, biofeedback, meditation, yoga, homeopathy, and creative arts (music, art, and dance) therapies. The research evidence for these and other CAM techniques varies in quality and quantity.

POPULAR USE OF CAM

Studies demonstrate that substantial proportions of persons with mental disorders, in the United States use one or more CAM remedies. One large population-based survey conducted in 1997 and 1998 revealed that 22.4 percent of Americans with major depression used one or more CAM therapies. The corresponding proportions of Americans with panic disorder (a condition marked by sudden surges of extreme anxiety), generalized anxiety disorder (a condition marked by high levels of nervousness across many situations), and either mania or psychosis (conditions often marked by a loss of contact with reality) were 32.0, 20.5, and 22.3 percent respectively. Persons with major depression and those with panic disorder were significantly more likely to use CAM treatments than other persons in the general population.

The study also found that people with mental disorders who used CAM treatments were as likely as those without mental disorders to seek conventional mental health treatments, such as psychotherapy and psychotropic medication. This information is important because certain herbal remedies can interfere with the effects of some widely used medications.

The results of another U.S. study from the same time period yielded higher percentages than did the 1997/1998 study. The study's investigative team found that 53.6 percent of persons with major depression had obtained CAM therapies in the year before the study; the corresponding number for persons with panic attacks was 56.7 percent. Among the most widely used CAM therapies (the percentage in parentheses refers to the proportion of people with major depression and panic attacks, respectively, using these therapies) were spiritual healing (10.5 and 9.9), energy healing (5.4 and 2.8), herbal remedies (4.3 and 3.3), megavitamins (3.4 and 3.6), aromatherapy (3.7 and 2.6), and hypnosis (1.8 and 3.0). Most people with major depression (63.9 percent) and with panic attacks (51.9 percent) who used CAM treatments also obtained conventional treatments. These latter percentages indicate, however, that large minorities of persons with mental disorders use CAM treatments in an alternative rather than complementary fashion. The data are worrisome given that a number of the CAM treatments used by respondents, such as energy therapies, megavitamins, and aromatherapy, are not empirically supported for the treatment of either mood or anxiety disorders.

Later systematic survey data on CAM use among persons with mental disorders is lacking. Nevertheless, the data from the late 1990s study suggest that

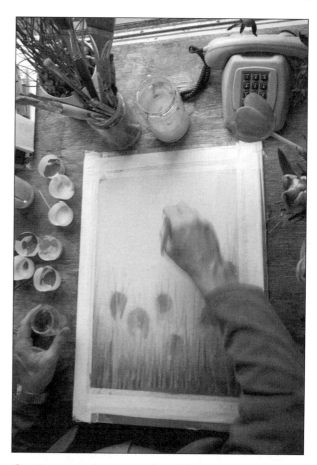

Creative arts therapy session. (Arno Massee/Photo Researchers, Inc.)

CAM use is prevalent among people with psychological problems, at least in the United States. As a consequence, it is essential to ascertain whether CAM treatments are effective for psychological problems and whether any could be harmful. The sections that follow briefly examine the scientific evidence concerning four commonly used CAM treatments for mental illness: acupuncture, herbal remedies, yoga and meditation, and creative arts therapies.

TREATMENTS AND TECHNIQUES

Acupuncture. Several investigators have examined the efficacy of acupuncture for clinical depression. A few early studies suggested that acupuncture may alleviate the symptoms of depression, but most of these studies were not conducted in a double-blind fashion and, therefore, may have been influenced by the expectations of treatment providers or patients, or both.

The most methodologically rigorous study, published in 2006, randomly assigned 151 persons with major depression to one of three "conditions" lasting eight weeks: traditional Chinese medicine acupuncture (condition 1), a sham acupuncture condition involving needles inserted into the "wrong" areas (condition 2), and a wait-list control condition (condition 3). The results revealed that both conditions (1) and (2) outperformed (3), but that (1) and (2) did not differ significantly from each other. Moreover, the effects of both genuine and sham acupuncture on depressive symptoms were relatively weak. These findings raise questions concerning the efficacy of acupuncture for depression and suggest that the effects of acupuncture on mood may be attributable to nonspecific influences, such as placebo effects; that is, improvement was caused by the mere expectation of improvement.

Herbal remedies. Although numerous herbal remedies are available for treating psychological problems, perhaps the two best known are St. John's wort (*Hypericum perforatum*) and kava (*Piper methysticum*). Following the passage of the Dietary Supplement Health and Education Act by the U.S. Congress in 1994, these and other herbal remedies for mood have not been regulated by the U.S. Food and Drug Administration. Therefore, mental health consumers in the United States take them at their own risk.

The data on the efficacy of St. John's wort for mood disorders have been inconsistent. A 2005 meta-analysis (quantitative review) revealed that St. John's wort exerted positive effects relative to a placebo among persons with mild to moderate depression. Nevertheless, the analysis also indicated that St. John's wort may be largely or entirely ineffective relative to placebo for persons with major depression and for those with prolonged depression. The study also found no evidence that St. John's wort is more effective than standard antidepressants, such as the selective serotonin reuptake inhibitors Prozac and Paxil.

A 2010 randomized-controlled trial of 189 persons suggested that St. John's wort may be more effective than placebo among persons with atypical depression, namely, among those persons who exhibit "reversed" features, such as overeating and oversleeping. Overall, the findings for St. John's wort point to potential positive effects on mild to moderate depres-

sion, and perhaps atypical depression, but offer little or no support for its use for severe depression.

Moreover, persons who take St. John's wort should be certain to inform their physicians, because the remedy can interfere with the effects of other medications. For example, St. John's wort can impede the effectiveness of chemotherapy medications and those used to treat human immunodeficiency virus infection. Evidence also exists that St. John's wort can interfere with the effects of birth control pills, anticoagulants (blood thinners), and antidepressants.

Kava is an herbal remedy that has been used medicinally in the South Pacific to reduce anxiety. The practice of using kava as an anxiolytic has spread to other regions. A 2009 study revealed that kava is more effective than placebo for generalized anxiety. Other evidence suggests that kava is not more effective than buspirone, an antianxiety agent.

Kava has been deemed unsafe because of its potential to create toxic liver reactions. Researchers have been assessing the efficacy of an aqueous extract of kava to create a mixture that reduces the toxicity of the herb. Further inquiry is required to ascertain this extract's safety and efficacy.

Meditation. Meditation comprises a heterogeneous array of self-control techniques, stemming largely from Buddhist and Hindu traditions and designed to enhance awareness and attention. A 2010 review of more than sixty studies (spanning thirty-five years) examined the effects of meditation techniques on a host of mental health difficulties, including mood, anxiety, and sleeping problems.

Although several of the studies in the review reported negative findings, most yielded preliminary evidence that various forms of meditation exert beneficial effects across a variety of psychological outcome variables. However, the overall quality of the research was limited, rendering any conclusions tentative. For example, many of the studies neglected to include control groups or included control groups of questionable adequacy. In addition, few of the studies incorporated adequate safeguards against client or therapist expectancy effects. In addition, it remains unclear whether meditation exerts positive effects above and beyond simpler interventions, such as relaxation.

Yoga. Yoga consists of a variety of physical and psychological techniques designed to heighten awareness. Hatha yoga, which originated in India but has

Mindfulness Meditation and Structural Changes in the Brain

Earlier scientific research has demonstrated that mindfulness mediation may reduce symptoms of anxiety, depression, and chronic pain, but little is known about meditation's effects on the brain. According to a 2011 study published in the journal Psychiatry Research: Neuroimaging, *practicing mindfulness meditation appears to be associated with measurable changes in the brain regions involved in memory, learning, and emotion. Mindfulness meditation focuses attention on breathing to develop increased awareness of the present.*

In this study, researchers took magnetic resonance images of the brains of sixteen participants two weeks before and after they joined the meditation program. (Participants were physician- and self-referred individuals seeking stress reduction.) Researchers also took brain images of a control group of seventeen non-meditators over a similar time period. Participants in the meditation group attended weekly sessions that included mindfulness training exercises and received audio recordings for guided meditation practice at home. They also kept track of how much time they practiced each day. Members of both groups completed a questionnaire, before and after joining the group, which measured five aspects of mindfulness: observing, describing, acting with awareness, nonjudging of inner experience, and nonreactivity to inner experience.

Brain images in the meditation group revealed increases in gray matter concentration in the left hippocampus. The hippocampus is an area of the brain involved in learning, memory, and emotional control and is suspected of playing a role in producing some of the positive effects of meditation. Gray matter also increased in four other brain regions (though not in the insula, a region that has shown changes in other meditation studies) in the meditation group. Responses to the questionnaire indicated improvements in three of the five aspects of mindfulness in the meditators, but not in the control group. The researchers concluded that these findings may represent an underlying brain mechanism associated with mindfulness-based improvements in mental health.

depression. Researchers also revealed that the studies varied considerably in the severity of the depression and nature of the yoga intervention delivered, and often omitted crucial methodological details.

As a consequence, the literature precludes strong conclusions regarding yoga's potential effectiveness for depression. Moreover, it remains unclear if any beneficial effects of yoga on depression, anxiety, or other psychological difficulties are attributable to yoga per se or to the relaxation or exercise associated with it.

Creative arts therapies. Creative arts therapies encompass a plethora of CAM treatments and are used in various guises to enhance mental health and to improve creativity, productivity, and interpersonal relations. Such therapies include those of art, music, dance, and poetry.

A 1997 review showed that most of the research on the effects of creative arts therapies on mental disorders has been limited in quality and quantity, and few studies have controlled for placebo effects or the nonspecific effects of attention from mental health professionals. Moreover, most investigations of creative arts therapies demonstrate short-term elevating effects on mood rather than improvements in the core features of mental disorders such as schizophrenia, autism, or major depression.

Of all creative arts therapies, music therapy has been perhaps the most extensively investigated. A 2006 review of three studies of music therapy for autism spectrum disorders yielded mixed results. They found positive effects of music therapy on the communicative and gestural deficits of autism, but no significant effects on its behavioral deficits. Still, the small sample sizes (the total number of participants across all three investigations was only twenty-four) and the paucity of long-term follow-up studies make it impossible to draw clear, strong inferences. A 2008 review of five studies of music therapy on depression revealed low rates of dropout and positive results in four of the studies. Nevertheless, as the study's authors noted, the substantial variations in the populations studied, the nature of the interventions, and the outcome measures administered again render any conclusions tentative.

CONCLUSIONS

Survey data demonstrate that large percentages, and perhaps majorities, of people with mental health

substantially influenced Western forms of yoga, comprises postures (such as bending and balancing the body), breathing exercises, and meditation. A 2005 review of five randomized-controlled trials concluded that yoga shows some promise as an intervention for problems, including mood and anxiety disorders, seek CAM therapies. These findings are troubling, given that most CAM therapies have been insufficiently investigated for such problems. However, preliminary evidence suggests that certain CAM therapies, including some herbal remedies (such as St. John's wort and kava), meditation, yoga, and music therapy, hold promise for certain psychological difficulties. Still, even these interventions must be regarded as only promising, and all require additional research before they can be regarded as empirically supported and, in the case of herbal remedies, safe for widespread public consumption.

A variety of other widely used CAM methods, including homeopathy, chiropractic, energy therapies, chelation therapy, and craniosacral therapy, are not empirically supported for mental health problems. Therefore, they should not be used in lieu of treatments of established effectiveness.

Mental health consumers should be aware that a host of factors may contribute to erroneous beliefs in the effectiveness of certain CAM treatments for psychological problems. In particular, many emotional difficulties, such as depression, panic disorder, and sleep, sexual, and eating disorders, often wax and wane in severity over relatively short time periods. As a consequence, persons with mental health problems may mistakenly attribute naturally occurring improvement in their symptoms to CAM interventions. In addition, the placebo effect can generate improvement that is independent of the ingredients of the CAM treatments themselves. For these and other reasons, one should rely on controlled studies, rather than subjective judgments or anecdotes, to ascertain whether these treatments are effective.

Scott Lilienfeld and Andrea Bozja

FURTHER READING

Hughes, Brian M. "How Should Clinical Psychologists Approach Complementary and Alternative Medicine? Empirical, Epistemological, and Ethical Considerations." *Clinical Psychology Review* 28 (2008): 657-675. A critical review of how clinical psychologists should evaluate CAM practices, including ethical, empirical, and epistemological perspectives on CAM.

Kessler, Ronald C., et al. "The Use of Complementary and Alternative Therapies to Treat Anxiety and Depression in the United States." *American Journal of Psychiatry* 158 (2001): 289-294. A comprehensive survey of CAM treatments for anxiety and depression, including data on how many participants used CAM treatments in lieu of conventional therapies and the perceived helpfulness of these treatments.

Sarris, Jerome. "Kava and St. John's Wort: Current Evidence for Use in Mood and Anxiety Disorders." *Journal of Alternative and Complementary Medicine* 15 (2009): 827-836. A helpful summary of research on the efficacy of kava and St. John's wort on anxiety and depression, respectively.

See also: Alzheimer's disease and non-Alzheimer's dementia; Anxiety and panic attacks; Art therapy; Autism spectrum disorder; Bipolar disorder; Color therapy; Compulsive overeating; Dance movement therapy; Depression, mild to moderate; Eating disorders; Humor and healing; Hypnotherapy; Memory and mental function impairment; Music therapy; Obsessive-compulsive disorder (OCD); Schizophrenia; Seasonal affective disorder; Tricyclic antidepressants.

Meridians

CATEGORY: Therapies and techniques

RELATED TERMS: Acupoints, acupressure vessels, acupuncture points, energy channels, *jing luo*

DEFINITION: Invisible pathways that circulate energy and maintain balance and harmony throughout the body.

PRINCIPAL PROPOSED USES: Acupressure, acupuncture, massage

OTHER PROPOSED USES: Jin Shin Jyutsu, meridian tapping techniques, moxibustion, plum blossom therapy, qigong, reflexology, Reiki, shiatsu, therapeutic touch, tuina

OVERVIEW

According to traditional Chinese medicine, the meridian system is the energy system of the body and is essential for maintaining good health and harmony. Each of the twelve main meridians, or pathways, relates to a yin, or solid organ (heart, lungs, liver, spleen, kidneys, pericardium), or to a yang, or hollow organ (small intestine, large intestine, gallbladder, stomach, urinary bladder, triple heater). Meridian pathways transport vital energy (*qi*) throughout the body. These high-energy areas act as guides in pressure-point therapies such as acupuncture to help diagnose and treat illnesses.

MECHANISM OF ACTION

Meridians are said to distribute vital life energy and to unify, link, and regulate all areas and activities of the body. Each meridian is associated with a unique set of disease symptoms. Pain occurs when the flow of energy along the meridian pathway is disrupted. Energy access points, known as acupoints or acupuncture points, are functional sites located on the surface of the skin along the meridian pathways. Stimulation at the appropriate site helps to restore the flow of energy, eliminate blockages, and promote healing at the affected area.

USES AND APPLICATIONS

Meridians are used in many forms of pressure-point therapies to help heal, maintain harmony, and prevent imbalances. Meridians are most often used in acupuncture, acupressure, and massage techniques.

SCIENTIFIC EVIDENCE

Although the use of meridians in ancient Chinese healing has existed for centuries, the concept remains controversial. The scientific basis for meridians is unknown. Most evidence supporting meridians is anecdotal because of a lack of scientific validation by Western standards. Regardless, energy-based techniques have gained widespread interest and acceptance.

Researchers have been unable to find an anatomical structure corresponding to the meridian. Some studies have linked meridians to neurovascular bundles, trigger points, and connective tissue spaces. Other studies suggest that meridians run along a fluid pathway and are associated with areas of lower electrical resistance and greater conductivity on the body. Results of these multiple studies were limited by inadequate research design, nonstandardized acupoint locations, small sample sizes, and a lack of rigorous statistical analysis. Although these studies provide possible insight into the meridian system, the results remain inconclusive.

Because of the elusive nature of meridians and acupoints, it is difficult to design an appropriate placebo control group and proper double-blind procedures. More rigorous research is needed to quantify the importance of the meridian healing network as a beneficial form of medical intervention.

CHOOSING A PRACTITIONER

Persons interested in meridian-based therapies should choose a qualified, trained practitioner.

Rose Ciulla-Bohling, Ph.D.

FURTHER READING

Filshie, Jacqueline, and Adrian White, eds. *Medical Acupuncture: A Western Scientific Approach.* New York: Churchill Livingstone/Elsevier, 2006.

Freeman, Lyn. *Mosby's Complementary and Alternative Medicine: A Research-Based Approach.* 3d ed. St. Louis, Mo.: Mosby/Elsevier, 2009.

Kohn, Livia. *Health and Long Life: The Chinese Way.* Cambridge, Mass.: Three Pines Press, 2005.

Koopsen, Cyndie, and Caroline Young. *Integrative Health: A Holistic Approach for Health Professionals.* Sudbury, Mass.: Jones and Bartlett, 2009.

See also: Acupressure; Acupuncture; Integrative medicine; Qigong; Reflexology; Reiki; Shiatsu; Therapeutic touch; Traditional healing.

Mesoglycan

CATEGORY: Herbs and supplements

RELATED TERMS: Aortic GAGs, aortic glycosaminoglycans, chondroitin polysulphate, chondroitin sulfate A, glycosaminoglycans, mucopolysaccharide

DEFINITION: Natural substance used as a dietary supplement for specific health benefits.

PRINCIPAL PROPOSED USES: Atherosclerosis, intermittent claudication, varicose veins

OTHER PROPOSED USES: Hemorrhoids, high cholesterol, kidney stones, osteoarthritis, phlebitis

OVERVIEW

Mesoglycan is a type of substance found in many tissues in the body, including the joints, the intestines, and the lining of blood vessels. Chemically, mesoglycan is related to the blood-thinning drug heparin and the supplement chondroitin. Unlike chondroitin, mesoglycan is primarily used to treat diseases of blood vessels. Preliminary evidence suggests that mesoglycan may be helpful for atherosclerosis, varicose veins, hemorrhoids, and phlebitis. (One should not self-treat phlebitis. It is a potentially deadly disease.)

SOURCES

Mesoglycan is not an essential nutrient because the body usually manufactures it from scratch. For supplement purposes, mesoglycan is commercially extracted from the intestines of pigs. Similar substances can be produced from cartilage, bone, and the lining of large blood vessels and are often used interchangeably.

THERAPEUTIC DOSAGES

The usual dosage of mesoglycan is 100 milligrams (mg) daily.

THERAPEUTIC USES

Most proposed uses of mesoglycan involve diseases of blood vessels. For example, evidence suggests that mesoglycan may slow the development of hardening of the arteries, perhaps by lowering cholesterol levels, thinning the blood, or through other effects.

People with severe hardening of the arteries sometimes develop blockage in the arteries of the legs, a condition called intermittent claudication. This condition limits the ability to walk by causing intense, cramping pain after walking a relatively short distance. There is some evidence that mesoglycan may help.

The conditions just discussed involve arteries. Mesoglycan may also be useful for various diseases of the veins, including varicose veins/venous insufficiency, hemorrhoids, and phlebitis.

One study suggests that a substance related to mesoglycan, hyaluronic acid, might be helpful for asthma when taken by inhalation. Preliminary evidence suggests mesoglycan may also be useful in treating kidney stones.

The substance chondroitin is used for the treatment of osteoarthritis. Based on the chemical similarities between chondroitin and mesoglycan, researchers conducted a large (almost four-hundred-participant) five-year, double-blind, placebo-controlled study of injected mesoglycan for slowing the progression of osteoarthritis. However, no benefits were seen.

SCIENTIFIC EVIDENCE

Intermittent claudication. A twenty-week, double-blind, placebo-controlled trial that enrolled 242 people evaluated the effects of mesoglycan (100 mg a

day orally, after a short course of injected treatment) for treating intermittent claudication. Significantly more participants in the mesoglycan group responded to treatment (defined as a greater than 50 percent improvement in walking distance) than in the placebo group.

Atherosclerosis in general. In a double-blind comparative study, men with atherosclerosis in the arteries of the heart (coronary artery disease) were given either 200 mg daily of mesoglycan or no extra treatment. After eighteen months, the layering of the vessel lining was 7.5 times greater in the untreated group than in the mesoglycan group, a significant difference. However, because this was not a double-blind, placebo-controlled trial, the results cannot be taken as truly reliable. Additional preliminary evidence that mesoglycan might help atherosclerosis comes from other studies in animals and humans.

It is not known for certain how mesoglycan might help atherosclerosis. There is some evidence that it can reduce cholesterol levels and also thin the blood.

Vein diseases. Several studies suggest that mesoglycan may be helpful in the treatment of vein problems, such as varicose veins/venous insufficiency, phlebitis, and hemorrhoids. For example, in a double-blind, placebo-controlled trial, 183 persons with leg ulcers caused by poor vein function were treated with either placebo or mesoglycan (first by injection and then orally) for twenty-four weeks. The results of this double-blind study suggest that mesoglycan significantly improved the rate at which the leg ulcers healed.

SAFETY ISSUES

Mesoglycan is essentially ground pig intestines and is believed to be safe, even if taken in large quantities. However, because mesoglycan appears to decrease blood clotting, it should not be combined with prescription blood thinners such as warfarin (Coumadin), clopidogrel (Plavix), ticlopidine (Ticlid), pentoxifylline (Trental), or heparin, or with drugs in the aspirin family. Maximum safe dosages for young children, pregnant or nursing women, or those with severe liver or kidney disease have not been determined.

EBSCO CAM Review Board

FURTHER READING

Arosio, E., et al. "A Placebo-Controlled, Double-Blind Study of Mesoglycan in the Treatment of Chronic Venous Ulcers." *European Journal of Vascular and En-*

dovascular Surgery 22 (2001): 365-372.

Nenci, G. G., et al. "Treatment of Intermittent Claudication with Mesoglycan." *Thrombosis and Haemostasis* 86 (2001): 1181-1187.

Petrigni, G., and L. Allegra. "Aerosolised Hyaluronic Acid Prevents Exercise-Induced Bronchoconstriction, Suggesting Novel Hypotheses on the Correction of Matrix Defects in Asthma." *Pulmonary Pharmacology and Therapeutics* 19, no. 3 (2006): 166-171.

See also: Asthma; Atherosclerosis and heart disease prevention; Cholesterol, high; Chondroitin; Heart attack; Heparin; Intermittent claudication; Phlebitis and deep vein thrombosis; Varicose veins; Venous insufficiency: Homeopathic remedies.

Metabolic syndrome

CATEGORY: Condition

RELATED TERM: Syndrome X

DEFINITION: Treatment of the development of several cardiovascular disease risk factors in a single person.

PRINCIPAL PROPOSED NATURAL TREATMENTS: All treatments related to diabetes, high cholesterol, high triglycerides, hypertension, and weight loss

OTHER PROPOSED NATURAL TREATMENTS: Chromium, conjugated linoleic acids, garlic, ginger, nopal cactus, vitamin E

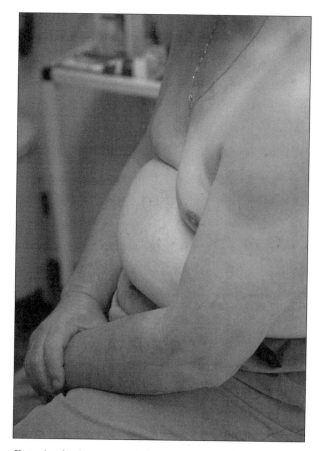

Excessive fat tissue around the abdomen is a risk factor for metabolic syndrome. (Philippe Garo/Photo Researchers, Inc.)

INTRODUCTION

Metabolic syndrome, also called syndrome X, is a poorly understood condition in which several cardiovascular disease risk factors develop in a single person. These risk factors include abdominal obesity, the excessive fat tissue in and around the abdomen. They also include an unhealthy cholesterol profile, that is, some elements of the following: low HDL, or good, cholesterol; high LDL, or bad, cholesterol; and high triglycerides. Other risk factors are high blood pressure, insulin resistance (either type 2 diabetes or prediabetes), a prothrombotic state (increased risk of blood clots), and a proinflammatory state (elevated levels of C-reactive protein, associated with increased rate of hardening of the arteries). All of these risk factors are separately associated with an increased rate of atherosclerosis, leading to angina, heart attacks, strokes, intermittent claudication, and related conditions. When they occur together, the risk is even higher.

Metabolic syndrome has become increasingly common in the United States; according to the American Heart Association, as many as 50 million Americans may have it. Although the causes of the syndrome are not clear, researchers believe that abdominal obesity plays a primary role. Abdominal obesity leads directly to high blood pressure. It also appears to cause insulin resistance, a condition in which the body does not respond properly to its own insulin. The first signs of insulin resistance include high levels of insulin in the body, impaired glucose tolerance, and disturbances in cholesterol profile. In time, frank diabetes of the type 2 variety can develop. Other elements of the metabolic syndrome may follow.

Defining Factors for Metabolic Syndrome

A person with three or more of the following factors is considered to have metabolic syndrome:

- Large waist measurement: 35 inches or more for women, 40 inches or more for men; this measurement also determines whether a person needs to lose weight
- Triglyceride level of 150 milligrams per deciliter (mg/dl) or higher
- HDL cholesterol of less than 50 mg/dl in women and of less than 40 mg/dl in men
- Blood pressure of 130/85 millimeters of mercury (mmHg) or higher (either number counts as a raised blood pressure)
- Fasting blood sugar of 100 mg/dl or higher

Exercise and weight loss can reduce insulin resistance; therefore, these two lifestyle treatments are the most important for addressing metabolic syndrome. Evidence does suggest that deliberate weight loss through dietary change, accompanied by increased levels of exercise, can help control metabolic syndrome. While any diet that effectively reduces weight would presumably work, there is some evidence that a Mediterranean-style diet, one that is low in refined carbohydrates, high in fiber, moderately high in vegetable proteins, and high in unsaturated fats, is particularly well suited for persons with this condition. Beyond diet, the surgical treatment for obesity (such as bypass surgery) has also been shown to effectively treat metabolic syndrome.

It has also been suggested that deficiency of the mineral chromium may play a role in the development of metabolic syndrome, and that supplementation may help. However, a study of sixty-three obese, nondiabetic adults with metabolic syndrome found that sixteen weeks of supplementation with 1,000 mg of chromium picolinate did not improve their insulin sensitivity, glucose metabolism, body weight, serum lipids, or inflammatory state. One preliminary placebo-controlled trial suggests that a cinnamon extract may modestly lower blood sugar and blood pressure and raise lean body weight in persons with metabolic syndrome. However, the reliability of these results must be questioned because, even at much higher doses, cinnamon has not consistently been shown to lower blood sugar in diabetics, and there is no other evidence of its favorable effects in high blood pressure.

Another preliminary placebo-controlled study tested a proprietary extract of freshwater algae in sixty people with the syndrome and found some evidence of overall benefit. In addition, a proprietary formulation of nopal cactus tested on fifty-nine overweight women showed some benefit for their metabolic syndrome. Another study failed to find that the supplement conjugated linoleic acid was helpful for metabolic syndrome.

EBSCO CAM Review Board

FURTHER READING

Bo, S., et al. "Effectiveness of a Lifestyle Intervention on Metabolic Syndrome." *Journal of General Internal Medicine* 22 (2007): 1695-1703.

Giugliano, D., A. Ceriello, and K. Esposito. "Are There Specific Treatments for the Metabolic Syndrome?" *American Journal of Clinical Nutrition* 87 (2008): 8-11.

Iqbal, N., et al. "Chromium Picolinate Does Not Improve Key Features of Metabolic Syndrome in Obese Nondiabetic Adults." *Metabolic Syndrome and Related Disorders* 7 (2009): 143-150.

Ziegenfuss, T. N., et al. "Effects of a Water-Soluble Cinnamon Extract on Body Composition and Features of the Metabolic Syndrome in Pre-diabetic Men and Women." *Journal of the International Society of Sports Nutrition* 3 (2006): 45-53.

See also: Cholesterol, high; Hypertension; Triglycerides, high.

Metamorphic technique

CATEGORY: Therapies and techniques

RELATED TERMS: Life force energy, reflex points, reflexology

DEFINITION: A gentle touch technique applied to the feet, hands, and head.

PRINCIPAL PROPOSED USES: General health, personal growth and development, relaxation, self-awareness, self-healing, stress reduction

OTHER PROPOSED USE: Behavior

OVERVIEW

The metamorphic technique was developed in the 1960s by Robert St. John, a British naturopath and reflexologist, to promote self-healing and personal development. The Metamorphic Association was founded in the late 1970s by one of his students, Gaston Saint-Pierre. The metamorphic technique is based on reflexology and uses gentle massage of the feet, hands, and head to help the body's vital energy or life force, called qi, to flow freely, enabling personal metamorphosis. The metamorphic technique assumes that all physical, mental, and emotional behaviors relate to energy pathways established during experiences in the womb, from conception to birth; it does not focus on specific symptoms or problems.

MECHANISM OF ACTION

The metamorphic technique is based on applying a gentle pressure on points known as spinal reflex points in the feet, hands, and head to release "stuck" energy created from earlier experiences. Manipulation of these areas triggers pattern shifts, freeing vital life energy and allowing a person to overcome limitations such as negative attitudes, emotions, and behaviors, and illnesses. This technique uses a person's inner intelligence to guide the life force toward healing, transformation, and realizing her or his full potential.

USES AND APPLICATIONS

The metamorphic technique promotes stress reduction, relaxation, well-being, and good health. It is a tool for personal growth and development; it enables positive change through self-awareness and self-transformation. The metamorphic technique can be used alone or with conventional or alternative and complementary therapies.

SCIENTIFIC EVIDENCE

Although many ancient healing therapies are guided by the life force energy, the concept remains controversial. Most evidence supporting the metamorphic technique is anecdotal.

The metamorphic technique's effectiveness in promoting relaxation and self-healing has not been validated by Western standards through randomized, double-blind, placebo-controlled clinical trials.

Studying the effectiveness of this gentle touch therapy is difficult because of the elusive nature of the life force and energy pathways. Problems arise in designing an appropriate placebo control group and proper double-blind procedures to ensure that both patient and practitioner are "blinded" during treatment.

Regardless, the metamorphic technique has gained widespread interest as a complementary treatment option because it pleasantly induces relaxation. However, more rigorous research is needed to properly assess its clinical effectiveness.

CHOOSING A PRACTITIONER

Although the metamorphic technique is easily learned, it is best if one chooses an experienced practitioner.

SAFETY ISSUES

The metamorphic technique is considered gentle, noninvasive, and safe for everyone.

Rose Ciulla-Bohling, Ph.D.

FURTHER READING

"About the Metamorphic Technique." Available at http://www.gastonsaintpierre.org.uk/metatech.htm.

Knight, Katherine L. "Metamorphic Technique: Tools for Inner Change." *Positive Health* 78 (2002): 51-53. Also available at http://www.positivehealth.com/issue/issue-78-july-2002.

So, P. S., Y. Jiang, and Y. Qin. "Touch Therapies for Pain Relief in Adults." *Cochrane Database of Systematic Reviews* (2008): CD006535. Available through EBSCO DynaMed Systematic Literature Surveillance at http://www.ebscohost.com/dynamed.

Saint-Pierre, Gaston. *The Universal Principles and the Metamorphic Technique: The Keys to Healing and Enlightenment.* New York: O Books, 2004.

Metamorphic Association. "What Is the Metamorphic Technique?" Available online at http://www.metamorphicassociation.org/faq.html.

See also: Acupressure; Biodynamic massage; Energy medicine; Manipulative and body-based practices; Massage therapy; Pain management; Progressive muscle relaxation; Qigong; Reflexology; Relaxation therapies; Shiatsu; Stress; Therapeutic touch.

Methotrexate

RELATED TERMS: Amethopterin, MTX

CATEGORY: Drug interactions

DEFINITION: Used in cancer chemotherapy and for treating inflammatory diseases such as rheumatoid arthritis and psoriasis.

INTERACTIONS: Citrate, dong quai, folate, ipriflavone, potassium citrate, St. John's wort, white willow

TRADE NAMES: Folex PFS, Immunex, Rheumatrex

POTASSIUM CITRATE

Effect: Possible Harmful Interaction

Potassium citrate and other forms of citrate (such as calcium citrate and magnesium citrate) may be used to prevent kidney stones. These agents work by making the urine less acidic. This effect on the urine may lead to decreased blood levels and therapeutic effects of methotrexate. It may be advisable to avoid these citrate compounds during methotrexate therapy except under medical supervision.

ST. JOHN'S WORT, DONG QUAI

Effect: Possible Harmful Interaction

St. John's wort (*Hypericum perforatum*) is used primarily to treat mild to moderate depression. The herb dong quai (*Angelica sinensis*) is often recommended for menstrual disorders such as dysmenorrhea, premenstrual syndrome (PMS), and irregular menstruation. Methotrexate has been reported to cause increased sensitivity to the sun, amplifying the risk of sunburn or skin rash. Because St. John's wort and dong quai may also cause this problem, taking these herbal supplements during methotrexate therapy might add to this risk. It may be a good idea to use sunscreen or to wear protective clothing during sun exposure if taking one of these herbs while using methotrexate.

WHITE WILLOW

Effect: Possible Harmful Interaction

The herb white willow (*Salix alba*), also known as willow bark, is used to treat pain and fever. White willow contains a substance that is converted by the body into a salicylate similar to aspirin. Case reports suggest that salicylates can increase methotrexate blood levels and toxicity. For this reason, one should avoid combining white willow with methotrexate.

IPRIFLAVONE

Effect: Possible Harmful Interaction

The supplement ipriflavone is used to treat osteoporosis. A three-year double-blind trial of almost five hundred women, as well as a small study, found worrisome evidence that ipriflavone can reduce white blood cell count in some people. For this reason, anyone taking medications that suppress the immune system should avoid taking ipriflavone.

CITRATE

Effect: Possible Harmful Interaction

Potassium citrate, sodium citrate, and potassium-magnesium citrate are sometimes used to prevent kidney stones. These supplements reduce urinary acidity and can therefore lead to decreased blood levels and effectiveness of methotrexate.

FOLATE

Effect: Supplementation Possibly Helpful

Folate (also known as folic acid) is a B vitamin that plays an important role in many vital aspects of health, including preventing neural tube birth defects and possibly reducing the risk of heart disease. Because inadequate intake of folate is widespread, if one is taking any medication that depletes or impairs folate even slightly, one may need supplementation.

Methotrexate is called a folate antagonist because it prevents the body from converting folate to its active form. In fact, this inactivation of folate plays a role in methotrexate's therapeutic effects. This leads to an interesting Catch-22: Methotrexate use can lead to folate deficiency, but taking extra folate could theoretically prevent methotrexate from working properly. However, evidence suggests that people who take methotrexate for rheumatoid arthritis, juvenile rheumatoid arthritis, or psoriasis can safely use folate supplements. Not only does the methotrexate continue to work properly, but also its usual side effects may decrease.

For example, in a forty-eight-week double-blind, placebo-controlled trial of 434 persons with active rheumatoid arthritis, use of folate helped prevent liver inflammation caused by methotrexate. Other side effects did not improve. A slightly higher dose of methotrexate was needed to reach the same level of benefit as taking methotrexate alone, but researchers felt this was worth it.

In the study just described, folate supplements did not help reduce the incidence of mouth sores and nausea. However, in other studies, folate supplements did reduce these side effects, both in persons receiving methotrexate for rheumatoid arthritis and in those with psoriasis. In addition, two studies of persons with rheumatoid arthritis found that use of folate supplements corrected the methotrexate-induced rise in homocysteine without affecting disease control.

Folate supplements have been found safe only as supportive treatment in the specific conditions noted above. It is not known, for example, whether folate supplements are safe for use by persons taking methotrexate for cancer treatment.

EBSCO CAM Review Board

FURTHER READING

Alexandersen, P., et al. "Ipriflavone in the Treatment of Postmenopausal Osteoporosis." *Journal of the American Medical Association* 285 (2001): 1482-1488.

Griffith, S. M., et al. "Do Patients with Rheumatoid Arthritis Established on Methotrexate and Folic Acid 5 Mg Daily Need to Continue Folic Acid Supplements Long Term?" *Rheumatology* 39 (2000): 1102-1109.

Hunt. P. G., et al. "The Effects of Daily Intake of Folic Acid on the Efficacy of Methotrexate Therapy in Children with Juvenile Rheumatoid Arthritis." *Journal of Rheumatology* 24 (1997): 2230-2232.

Van Ede, A. E., et al. "Effect of Folic or Folinic Acid Supplementation on the Toxicity and Efficacy of Methotrexate in Rheumatoid Arthritis." *Arthritis and Rheumatology* 44 (2001): 1515-1524.

_____. "Homocysteine and Folate Status in Methotrexate-Treated Patients with Rheumatoid Arthritis." *Rheumatology* 41, no. 6 (2002): 658-665.

See also: Citrate; Dong quai; Folate; Food and Drug Administration; Ipriflavone; Potassium citrate; St. John's wort; Supplements: Introduction; White Willow.

Methoxyisoflavone

CATEGORY: Functional foods
RELATED TERM: 5-methyl-7-methoxyisoflavone
DEFINITION: Natural product used as a dietary supplement for specific health benefits.

PRINCIPAL PROPOSED USE: Sports and fitness enhancement

OVERVIEW

Isoflavones are naturally occurring, hormonally active substances found in soy and other foods. Chemical modifications of isoflavones have been studied as possible alternative treatments for various conditions. One of these modifications, ipriflavone, was developed primarily for treating osteoporosis. Methoxyisoflavone is a chemical derivative of ipriflavone, but it is marketed as a bodybuilding acquired immunodeficiency syndrome

SOURCES

Methoxyisoflavone is not a nutrient and is not supplied to any meaningful extent in food. However, it is possible that, once in the body, natural isoflavones, such as daidzein, may be converted into methoxyisoflavone.

THERAPEUTIC DOSAGES

A typical recommended dose of methoxyisoflavone is 200 to 400 milligrams (mg) taken twice daily.

THERAPEUTIC USES

Methoxyisoflavone is marketed as an anabolic steroid, said to increase muscle mass without causing androgenic (testosterone-like) effects. However, there is no meaningful evidence that it actually works.

The use of methoxyisoflavone in the United States began with two U.S. patents established in the late 1970s. The patent applications report a few research studies performed by the Hungarian pharmaceutical company Chinoin. None of these studies were published in peer-reviewed journals; furthermore, even as described, this research is altogether inadequate to demonstrate effectiveness, consisting as it does only of animal studies and exceedingly preliminary studies on humans. Proof of effectiveness is not required to establish a patent.

One placebo-controlled human trial on methoxyisoflavone was published in abstract form in 2001. Apparently, this study found that athletes who took 800 mg per day of methoxyisoflavone for eight weeks experienced a significantly greater increase in muscle mass than those who took placebo. However, despite claims made by methoxyisoflavone retailers and proponents, this study was not published in a prestigious journal. Rather, it appeared in what is a called a "supplement" published in association with a fairly prestigious journal. Supplements are special editions printed by a journal for extra income; they explicitly lack the supervision, approval, review, or imprimatur of the journal itself. For this reason, all studies published in journal supplements must be carefully considered. This is particularly so in cases such as that of methoxyisoflavone, in which only an abstract of the study was published, rather than the full text of the study itself.

Another oft-repeated claim regarding methoxyisoflavone is that it is widely utilized in the livestock industry to enhance lean mass. However, if livestock breeders are using methoxyisoflavone, they are keeping that use quiet: A Web search for "methoxyflavone" and "livestock" turned up numerous sites that sell supplements to humans (and make this claim to support the sales of their product) but not a single site by or for livestock breeders. There is no meaningful evidence to indicate that methoxyisoflavone is useful as a sports supplement for performance enhancement.

SAFETY ISSUES

Methoxyflavone has not undergone comprehensive safety testing. Those who take it do so at their own risk.

EBSCO CAM Review Board

FURTHER READING

American Dietetic Association et al. "American College of Sports Medicine Position Stand: Nutrition and Athletic Performance." *Medicine and Science in Sports and Exercise* 41 (2009): 709-731.

Incledon, T., D. van Gammeren, and J. Antonio. "The Effects of 5-Methyl-7-Methoxyisoflavone on Body Composition and Performance in College-Aged Men." *Medicine and Science in Sports and Exercise* 33, suppl. 5 (2001): S338.

Manore, M., et al. "BJSM Reviews: A-Z of Nutritional Supplements: Dietary Supplements, Sports Nutrition Foods, and Ergogenic Aids for Health and Performance." *British Journal of Sports Medicine* 45 (2011): 73-74.

See also: Sports and fitness support: Enhancing performance.

Methyldopa

CATEGORY: Drug interactions
DEFINITION: A medication sometimes used to control hypertension.
INTERACTIONS: Coenzyme Q_{10}, iron
TRADE NAME: Aldomet

COENZYME Q_{10} (CoQ$_{10}$)

Effect: Supplementation Possibly Helpful

There is some evidence that methyldopa might impair the body's ability to manufacture the substance CoQ_{10}. Taking CoQ_{10} supplements might make sense as a general precaution, but no specific benefit has been established.

IRON

Effect: Take at a Different Time of Day

Iron supplements can interfere with the absorption of methyldopa, so persons should be sure not to take iron during the two hours before or after using methyldopa.

EBSCO CAM Review Board

FURTHER READING

Campbell, N. R., and B. B. Hasinoff. "Iron Supplements: A Common Cause of Drug Interactions." *British Journal of Clinical Pharmacology* 31 (1991): 251-255.

_____, V. Paddock, and R. Sundaram. "Alteration of Methyldopa Absorption, Metabolism, and Blood Pressure Control Caused by Ferrous Sulfate and Gluconate." *Clinical Pharmacology and Therapeutics* 43 (1988): 381-386.

See also: Coenzyme Q_{10}; Food and Drug Administration; Hypertension; Iron; Supplements: Introduction.

Methyl sulfonyl methane

CATEGORY: Herbs and supplements
RELATED TERM: Dimethyl sulfone
DEFINITION: Natural substance used to treat specific health conditions.
PRINCIPAL PROPOSED USE: Osteoarthritis
OTHER PROPOSED USES: Improving growth of nails and hair, interstitial cystitis, rheumatoid arthritis, rosacea, snoring, sports injuries

OVERVIEW

Methyl sulfonyl methane (MSM) is a sulfur-containing compound normally found in many foods. It is chemically related to DMSO (dimethyl sulfoxide), a popular (although unproven) treatment for arthritis. When DMSO is applied on the skin or taken orally, about 15 percent of it breaks down in the body to form MSM.

Some researchers have suggested that the resulting MSM could be responsible for the benefits attributed to DMSO. If so, MSM might be preferable as a treatment, because it does not cause some of the unpleasant side effects associated with DMSO treatment, such as body odor and bad breath. In addition, as a natural substance found in food, MSM would be expected to have a good safety profile. However, there is no more than preliminary evidence that MSM is useful for any medical condition.

REQUIREMENTS AND SOURCES

There is no dietary requirement for MSM. However, it occurs naturally in cow's milk, meat, seafood, vegetables, fruits, and even coffee, tea, and chocolate. MSM supplements are sold in health food stores and some pharmacies. Although creams and lotions containing MSM are also available, it is difficult to see the purpose of these topical products because MSM, unlike DMSO, is not absorbed through the skin.

MSM supplies sulfur. Some advertisements for MSM claim that sulfur deficiency is widespread and that for this reason alone MSM will improve the health of almost everybody who takes it. However, there are numerous other dietary sources of sulfur, including, most prominently, many forms of ordinary protein.

THERAPEUTIC DOSAGES

Dosages of oral MSM used for therapeutic purposes range from 1,500 to 10,000 milligrams (mg) daily, usually divided up into three daily doses.

THERAPEUTIC USES

Two small double-blind, placebo-controlled studies indicate that MSM may be helpful for osteoarthritis. In one small, placebo-controlled trial, the topical application of methylsulfonylmethane with silymarin (milk thistle) for one month appeared to be effective in the treatment of forty-six subjects with the skin condition rosacea.

MSM for Arthritis Pain: A Study

Many drugs have arisen in an attempt to alleviate pain and disability, including acetaminophen; nonsteroidal anti-inflammatory drugs (NSAIDs) such as cyclooxygenase-2 (COX-2) inhibitors; and others. Knee osteoarthritis (OA) patients have also turned to surgical interventions and complementary and alternative medicine as these have some ameliorating effects as well. Due to recent safety concerns regarding COX-2 selective drugs, patients have turned to over-the-counter (OTC) dietary supplements that claim to be safer in the long-term treatment of OA. These include glucosamine and chondroitin sulfate, both of which have been examined in previous studies. Methylsulfonylmethane (MSM) is another OTC drug that is often sold in combination with glucosamine and chondroitin sulfate. MSM can be bought at health food stores and on the Internet in products such as creams and capsules.

MSM is an organosulfur molecule that can be synthesized commercially from dimethylsulfoxide (DMSO). MSM is also naturally present in the human body, because as it is metabolized from ingested DMSO. Many properties have been attributed to MSM, some of which include chemopreventive properties, anti-inflammatory activities, anti-atherosclerotic action, prostacyclin (PGI2) synthesis inhibition, and free radical scavenging activity. Nevertheless, conclusive data on the biochemical effects and mechanism of action of MSM are minimal. Even less is known about how these effects may benefit patients with OA of the knee.

Source: Eytan M. Debbi et al. "Efficacy of Methylsulfonylmethane Supplementation on Osteoarthritis of the Knee." *BMC Complementary and Alternative Medicine* 11 (2011). This open-access article is available at http://www.biomedcentral.com/1472-6882/11/50.

Small unpublished trials have been used to claim that MSM is effective for the treatment of snoring, aiding the growth of nails and hair, and assisting in recovery from sports injuries. However, the design of each of these studies was substandard, and the results were not subjected to any proper statistical analysis; therefore, they cannot be taken as meaningful evidence of efficacy.

One study in mice found positive effects of MSM in the treatment of rheumatoid arthritis. Other animal studies hint that MSM might have cancer-preventive properties. Human studies on these potential uses of MSM have not been reported.

MSM has also been proposed as a treatment for interstitial cystitis, an inflammation in the wall of the bladder that causes frequent and painful urination. When prescribed for this condition, MSM is usually placed directly into the bladder, although oral use has also been suggested. However, no clinical studies on this use have been performed: The only evidence for this treatment comes from case studies and anecdotal reports. Since interstitial cystitis is known to respond very positively to placebos, these reports mean little. MSM has also been advocated for allergies (including drug allergies), scleroderma, excess stomach acid, and constipation, but there is no meaningful evidence whatsoever to support these proposed uses.

SCIENTIFIC EVIDENCE

In a double-blind, placebo-controlled study performed in India, 118 people with osteoarthritis of the knee were given one of the following four treatments: glucosamine (500 mg, three times daily), MSM (500 mg, three times daily), a combination of glucosamine and MSM, or a placebo. The study ran for twelve weeks. The results showed that both MSM and glucosamine improved arthritis symptoms compared with a placebo, and that the combination of MSM and glucosamine was more effective than either one alone. Benefits were also seen in a twelve-week double-blind, placebo-controlled trial of fifty people with osteoarthritis, utilizing MSM at a dose of 3 grams (g) twice daily.

However, in a comprehensive review of six studies involving 681 patients with osteoarthritis of the knee, researchers concluded that it is not possible to convincingly determine whether either DMSO or MSM is beneficial.

SAFETY ISSUES

MSM is a natural component of the foods people normally eat and is not believed to be toxic. A laboratory study examining doses up to 8 g per kilogram of body weight per day (about 250 times the highest dose normally used by humans) reported that no toxic effects were seen. Maximum safe doses for young children, pregnant or nursing women, and people with liver or kidney disease are not known. Possible drug interactions are also not known.

EBSCO CAM Review Board

FURTHER READING

Berardesca, E., et al. "Combined Effects of Silymarin and Methylsulfonylmethane in the Management of Rosacea: Clinical and Instrumental Evaluation." *Journal of Cosmetic Dermatology* 7 (2008): 8-14.

Brien, S., et al. "Systematic Review of the Nutritional Supplements Dimethyl Sulfoxide (DMSO) and Methylsulfonylmethane (MSM) in the Treatment of Osteoarthritis." *Osteoarthritis Cartilage* 16, no. 11 (2008): 1277-1288.

Kim, L. S., et al. "Efficacy of Methylsulfonylmethane (MSM) in Osteoarthritis Pain of the Knee." *Osteoarthritis Cartilage* 14, no. 3 (2006): 286-299.

Usha, P. R., and M. U. R. Naidu. "Randomised, Double-Blind, Parallel, Placebo-Controlled Study of Oral Glucosamine, Methylsulfonylmethane, and Their Combination in Osteoarthritis." *Clinical Drug Investigation* 24 (2004): 353-363.

See also: Herbal medicine; Milk thistle; Osteoarthritis.

Migraines

CATEGORY: Condition

DEFINITION: Treatment of a class of severe headaches that share characteristic symptoms, including visual disturbances.

PRINCIPAL PROPOSED NATURAL TREATMENTS: Butterbur, feverfew, 5-hydroxytryptophan, magnesium

OTHER PROPOSED NATURAL TREATMENTS: Acupuncture, biofeedback, chiropractic, coenzyme Q_{10}, fish oil, food allergen avoidance, lipoic acid, magnet therapy, massage, relaxation therapies, soy isoflavones (combined with black cohosh and dong quai), vitamin B_2 (riboflavin), yoga

INTRODUCTION

The term "migraine" refers to a class of headaches sharing certain characteristic symptoms. Headache pain usually occurs in the forehead or temples, often on one side only and typically accompanied by nausea and a preference for a darkened room. Headache attacks last for several hours, up to a day or more. They are usually separated by completely pain-free intervals. In some cases, headache pain is accompanied by a visual (or occasionally nonvisual) disturbance known as an aura. Migraines are classified as migraine with aura or migraine without aura.

Migraines can be set off by a variety of triggers, including fatigue, stress, hormonal changes, and foods such as alcoholic beverages, chocolate, peanuts, and avocados. When people with migraine headaches first consult a physician, they are generally advised to identify such triggers and to avoid them if possible. However, migraines quite frequently occur with no obvious avoidable triggering factor.

The underlying cause of migraine headaches has been a subject of continuing controversy for more than a century. Opinion has swung back and forth between two primary beliefs: that migraines are related to epileptic seizures and originate in the nervous tissue of the brain or that blood vessels in the skull cause headache pain when they dilate or contract

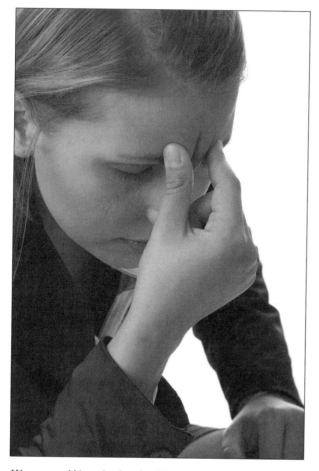

Woman rubbing forehead with migraine headache pain. (© Piotr Marcinkski/Dreamstime.com)

(vascular headaches). Most likely, several factors are involved, and more than one stimulus can trigger a migraine attack.

Conventional treatment of acute migraines has been revolutionized by drugs in the triptan family. These medications can completely abort a migraine headache in many persons. They work by imitating the action of serotonin on blood vessels, causing them to contract. However, although they are dramatically effective for the majority of people with migraines, a substantial minority do not respond, for reasons that are unclear.

People interested in prevention of migraines have a great variety of options, including ergot drugs, antidepressants, beta-blockers, calcium channel blockers, and antiseizure medications. Picking the best one is mostly a matter of trial and error. Most people can find some medication that will work.

Serious diseases may occasionally first present themselves as migraine-type headaches, so if a person suddenly starts having migraines without a previous history, or if the pattern of the migraines changes significantly, it is essential to seek medical evaluation.

PRINCIPAL PROPOSED NATURAL TREATMENTS

Several herbs and supplements have shown considerable promise for helping to prevent migraines.

Butterbur. Two double-blind, placebo-controlled studies suggest that an extract of the herb butterbur may be helpful for preventing migraines. Butterbur extract was tested as a migraine preventive in a double-blind, placebo-controlled study involving sixty men and women who experienced at least three migraines per month. After four weeks without any conventional medications, participants were randomly assigned to take either 50 milligrams (mg) of butterbur extract or placebo twice daily for three months. The results were positive: Both the number of migraine attacks and the total number of days of migraine pain were significantly reduced in the treatment group compared with the placebo group. Three of four persons taking butterbur reported improvement, compared to one of four in the placebo group. No significant side effects were noted.

In another double-blind, placebo-controlled study performed by different researchers, 202 people with migraine headaches received either 50 mg twice daily of butterbur extract, 75 mg twice daily, or placebo. In the three months of the study, the frequency of migraine attacks gradually decreased in all three groups. However, the group receiving the higher dose of butterbur extract showed significantly greater improvement than those in the placebo group. The lower dose of butterbur failed to prove significantly more effective than placebo.

Based on these two studies, it does appear that butterbur extract is helpful for preventing migraines, and that 75 mg twice daily is more effective than 50 mg twice daily. However, further research is necessary to establish this with certainty.

Feverfew. Five meaningful, double-blind, placebo-controlled studies have evaluated feverfew's effectiveness as a preventive treatment for migraines, but the results have been inconsistent. The best of the positive trials used a feverfew extract made by extracting the herb with liquid carbon dioxide. Two other trials that used whole feverfew leaf also found it effective; however, two studies that used feverfew extracts did not find benefit.

In a well-conducted, sixteen-week, double-blind, placebo-controlled study of 170 people with migraines, the use of a feverfew product made via liquid carbon dioxide extraction resulted in a significant decrease in headache frequency compared to the effect of the placebo treatment. In the treatment group, headache frequency decreased by 1.9 headaches per month, compared to a reduction of 1.3 headaches per month in the placebo group. The average number of headaches per month before treatment was 4.76. An earlier study using the same extract had failed to find benefit, but it primarily enrolled people who were less prone to migraines.

Two other studies used whole feverfew leaf and found benefit. The first followed fifty-nine people for eight months. For four months, one-half received a daily capsule of feverfew leaf and the other half received placebo. The groups were then switched and followed for an additional four months. Treatment with feverfew produced a 24 percent reduction in the number of migraines and a significant decrease in nausea and vomiting during the headaches. A subsequent double-blind study of fifty-seven people with migraines found that the use of feverfew leaf could decrease the severity of migraine headaches. This trial did not report whether there was any change in the frequency of migraines. Another study used an alcohol extract but failed to find benefit.

Magnesium. Magnesium is another natural treatment that has shown promise for the prevention of migraine headaches. A twelve-week double-blind study followed eighty-one people with recurrent migraines. One-half received 600 mg of magnesium daily (in the rather unusual form of trimagnesium dicitrate), and the other half received placebo. By the final three weeks of the study, the frequency of migraine attacks was reduced by 41.6 percent in the treated group, compared to 15.8 percent in the placebo group. The only side effects observed were diarrhea (18.6 percent) and digestive irritation (4.7 percent). Preliminary studies also suggest that magnesium may be helpful for migraines triggered by hormonal changes occurring with the menstrual cycle.

5-hydroxytryptophan. The body manufactures 5-hydroxytryptophan (5-HTP) on its way to making serotonin. When 5-HTP is taken as a supplement, the net result may be increased serotonin production. Because a number of drugs that affect serotonin are used to prevent migraine headaches, 5-HTP has been tried too. Some evidence suggests that it may work when taken at a dosage of 400 to 600 mg daily. Lower doses may not be effective.

In a six-month trial of 124 people, 5-HTP (600 mg daily) proved just as effective as the standard drug methysergide. The most dramatic benefit seen was a reduction in the intensity and duration of migraines. Because methysergide has been proven better than placebo for migraine headaches in earlier studies, the study results provide meaningful, although not airtight, evidence that 5-HTP is also effective.

Similarly good results were seen in another comparative study that used a different medication and 5-HTP (at a dose of 400 mg daily). However, in another study, 5-HTP (up to 300 mg daily) was less effective than the drug propranolol. Also, in a study involving children, 5-HTP failed to demonstrate benefit. Other studies that are sometimes quoted as evidence that 5-HTP is effective for migraines actually enrolled adults or children with many different types of headaches (including migraines).

Putting all this evidence together, it appears that 5-HTP can help people with frequent migraine headaches if taken in sufficient doses, but further research needs to be done. In particular, a large double-blind study is needed that compares 5-HTP with placebo over a period of several months.

Mitochondrial enhancers. Mitochondria are the energy-producing subunits of cells. Based on the highly speculative theory that mitochondrial dysfunction may play a role in migraines, three substances have been tried for migraine prevention: vitamin B_2 (riboflavin), coenzyme Q_{10} (CoQ_{10}), and lipoic acid. Results have been a bit promising.

A three-month, double-blind, placebo-controlled study of fifty-five people with migraines found that vitamin B_2 (at a daily dose of 400 mg) significantly reduced the frequency and duration of migraine attacks. The majority of the participants experienced a greater than 50 percent decrease in the number of migraine attacks and in the total days with headache pain. A subsequent study failed to find benefit with a combination of vitamin B_2, magnesium, and feverfew; however, it is possible that the 25-mg daily dose of vitamin B_2 used as the placebo confused the issue by providing some benefits on its own.

Another small, double-blind, placebo-controlled trial found benefit with CoQ_{10} (100 mg three times daily). In this study, about 50 percent of the people taking this supplement had a significant decrease in migraine frequency, compared to 15 percent in the placebo group. A similar study of lipoic acid hinted at benefit, but the results failed to pass tests of statistical significance.

OTHER PROPOSED NATURAL TREATMENTS

In a twenty-four-week double-blind study, forty-nine women with menstrual migraines received either placebo or soy isoflavones combined with dong quai and black cohosh extracts. Beginning at the twentieth week, the use of the herbal supplement resulted in decreased severity and frequency of headaches compared with placebo. It is not clear which of the ingredients in the combination was helpful; contrary to what is stated in this research report, the newest consensus is that neither black cohosh nor dong quai is a phytoestrogen, but that they may have other effects.

Despite promising results in an earlier and widely publicized study, a much larger and longer study of fish oil for migraines failed to find benefit. In this sixteen-week, double-blind, placebo-controlled study of 167 persons with recurrent migraines, the use of fish oil did not significantly reduce headache frequency or severity. Another small, double-blind, placebo-controlled study failed to find statistically significant evidence of benefit. Calcium, chromium, folate, ginger, and vitamin C have also been reported to be helpful for migraines, but there is no meaningful scientific evidence for any of these natural products. Identifying and eliminating allergenic foods from one's diet might be helpful for reducing the frequency of migraine attacks.

Evidence is inconsistent or incomplete regarding the potential benefit of chiropractic manipulation or acupuncture for the treatment and prevention of migraines. Biofeedback, massage, yoga, and a form of magnet treatment called pulsed electromagnetic field therapy have shown some promise for migraines. A careful review of twenty-nine trials found psychological interventions such as cognitive behavioral therapy, biofeedback, relaxation, and coping associated with reduced chronic headache or migraine pain in 589 children. These treatments were compared with placebo, standard treatment, waiting list control, or other active treatments.

HERBS AND SUPPLEMENTS TO USE WITH CAUTION

Various herbs and supplements may interact adversely with drugs used to treat migraine headaches, so one should be cautious when considering the use of herbs and supplements.

EBSCO CAM Review Board

FURTHER READING

Alecrim-Andrade, J., et al. "Acupuncture in Migraine Prevention." *Clinical Journal of Pain* 24 (2008): 98-105.

Diener, H. C., et al. "Efficacy of Acupuncture for the Prophylaxis of Migraine." *Lancet Neurology* 5 (2006): 310-316.

Eccleston, C., et al. "Psychological Therapies for the Management of Chronic and Recurrent Pain in Children and Adolescents." *Cochrane Database of Systematic Reviews* (2009): CD003968. Available through *EBSCO DynaMed Systematic Literature Surveillance* at http://www.ebscohost.com/dynamed.

Gottschling, S., et al. "Laser Acupuncture in Children with Headache." *Pain* 137 (2008): 405-412.

Jena, S., et al. "Acupuncture in Patients with Headache." *Cephalalgia* 28 (2008): 969-979.

John, P. J., et al. "Effectiveness of Yoga Therapy in the Treatment of Migraine Without Aura." *Headache* 47 (2007): 654-661.

Lawler, S. P., and L. D. Cameron. "A Randomized, Controlled Trial of Massage Therapy as a Treatment for

Migraine." *Annals of Behavioral Medicine* 32 (2006): 50-59.

Lipton, R. B., et al. "*Petasites hybridus* Root (Butterbur) Is an Effective Preventive Treatment for Migraine." *Neurology* 63 (2004): 2240-2244.

Magis, D., et al. "A Randomized, Double-Blind, Placebo-Controlled Trial of Thioctic Acid in Migraine Prophylaxis." *Headache* 47 (2007): 52-57.

Nestoriuc, Y., et al. "Biofeedback Treatment for Headache Disorders." *Applied Psychophysiology and Biofeedback* 33 (2008): 125-140.

See also: Butterbur; Feverfew; 5-hydroxytryptophan; Headache, cluster; Headache, tension; Magnesium; Pain management; Stress.

Migraines: Homeopathic remedies

CATEGORY: Homeopathy

DEFINITION: Homeopathic treatment of headaches characterized by severe pain, visual disturbances, light sensitivity, nausea, and other symptoms.

STUDIED HOMEOPATHIC REMEDIES: Belladonna, *Cyclamen*, *Gelsemium*, ignatia, *Lachesis*, *Natrum muriaticum*, silicea, sulphur

INTRODUCTION

The term "migraine" refers to a class of headaches that share certain characteristic symptoms. Migraine pain may be preceded or accompanied by visual changes or other symptoms, such as severe sensitivity to light or sound, heart palpitations, faintness, nausea, or vomiting. Symptoms that precede the onset of a migraine attack are known as prodromal symptoms.

In migraines, headache pain usually occurs in the forehead or temples, often on one side only and typically accompanied by nausea and a preference for a darkened room. Headache attacks last for several hours up to one day or more. They are usually separated by completely pain-free intervals. In some cases, headache pain is accompanied by a visual (or occasionally nonvisual) disturbance known as an aura. Migraines are classified as migraine with aura or migraine without aura.

Migraines can be triggered by a variety of causes, including fatigue, stress, hormonal changes, and foods such as alcohol, chocolate, peanuts, and avocados. However, in many people, migraines occur with no obvious triggering factor.

SCIENTIFIC EVALUATIONS OF HOMEOPATHIC REMEDIES

Four double-blind, placebo-controlled studies have evaluated the use of classical homeopathic approaches to treat migraines and other forms of headache. One study found significant evidence of benefit, while the others did not.

In the positive study, sixty people who suffered from migraines were given either a classical homeopathic remedy or placebo. At the start of the study, researchers evaluated each person and, based on classical homeopathy, prescribed one or two of the following remedies: belladonna, ignatia, *Lachesis*, silicea, *Gelsemium*, *Cyclamen*, *Natrum muriaticum*, or sulphur, each in 30c (centesimal) potency. Once an appropriate remedy was determined for each participant, researchers randomly divided participants into treatment and control groups.

At the conclusion of the four-month study, the treatment group showed statistically significant reduction in the intensity, duration, and frequency of migraine attacks, compared with the placebo group.

Another four-month, double-blind, placebo-controlled trial of about the same size also evaluated the effects of individualized homeopathic treatment on migraines, but with less positive results. On most measurements of headache severity, no statistically significant differences were seen between the treated group and the placebo group.

Lack of benefit was seen in two other trials, each involving individualized homeopathic treatment and enrolling a total of more than 150 people. The larger of these two trials, however, included people with various forms of headache, not just migraines.

TRADITIONAL HOMEOPATHIC TREATMENTS

Classical homeopathy offers many possible homeopathic treatments for migraine headaches. These therapies are chosen based on various specific details of the person seeking treatment.

If the headache is throbbing and the pain increases from the slightest disturbance of light, motion, or noise, and the condition worsens in the afternoon, the affected person may fit the symptom picture for the remedy belladonna. Other features for this symptom picture include a flushed, hot face and cold hands and feet.

If the headache is situated on the left side of the head and the pain is congested and pulsing, the affected person may be a candidate for the homeopathic remedy *Lachesis.* Other characteristics of the symptom picture include a flushed or blotchy face, pain that is worse from sleeping (during the day or night), and pain that is sometimes worse from heat. For women, the pain is worse before the menstrual period and better once the flow begins.

If the migraine occurs after mental exertion or near the menstrual period and the affected person is especially nervous and chilly, then the remedy silicea may be indicated. Headaches associated with this remedy are usually on the right side, starting at the back of the skull and extending to the forehead.

EBSCO CAM Review Board

FURTHER READING

Owen, J. M., and B. N. Green. "Homeopathic Treatment of Headaches." *Journal of Chiropractic Medicine* 3 (2004): 45-52.

Schiapparelli, P., et al. "Non-pharmacological Approach to Migraine Prophylaxis." *Neurological Sciences* 31, suppl. 1 (2010): S137-S139.

Straumsheim, P., et al. "Homeopathic Treatment of Migraine." *British Homeopathic Journal* 89 (2000): 4-7.

Whitmarsh, T. E., D. M. Coleston-Shields, and T. J. Steiner. "Double-Blind, Randomized, Placebo-Controlled Study of Homeopathic Prophylaxis of Migraine." *Cephalgia* 17 (1997): 600-604.

Witt, C. M., R. Lüdtke, and S. N. Willich. "Homeopathic Treatment of Patients with Migraine." *Journal of Complementary and Alternative Medicine* 16 (2010): 347-355.

See also: Headaches, cluster; Headaches, tension; Nausea; Stress; Vertigo.

Milk thistle

CATEGORY: Herbs and supplements

RELATED TERMS: Holy thistle, Mary thistle, Silibinin, *Silybum marianum*, silymarin, wild artichoke

DEFINITION: Natural plant product used to treat specific health conditions.

PRINCIPAL PROPOSED USES: Alcoholic hepatitis, liver cirrhosis, mushroom poisoning (special intravenous form only), protection from liver-toxic medications, rosacea, viral hepatitis

OTHER PROPOSED USES: Diabetes, obsessive-compulsive disorder

OVERVIEW

The milk thistle plant commonly grows from two to seven feet in height, with spiny leaves and reddish-purple, thistle-shaped flowers. It has also been called wild artichoke, holy thistle, and Mary thistle. Native to Europe, milk thistle has a long history of use as both a food and a medicine. At the turn of the twentieth century, English gardeners grew milk thistle to use its leaves like lettuce (after cutting off the spines), the stalks like asparagus, the roasted seeds like coffee, and the roots (soaked overnight) like oyster plant. The seeds and leaves of milk thistle were used for medicinal purposes as well, such as treating jaundice and increasing breast milk production.

German researchers in the 1960s were sufficiently impressed with the history and clinical effectiveness of milk thistle to begin examining it for active constituents. In 1986, Germany's Commission E approved an oral extract of milk thistle as a treatment for liver disease. However, the evidence that it really works remains incomplete and inconsistent.

THERAPEUTIC DOSAGES

The standard dosage of milk thistle is 200 milligrams (mg) two to three times a day of an extract standardized to contain 70 percent silymarin. There is some evidence that silymarin bound to phosphatidylcholine may be better absorbed. This form should be

Milk thistle seeds. (Scimat/Photo Researchers, Inc.)

taken at a dosage of 100 to 200 mg twice a day. Considering the severe nature of liver disease, a doctor's supervision is essential. Also, milk thistle preparations that are designed for oral use should not be injected.

THERAPEUTIC USES

Based on the extensive folk use of milk thistle in cases of jaundice, European medical researchers began to investigate its medicinal effects. It is currently used to treat alcoholic hepatitis, liver cirrhosis, liver poisoning, and viral hepatitis, as well as to protect the liver in general from the effects of liver-toxic medications. However, despite this wide usage, there is no definitive evidence that it is effective.

Standardized milk thistle extract is known as silymarin. Silymarin itself is a mixture of at least seven chemicals. The most active of these chemicals is commonly known as silibinin. However, silibinin too is, in fact, a mixture, comprising the two related substances silibinin A and silibinin B. When injected intravenously, silibinin is thought to act as an antidote to poisoning by the deathcap mushroom, *Amanita phalloides*. Animal studies suggest that milk thistle extracts can also protect against many other poisonous substances, from toluene to the drug acetaminophen. One animal study suggests that milk thistle can also protect against fetal damage caused by alcohol.

Silibinin is hypothesized to function by displacing toxins that might bind to the liver, as well as by causing the liver to regenerate more quickly. It may also act as an antioxidant and also stabilize liver cell membranes.

In Europe, milk thistle is often added as extra protection when patients are given medications known to cause liver problems. However, milk thistle failed to prove effective for preventing liver inflammation caused by the Alzheimer's drug Cognex (tacrine).

Milk thistle is also used in a vague condition known as minor hepatic insufficiency, or sluggish liver. This term is mostly used by European physicians and American naturopathic practitioners (conventional physicians in the United States do not recognize it). Symptoms are supposed to include aching under the ribs, fatigue, unhealthy skin appearance, general malaise, constipation, premenstrual syndrome, chemical sensitivities, and allergies.

One small but apparently well-conducted, double-blind trial found evidence that milk thistle might improve blood sugar control in type 2 diabetes. Milk thistle may also offer some protection to the kidney.

Highly preliminary evidence hints that milk thistle might help reduce breast cancer risk. Milk thistle is sometimes recommended for gallstones and psoriasis, but there is little to no evidence that it really helps these conditions.

In one small, placebo-controlled trial, the topical application of milk thistle with methylsulfonylmethane (MSM) for one month appeared to be effective in the treatment of forty-six subjects with the skin condition rosacea.

A small preliminary study investigated whether milk thistle can help to relieve obsessive-compulsive disorder (OCD). Thirty-five adults with OCD were randomized to receive milk thistle (600 mg per day) or the medication fluoxetine (30 mg per day), which is commonly used to treat OCD. At the end of the eight-week trial, researchers did not find any significant differences between the two groups.

SCIENTIFIC EVIDENCE

As noted above, there is considerable evidence from studies in animals that milk thistle can protect the liver from numerous toxins. However, human studies of people suffering from various liver diseases have often yielded mixed results. A 2007 review of published and unpublished studies on milk thistle as a treatment for liver disease caused by alcohol or viral hepatitis concluded that benefits were seen only in low-quality trials, and even in those, milk thistle did not show more than a slight benefit.

Acute viral hepatitis. A twenty-one-day double-blind, placebo-controlled study of 57 people with acute viral hepatitis found significant improvements in the group receiving milk thistle. In another study, 105 people with acute hepatitis receiving milk thistle (140 mg, three times daily) showed modest improvement in some symptoms compared with those taking a placebo for four weeks. On the other hand, a thirty-five-day study of 151 individuals thought to have acute hepatitis found no benefit with milk thistle, but this study has been criticized for failing to document that the participants actually had acute hepatitis.

Chronic viral hepatitis. Inconsistent evidence exists regarding whether milk thistle is helpful for chronic viral hepatitis B or C. The herb does not appear to affect levels of virus in the body, but it might help protect the liver from damage and improve some symptoms.

Alcoholic hepatitis. A double-blind, placebo-controlled study performed in 1981 followed 106 Finnish soldiers with alcoholic liver disease over a period of four weeks. The treated group showed a significant decrease in elevated liver enzymes and improvement in liver histology (the microscopic structure of liver tissue), as evaluated by biopsy in 29 subjects.

Two similar studies provided essentially equivalent results. However, a three-month, randomized, double-blind study of 116 people showed little to no additional benefit, perhaps because most participants reduced their alcohol consumption and almost half stopped drinking entirely. Another study found no benefit in 72 patients followed for fifteen months. It is more effective for people with alcoholism to quit drinking than to continue drinking and take milk thistle.

Liver cirrhosis. A double-blind, placebo-controlled study of 170 people with alcoholic or nonalcoholic cirrhosis found that in the group treated with milk thistle, the four-year survival rate was 58 percent compared with only 38 percent in the placebo group. This difference was statistically significant.

A double-blind, placebo-controlled trial that enrolled 172 people with cirrhosis for four years also found reductions in mortality, but it just missed the conventional cutoff for statistical significance. A two-year double-blind, placebo-controlled study of 200 individuals with alcoholic cirrhosis found no reduction in mortality attributable to the use of milk thistle. However, in a analysis of nineteen randomized trials, researchers concluded that milk thistle was significantly more effective at reducing mortality from liver cirrhosis (mostly alcohol-related) compared with a placebo, but no more effective at reducing mortality from any cause.

Other double-blind studies of people with various forms of cirrhosis have looked at changes in tests of liver function rather than mortality. Some found benefit, while others did not.

Protection from medications that damage the liver. Numerous medications can injure or inflame the liver. Preliminary evidence suggests that milk thistle might protect against liver toxicity caused by drugs such as acetaminophen, alcohol, phenothiazines, and phenytoin (Dilantin). However, according to a twelve-week, double-blind study of 222 people, milk thistle does not seem to prevent the liver inflammation caused by the Alzheimer's drug tacrine (Cognex).

SAFETY ISSUES

Milk thistle is believed to possess very little toxicity. Animal studies have not shown any negative effects even when high doses were administered over a long period of time. A study of 2,637 participants reported in 1992 showed a low incidence of side effects, limited mainly to mild gastrointestinal disturbance. However, on rare occasions severe abdominal discomfort may occur.

On the basis of its extensive use as a food, milk thistle is believed to be safe for pregnant or nursing women, and researchers have enrolled pregnant women in studies. However, safety in young children, pregnant or nursing women, and individuals with severe renal disease has not been formally established.

IMPORTANT INTERACTIONS

Milk thistle might have a protective function in persons taking medications that could damage the liver, such as acetaminophen, phenytoin (Dilantin), alcohol, and phenothiazines. One report has noted that silibinin can inhibit a bacterial enzyme called beta-glucuronidase, which plays a role in the activity of certain drugs, such as oral contraceptives. This could theoretically reduce the effectiveness of oral contraceptives.

EBSCO CAM Review Board

FURTHER READING

Berardesca, E., et al. "Combined Effects of Silymarin and Methylsulfonylmethane in the Management of Rosacea: Clinical and Instrumental Evaluation." *Journal of Cosmetic Dermatology* 7 (2008): 8-14.

El-Kamary, S. S., et al. "A Randomized Controlled Trial to Assess the Safety and Efficacy of Silymarin on Symptoms, Signs and Biomarkers of Acute Hepatitis." *Phytomedicine* 16, no. 5 (2009): 391-400.

Huseini, H. F., et al. "The Efficacy of *Silybum marianum (L.) Gaertn.* (Silymarin) in the Treatment of Type II Diabetes." *Phytotherapy Research* 20, no. 12 (2006): 1036-1039.

Hutchinson, C., A. Bomford, and C. A. Geissler. "The Iron-Chelating Potential of Silybin in Patients with Hereditary Haemochromatosis." *European Journal of Clinical Nutrition* 64, no. 10 (2010): 1239-1241.

Kroll, D. J., H. S. Shaw, and N. H. Oberlies. "Milk Thistle Nomenclature: Why It Matters in Cancer Research and Pharmacokinetic Studies." *Integrative Cancer Therapies* 6 (2007): 110-119.

Rambaldi, A., B. Jacobs, and C. Gluud. "Milk Thistle for Alcoholic and/or Hepatitis B or C Virus Liver Diseases." *Cochrane Database of Systematic Reviews* 4 (2007): CD003620.

Saller, R., et al. "An Updated Systematic Review with Meta-analysis for the Clinical Evidence of Silymarin." *Forschende Komplementarmedizine* 15 (2008): 9-20.

Sayyah, M., et al. "Comparison of *Silybum marianum* (L.) *Gaertn.* with Fluoxetine in the Treatment of Obsessive-Compulsive Disorder." *Progress in Neuro-Psychopharmacology and Biological Psychiatry* 34, no. 2 (2010): 362-365.

See also: Hepatitis, alcoholic; Hepatitis, viral; Herbal medicine; Liver disease; Methyl sulfonyl methane; Rosacea.

Mind/body medicine

CATEGORY: Issues and overviews
DEFINITION: A type of traditional healing that emphasizes the interconnectedness of the mind and the body.

OVERVIEW

According to Hippocrates, "The natural healing force within each one of us is the greatest force in getting well." Ancient civilizations and the indigenous peoples of the Americas, for example, have known and practiced mind/body medicine for centuries. These ancient healing practices include traditional Chinese medicine, Ayurvedic medicine, and various forms of indigenous medicine. This conceptual framework of interdependence of the mind/body relationship is in sharp contrast to the theory of Western medicine, which separates the mind from the body and sees no interconnection between them.

MODERN INTERESTS

In the early 1960s came renewed interest in the possible connection between the mind and the body in the context of healing. George Solomon, a psychiatrist, knew that persons with rheumatoid arthritis had an exacerbation of symptoms when they were depressed. From this realization he developed a new field of medicine that incorporated the knowledge of psychology, neurology, and immunology: psychoneuroimmunology. Another physician, Herbert Benson, studied the affect of meditation on blood pressure levels. Psychologist Robert Ader further illustrated the relationship of mind and body and how this interplay could be affected by mental and emotional cues. He was interested in how this relationship affected the immune system. The mind/body connection, for the most part, is no longer viewed with suspicion. Indeed, its study is now part of the curricula of many medical schools worldwide.

MIND/BODY MEDICINE

Theoretically, mind/body medicine works through reducing stress levels, thereby decreasing the overload release of hormones such as cortisol, which affect the immune system. These hormones have a major affect on the cardiovascular system, and they also increase inflammation of organs and joints. By decreasing the release of these stressors, one can manage many chronic diseases. Experiments have shown not only a reduction in blood pressure but also a reduction in body temperature.

One has only to close one's eyes and open one's mind to visualize a Hindu monk, for example, performing such physical-mental feats. These acts of will, through self-control practiced through multiple forms of relaxation, can be performed by anyone with training.

Mind/Body Therapies

Progressive relaxation. Progressive relaxation is the tensing and relaxing of various voluntary muscle groups throughout the body in an orderly sequence. The theory is that when a person is emotionally tense, he or she unconsciously clenches or tightens muscles. Progressively relaxing the muscles releases both the physical and the mental tension.

Meditation. Meditation is the focusing of the mind continuously on one thought, word (mantra), object, or mental image for a period of time. It can also involve focusing on breathing or on sensations in the body. The goal of meditation is to quiet the mind.

Hypnosis. Hypnosis is a state of inner absorption, concentration, and focused attention. The unconscious mind is allowed to take over, and positive imagery and suggestions are used to help improve mental and physical health.

Yoga. Yoga is a practice that includes physical exercises, postures, balancing, breathing techniques, and meditation.

Karen Schroeder, M.S., RD; reviewed by Brian P. Randall, M.D.

Meditation, yoga, guided visualization, relaxation techniques, biofeedback, and cognitive behavioral therapy are methods employed in mind/body medicine.

Conditions that have been improved by choosing an appropriate modality include asthma, coronary heart disease, hypertension (high blood pressure), anxiety, insomnia, fibromyalgia, menopausal symptoms, and the nausea and vomiting associated with chemotherapy. By choosing the preferred modality, a participant enhances the chance for success.

Hypnosis is another form of mind/body medicine that has gained favor. It has been shown to be advantageous in multiple situations, including dental treatments, minor surgery, and treatment for phobias. Although this is a proven modality, it may not work for everybody.

David Spiegel of Stanford University School of Medicine treated eighty-six women with late-stage breast cancer; one-half received standard recommended treatments, the other half received, in addition to the standard treatment, weekly support sessions in which the women shared personal triumphs and grief. The women who participated in these support groups lived twice as long as those who did not have this social support. Other clinical trails have shown that meditation and laughter affect mood and improve the quality of life.

Practice

As with any form of medical therapy, treatments should be rendered by licensed professionals only. Mind/body medicine does not provide curative measures as such. It is a form of integrative medicine, complementary to well-established medical treatments.

Also, it is important to have ongoing evaluation of the success or failure of treatment. Re-evaluation, which can be curative in its own right, is an ongoing process that should be incorporated into the routine activities of the person seeking care.

Motivation of the patient and the trust instilled by the practitioner are as much a part of mind/body medicine as the treatment itself. As with any form of healing, the interplay among those involved needs to be established at the start of treatment. The greatest satisfaction a practitioner can achieve is attainment of the goals set by both the practitioner and the person being treated.

M. Barbara Klyde, Ph.D.P.H., PA-C

Further Reading

Ader, R., and N. Cohen. "Psychoneuroimmunology: Conditioning and Stress." *Annual Review of Psychology* 44 (1993): 53-85.

Lando, J., and S. M. Williams. "Uniting Mind and Body in Our Health Care and Public Health Systems." *Preventing Chronic Disease* 3, no. 2 (2006): A31.

McMillan, T. L., and S. Mark. "Complementary and Alternative Medicine and Physical Activity for Menopausal Symptoms." *Journal of the American Medical Women's Association* 59, no. 4 (2004): 270-277.

See also: Biofeedback; Energy medicine; Faith healing; Guided imagery; Humor and healing; Integrative medicine; Meditation; Mental health; Relaxation therapies; Spirituality; Stress; Traditional healing; Transcendental Meditation; Walking, mind/body; Whole medicine; Yoga.

Mistletoe

Category: Herbs and supplements
Related terms: European mistletoe, *Viscum album*
Definition: Natural plant product used to treat specific health conditions.
Principal proposed use: Cancer treatment support
Other proposed uses: Colds and flu, diabetes, hypertension

Overview

European mistletoe, famous during the Christmas season, is a semiparasitic plant that grows on trees in Europe and Asia. Its young leafy twigs and flowers were used as an all-heal or panacea, said to be helpful for virtually all diseases. The herb is also said to have played a role in Celtic religious celebrations. American mistletoe, *Phoradendron leucarpum*, is related to European mistletoe, but it is thought to be more toxic and has not been well studied.

Therapeutic Dosages

Injectible mistletoe extracts should be used only under the supervision of a physician. Mistletoe tea can be made by soaking 10 to 20 grams (g) of chopped leaves in 2 cups of water for eight hours. A typical dose is 1 to 3 cups daily.

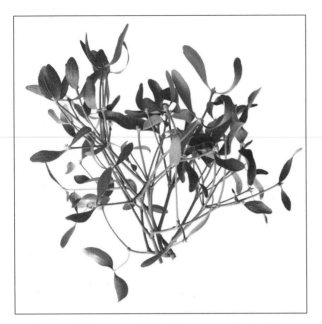

In the twentieth century, mistletoe became popular in Germany through the advocacy of mystic and philosopher Rudolf Steiner, who recommended injectable forms of mistletoe as a treatment for cancer. (© Witold Krasowski/Dreamstime.com)

THERAPEUTIC USES

In the twentieth century, mistletoe became popular in Germany through the advocacy of mystic and philosopher Rudolf Steiner. The school of medicine he founded, anthroposophical medicine, recommended injectable forms of mistletoe as a treatment for cancer. The initial basis for this use was Steiner's so-called clairvoyant insight. Scientific tests were subsequently conducted with somewhat positive results, but current evidence is far from definitive.

Mistletoe extracts show anticancer effects in the test tube. However, test-tube studies cannot show a treatment effective; only controlled clinical trials can do that. A 2003 review found ten human trials of injected mistletoe for cancer that met at least minimal scientific standards. Even these studies generally suffered from significant weaknesses in design. The review authors noted that the better-designed studies failed to find evidence of any benefit, in terms of lengthened remission, improved quality of life, or chance of survival. Subsequent human trials have also failed to reach adequate levels of scientific rigor or clinical relevance and have, therefore, failed to clarify matters. Another review of twenty-one clinical trials found no convincing evidence that mistletoe was effective for cancer survival, tumor response, quality of life, psychological distress, or any other favorable outcomes. However, two of the better designed studies did suggest some benefit for breast cancer patients undergoing chemotherapy. A more recent review of forty-nine studies found that the addition of mistletoe to standard cancer treatment was associated with improved survival in cancer patients. An analysis restricted to randomized controlled trials, however, showed less of an overall effect.

Oral uses of mistletoe have not undergone significant study. Weak evidence, too weak to rely upon, hints that constituents of mistletoe might potentially offer benefit in diabetes and colds and flu. It is commonly stated that oral mistletoe products reduce blood pressure, but there is no scientific evidence to support this belief.

SAFETY ISSUES

In large clinical trials, use of injected pharmaceutical-grade mistletoe products has not been associated with serious adverse effects, although pain at the injection site and mild flulike symptoms are common. Severe allergic reactions may occur rarely.

Oral use of a mistletoe product has been associated with hepatitis. Mistletoe berries and perhaps the leaves can cause severe toxicity, especially in children. American mistletoe may be more toxic than European mistletoe. Mistletoe is not recommended for use in young children, pregnant or nursing women, or people with severe liver or kidney disease.

EBSCO CAM Review Board

FURTHER READING

Grossarth-Maticek, R., and R. Ziegler. "Prospective Controlled Cohort Studies on Long-term Therapy of Cervical Cancer Patients with a Mistletoe Preparation (Iscador)." *Forschende Komplementarmedizine* 14 (2007): 140-147.

_____. "Randomized and Non-randomized Prospective Controlled Cohort Studies in Matched Pair Design for the Long-term Therapy of Corpus Uteri Cancer Patients with a Mistletoe Preparation (Iscador)." *European Journal of Medical Research* 13 (2008): 107-120.

Horneber, M. A., et al. "Mistletoe Therapy in Oncology." *Cochrane Database of Systematic Reviews* 2 (2008): CD003297.

Karagoz, A., et al. "Antiviral Potency of Mistletoe (*Viscum album* ssp. *album*) Extracts Against Human Parainfluenza Virus Type 2 in Vero Cells." *Phytotherapy Research* 17 (2003): 560-562.

Klopp, R., et al. "Influence of Complementary *Viscum album* (Iscador) Administration on Microcirculation and Immune System of Ear, Nose, and Throat Carcinoma Patients Treated with Radiation and Chemotherapy." *Anticancer Research* 25 (2005): 601-610.

Kovacs, E. "Effects of *Viscum album* Extract Therapy in Patients with Cancer: Relation with Interleukin-6, Soluble Interleukin-6 Receptor, and Soluble gp130." *Journal of Alternative and Complementary Medicine* 10 (2004): 241-246.

Ostermann, T., C. Raak, and A. Büssing. "Survival of Cancer Patients Treated with Mistletoe Extract (Iscador): A Systematic Literature Review." *BMC Cancer* 9 (2009): 451.

Schink, M., et al. "Mistletoe Extract Reduces the Surgical Suppression of Natural Killer Cell Activity in Cancer Patients." *Forschende Komplementarmedizine* 14 (2007): 9-17.

See also: Cancer treatment support; Herbal medicine.

Mitral valve prolapse

CATEGORY: Condition

RELATED TERMS: Dysautonomia, mitral valve prolapse syndrome

DEFINITION: Treatment of the condition caused by the prolapse, or misalignment, of one of the valves of the heart.

PRINCIPAL PROPOSED NATURAL TREATMENT: Magnesium

OTHER PROPOSED NATURAL TREATMENTS: Acetyl-L-carnitine, acupuncture, arginine, CoQ_{10}, creatine, 5-hydroxytryptophan, gamma-linolenic acid, hawthorn, hops, kava, L-carnitine, lemon balm, lipoic acid, melatonin, multivitamin-multimineral supplements, oligomeric proanthocyanidins, passionflower, taurine, valerian, vitamin B_1, vitamin E

INTRODUCTION

Mitral valve prolapse (MVP) affects about 2 percent of people in the United States. (Past estimates were higher because of errors in diagnosis.) As the name suggests, MVP involves prolapse (misalignment or the falling out of place) of one of the valves of the heart, the mitral valve.

The mitral valve sits at the opening between the left atrium and left ventricle and opens and closes so that blood flows only in one direction (atrium to ventricle). In MVP, the mitral valve fails to make a proper snug fit and instead billows (prolapses) back into the atrium, making a sound that can be heard through a stethoscope.

MVP is generally benign. Sometimes, however, the mitral valve fits so poorly that a large amount of blood leaks back from the ventricle to the atrium. This is called mitral regurgitation, and it can be dangerous, eventually requiring surgery.

In the past, a set of symptoms called dysautonomia was thought to frequently occur in association with MVP. Dysautonomia involves malfunction of the autonomic nervous system (the part of the nervous system that is not under conscious control). MVP plus dysautonomia used to be called mitral valve prolapse syndrome. Symptoms were said to include chest pain with no apparent medical cause, panic attacks and anxiety, heart palpitations, sweating, dizziness, lightheadedness, weakness, balance problems, hypersensitive startle reflex, shortness of breath, numbness or tingling in the fingers or toes, hyperventilation, and sensitivity to caffeine and other stimulants. However, more recent evidence indicates that symptoms of dysautonomia occur with no greater frequency in people with MVP than in people without MVP. In other words, there is probably no connection between the two conditions. People who were previously diagnosed with MVP syndrome are now said to have two separate conditions: MVP plus symptoms of dysautonomia. The cause of these dysautonomic symptoms is not clear, but it probably involves a response to stress.

Conventional treatment for MVP involves regular monitoring for mitral regurgitation and maintenance of normal weight and blood pressure to avoid excess strain on the valve. In addition, people with MVP are given antibiotics before surgical or dental procedures. Those procedures may release bacteria into the bloodstream, and in people with MVP, bacteria may stick to the valves and cause infection (a condition called endocarditis). Antibiotic treatment can prevent this. People with MVP who also have symptoms of dysautonomia may be separately treated for those symptoms too.

PRINCIPAL PROPOSED NATURAL TREATMENTS

Low levels of magnesium can cause some symptoms similar to dysautonomia. One study evaluated 141 people with MVP and dysautonomia and found that 60 percent of them had low levels of magnesium in the blood. This subgroup of people with low magnesium were then enrolled in a ten-week, double-blind, placebo-controlled crossover trial. (They received placebo or magnesium supplements for five weeks, and then were "crossed over" to the other group.) People receiving magnesium experienced a significant reduction in dysautonomic symptoms, such as chest pain, palpitations, anxiety, and shortness of breath.

Note that it is unlikely that these people had magnesium deficiency. Magnesium deficiency is thought to be a rare condition. More likely, low magnesium levels are a consequence of some other factor that also causes dysautonomia symptoms. Regardless, magnesium supplementation could help treat such symptoms. However, more studies are necessary to validate this promising possibility.

OTHER PROPOSED NATURAL TREATMENTS

Various herbs and supplements that are thought to help the heart in miscellaneous ways (such as treating congestive heart failure or preventing coronary artery disease) are often recommended for MVP too, on general principles. These herbs and supplements include arginine, CoQ_{10}, creatine, hawthorn, L-carnitine, oligomeric proanthocyanidins, taurine, vitamin B_1, and vitamin E. However, there is no scientific reason to believe that any of these natural treatments would help MVP.

A variety of other natural treatments are used to treat anxiety-related dysautonomia symptoms. These treatments include 5-hydroxytryptophan, acupuncture, hops, kava, lemon balm, melatonin, multivitamin-multimineral supplements, passionflower, and valerian. Natural treatments used for stress also may be helpful.

A serious form of autonomic nervous system dysfunction can occur in people with diabetes. The supplements lipoic acid, acetyl-L-carnitine, and gamma-linolenic acid have shown some promise for this condition, and for this reason they have been recommended for the treatment of dysautonomic symptoms.

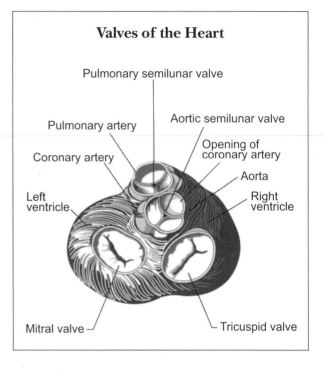

Valves of the Heart

Pulmonary semilunar valve
Pulmonary artery
Coronary artery
Left ventricle
Mitral valve
Aortic semilunar valve
Opening of coronary artery
Aorta
Right ventricle
Tricuspid valve

HERBS AND SUPPLEMENTS TO USE WITH CAUTION

Numerous herbs and supplements may interact adversely with drugs used to treat mitral valve prolapse.

EBSCO CAM Review Board

FURTHER READING

Bobkowski, W., A. Nowak, and J. Durlach. "The Importance of Magnesium Status in the Pathophysiology of Mitral Valve Prolapse." *Magnesium Research* 18 (2005): 35-52.

Freed, L. A., et al. "Prevalence and Clinical Outcome of Mitral-Valve Prolapse." *New England Journal of Medicine* 341 (1999): 1-7.

Lichodziejewska, B., et al. "Clinical Symptoms of Mitral Valve Prolapse Are Related to Hypomagnesemia and Attenuated by Magnesium Supplementation." *American Journal of Cardiology* 79 (1997): 768-772.

Zipes, Douglas P., et al., eds. *Braunwald's Heart Disease: A Textbook of Cardiovascular Medicine*. 8th ed. Philadelphia: Saunders/Elsevier, 2008.

See also: Cardiomyopathy; Heart attack; Magnesium.

Molybdenum

Category: Herbs and supplements
Related term: Mo
Definition: Natural food and water substance used to treat specific health conditions.
Principal proposed uses: None
Other proposed uses: Female sexual dysfunction, general well-being, insomnia, male sexual dysfunction, tooth decay prevention, weight loss

Overview

Molybdenum is an essential trace mineral. Deficiency of molybdenum is rare but may occur in certain parts of the world. Current marketing of molybdenum products for the treatment of medical conditions is not founded on any meaningful scientific evidence.

Requirements and Sources

Molybdenum is found in a variety of foods, including dark green leafy vegetables, legumes, and whole grains. Mineral water and hard tap water may also supply significant amounts of molybdenum.

Deficiency of molybdenum is believed to be rare. Although accurate recommended daily intake levels for molybdenum have not been determined, less precise safe and adequate intake levels have been set in the United States as follows: 15 to 50 micrograms (mcg) for persons up to three years of age, 30 to 75 mcg for those from four to six years old, 50 to 150 mcg for those seven to ten years old, and 75 to 250 mcg for those aged eleven and older.

Therapeutic Dosages

There are no known uses of molybdenum that would suggest doses other than the safe and adequate levels noted in the previous section. Molybdenum is marketed both as a tablet and as a liquid supplement containing the mineral in dissolved form. Despite widespread claims, there is no evidence that any form of molybdenum is absorbed to a markedly superior extent.

Therapeutic Uses

Web sites that advocate molybdenum products make numerous health claims that lack scientific foundation. Some of these unsupported claims include that molybdenum regulates the body's pH, enhances the body's ability to burn fat, eliminates toxins, promotes general well-being, prevents tooth decay, aids sleep, reduces allergic reaction to chemicals such as MSG and sulfites, and increases male and female libido. None of these claims have any scientific support, and some (such as regulating the body's pH) make no sense from a scientific point of view.

Additionally, it is often stated by some manufacturers of molybdenum products that a variety of disease are commonly caused or worsened by molybdenum deficiency. These include acne, allergies, asthma, athlete's foot, Bell's palsy, bladder infection, candidiasis, canker sores, depression, diabetes, eczema, Gulf War syndrome, viral hepatitis, herpes simplex, liver cirrhosis, lupus, Lyme disease, multiple sclerosis, and prostatitis. However, all of these claims lack even the bare minimum of foundation.

In certain areas of China, molybdenum deficiency may occur relatively commonly. There are higher rates of some forms of cancer in these regions; however, when molybdenum supplementation was tried, it failed to make a difference, perhaps because other, unidentified deficiencies were involved as well.

Safety Issues

When taken at recommended dosages, molybdenum should be safe. Excessive intake of molybdenum could in theory lead to copper deficiency. People with serious kidney disease should also avoid taking molybdenum (or any other supplement) except on the advice of a physician. One isolated report hints that excessive molybdenum intake can cause symptoms of psychosis.

EBSCO CAM Review Board

Further Reading

Blot, W. J., et al. "Nutrition Intervention Trials in Linxian, China: Supplementation with Specific Vitamin/Mineral Combinations, Cancer Incidence, and Disease-Specific Mortality in the General Population." *Journal of the National Cancer Institute* 85 (1993): 1483-1492.

Brewer, G. J. "Practical Recommendations and New Therapies for Wilson's Disease." *Drugs* 50 (1995): 240-9.

Momcilovic, B. "A Case Report of Acute Human Molybdenum Toxicity from a Dietary Molybdenum Supplement: A New Member of the *Lucor metallicum* Family." *Arhiv za Higijenu Rada I Toksikologiju* 50 (1999): 289-297.

See also: Herbal medicine.

Monoamine oxidase (MAO) inhibitors

CATEGORY: Drug interactions
DEFINITION: A group of antidepressant drugs.
INTERACTIONS: Ephedra, green tea, ginseng, 5-hydroxy-tryptophan (5-HTP), S-adenosylmethionine (SAMe), St. John's wort, scotch broom
DRUGS IN THIS FAMILY: Furazolidone (Furoxone), isocarboxazid (Marplan), phenelzine sulfate (Nardil), tranylcypromine sulfate (Parnate)

EPHEDRA
Effect: Dangerous Interaction
Because it contains the stimulant ephedrine, combining the herb ephedra with monoamine oxidase (MAO) inhibitors can rapidly produce a severe, dangerous interaction and should be avoided. In the United States, it is illegal to sell products containing ephedra.

SCOTCH BROOM
Effect: Dangerous Interaction
The herb scotch broom contains high levels of tyramine, so it should not be taken with MAO inhibitors.

GREEN TEA
Effect: Probable Dangerous Interaction
Because it contains caffeine, green tea should not be combined with MAO inhibitors.

GINSENG
Effect: Possible Dangerous Interaction
According to one report, the combination of ginseng and the MAO inhibitor phenelzine caused worrisome symptoms. While this may have been caused by caffeine contamination of the ginseng, experts recommend avoiding ginseng-MAO inhibitor combinations.

ST. JOHN'S WORT
Effect: Possible Dangerous Interaction
Current thinking suggests that St. John's wort functions somewhat similarly to SSRI (selective serotonin-reuptake inhibitor) antidepressants. Because SSRIs should not be combined with MAO inhibitors, St. John's wort probably should not be combined with them either.

5-HYDROXYTRYPTOPHAN (5-HTP), S-ADENOSYLMETHIONINE (SAMe)
Effect: Possible Dangerous Interactions
Based on one case report and on current thinking about how they work, SAMe and 5-HTP should not be combined with MAO inhibitors.

EBSCO CAM Review Board

FURTHER READING
Brinker, F. "Interactions of Pharmaceutical and Botanical Medicines." *Journal of Naturopathic Medicine* 7 (1997): 14.
Iruela, L. M., et al. "Toxic Interaction of S-adenosylmethionine and Clomipramine." *American Journal of Psychiatry* 150 (1993): 522.
Jones, B. D., and A. M. Runikis. "Interaction of Ginseng with Phenelzine." *Journal of Clinical Psychopharmacology* 7 (1987): 201-202.

See also: Depression, mild to moderate; Ephedra; 5-hydroxytryptophan; Food and Drug Administration; Green tea; Ginseng; Mental health; SAMe; St. John's wort; SSRIs; Tricyclic antidepressants.

Morning sickness

CATEGORY: Condition
RELATED TERMS: Hyperemesis gravidarum, nausea of pregnancy
DEFINITION: Treatment of nausea and vomiting associated with pregnancy.
PRINCIPAL PROPOSED NATURAL TREATMENTS: Acupressure, ginger, vitamin B_6
OTHER PROPOSED NATURAL TREATMENTS: Red raspberry, vitamin C, vitamin K

INTRODUCTION
Nausea afflicts the majority of women during the first trimester of pregnancy. However, this is also the precise period in which drug therapy is most worrisome because of the extreme vulnerability of the fetus. For this reason, conventional medicine has to some extent welcomed alternative medicine's quest for safe, natural treatment options.

PRINCIPAL PROPOSED NATURAL TREATMENTS
Two natural therapies, vitamin B_6 and ginger, have some evidence supporting their use in the treatment

of nausea in pregnancy. In addition, acupressure may be helpful.

Vitamin B6. For many years, conventional practitioners have recommended vitamin B_6 supplements to treat morning sickness. In 1995, a large double-blind, placebo-controlled study validated this use. In this trial, 342 pregnant women were given placebo or 30 milligrams (mg) of vitamin B_6 daily. Participants then graded their symptoms by noting the severity of their nausea and recording the number of vomiting episodes. The women in the vitamin B_6 group experienced significantly less nausea than the placebo group, suggesting that regular use of vitamin B_6 can be helpful for morning sickness. However, despite the benefits for nausea, vomiting episodes were not significantly reduced. At this dose (30 mg daily), vitamin B_6 is believed to be entirely safe.

Ginger. Ginger is a nausea remedy recommended by many in conventional medicine and by traditional healers from around the world. In 2001, a relatively well-designed double-blind, placebo-controlled trial of seventy pregnant women evaluated the effectiveness of ginger for morning sickness. Participants received either placebo or 250 mg of powdered ginger three times daily for four days. The results showed that ginger significantly reduced nausea and vomiting. No significant side effects occurred.

One study of 138 women and another of 291 women found ginger just as effective for morning sickness as vitamin B_6. However, a third study of 70 women found ginger to be somewhat better than B_6. None these studies used a placebo group.

Acupressure. Several studies have evaluated the potential benefits for morning sickness of treatment on a single acupuncture point (P6), traditionally thought to be effective for relief of nausea and vomiting, by the use of acupressure. This point is located on the inside of the forearm, about two inches above the wrist crease. Most positive trials have investigated the effects of pressure on this point (acupressure), rather than needling. The most common means used involve a wristband with a pearl-sized bead, situated over the P6 point. The wristband exerts pressure as it is worn, and the wearer can also press on it for extra stimulation.

In general, acupressure has shown good results. For example, a double-blind, placebo-controlled study of ninety-seven women that was reported in 2001 found evidence that wristband acupressure may

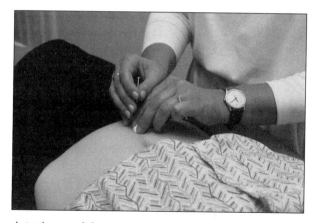

A patient receiving an acupuncture treatment for morning sickness. (Francoise Sauze/Photo Researchers, Inc.)

help relieve symptoms of morning sickness. Participants wore either a real wristband or a fake one that appeared identical. Both real and fake acupressure caused noticeable improvement in more than one-half of the participants. However, women using the real wristband showed significantly greater improvement. Benefits were also reported the same year in a double-blind, placebo-controlled study of sixty women.

These results are consistent with previous studies that also found benefit. Furthermore, a double-blind, placebo-controlled study of sixty pregnant women found that ten minutes of self-applied manual acupressure on either P6 or a sham point four times daily improved symptoms. However, two studies failed to find benefit for severe morning sickness.

OTHER PROPOSED NATURAL TREATMENTS

Multivitamin-multimineral tablets have shown promise for morning sickness, possibly because of their vitamin B_6 content. A combination of vitamin K (at a dose of 5 mg–much higher than nutritional needs) and vitamin C (25 mg) is sometimes recommended for morning sickness, based on an uncontrolled study conducted in the 1950s. Red raspberry is also frequently recommended, but there is no evidence that it works.

Pregnant women commonly develop iron deficiency anemia. Iron supplements, however, can cause unpleasant stomach pain, thereby aggravating morning sickness. One study found evidence that a fairly low supplemental dose of iron (20 mg daily) is nearly as effective for treating anemia of pregnancy as

40 mg or even 80 mg daily, and it is less likely to cause gastrointestinal side effects.

EBSCO CAM Review Board

FURTHER READING

Ensiyeh, J., and M. A. Sakineh. "Comparing Ginger and Vitamin B6 for the Treatment of Nausea and Vomiting in Pregnancy." *Midwifery* 25 (2009): 649-653.

Heazell, A., et al. "Acupressure for the In-Patient Treatment of Nausea and Vomiting in Early Pregnancy." *American Journal of Obstetrics and Gynecology* 194 (2006): 815-820.

Hsu, E., et al. "A Prospective Randomized Controlled Trial of Acupressure vs. Sham for Pregnancy-Related Nausea and Vomiting in the Emergency Department." *Academy of Emergency Medicine* 10 (2003): 437.

Keating, A., and R. A. Chez. "Ginger Syrup as an Antiemetic in Early Pregnancy." *Alternative Therapies in Health and Medicine* 8 (2002): 89-91.

Smith, C., et al. "A Randomized Controlled Trial of Ginger to Treat Nausea and Vomiting in Pregnancy." *Obstetrics and Gynecology* 103 (2004): 639-645.

Werntoft, E., and A. K. Dykes. "Effect of Acupressure on Nausea and Vomiting During Pregnancy." *Journal of Reproductive Medicine* 46 (2001): 835-839.

Zhou, S. J., et al. "Should We Lower the Dose of Iron When Treating Anaemia in Pregnancy?" *European Journal of Clinical Nutrition* 63 (2009): 183-190.

See also: Acupressure; Acupuncture; Biotin; Ginger; Iron; Nausea; Pregnancy support; Vitamin B$_6$; Women's health.

Motherwort

CATEGORY: Herbs and supplements

RELATED TERMS: *Leonurus artemisia, Leonurus cardiaca*

DEFINITION: Natural plant product used to treat specific health conditions.

PRINCIPAL PROPOSED USES: None

OTHER PROPOSED USES: Irregular or rapid heartbeat, uterine stimulant, pregnancy support

OVERVIEW

As its Latin name *cardiaca* suggests, motherwort has traditionally been used to treat heart conditions. The ancient Greeks and Romans employed motherwort to treat heart palpitations as well as depression, which they considered a problem of the heart. Centuries later, Europeans would believe motherwort helpful for infirmities of the heart but also considered the herb to have strengthening and stimulating effects on the uterus, using it to bring on a delayed menstrual period, as an aid during labor, and to relax a woman's womb after childbirth.

These uses of motherwort correspond well with those in traditional Chinese medicine, which employs the Asian variety, *Leonurus artemisia*, to treat menstrual disorders or to help a woman expel a dead fetus and placenta from her womb. In eastern China, women still drink a syrup made from motherwort to promote the recovery of the uterus after childbirth; the herb has a strong bitter taste, so visitors to a recovering mother often bring along sugar as a gift.

THERAPEUTIC DOSAGES

Germany's Commission E recommends a dose of 4.5 grams (g) of dried herb daily, or the equivalent, for the treatment of irregular or rapid heartbeat and in the treatment of hyperthyroidism (an overactive thyroid). Because these symptoms can be a sign of serious medical illness, motherwort should not be used except under medical supervision. Also, motherwort should not be combined with other heart medications, as they might interact unpredictably.

THERAPEUTIC USES

Germany's Commission E has authorized motherwort for the treatment of rapid or irregular heartbeat caused by anxiety and stress, and part of an overall treatment plan for hyperthyroidism, a condition that also causes irregular heartbeat. However, there is no real evidence to support these uses of the herb. The best that can be said is that in one test-tube study, motherwort slowed the beating of normal rat heart cells and inhibited the effects of substances that usually speed up heart cell contractions.

Two other test-tube studies suggest that leonurine, a compound found in some species of motherwort, may affect the uterus. One of these studies found that low concentrations of leonurine induced uterine contractions, but that higher concentrations inhibited contractions. These opposing effects might explain how motherwort could induce both labor and menstruation and yet could also relax the uterus after childbirth (as it is traditionally said to do). However,

COMPLEMENTARY AND ALTERNATIVE MEDICINE

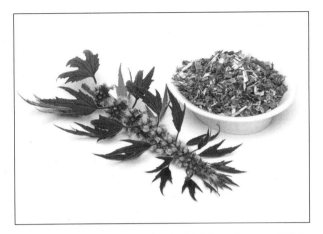

Motherwort stem next to a bowl of dried motherwort. (Bilda-gentur-online/TH Foto-Werbung /Photo Researchers, Inc.)

FURTHER READING

Blumenthal, M., ed. *The Complete German Commission E Monographs, Therapeutic Guide to Herbal Medicines.* Austin, Tex.: American Botanical Council, 1998.

Zou, Q. Z., et al. "Effect of Motherwort on Blood Hyperviscosity." *American Journal of Chinese Medicine* 17 (1989): 65-70.

See also: Chinese medicine; Herbal medicine.

until properly designed human studies are performed, it will be impossible to determine whether motherwort is actually safe or effective for these traditional uses.

One poorly designed study suggests that motherwort might improve blood circulation. Another study of equally low quality hints that motherwort might protect brain tissue in people who have had a stroke. One component of motherwort, ursolic acid, has been found to possess possible antiviral and antitumor properties; however, this extremely preliminary information should not be taken to mean that motherwort can fight viral infections or help treat cancer.

SAFETY ISSUES

The safety of motherwort has not been well studied; however, obvious side effects appear to be rare, except for occasional allergic reactions and gastrointestinal distress. Because of the herb's traditional use for uterine stimulation and the corroborating results of some test-tube studies, motherwort should not be used by pregnant women until further scientific investigation has been performed. In addition, preliminary animal evidence suggests that women with a history of breast cancer or those at high risk for developing it should avoid motherwort. Safety in young children, nursing women, or people with severe liver or kidney disease has not been established.

EBSCO CAM Review Board

Muira puama

CATEGORY: Herbs and supplements
RELATED TERMS: Potency wood, *Ptychopetalum olacoides, P. uncinatum, P. guyanna*
DEFINITION: Natural plant product used to treat specific health conditions.
PRINCIPAL PROPOSED USE: Male sexual dysfunction
OTHER PROPOSED USE: Enhancing mental function

OVERVIEW

Muira puama is a bush that is native to the Brazilian Amazon rainforest. Its bark and roots have been used traditionally for a variety of medicinal purposes, including impotence in men, loss of libido in women, nerve problems (including paralysis and tremor), anxiety, digestive problems, and arthritis.

THERAPEUTIC DOSAGES

Muira puama is generally taken in the form of a liquid alcohol extract. Label instructions for dosage should be followed.

THERAPEUTIC USES

Explorers brought muira puama to Europe, where it became popular primarily as a treatment for impotence. However, there has been no reliable scientific evaluation of the effectiveness of this herb. One study is commonly cited as showing that muira puama is more effective for impotence than the drug yohimbine (from the herb yohimbe). However, this study actually shows nothing. It was an open trial, in which all participants took muira puama. The researchers simply compared the benefits seen in this trial to the benefits seen in other trials in which people took yohimbine. From a scientific perspective, this is not permissible. The placebo effect is strong and varies from study to study. One can assume without even performing the experiment that if men with sexual dysfunction are given a treatment that they believe might help them, they will be helped. To determine whether muira puama is helpful for impotence would require a double-blind, placebo-controlled study. To determine whether it is more effective than yohimbine would require a double-blind study in which some people took muira puama and some took yohimbine. Because no double-blind studies of muira puama have been reported, use of this herb has to be regarded as entirely speculative.

Weak evidence hints that muira puama may be helpful for enhancing mental function by increasing brain levels of acetylcholine, but this evidence is far too preliminary to indicate effectiveness.

Safety Issues

From the limited evidence that is available, it does not appear that use of muira puama commonly causes significant side effects. However, comprehensive formal safety evaluation has not been conducted. For this reason, muira puama should not be used by pregnant or nursing women, young children, or individuals with severe liver or kidney disease.

EBSCO CAM Review Board

Further Reading

Siqueira, I. R., et al. "*Ptychopetalum olacoides*, a Traditional Amazonian 'Nerve Tonic,' Possesses Anticholinesterase Activity." *Pharmacology, Biochemistry, and Behavior* 75 (2003): 645-650.

See also: Herbal medicine; Sexual dysfunction in men.

Mullein

Category: Herbs and supplements
Related term: Grandmother's flannel, *Verbascum thapsus*
Definition: Natural plant product used to treat specific health conditions.
Principal proposed uses: None
Other proposed uses: Asthma, colds, cough, ear infection (topical, in combination with other herbs), sore throat

Overview

Also called grandmother's flannel for its thick, soft leaves, mullein is a common wildflower that can grow almost anywhere. It reaches several feet tall and puts up a spike of densely packed tiny yellow flowers. Mullein has served many purposes over the centuries, from making candlewicks to casting out evil spirits, but as medicine it was primarily used to treat diarrhea, respiratory diseases, and hemorrhoids.

Therapeutic Dosages

Mullein tea is made by adding 1 to 2 teaspoons of dried leaves and flowers to 1 cup of boiling water and steeping for ten minutes. The tea must be strained before drinking because fuzzy bits of the herb can stick in one's throat and cause an irritating tickle. Instead of drinking the tea, one can also breathe the steam from a boiling pot of mullein tea.

Mullein seeds contain the potentially toxic substance rotenone. For this reason, it is advisable to make sure there are no seeds in the mullein flowers used, or, alternatively, to use only the mullein leaf.

For ear infection pain, mullein oil products are brought to room temperature and dripped into the ear canal. However, it is advisable to make sure the eardrum is not punctured before dripping mullein oil into the ear.

Therapeutic Uses

Mullein contains a high proportion of mucilage (large sugar molecules); mucilage is generally thought to have a soothing effect. Mullein also contains saponins that may help loosen mucus. On this basis, mullein has been suggested as a treatment for asthma, colds, coughs, and sore throats. However, there is no meaningful evidence that it is useful for any of these conditions.

Mullein is traditionally combined with other herbs in oil preparations to soothe the pain of ear infections (otitis media, or middle ear infection, but not swimmer's ear, an external ear infection), and one study provides preliminary support for this use.

As with many herbs, test-tube studies have found that mullein can kill viruses on contact. In addition, an interesting but highly preliminary study suggests that mullein might help certain medications used for influenza work better. These findings, however, are far too scant to show that internal use of mullein will fight viral infections.

Oral mullein is said to be most effective when combined with other herbs of similar qualities, such as yerba santa, marshmallow, cherry bark, and elecampane, but there is no evidence to support this belief.

SCIENTIFIC EVIDENCE

Two double-blind trials enrolling a total of more than 250 children with eardrum pain caused by middle ear infection compared the effectiveness of an herbal preparation containing garlic, St. John's wort, and calendula against a standard anesthetic ear drop product (ametocaine and phenazone). The results indicated that the two treatments reduced pain to an equivalent extent. However, due to the strong placebo response in pain conditions, this study would have needed a placebo group to provide truly dependable evidence that the herb is effective. While herbal ear products may reduce pain, it is somewhat unlikely that they have any actual effect on the infection because of the barrier formed by the eardrum.

SAFETY ISSUES

Mullein leaves and flowers are on the U.S. Food and Drug Administration's list of substances generally recognized as safe (GRAS), and there have been no credible reports of serious adverse effects. However, mullein seeds contain the insecticide and fish poison rotenone. While rotenone is relatively safe in humans, it does present some risks. If mullein leaf products are contaminated with mullein seeds, long-term use might be harmful. For this reason, as well as a complete lack of formal safety investigation of mullein, young children, pregnant or nursing women, and those with severe liver or kidney disease should not use mullein for a prolonged period of time.

EBSCO CAM Review Board

FURTHER READING

Sarrell, E. M., H. A. Cohen, and E. Kahan. "Naturopathic Treatment for Ear Pain in Children." *Pediatrics* 111 (2003): E574-579.

Sarrell, E. M., A. Mandelberg, and H. A. Cohen. "Efficacy of Naturopathic Extracts in the Management of Ear Pain Associated with Acute Otitis Media." *Archives of Pediatric and Adolescent Medicine* 155 (2001): 796-799.

Serkedjieva, J. "Combined Antiinfluenza Virus Activity of *Flos verbasci* Infusion and Amantadine Derivatives." *Phytotherapy Research* 14 (2000): 571-574.

See also: Calendula; Ear infections; Elecampane; Garlic; Herbal medicine; Marshmallow; St. John's wort; Yerba santa.

Multiple sclerosis (MS)

CATEGORY: Condition
DEFINITION: Treatment of a disease that affects the fatty sheath that covers nerve fibers in the brain and spinal cord and leads to the slowing or blocking of nerve signals.
PRINCIPAL PROPOSED NATURAL TREATMENTS: None
OTHER PROPOSED NATURAL TREATMENTS: Bee venom, evening primrose oil, fish oil, ginkgo, linoleic acid, magnet therapy, neural therapy, phenylalanine, reflexology, threonine, vitamin B_{12}, vitamin D

INTRODUCTION

Multiple sclerosis (MS) is a disease affecting the fatty sheath that covers nerve fibers in the brain and spinal cord. This sheath, made of a substance called myelin, normally insulates the nerve fibers, allowing nerve impulses to move swiftly and efficiently between brain, spinal cord, and body. In MS, patchy areas of this insulating material are destroyed and replaced by scar tissue, which results in the slowing or blocking of nerve signals.

People with MS may experience symptoms such as blurred vision, muscle weakness and spasticity, difficulty walking, poor coordination, bladder problems, numbness, and fatigue. In its most common form, the disease begins between the ages of twenty and forty with an initial attack of symptoms followed by partial or complete remission. Further attacks usually follow and can eventually lead to progressive disability. Another form of the disease progresses more quickly.

Although the exact cause of MS is not known, scientists generally assume that MS is an autoimmune disease in which the immune system attacks the body's own myelin cells. Scientists theorize that something, perhaps a toxin or virus, triggers this autoimmune response in susceptible people. It appears that not all people are equally susceptible. Gene studies suggest that genetics plays a role in who gets the disease, but other factors too seem to be important. For example, MS tends to be more common the farther one travels from the equator. The disease is also more prevalent

---

Fats and MS

The Swank diet, in which unsaturated fats replace most saturated fat, is summarized here as an alternative treatment for MS.

- Saturated fat intake should not exceed 15 grams per day.
- Unsaturated fat (oils) should be kept to 20 to 50 grams per day.
- Avoid red meat for the first year of the diet.
- After the first year of the diet, 3 ounces of red meat can be consumed once per week.
- Dairy products must contain 1 percent or less butterfat, unless otherwise noted.
- Avoid processed foods containing saturated fat.
- Cod liver oil (1 teaspoon or equivalent capsules) and a multivitamin and mineral supplement are recommended daily.

Source: Adapted from http://www.swankmsdiet.org.

---

in societies with greater dietary intake of meat and animal fat, lower intake of unsaturated fats compared to saturated fats, and lower intake of fish. Not everyone agrees that all of these factors actually contribute to the disease. Some factors may simply be statistically associated with the actual cause.

There is no cure for MS, but several newer drugs, including two forms of the substance interferon (Avonex and Betaseron) and an unrelated drug, glatiramer acetate (Copaxone), appear able to reduce the frequency of relapses in people with certain forms of MS and slow the rate of progression of the disease. Other medications reduce the severity of acute attacks or treat specific symptoms such as muscle spasticity.

PROPOSED NATURAL TREATMENTS

While there are no well-documented natural treatments for multiple sclerosis, there are a few options that may provide some help. There is some evidence that changing the type and amount of fat in the diet might alter the course of MS. Based on observations from population studies linking diets lower in fat or saturated fat to lower rates of MS, physician R. L. Swank developed a special low-fat diet for MS in which unsaturated fats replace most saturated fat. This ap-

proach, called the Swank diet, has been used by many people with MS. When he analyzed the long-term effects of the diet on his patients, Swank found that those adhering closely to the diet for twenty to thirty-four years developed significantly less disability than those who ate more saturated fat. Because these were not controlled trials, they do not actually prove that the Swank diet works. Nonetheless, the possible connection between MS and fatty acids continues to arouse interest, and a variety of essential fatty acids have been proposed as possible treatments for MS. Although a link between fat intake and MS is intriguing, research has not provided clear-cut evidence that any of these treatments help.

Linoleic acid. One of the omega-6 essential fatty acids, linoleic acid, is found in high concentration in sunflower and safflower oil and in lower concentrations in most other vegetable oils. Several researchers have investigated whether linoleic acid in the form of sunflower seed oil can help MS, but the results of their research were equivocal.

Three groups of investigators performed double-blind studies, using olive oil as a placebo, to see if linoleic acid supplements could affect the symptoms or course of MS. Two of these studies (one involving 75 people, the other 116) found that those taking linoleic acid had shorter and less-severe attacks of MS compared to those taking placebo. However, in the two years of the trials, the frequency of attacks and overall levels of disability were not significantly affected. The third study of seventy-six people found that linoleic acid had no effects on either MS attacks or degrees of disability in 2.5 years, compared to olive oil.

Another researcher suggests that these studies may have been too short and that it may take far longer than two years for linoleic acid to exert its effects on myelin. Olive oil also contains important fatty acids; others have wondered if the olive oil could have been an effective treatment on its own, thereby obscuring the benefits of linoleic acid. Finally, another researcher who carefully examined the study reports found that linoleic acid might have been effective in those persons with less severe MS symptoms.

Although interesting, this type of after-the-fact analysis must be interpreted with caution. More studies are needed to confirm whether linoleic acid, taken early in the course of MS or at other times, has the power to prevent, delay, or improve disability. In the three double-blind studies, participants received

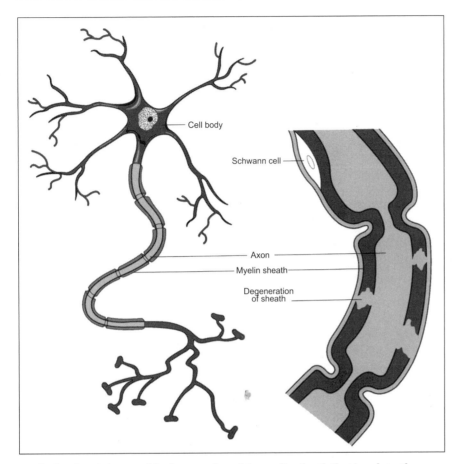

Multiple sclerosis is caused by degeneration of the myelin sheath that insulates the axons of nerve cells; a nerve cell is shown on the left.

17 to 20 grams (g) of linoleic acid per day, the equivalent of one ounce of sunflower seed oil.

Other essential fatty acids. There has been much excitement about other essential fatty acids as treatments for MS, including those found in fish oil (omega-3) and evening primrose oil (omega-6). However, evidence does not support this concept.

Blood tests among people with MS have found lower levels of omega-3 fatty acids in their body fluids and tissues compared to those without MS. This hints, but does not prove, that taking extra omega-3 fatty acids might help. Only double-blind, placebo-controlled studies can show that treatments actually work.

The only meaningful double-blind study of fish oil for MS failed to find evidence of benefit. In this two-year study of 292 people with MS, comparing fish oil's omega-3 fatty acids with an olive oil placebo, no sig-

nificant differences were seen between the two groups. Another study did find possible benefit with fish oil compared to olive oil in the relapsing-remitting form of MS. When fish oil was used in combination with a low-fat diet, participants showed benefits on some measures. However, the study was small, and the results were far from definitive. Similarly, while some researchers have suggested that gamma-linolenic acid might be beneficial in MS, what little evidence there is remains more negative than positive.

Threonine. Early evidence suggests that threonine, a naturally occurring amino acid, might be able to decrease the muscle spasticity that often occurs with MS. Two small double-blind studies found a modest but statistically significant improvement in muscle spasticity among people who took threonine compared to those who took placebo. In one study of twenty-six people with MS, the improvement was so slight after eight weeks of treatment that it was detectable by doctors but not by the participants themselves. In the other study, both researchers and a few of the thirty-three participants noticed improvement after two weeks of treatment, with some persons reporting fewer spasms and milder pain. This shorter trial that showed more improvement also used lower doses: 6 g daily of L-threonine, as opposed to 7.5 g daily of threonine. No significant side effects were noted in either study.

Vitamin B$_{12}$. Because several studies have found MS to be occasionally associated with vitamin B$_{12}$ deficiency, and lack of B$_{12}$ can cause neurological problems on its own, some doctors recommend that people with MS be screened for this condition. One preliminary study suggested that massive doses of B$_{12}$ could improve certain test results ("evoked potentials") but not disability in people with chronic progressive MS. A double-blind study of fifty people with MS found that high doses of injected hydroxocobalamin, a form of B_{12}, did not affect the course of disease or number of relapses.

Vitamin D. The human body normally obtains vitamin D in one of two ways: through diet or through exposure to the sun. More than one group of researchers has noted that populations in areas with less sunshine tend to have a higher incidence of MS, unless the residents of these areas commonly eat more fish that is rich in vitamin D. This has led to a theory that vitamin D might confer some protection against MS. No human studies have adequately tested this hypothesis, although one poorly designed study did investigate a combination of calcium, magnesium, and vitamin D given in the form of cod liver oil; the study found some benefit.

Phenylalanine and TENS. Phenylalanine is an essential amino acid, meaning that it is essential for life and that the human body cannot manufacture it from other chemicals. Humans normally obtain all the phenylalanine needed for nutritional purposes from high-protein foods. Supplemental phenylalanine has been studied for MS only in combination with another treatment called transcutaneous nerve stimulation (TENS), a portable electrical device used to decrease pain and muscle spasticity.

Two small double-blind trials compared phenylalanine to placebo among a total of sixteen people with MS being treated with TENS. In both studies, those treated with phenylalanine and TENS experienced less muscle spasticity, fewer bladder symptoms, and less depression after four weeks of treatment than those treated with TENS and placebo. These findings are somewhat difficult to interpret, but they tend to suggest that phenylalanine may be helpful in MS.

Other treatments. A special form of magnet therapy called PEMF (pulsed electromagnetic field therapy) has shown some promise for MS. In a two-month, double-blind, placebo-controlled study, thirty people with multiple sclerosis applied a real or a fake PEMF device to one of three acupuncture points on the shoulder, back, or hip. The study found statistically significant improvements in the treatment group, most notably in bladder control, hand function, and muscle spasticity.

One small double-blind trial suggests that neural therapy, a treatment related to acupuncture, might be helpful for MS. In addition, weak evidence hints that reflexology might be helpful.

The use of bee stings or injected bee venom for MS has generated a great deal of interest over the years, despite a lack of reliable research supporting its use. The one meaningful study, reported in 2005, failed to find any benefit. Other treatments suggested for MS include adenosine monophosphate, biotin, glycine, proteolytic enzymes, selenium, and vitamins B_1, C, and E, but little evidence supports these recommendations.

Although the herb ginkgo is sometimes suggested as a treatment for MS, there is no meaningful evidence that it works. One study reported as showing benefit was actually too small to provide meaningful results. Another double-blind study examined ginkgolide B, a chemical in ginkgo, for treating MS attacks, but it found no evidence of benefit.

EBSCO CAM Review Board

FURTHER READING

Johnson, S. K., et al. "The Effect of *Ginkgo biloba* on Functional Measures in Multiple Sclerosis." *Explore* (New York) 2 (2006): 19-24.

Lambert, C. P., et al. "Influence of Creatine Monohydrate Ingestion on Muscle Metabolites and Intense Exercise Capacity in Individuals with Multiple Sclerosis." *Archives of Physical Medicine and Rehabilitation* 84 (2003): 1206-1210.

Siev-Ner, I., et al. "Reflexology Treatment Relieves Symptoms of Multiple Sclerosis." *Multiple Sclerosis* 9 (2003): 356-361.

Weinstock-Guttman, B., et al. "Low Fat Dietary Intervention with Omega-3 Fatty Acid Supplementation in Multiple Sclerosis Patients." *Prostaglandins, Leukotrienes, and Essential Fatty Acids* 73 (2005): 397-404.

Wesselius, T., et al. "A Randomized Crossover Study of Bee Sting Therapy for Multiple Sclerosis." *Neurology* 65 (2005): 1764-1768.

See also: Fish oil; Gamma-linolenic acid; Phenylalanine; Vitamin B_{12}; Vitamin D.

Music therapy

CATEGORY: Therapies and techniques
RELATED TERMS: Music intervention, music intonation therapy

DEFINITION: The clinical and evidence-based use of music, including playing instruments and singing, in therapeutic practice.

PRINCIPAL PROPOSED USES: Aggressive behavior in children, autism, dementia, frontal lobe syndromes, language disabilities, movement disorders, stress, Tourette's syndrome

OTHER PROPOSED USES: Depression following brain surgery, post-traumatic stress disorder, stroke

OVERVIEW

The usefulness of music in medical settings has been recognized for more than two hundred years. It was initially used to distract patients from the monotony of a hospital stay, but the medical utility of music therapy is now being investigated as knowledge of the human brain increases. The National Association for Music Therapy and the American Music Therapy Association oversee professionals in the field of music therapy. In the United States, music-therapy education programs include multiple areas of study, clinical internships, and a national board certification examination.

Music therapy is frequently used in the treatment of persons with language deficits and in those persons recovering from strokes or traumatic brain injuries. Studies of healthy volunteers have identified the area of the brain that responds to and processes music; it is located within the right hemisphere. Other structures involved in experiencing music include the frontal lobe, limbic system, and imagery-related cortical regions of the temporal, parietal, and occipital lobes. The frontal lobe and the limbic system are also important structures in the formation of emotions, so the use of music may help persons with neurological conditions express themselves through means other than language.

As is well known, the left hemisphere of the brain controls language functions. Experts believe that music

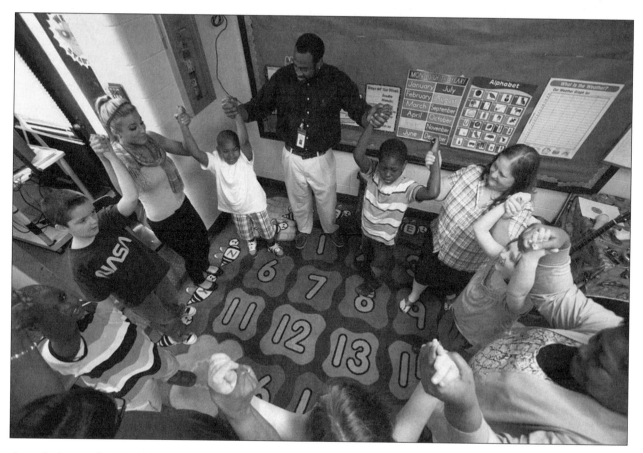

A music-therapy class for children with autism. (AP Photo)

intonation therapy (MIT), which combines music with singing, may help children with autism develop language skills. (Many children with autism have musical ability, so association of music with language may assist in the advancement of their language skills.) In the practice of MIT, the music component is removed after speech begins or improves; it is hoped that the child continues to develop. It is difficult, however, to determine if the development of language skills comes from music therapy or from the maturation of the child. Using the same MIT techniques, persons recovering from strokes or traumatic brain injuries who have suffered left-hemisphere damage may relearn speech using the right hemisphere of the brain.

Music therapy is also used with physical rehabilitation therapy and to alleviate symptoms similar to those of Parkinson's disease. During physical therapy, the rhythm of the music helps the person anticipate his or her next movement and move in a more smooth and natural manner. Persons with neurologic disorders suffering from shaking or spasms may be able to regain some control over their movements using rhythm to help them focus on regulating their movements.

Music therapy is often used as a pain management tool and in complex medical procedures in which the person must remain conscious. Music may alleviate mild to moderate pain through distraction, but it has not been effective for more painful procedures. It is unclear what, if any, effect music has on pain-detecting mechanisms in the brain. Alternative theories suggest that music therapy simply provides a distraction for a person with painful physical symptoms.

MECHANISM OF ACTION

Although the exact mechanism of action of music therapy on the brain has yet to be elucidated, it is believed to affect areas of the brain controlling the autonomous nervous system. Music may help regulate the endocrine system and the autonomic nervous system. There is evidence that music affects areas of the temporal lobe of the brain associated with seizures, because persons with epilepsy have occasionally had seizures induced by music or have had audio hallucinations preceding a seizure.

USES AND APPLICATIONS

In active music therapy, the therapist and patient participate in playing music, using instruments, or singing. In passive music therapy, music is played while the patient is in a relaxed state. There are five types of music therapy that may be used alone or in combination: receptive (listening to music to draw out an emotional response); compositional (the patient writes an original musical composition); improvisational (the music therapist and the patient spontaneously create music); re-creative (the patient learns to play an instrument); and activity (the patient and the therapist play musical games).

SCIENTIFIC EVIDENCE

The benefits of music therapy are difficult to quantify because each patient's treatment is customized based on the type and severity of disability or injury. No studies have compared the results of music therapy with other types of therapy, but there is a growing body of evidence in the form of controlled clinical studies seeming to support the effectiveness of music therapy.

In a study of forty-eight children with violent or aggressive behavior, twenty-four had participated in a music intervention program and twenty-four did not take part in any therapy. The music intervention therapy comprised two music classes each week for fifteen weeks and was conducted by a certified music therapist in a group setting. At the end of the study, children who participated in the music therapy sessions demonstrated statistically significant improvements in aggressive behavior and self-esteem, as measured by questionnaires completed by parents and teachers.

Another study evaluated eighty-seven elderly, institutionalized persons with cerebrovascular disease; fifty-five persons received music therapy for forty-five minutes each week for a minimum of ten weeks, and twenty-two persons received no therapy. At the conclusion of the study, persons in the music-therapy group demonstrated statistically significant decreases in acute chronic heart failure and in plasma levels of cytokines, adrenaline, and noradrenaline. These results suggest that music therapy may be a useful tool in preventing heart failure in persons with cerebrovascular disease.

CHOOSING A PRACTITIONER

Music therapists usually practice in conjunction with a medical or rehabilitation team. Music therapists in private practice receive clients through recommendations from either medical doctors or psychologists/psychiatrists.

SAFETY ISSUES

No adverse events have been reported in cases using music therapy.

Deborah A. Appello, M.S.

FURTHER READING

Accordino, Robert, Ronald Comer, and Wendy B. Heller. "Searching for Music's Potential: A Critical Examination of Research on Music Therapy with Individuals with Autism." *Research in Autism Spectrum Disorders* 1 (2007): 101-115.

American Music Therapy Association. "Music Therapy Makes a Difference." Available at http://www.musictherapy.org.

Bensimon, Moshe, Dorit Armir, and Yuval Wolf. "Drumming Through Trauma: Music Therapy with Post-traumatic Soldiers." *Arts in Psychotherapy* 35 (2008): 34-48.

Choi, Ae-Na, Myeong Soo Lee, and Jung-Sook Lee. "Group Music Intervention Reduces Aggression and Improves Self-Esteem in Children with Highly Aggressive Behavior." *Complementary and Alternative Medicine* 7, no. 2 (2008): 213-217.

Codding, Peggy, and Suzanne Hanser. "Music Therapy." In *Complementary and Integrative Medicine in Pain Management*, edited by Michael I. Weintraub. New York: Springer, 2008.

Okada, Kaoru, et al. "Effects of Music Therapy on Autonomic Nervous System Activity, Incidence of Heart Failure Events, and Plasma Cytokine and Catecholamine Levels in Elderly Patients with Cerebrovascular Disease and Dementia." *International Heart Journal* 50 (2009): 95-110.

Sacks, Oliver. "The Power of Music." *Brain* 129 (2006): 2528-2532.

See also: Aging; Aromatherapy; Art therapy; Autism spectrum disorders; Ayurveda; Color therapy; Crystal healing; Dance movement therapy; Energy medicine; Hypnotherapy; Magnet therapy; Mind/body medicine; Polarity therapy; Relaxation therapies; Stress; Traditional healing.

Myrrh

CATEGORY: Herbs and supplements
RELATED TERMS: *Commiphora molmol, Commiphora myrrha*

DEFINITION: Natural plant product used to treat specific health conditions.
PRINCIPAL PROPOSED USES: Mouth diseases (canker sores, gingivitis, halitosis, and sore throat)
OTHER PROPOSED USES: Eczema, schistosomiasis, ulcers

OVERVIEW

Myrrh is the dried resin of the tree *Commiphora myrrha*. Native to Somalia and eastern Ethiopia, myrrh has a long history of traditional use in perfumes and incense. Additionally, it has perhaps an equally long history as a medicinal treatment, primarily for conditions of the mouth, such as canker sores, gum disease, halitosis, and sore throat.

C. myrrha is not the same plant as the similarly named *C. mukul*. The latter is the source of guggulsterones, which have been proposed for use in treating elevated cholesterol.

THERAPEUTIC DOSAGES

When used for mouth conditions, tincture of myrrh may be applied directly to canker sores or inflamed gums. It can also be diluted in water and used as a gargle. When taken internally, a typical dose of myrrh is 1 gram (g) of resin three times daily.

THERAPEUTIC USES

Modern herbalists continue to use myrrh for its traditional uses related to the mouth. In addition, it has been advocated for treatment of eczema and stomach ulcers. However, there is no meaningful scientific evidence that the herb provides any benefits when used for these or any other purposes.

Beginning in 2001, a pharmaceutical-grade myrrh product known as Mirazid was marketed for treatment of the disease schistosomiasis. Caused by a type of flatworm, schistosomiasis is common in Africa as well as parts of Asia and South America. It is a seriously debilitating illness, and considerable attention has been devoted to addressing it. China, for example, eliminated the illness within its borders by means of a massive countrywide effort involving much of the country's human population; working by hand, the Chinese people destroyed the entire population of the snail species that carries schistosomiasis. However, while this approach was successful, use of myrrh was not. It appears that the marketing of Mirazid as a schistosomiasis treatment was premature. A few highly preliminary studies had shown benefit, but subsequent full-scale trials found it to be far less effective than conventional treatment, and perhaps not effective at all.

SAFETY ISSUES

In studies of myrrh for treatment of schistosomiasis, no significant side effects were identified. However, comprehensive safety studies have not been performed. Maximum safe doses in pregnant or nursing women, or people with severe liver of kidney disease have not been determined.

EBSCO CAM Review Board

FURTHER READING

Barakat, R., H. Elmorshedy, and A. Fenwick. "Efficacy of Myrrh in the Treatment of Human Schistosomiasis Mansoni." *American Journal of Tropical Medicine and Hygiene* 73 (2005): 365-367.

Botros, S., et al. "Efficacy of Mirazid in Comparison with Praziquantel in Egyptian Schistosoma Mansoni-Infected School Children and Households." *American Journal of Tropical Medicine and Hygiene* 72 (2005): 119-123.

See also: Herbal medicine.

N

N-acetyl cysteine

CATEGORY: Herbs and supplements

RELATED TERMS: NAC, N-acetylcysteine

DEFINITION: Natural substance of the human body used as a supplement to treat specific health conditions.

PRINCIPAL PROPOSED USES: Angina pectoris (in combination with conventional treatment), chronic bronchitis, preventing influenza

OTHER PROPOSED USES: Chemical dependency (cocaine), chemotherapy support, chronic blepharitis, colon cancer prevention, female infertility caused by polycystic ovary syndrome, human immunodeficiency virus support, liver failure, pathological gambling (gambling addiction), protection against kidney damage caused by contrast agents, schizophrenia, Sjögren's syndrome

OVERVIEW

N-acetyl cysteine (NAC) is a specially modified form of the dietary amino acid cysteine. When taken orally, NAC is thought to help the body make the important antioxidant enzyme glutathione. It has shown promise for a number of conditions, especially chronic bronchitis.

REQUIREMENTS AND SOURCES

There is no daily requirement for NAC, and it is not found in food.

THERAPEUTIC DOSAGES

Optimal levels of NAC have not been determined. The amount used in studies has varied from 250 to 1,500 milligrams (mg) daily.

It has been suggested that NAC may increase excretion of trace minerals; some evidence, however, suggests that this effect is too minimal to make a real difference. Prudence suggests that individuals taking NAC for an extended period of time should also consider taking a standard multivitamin-multimineral supplement.

THERAPEUTIC USES

Significant but not entirely consistent evidence suggests that regular use of NAC is helpful for individuals with chronic bronchitis (a condition commonly associated with smoking and emphysema) in reducing frequency of acute flare-ups of the condition. Regular use of NAC may help prevent influenza, possibly by stimulating immunity.

One substantial study found evidence that NAC may augment the effectiveness of clomiphene, a drug used for female infertility, in women with polycystic ovary syndrome. Another study found NAC far less effective for this purpose than the drug metformin; however, it still could have provided some benefit.

Mixed evidence suggests that NAC may also enhance the effectiveness of the drug nitroglycerin, used for the treatment of angina. However, severe headaches can develop as a side effect. NAC may be helpful in a life-threatening condition called acute respiratory distress syndrome. Very high dosages of NAC are used in hospitals as a conventional treatment for acetaminophen poisoning. One should not attempt to self-treat angina, acute respiratory distress syndrome, or acetaminophen poisoning. Medical supervision is absolutely essential because of the very real risk of death in these conditions. According to some, but not all, studies, NAC may be helpful for preventing complications that occur during cardiac surgery.

Some research has also suggested that NAC may be helpful for Sjögren's syndrome (a disease that causes dry eyes, among other symptoms), chronic blepharitis (ongoing infections of the eyelid), severe liver disease, and reducing the side effects of the cancer chemotherapy drug ifosfamide. Other evidence hints that NAC might help offset the carcinogenic effects of smoking and reduce colon cancer risk. Weak evidence hints that NAC might reduce some side effects (specifically, cardiac toxicity and hair loss) caused by the cancer chemotherapy drug doxorubicin.

NAC has been proposed as supportive therapy for

HIV. Despite some intriguing results, overall the evidence is inconsistent at best. Several studies have suggested that NAC may be beneficial as an aid to treating various mental health disorders, including schizophrenia, cocaine dependence, and even pathological gambling.

To get more information from certain types of X rays, radiologists often administer substances called contrast agents. However, contrast agents can damage the kidney. It has been suggested that NAC can help protect the kidney from such damage; however, the most recent and best-designed study failed to find any benefit.

One double-blind trial failed to find NAC helpful for head and neck or lung cancer. Studies have also failed to find NAC helpful for treating viral hepatitis or preeclampsia, or enhancing sports performance.

SCIENTIFIC EVIDENCE

Chronic bronchitis. Individuals who have smoked cigarettes for many years eventually develop deterioration in their lungs leading to various symptoms, including chronic production of thick mucus. This so-called chronic bronchitis (closely related to chronic obstructive pulmonary disease) tends to flare up periodically into severe acute attacks possibly requiring hospitalization.

Regular use of NAC may diminish the number of these attacks. A review and meta-analysis selected eight double-blind, placebo-controlled trials of NAC for chronic bronchitis. The results of these studies, involving a total of about 1,400 individuals, suggest that NAC taken daily at a dose of 400 to 1,200 mg can reduce the number of acute attacks of severe bronchitis. However, the largest and best of these studies, a three-year double-blind, placebo-controlled trial of 523 people, failed to find that use of NAC at a dose of 600 mg daily reduced exacerbations or delayed the typical progressive worsening of lung function. It is not clear how NAC works (if it does); the old concept that it acts by thinning mucus may not be correct.

Influenza. In a double-blind, placebo-controlled study of 262 seniors, regular use of NAC at dose of 600 mg twice daily helped prevent the development of influenza-like illnesses. Over the six-month study period, only 25 percent of participants taking NAC developed flulike symptoms, compared with 79 percent in the placebo group, a statistically significant difference.

Blood tests suggested that NAC did not prevent influenza infection; about as many people showed antibodies indicating influenza infection in the NAC group as in the placebo group. Rather, the supplement seemed to reduce the rate at which influenza infection became severe enough to cause noticeable symptoms. Tests of immune function hinted that NAC functioned by increasing the strength of the immune response.

Angina pectoris. Angina pectoris is a squeezing feeling in the chest caused by inadequate blood supply to the heart. It can be a precursor of heart attacks. People with angina often use the drug nitroglycerin to relieve symptoms. One four-month double-blind, placebo-controlled study of two hundred people with heart disease found that the combination of nitroglycerin and NAC significantly reduced the incidence of heart attacks and other severe heart problems. NAC alone and nitroglycerin alone were not as effective. The only problem was that the combination of nitroglycerin and NAC caused severe headaches in many participants. This effect has been seen in other studies as well.

NAC may also help in cases of nitroglycerin tolerance, a condition in which the drug becomes less effective over time. In a small double-blind study of thirty-two people with angina, tolerance developed in fifteen of sixteen individuals who took nitroglycerin only, but in just five of sixteen individuals who took nitroglycerin plus 2 grams of NAC daily. However, other studies have found no benefit.

Female infertility. In a double-blind, placebo-controlled study of 150 women suffering from infertility who had not responded to treatment with the fertility drug clomiphene, use of NAC at 1,200 mg daily significantly augmented the effectiveness of clomiphene. Treatment was begun on day three of the menstrual cycle and continued for five days. About 20 percent of women in the NAC plus clomiphene group became pregnant, compared with 0 percent in the placebo plus clomiphene group.

Acute respiratory distress syndrome. A double-blind, placebo-controlled clinical trial compared the effectiveness of NAC, Procysteine (a synthetic cysteine building-block drug), and a placebo in forty-six people with acute respiratory distress syndrome. This catastrophic lung condition can occur when an unconscious person inhales a small amount of his or her own vomit. Both NAC and Procysteine reduced the severity of the condition in some people (compared with a placebo). However, overall it did not reduce the number of deaths.

Colon cancer prevention. A preliminary double-blind, placebo-controlled study of NAC enrolled sixty-two individuals, each of whom had had a polyp removed from the colon. The abnormal growth of polyps is closely associated with the development of colon cancer. In this study, the potential anticancer benefits of NAC treatment were evaluated by taking a biopsy of the rectum. Individuals taking NAC at 800 mg daily for twelve weeks showed more normal cells in the biopsied tissue compared with those in the placebo group.

SAFETY ISSUES

NAC appears to be a very safe supplement when taken alone, although one study in rats suggests that sixty to one hundred times the normal dose can cause liver injury. The combination of nitroglycerin and NAC can cause severe headaches. Safety in young children, women who are pregnant or nursing, and individuals with severe liver or kidney disease has not been established.

EBSCO CAM Review Board

FURTHER READING

Cakir, O., et al. "N-acetylcysteine Reduces Lung Reperfusion Injury After Deep Hypothermia and Total Circulatory Arrest." *Journal of Cardiac Surgery* 19 (2004): 221-225.

Dhalla, N. S., et al. "Status of Myocardial Antioxidants in Ischemia-Reperfusion Injury." *Cardiovascular Research* 47 (2000): 446-456.

Eren, N., et al. "Effects of N-acetylcysteine on Pulmonary Function in Patients Undergoing Coronary Artery Bypass Surgery with Cardiopulmonary Bypass." *Perfusion* 18 (2003): 345-350.

Fischer, U. M., et al. "Myocardial Apoptosis Prevention by Radical Scavenging in Patients Undergoing Cardiac Surgery." *Journal of Thoracic and Cardiovascular Surgery* 128 (2004): 103-108.

Fischer, U. M., P. Tossios, and U. Mehlhorn. "Renal Protection by Radical Scavenging in Cardiac Surgery Patients." *Current Medical Research and Opinion* 21 (2005): 1161-1164.

Larowe, S. D., et al. "Is Cocaine Desire Reduced by N-acetylcysteine?" *American Journal of Psychiatry* 164 (2007): 1115-1117.

Tossios, P., et al. "N-acetylcysteine Prevents Reactive Oxygen Species-Mediated Myocardial Stress in Patients Undergoing Cardiac Surgery." *Journal of Thoracic and Cardiovascular Surgery* 126 (2003): 1513-1520.

See also: Angina; Bronchitis; Cancer risk reduction; Herbal medicine; Infertility, female.

Nails, brittle

CATEGORY: Condition
RELATED TERMS: Onychorrhexis, onychoschisis, onychoschizia
DEFINITION: Treatment of a condition of the fingernails that leads to brittleness.
PRINCIPAL PROPOSED NATURAL TREATMENT: Biotin
OTHER PROPOSED NATURAL TREATMENTS: Calcium, cysteine, gelatin, horsetail (*Equisetum arvense*), iron, silicon, vitamin A, zinc

INTRODUCTION

Brittle fingernails are a common condition, occurring in about 20 percent of people and more commonly in women. Brittle nails usually break or peel off in horizontal layers, starting at the nail's free end. The term "brittle nails" can also refer to a condition in which lengthwise splits appear in the nail. In either case, the nail's structure is faulty.

Brittleness in the nail may be caused by trauma, such as repeated wetting and drying, repeated exposure to detergents and water, and excessive exposure to harsh solvents, such as those found in nail polish remover. If the nails are regularly exposed to such stresses, it may be worth trying protective gloves when washing dishes and doing other chores. In the case of nail polish remover, gentler, less toxic brands are available. One should check with retailers of natural cosmetic products.

Nail brittleness may also be caused by an underlying medical condition such as Raynaud's disease, by low thyroid function (hypothyroidism), or by lung conditions. Other possible causes include skin diseases (psoriasis, lichen planus, alopecia areata) and

The Anatomy of a Nail

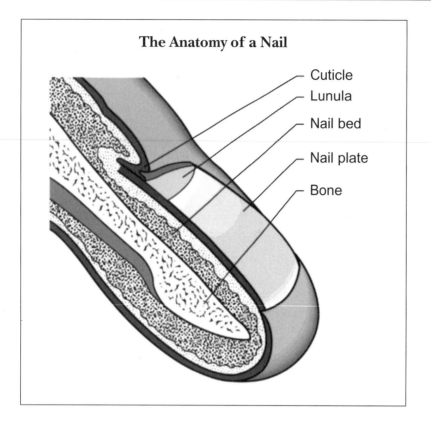

- Cuticle
- Lunula
- Nail bed
- Nail plate
- Bone

prove their microscopic structure. To arrive at their results, the researchers used a scanning electron microscope to examine the effects of biotin in eight women with brittle nails who were given 2.5 milligrams (mg) of biotin daily for six to nine months. An additional twenty-four persons were also studied; ten served as controls and fourteen were examined in a way that makes the interpretation of their results questionable. Because all nail clippings were examined without the researchers being aware of whose clippings they were looking at, these results have some validity. However, the study was too small to allow definitive conclusions.

Two small open studies also reported benefits with biotin supplementation. However, because there was no control group in either study, the results cannot be taken as reliable.

OTHER PROPOSED NATURAL TREATMENTS

The mineral silicon has been widely marketed for decades as a treatment for brittle nails, brittle hair, and aging skin. However, the first potentially meaningful clinical trial was not reported until 2004. In this double-blind, placebo-controlled study of fifty women, the use of 10 mg daily of silicon (as orthosilicic acid) for twenty weeks did appear to improve the condition of the women's nails. However, this study, performed by the manufacturer of a silicon product, leaves much to be desired in design and reporting.

The herb horsetail (*Equisetum arvense*), naturally high in silicon, is also sometimes mentioned as a treatment for brittle nails A number of other nutritional therapies also have been tried, including calcium, cysteine, gelatin-containing preparations, iron, vitamin A, and zinc. However, there is no evidence that any of these treatments are effective.

EBSCO CAM Review Board

endocrine disorders, tuberculosis, Sjögren's syndrome, and malnutrition. Selenium poisoning can also cause brittle nails.

Because of all these possibilities, it is important to rule out a serious underlying problem before trying nutritional or herbal treatments for brittle nails. If a medical cause for this condition is not found, it may be worth considering some of the approaches described here.

PRINCIPAL PROPOSED NATURAL TREATMENTS

Although no herb or supplement has been proven effective for brittle nails, there is some evidence that the B vitamin biotin might help. Animal studies suggest that biotin supplementation can be helpful for deformed hooves in horses and pigs. Because animal hooves are made of keratin, the same substance from which human nails are made, these findings have encouraged researchers to study the effects of biotin on brittle nails in humans.

Preliminary evidence from a small controlled study suggests that biotin may increase the thickness of brittle nails, reduce their tendency to split, and im-

FURTHER READING

Baran, R., et al., eds. *Baran and Dawber's Diseases of the Nails and Their Management*. 3d ed. Malden, Mass.: Blackwell Science, 2001.

Biotin Food Sources

Food	Serving Size	Biotin (micrograms)
Yeast	1 packet (7 grams)	1.4-14
Bread, whole wheat	1 slice	0.02-6
Egg, cooked	1 large	13-25
Cheese, cheddar	1 ounce	0.4-2
Liver, cooked	3 ounces	27-35
Pork, cooked	3 ounces	2-4
Salmon, cooked	3 ounces	4-5
Avocado	1 whole	2-6
Raspberries	1 cup	0.2-2
Cauliflower, raw	1 cup	0.2-4

Barel, A., et al. "Effect of Oral Intake of Choline-Stabilized Orthosilicic Acid on Skin, Nails, and Hair in Women with Photodamaged Skin." *Archives of Dermatological Research* 297 (2005): 147-153.

Hochman, L. G., R. K. Scher, and M. S. Meyerson. "Brittle Nails: Response to Daily Biotin Supplementation." *Cutis* 51 (1993): 303-305.

See also: Biotin; Calcium; Hypothyroidism; Raynaud's phenomenon.

Narcotic addiction

CATEGORY: Condition

RELATED TERMS: Drug addiction, cocaine addiction, cocaine dependency, heroin addiction, heroin dependency, methamphetamine addiction

DEFINITION: Treatment of addictions to narcotics, including cocaine, heroine, and methamphetamine.

PRINCIPAL PROPOSED NATURAL TREATMENTS: None

OTHER PROPOSED NATURAL TREATMENTS: Acupuncture, *Bacopa monniera* (brahmi), *Ginkgo biloba*, lobelia, N-acetylcysteine, passionflower, rosemary, velvet antler, yoga

INTRODUCTION

The family of drugs loosely known as narcotics includes chemicals in the opiate family, such as heroin, along with cocaine and variations of methamphetamine (or speed). All of these drugs produce intense psychological symptoms during withdrawal, and most cause physical symptoms, making them some of the most addictive substances known.

The process of overcoming narcotic addiction involves short-term assistance to ease the immediate withdrawal period, long-term psychological work to induce behavior change, and, in some cases, maintenance treatment with long-acting narcotics such as methadone. New classes of medications are under investigation for aiding withdrawal.

PROPOSED NATURAL TREATMENTS

There are no well-established natural treatments to aid the treatment of drug addiction, but some have shown some promise.

Passionflower. The herb passionflower is thought to have mild sedative properties and has been suggested as an aid to drug withdrawal. A fourteen-day double-blind trial enrolled sixty-five men addicted to opiate drugs and compared the effectiveness of a blend of passionflower and the drug clonidine to clonidine alone. Clonidine is used widely to assist in narcotic withdrawal. It effectively reduces physical symptoms, such as increased blood pressure. However, it does not help emotional symptoms, such as drug-craving, anxiety, irritability, agitation, and depression. These symptoms can be quite severe, and they often cause enrollees in drug treatment programs to end participation.

In this fourteen-day study, the use of passionflower with clonidine significantly eased the emotional aspects of withdrawal compared to the use of clonidine alone. However, more research is necessary to prove this treatment effective.

Acupuncture. Although some animal studies suggest that various forms of acupuncture may have some benefits for chemical dependency, study results in humans have been mixed at best, with the largest studies reporting no benefits. For example, while benefits were seen in a much smaller single-blind trial, a large placebo-controlled trial that evaluated 620 cocaine-dependent adults found acupuncture no more effective than sham acupuncture or relaxation training. Similarly, a single-blind, placebo-controlled study of 236 persons found no benefit from ear acupuncture for cocaine addiction. In a similar study involving heroin addicts, a high dropout rate made the results difficult to interpret. Finally, in a placebo-controlled trial involving eighty-three people addicted to drugs attending a methadone detoxification clinic, the addition of ear acupuncture did not improve withdrawal symptoms or cravings. Methadone, a relatively weak narcotic, is commonly used to treat narcotic addition over the long-term.

Other natural approaches. One study provides weak evidence that the substance N-acetylcysteine might be helpful for treating cocaine dependence. Similarly weak evidence hints at potential benefits for opiate addiction with the herbs brahmi (*Bacopa monniera*), rosemary, and velvet antler.

Weak evidence hints that the substance lobeline from the herb lobelia might offer benefit for methamphetamine addiction. Also, a ten-week double-blind trial failed to find ginkgo helpful for cocaine dependence. Another study failed to find hatha yoga helpful for enhancing the effectiveness of a methadone maintenance treatment for heroin addiction.

In a review of twenty-one studies involving almost three thousand persons, researchers concluded that Chinese herbal medicine was as effective as commonly prescribed medications for drug withdrawal symptoms in heroin addicts. They could not draw any conclusions, however, regarding what specific herbs were most beneficial.

EBSCO CAM Review Board

FURTHER READING

Akhondzadeh, S., et al. "Passionflower in the Treatment of Opiates Withdrawal." *Journal of Clinical Pharmacy and Therapeutics* 26 (2001): 369-373.

Bearn, J., et al. "Auricular Acupuncture as an Adjunct to Opiate Detoxification Treatment: Effects on Withdrawal Symptoms." *Journal of Substance Abuse Treatment* 36 (2009): 345-349.

Kampman, K., et al. "A Pilot Trial of Piracetam and *Ginkgo biloba* for the Treatment of Cocaine Dependence." *Addictive Behaviors* 28 (2003): 437-448.

Larowe, S. D., et al. "Is Cocaine Desire Reduced by N-acetylcysteine?" *American Journal of Psychiatry* 164 (2007): 1115-1117.

Liu, T. T., et al. "A Meta-analysis of Chinese Herbal Medicine in Treatment of Managed Withdrawal from Heroin." *Cellular and Molecular Neurobiology* 29 (2009): 17-25.

Margolin, A., et al. "Acupuncture for the Treatment of Cocaine Addiction." *Journal of the American Medical Association* 287 (2002): 55-57.

See also: Alcoholism; Benzodiazepine addiction and dependency; Mental health; Opioid addiction and dependency; Smoking addiction; Smoking and nutrition.

National Center for Complementary and Alternative Medicine (NCCAM)

CATEGORY: Organizations and legislation

DEFINITION: A U.S. government scientific and informational resource on the efficacy and safety of complementary and alternative medicine for consumers, practitioners, and policymakers.

DATE: Founded 1999

OVERVIEW

The National Center for Complementary and Alternative Medicine (NCCAM) is a resource for health consumers and practitioners for information and guidance on complementary and alternative medicine (CAM). NCCAM is a government agency, under the umbrella of the U.S. Department of Health and Human Services (DHHS) as part of the National Institutes of Health (NIH).

NCCAM's principal mission is to apply the scientific method of experimentation and verification to various CAM practices to best inform the public, health care providers, and lawmakers about the efficacy of CAM procedures and therapies. Scientific evidence enhances decision making, and the organization helps consumers make informed choices.

NCCAM'S WEB PRESENCE

The central mission of the organization is not clear in its name, but that mission becomes clear when one visits its Web site. For example, the home page presents several subsection links, including Topics A-Z, which is described as "research based info from acupuncture to zinc." Other subsections are What Is CAM?; Be Informed, to "learn how to find out what's safe and effective"; and Herbs at a Glance, "presenting the uses and side effects of herbs and botanicals." Another section provides Resources for Health Professionals. Information in Spanish is available by selecting that option.

A news menu links visitors to CAM-related news articles. Referenced articles include "Beware of Fraudulent Dietary Supplements and Tea Tree Oil: Uses, Side Effects, Research." Other highlighted resources focus on hepatitis C, chronic pain, and colds and influenza. Other articles include "Mindfulness Meditation Is Associated with Structural Changes in the Brain" and "Analysis of National Survey Shows CAM Use in People with Pain or Neurological Conditions." The page also features advanced research options, so that users can search by topic or date, or both

Most of the linked resources present on the home page reflect the organization's mission. The site's interface is well organized, and it highlights significant information on the role of science in CAM.

Information on the site can be shared by users through links to social media such as Twitter, Facebook, Myspace, StumbleUpon, Digg, and Delicious. Users can receive CAM-related information updates through email, RSS (real simple syndication), Twitter, or Facebook. A search function allows for keyword searches of all NCCAM sections and databases.

FUNDING AND OTHER CONSIDERATIONS

NCCAM is a federally funded organization that has been authorized by the U.S. Congress to accept tax-deductible donations. Funding sources can be potential influences on an organization's point of view. Detailed funding information helps determine the role, if any, of the direction and goals of NCCAM. Transparency about donors, donation amounts, and NCCAM policy regarding donations would help clarify whether potential conflicts of interest exist or could arise.

SCIENCE AND NCCAM

NCCAM's emphasis on science helps to legitimize CAM practices. The science appeals to health care professionals and consumers who desire a critical analysis of CAM treatments. Rigorous scientific methodology includes asking a question or stating a hypoth-

esis, testing the hypothesis through experimentation, collecting data, and applying the experiment's results to the hypothesis or original question. Questions can be answered, and a better approximation of the truth of a situation can be formulated, if the experimental results are reproducible and if they support the original hypothesis.

The research section of the Web site includes subsections with information on policies, clinical trials, and sponsored research. Clicking on the sponsored research section brings up information on NCCAM-funded research for a given fiscal year.

The grants section includes subsections on award types, types of research funded, and funding opportunities. Selecting the funding options brings up information related to the NIH "Guide for Grants and Contracts." Research funding priorities include certain areas of special interest, such as CAM use for chronic pain, CAM's role in improving health and wellness, and the role of CAM in quality-of-life issues.

The training section includes subsections for online lectures and continuing education. Online lecture topics include herbs and other dietary supplements, mind/body medicine, aging, and the effects of natural products. Each lecture is accompanied by transcripts, online tests, additional resource links, and a certificate of completion. Medical professionals, including doctors and nurses, can register to earn continuing education credits after completing activities and testing related to materials available in the training section.

The site's information is presented as either supported by science or rejected by science. The site also lists potential alternative therapies and identifies areas requiring more study and investigation. The site is comprehensive, covering herbs, therapies, and treatments.

The site also provides links to scientific literature reviews, systematic reviews, meta-analyses, and relevant articles from well-regarded medical journals. For acupuncture, articles include "Acupuncture for Chronic Low-Back Pain" from the *New England Journal of Medicine* and "Integrative Oncology in Lung Cancer" from *Chest*.

CONCLUSION

NCCAM's mission is to "define, through rigorous scientific investigation, the usefulness and safety of complementary and alternative medicine

Important Events in the History of NCCAM

October 1991—The U.S. Congress passes legislation that provides $2 million in funding for fiscal year 1992 to establish an office within the National Institutes of Health (NIH) to investigate and evaluate promising unconventional medical practices.

September 1992—A Workshop on Alternative Medicine is convened to discuss the state of the art of major areas of alternative medicine and to direct attention to priority areas for future research.

June 1993—The NIH Revitalization Act of 1993 formally establishes the Office of Alternative Medicine (OAM) within the NIH to facilitate the study and evaluation of complementary and alternative medical (CAM) practices and to disseminate the resulting information to the public.

October 1996—A Public Information Clearinghouse is established.

November 1996—OAM is designated a World Health Organization Collaborating Center for Traditional Medicine.

October 1998—NCCAM is established by Congress under the Omnibus Appropriations Act of 1999. This bill amends Title IV of the Public Health Service Act and elevates the status of the OAM to an NIH Center.

February 1999—The U.S. Secretary of Health and Human Services (HHS) signs the organizational change memorandum creating NCCAM and making it the twenty-fifth independent component of NIH.

February 2001—NCCAM and the National Library of Medicine launch CAM on PubMed, a comprehensive Internet source of research-based information on CAM.

May 2004—NCCAM and the National Center for Health Statistics of the U.S. Centers for Disease Control and Prevention announce findings from the largest nationally representative survey to date on Americans'

use of CAM (part of the 2002 National Health Interview Survey).

January 2005—The National Academies' Institute of Medicine releases a report, *Complementary and Alternative Medicine in the United States*, which was requested by NCCAM and federal partners. The report focuses on the scientific and policy implications of the widespread use of CAM.

May 2007—NCCAM establishes a Complementary and Integrative Medicine Consult Service at the NIH Clinical Center.

June 2008—NCCAM launches "Time to Talk," an educational campaign to encourage health consumers and their health care providers to openly discuss the use of CAM.

December 2008—An NCCAM-supported supplement on CAM in the 2007 National Health Interview Survey yields the first nationally representative data on children's use of CAM and on trends in adult CAM use.

July 2009—The first nationally representative figures are released on how much Americans spend on CAM, from a nationwide government study cofunded by NCCAM. In 2007, Americans spent nearly $34 billion out-of-pocket on CAM, of which about two-thirds was for self-care.

September 2010—NCCAM launches the *Clinical Digest*, a monthly e-newsletter that offers evidence-based information on CAM, including scientific literature searches, summaries of NCCAM-funded research, and fact sheets for consumers.

February 2011—NCCAM releases its third strategic plan, *Exploring the Science of Complementary and Alternative Medicine: Third Strategic Plan 2011-2015*. The plan presents a series of goals and objectives to guide NCCAM in determining priorities for future research in CAM.

---

interventions and their roles in improving health and health care." By carrying out this mission, the organization plays a vital role in the health of consumers, in the education of practitioners, and in the making of health policy.

Richard P. Capriccioso, M.D.

FURTHER READING

Capriccioso, Richard P. "Complementary and Alternative Therapies." In *Salem Health: Cancer*, vol. 1, edited by Richard K. Wright. Pasadena, Calif.: Salem Press, 2008. A comprehensive review and survey of complementary and alternative categories and treatments, with cancer treatment emphasis. Some CAM organizational information adapted from NCCAM resources is utilized in this article.

Fontaine, K. L. *Complementary and Alternative Therapies for Nursing Practice.* 2d ed. Upper Saddle River, N.J.: Pearson/Prentice Hall, 2005. Integrated nursing practice and CAM sections are presented in this complementary and alternative medicine textbook. Alternative and complementary health care resources are compiled and can be used as supplements and/or alternative viewpoints to NCCAM information.

Kantor, M. "The Role of Rigorous Scientific Evaluation in the Use and Practice of Complementary and Alternative Medicine." *Journal of the American College of Radiology* 6, no. 4 (2009): 254-262. Evaluates the scope and mission of NCCAM and examines the need for scientific evaluation in CAM in general.

National Center for Complementary and Alternative Medicine. http://nccam.nih.gov.

See also: Alternative versus traditional medicine; American Academy of Anti-Aging Medicine; CAM on PubMed; Clinical trials; Codex Alimentarius Commission; Dietary Supplement Health and Education Act of 1994; Double-blind, placebo-controlled studies; Food and Drug Administration; National Health Federation; Office of Cancer Complementary and Alternative Medicine; Office of Dietary Supplements; Regulation of CAM; Scientific method.

National Health Federation

CATEGORY: Organizations and legislation

DEFINITION: A nonprofit organization that promotes health education for consumers and seeks to eliminate certain government restrictions on food, water, vitamins, supplements, and alternative medical techniques.

DATE: Founded in 1955

OVERVIEW

The mission of the National Health Federation (NHF) comprises twelve "health-freedom rights" that guide the organization. These rights, which are presented as basic human rights, include the right to control one's own body, to seek and receive alternative medicine, and to keep such information private. Central to these rights is personal freedom of choice, which includes the right to opt out of mandatory childhood vaccines, the right to utilize vitamins and supplements without prescription or regulation, and, ultimately, the right of every person to make health decisions without government restrictions.

MEMBERSHIP

NHF members receive a subscription to the quarterly magazine *Health Freedom News*, access to the NHF's alternative health care provider referral list, and representation from a Washington, D.C., lobbyist in pursuit of NHF health goals. Although NHF is primarily focused on health issues in the United States, its membership, affiliate organizations, and advisory board are international in scope. The NHF boasts of its elite membership in the Codex Alimentarius Commission, the highest international body on food standards and part of the United Nations. Although NHF believes the codex is misguided on dietary supplements (in favor of regulation and its ranking of supplements based on their efficacy), it believes that revised codex guidelines will become the international standard, replacing domestic legislation on health and nutrition.

To support its mission, the NHF Web site archives relevant articles, often written by third parties, and resources such as other Web sites and lists of alternative-based books.

ACTIVITIES

The NHF cites the passing of the Poultry Products Inspection Act of 1957, which requires federal regulation of interstate poultry commerce, as one of the organization's earliest successes. Other activities include opposition to the Dietary Supplement Safety Act of 2003, which would have required manufacturers of dietary supplements to report adverse events, such as the death of consumers from taking their respective products, to the federal government. The 2003 bill was, in part, an attempt to modify the Dietary Supplement Health and Education Act of 1994, which deregulated the manufacture and distribution of vitamins and supplements. In 2010, similar regulatory legislation was under review by the U.S. Senate Committee on Health, Education, Labor, and Pensions; NHF opposed this legislation as well.

Given its stance on common, long-term health practices in the United States, the NHF is not without controversy. In August 2010, the U.S. Food and Drug Administration (FDA) sent a warning letter to the manufacturer of an anti-inflammatory cream, which had been endorsed and named for an NHF holistic expert, because the product's labeling violated FDA rules on unproved remedies. Clashes between the founder of the NHF and the FDA predate the organization's creation. Conflict continued through the 1970s, when the NHF began an aggressive campaign to ban fluoride from drinking water. Perhaps most controversial is the NHF's push to eliminate what it believes are "unnecessary" and even "dangerous" childhood vaccines.

Regardless of the ongoing controversies, the NHF continues its tenuous relationship with the FDA and other regulatory agencies, as new therapies and techniques evolve and as health regulation continues to be legislated.

Dana K. Bagwell

FURTHER READING

National Health Federation. http://www.thenhf.com.
National Institutes of Health. Office of Dietary Supplements. http://www.ods.od.nih.gov.
U.S. Food and Drug Administration. "Tips for the Savvy Supplement User: Making Informed Decisions and Evaluating Information." Available at http://www.fda.gov/food/dietarysupplements/consumerinformation/ucm110567.htm.

See also: Dietary Supplement Health and Education Act of 1994; Food and Drug Administration; Health freedom movement; National Center for Complementary and Alternative Medicine; Office of Dietary Supplements; Regulation of CAM.

Naturopathy

CATEGORY: Therapies and techniques
RELATED TERMS: Adrenal support, natural medicine, naturopathic medicine
DEFINITION: Prevention and treatment of disease through natural remedies and healing, including nutrition, exercise, and detoxification.
PRINCIPAL PROPOSED USES: None

OVERVIEW

Naturopathy, or "natural medicine," is one of the most important branches of alternative medicine, exerting an influence far beyond the actual numbers of its formal practitioners. Popularized by medical practitioner Benedict Lust at the beginning of the twentieth century, naturopathy's immediate roots go back to the spa treatments of nineteenth-century Germany, but its founding principles are in the writings of Hippocrates and other healers of the ancient world.

The defining principle of naturopathy is *vis medicatrix naturae*, or "nature's healing power." From this perspective, disease is caused by departing from the natural way of living, and health is established by returning to it.

Much of conventional medicine's current interest in diet and lifestyle came into being through the influence of naturopathic practitioners. There is little doubt that their general recommendations are health-promoting: Eat a well-balanced diet rich in fruits and vegetables, exercise regularly, maintain a healthful weight, and avoid toxic habits, such as smoking. It is less clear, however, whether the more specific dietary suggestions sometimes made by naturopathic practitioners will actually enhance health. Some of these suggestions include drinking sixty-four ounces of water daily, eating organic fruits and vegetables, and avoiding certain food combinations (such as starches and protein).

Herbal medicine. Naturopathic medicine is also largely responsible for the resurgence in interest in herbal medicine. Growing scientific evidence suggests that some herbs have real healing properties.

Vitamins, minerals, and supplements. Naturopathic practitioners are also known for emphasizing the use of vitamins and supplements. Ironically, early practitioners of naturopathy were quite opposed to the use of vitamins and supplements, considering them refined, processed foods (which they are). Matters changed in the 1960s when Linus Pauling promoted vitamin C as a cure for many illnesses, leading to the development of orthomolecular medicine. This approach, now incorporated into naturopathy, believes that the roots of many diseases may be found in a subtle form of malnutrition caused by a combination of the following factors: poor diet, inability to absorb nutrients, increased need for nutrients, and difficulties metabolizing or using nutrients. When nutrient levels in the body are increased, the theory goes, the body will have the means to heal itself.

On this principle, naturopathic practitioners often recommend that people take relatively high doses of certain nutrients in the form of supplements. In addition, they believe that many non-nutrient substances found in plants can contribute to health.

Detoxification. Another traditional naturopathic principle is the concept of detoxification. This term refers to the belief that modern life, with its chemical pollutants, poor lifestyle habits, and psychological stresses, causes toxins to accumulate in the body. These toxins are said to be a major cause of disease, and removing them from the body is believed to promote health. Detoxification methods include adopting a healthful diet, drinking large quantities of water, using cleansing herbs and supplements, and undergoing special processes such as colon-cleansing, liver-flushing, and removal of mercury fillings. There is little scientific evidence that any of these methods enhance general health.

Immune support. Immune support is another characteristic naturopathic interest. Based on the indisputable fact that the body's susceptibility to illness is at least as important a factor as its accidental exposure to microorganisms, naturopathic practitioners utilize a number of treatments that they believe will enhance immunity. These treatments include a variety of herbs and supplements and the elimination of certain foods from the diet, such as white sugar. However, it has proved difficult to establish scientifically that any treatment does indeed boost immunity.

Adrenal support. Adrenal support is also commonly recommended by naturopathic practitioners. This method is based on classic studies performed in the early to mid-twentieth century that found a relationship among stress, illness, and adrenal function. Naturopathic practitioners frequently recommend treatments they believe will help the adrenals, including removing sugar and stimulants from the diet while adding adrenal supplements and other herbs and supplements said to strengthen adrenal function.

Adrenal support is said to be helpful for a variety of conditions, including allergies, anxiety, fatigue, and stress. However, the theory of adrenal support has a limited scientific foundation, and it does not by itself justify the common therapies used with the diagnosis. Furthermore, there is little specific scientific evidence to indicate that methods used to support the adrenals are beneficial for any disease.

Other treatments related to naturopathic medicine. Various other treatments have gathered under the umbrella of naturopathic medicine more for historical reasons than for a close connection to *vis medicatrix naturae.* These treatments include emphases on the following: food allergies; the belief that low (rather than high) stomach acid is a cause of many illnesses; an interest in the yeast *Candida* and other intestinal parasites; an interest in certain animal-based hormones, such as thyroid supplements; and an attitude of caution toward many interventions recommended by conventional medicine (such as vaccinations).

Diagnostic techniques. Besides its unique treatment approaches, naturopathic medicine also makes use of a number of characteristic diagnostic techniques, such as hair and saliva analysis, and a more fine-grained analysis of standard blood tests than conventional medicine believes to be warranted.

CHOOSING A PRACTITIONER

Principles of naturopathic medicine are applied by holistic medical doctors (M.D.'s) and doctors of osteopathy (D.O.'s), chiropractors, massage therapists, herbalists, and nutritionists. However, the premier practitioners of this form of medicine are naturopathic physicians (N.D.'s). Several states offer the N.D. licensure, and most major Canadian provinces also license N.D.'s. In states where the N.D. license is not granted, N.D.'s may still practice, although in something of a legal gray zone.

Also, some accredited colleges in North America grant the N.D. degree. These include Bastyr University (Kenmore, Washington), Boucher Institute of Naturopathic Medicine (New Westminister, British Columbia), Canadian College of Naturopathic Medicine (Toronto, Ontario), National College of Natural Medicine (Portland, Oregon), Southwest College of Naturopathic Medicine (Tempe, Arizona), and the University of Bridgeport, College of Naturopathic Medicine (Bridgeport, Connecticut).

EBSCO CAM Review Board

FURTHER READING

Busse, J. W., K. Wilson, and J. B. Campbell. "Attitudes Towards Vaccination Among Chiropractic and Naturopathic Students." *Vaccine* 26 (2008): 6237-6243.

Fleming, S. A., and N. C. Gutknecht. "Naturopathy and the Primary Care Practice." *Primary Care* 37 (2010): 119-136.

Herman, P. M., et al. "A Method for Describing and Evaluating Naturopathic Whole Practice." *Alternative Therapies in Health and Medicine* 12 (2006): 20-28.

Leung, B., and M. Verhoef. "Survey of Parents on the Use of Naturopathic Medicine in Children:

Characteristics and Reasons." *Complementary Therapies in Clinical Practice* 14 (2008): 98-104.

See also: Alternative versus traditional medicine; Chiropractic; Homeopathy; Lust, Benedict; Orthomolecular medicine; Osteopathic manipulation; Traditional healing.

Nausea

CATEGORY: Condition
RELATED TERMS: Car sickness, morning sickness, motion sickness, postsurgical nausea, sea sickness
DEFINITION: Treatment of nausea caused by motion sickness, pregnancy, surgery, and other factors.
PRINCIPAL PROPOSED NATURAL TREATMENTS:
- *Various forms of nausea:* Acupressure-acupuncture, ginger
- *Morning sickness:* Vitamin B_6

OTHER PROPOSED NATURAL TREATMENTS
- *Postsurgical nausea:* Peppermint
- *Morning sickness:* Low-fat diet, vitamin C, vitamin K

INTRODUCTION

Nausea can be caused by many factors, including stomach flu, viral infections of the inner ear (labyrinthitis), motion sickness, pregnancy, and chemotherapy. Unceasing nausea can be more disabling than chronic pain. Successful treatment can make an enormous difference in an affected person's quality of life.

The sensation of nausea can originate either in the nervous system or in the digestive tract itself. Most conventional treatments for nausea, such as Dramamine and Compazine, act on the nervous system, but products such as Pepto-Bismol soothe the digestive tract directly.

PRINCIPAL PROPOSED NATURAL TREATMENTS

The herb ginger has become a widely accepted treatment for nausea of various types. Vitamin B_6 may be helpful for the nausea of pregnancy.

Ginger. Limited scientific evidence suggests that the herb ginger can be helpful for various forms of nausea.

Nausea and vomiting during pregnancy. Four double-blind, placebo-controlled studies enrolling at total of 246 women found ginger more effective than placebo for the treatment of morning sickness. For example, a double-blind, placebo-controlled trial of seventy pregnant women evaluated the effectiveness of ginger for morning sickness. Participants received either placebo or 250 milligrams (mg) of powdered ginger three times daily for four days. The results showed that ginger significantly reduced nausea and vomiting. No significant side effects occurred. Benefits were also seen in a double-blind, placebo-controlled trial of twenty-seven women, and in a poorly designed double-blind, placebo-controlled trial of twenty-six women.

One study of 138 women and another of 291 women found ginger as effective for morning sickness as vitamin B_6. Neither of these studies, however, used a placebo group. Because there is only one study indicating that vitamin B_6 is effective, this vitamin is not quite ready to be used as a gold standard treatment. Comparing one unproven treatment to another without using a placebo group is inadequate for determining effectiveness. It should be noted that ginger has not been proven safe for pregnant women.

Motion sickness. A double-blind, placebo-controlled study of seventy-nine Swedish naval cadets found that 1 gram of ginger could decrease vomiting and cold sweating without significantly decreasing nausea and vertigo. Benefits were also seen in a double-blind study of thirty-six persons given ginger, dimenhydrinate, or placebo.

In addition, a double-blind comparative study that followed 1,489 people aboard a ship found ginger to be just as effective as various medications (cinnarizine, cinnarizine with domperidone, cyclizine, dimehydrinate with caffeine, meclizine with caffeine, and scopolamine). Another double-blind study found equivalent benefit of ginger at a dose of 500 mg every four hours and dimenhydrinate (100 mg every four hours) in a group of sixty passengers aboard a ship. Similar results were also seen in a small double-blind study involving children.

However, a 1984 study funded by the National Aeronautics and Space Administration found that ginger was not any more effective than placebo at reducing the symptoms of nausea caused by a vigorous nausea-provoking method. Negative results were also seen in another study that used a strong nausea stimulus. These studies, in effect, show that the foregoing treatments are somewhat effective for motion sickness but are not effective for severe nausea.

Postsurgical nausea. A British double-blind study compared the effects of ginger, placebo, and the drug metoclopramide in the treatment of nausea following gynecological surgery. The results in sixty women showed that both treatments produced similar benefits compared with placebo.

A similar British study followed 120 women receiving gynecological surgery. Whereas nausea and vomiting developed in 41 percent of participants given placebo, in the groups treated with ginger or metoclopramide (Reglan), these symptoms developed in only 21 percent and 27 percent, respectively. However, three other studies enrolling about four hundred people failed to find ginger more effective than placebo. A 2004 article that reviewed all this evidence concluded that, on balance, ginger is not effective for postsurgical nausea.

One should not use ginger either before or immediately after surgery or labor and delivery without a physician's approval. Not only is it important to have an empty stomach before undergoing anesthesia, but there are theoretical concerns that ginger may affect bleeding.

Acupressure and acupuncture. A single acupuncture point, P6, has traditionally been thought helpful for relief of various forms of nausea and vomiting. This acupuncture point is located on the inside of the forearm, about two inches above the wrist crease. Most studies have investigated the effects of pressure on this point (acupressure) rather than needling. The most common methods involve a wristband with a pearl-sized bead in it situated over P6. The band exerts pressure on the bead while it is worn, and the user can press on the bead for extra stimulation.

Although the research record is mixed, on balance it appears that P6 stimulation offers benefits for various types of nausea. This approach has been studied in anesthesia-induced nausea, the nausea and vomiting of pregnancy, and other forms of nausea.

Anesthesia-induced nausea. General anesthetics and other medications used for surgery frequently cause nausea. About eight controlled studies enrolling a total of more than 750 women who had gynecological surgery found that P6 stimulation reduced postsurgical nausea compared with placebo. On the negative side, a double-blind, placebo-controlled study of 410 women undergoing gynecological surgery failed to find P6 acupressure more effective than fake acupressure. (Both were more effective than no treatment). A small trial of

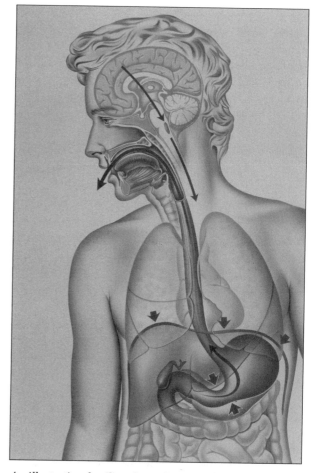

An illustration detailing the mechanism that causes vomiting. (John Bavosi/Photo Researchers, Inc.)

acupuncture in gynecological surgery also failed to find benefit, as did three studies of acupressure for women undergoing cesarean section. Studies of acupuncture or acupressure in other forms of surgery have produced about as many negative results as positive ones.

Nausea and vomiting during pregnancy. Several controlled studies have evaluated the benefits of acupressure or acupuncture for morning sickness. The results for acupressure have generally been more positive than for acupuncture.

For example, a double-blind, placebo-controlled study of ninety-seven women found evidence that wristband acupressure may work. Participants wore either a real wristband or a phony one that appeared identical. Both real and fake acupressure caused noticeable improvement in more than one-half of the participants. However, women using the real wrist-band showed better results in terms of the duration of nausea. The intensity of the nausea symptoms was not significantly different between groups. These results are consistent with previous studies of acupressure for morning sickness. However, two studies failed to find benefit for severe morning sickness.

One large trial of acupuncture instead of acupressure failed to find benefit. This single-blind, placebo-controlled study of 593 pregnant women with morning sickness compared the effects of traditional acupuncture, acupuncture at P6 only, acupuncture at "wrong" points (sham acupuncture), and no treatment. Women in all three treatment groups (including the fake acupuncture group) showed significant improvements in nausea and dry retching compared to the no-treatment group. However, neither form of real acupuncture proved markedly more effective than fake acupuncture.

Motion sickness. Studies are conflicting on whether acupressure is helpful for motion sickness.

Vitamin B₆. A large double-blind study (with almost 350 people) suggests that 30 mg daily of vitamin B_6 can reduce the sensation of nausea in morning sickness.

OTHER PROPOSED NATURAL TREATMENTS

Preliminary studies suggest peppermint oil may be able to reduce postoperative nausea. Multivitamin-multimineral tablets have also shown promise, possibly because of their vitamin B_6 content. On the basis of studies conducted in the 1950s, a combination of vitamin K (at the enormous dose, for vitamin K, of 5 mg daily) and vitamin C (25 mg daily) is sometimes recommended for morning sickness.

EBSCO CAM Review Board

FURTHER READING

Borrelli, F., et al. "Effectiveness and Safety of Ginger in the Treatment of Pregnancy-Induced Nausea and Vomiting." *Obstetrics and Gynecology* 105 (2005): 849-856.

Duggal, K. N., et al. "Acupressure for Intrathecal Narcotic-Induced Nausea and Vomiting After Caesarean Section." *International Journal of Obstetric Anesthesia* 7 (2004): 231-236.

Gan, T. J., et al. "A Randomized Controlled Comparison of Electro-Acupoint Stimulation or Ondansetron Versus Placebo for the Prevention of Postoperative Nausea and Vomiting." *Anesthesia and Analgesia* 99 (2004): 1070-1075.

Habib, A. S., et al. "Transcutaneous Acupoint Electrical Stimulation with the ReliefBand(R) for the Prevention of Nausea and Vomiting During and After Cesarean Delivery Under Spinal Anesthesia." *Anesthesia and Analgesia* 102 (2006): 581-584.

Heazell, A., et al. "Acupressure for the In-Patient Treatment of Nausea and Vomiting in Early Pregnancy." *American Journal of Obstetrics and Gynecology* 194 (2006): 815-820.

Manusirivithaya, S., et al. "Antiemetic Effect of Ginger in Gynecologic Oncology Patients Receiving Cisplatin." *International Journal of Gynecological Cancer* 14 (2004): 1063-1069.

Miller, K. E., and E. R. Muth. "Efficacy of Acupressure and Acustimulation Bands for the Prevention of Motion Sickness." *Aviation, Space, and Environmental Medicine* 75 (2004): 227-234.

Roscoe, J. A., et al. "Acustimulation Wrist Bands Are Not Effective for the Control of Chemotherapy-Induced Nausea in Women with Breast Cancer." *Journal of Pain Symptom Management* 29 (2005): 376-384.

Smith, C., et al. "A Randomized Controlled Trial of Ginger to Treat Nausea and Vomiting in Pregnancy." *Obstetrics and Gynecology* 103 (2004): 639-645.

See also: Acupuncture; Cancer treatment support; Ginger; Vitamin B_6.

Neck pain

CATEGORY: Condition
RELATED TERMS: Cervicalgia, cervical pain
DEFINITION: Treatment of soft-tissue pain of the neck.
PRINCIPAL PROPOSED NATURAL TREATMENTS: None
OTHER PROPOSED NATURAL TREATMENTS: Acupuncture, biofeedback, boswellia, butterbur, chiropractic, chondroitin, ginger, glucosamine, hypnosis, massage, osteopathic manipulation, prolotherapy, proteolytic enzymes, relaxation therapies, turmeric, white willow

INTRODUCTION

Neck pain is a common condition. In many cases, X rays do not show anything wrong with the neck, suggesting that the problem is a relatively subtle one involving soft tissues. (Conversely, X rays of people without neck pain often show arthritis; this suggests that even when positive X-ray results are found in people with neck pain, they may be unrelated.) Subtle or not in origin, the discomfort of neck pain can be severe and can lead to real disability.

The cause of soft-tissue neck pain is not known. Symptoms may follow a whiplash injury or simply arise, apparently, from bad posture or chronic tension. It is unclear that any conventional medicine intervention for neck pain or whiplash speeds recovery or produces any other long-term benefit.

PROPOSED NATURAL TREATMENTS

Although several alternative treatments for neck pain have shown promise, none has been scientifically substantiated.

Acupuncture. A 2006 review of the literature found ten controlled studies of acupuncture for chronic neck pain. The pooled results suggest that acupuncture may be more effective than fake acupuncture, at least in the short term. However, overall, the study quality was fairly low.

In a study of 177 people with chronic neck pain, fake acupuncture proved more effective than massage. In a pilot study, ten weeks of acupuncture combined with physical therapy appeared to be more effective than either acupuncture or physical therapy alone for chronic neck pain, at least over the short term. The most likely explanation for these contradictory reports is that acupuncture's effect on neck pain, if any, is fairly modest.

Chiropractic. Millions of people report that chiropractic spinal manipulation has relieved their neck pain, but there is little scientific evidence supporting the use of spinal manipulation for this purpose. Most studies have found manipulation (with or without related therapies, such as mobilization or massage) to be no more effective than placebo or no treatment. One large study (almost two hundred participants) found that a special exercise program called MedX was more effective than chiropractic spinal manipulation. However, a study that was reported in 2006 found that a single high-velocity, low-amplitude (that is, chiropractic-style) manipulation of the neck was more effective than a single mobilization procedure in improving range of motion and pain.

Other treatments. Osteopathic manipulation, a form of treatment often compared to chiropractic, is widely believed to help neck pain, but there is no meaningful

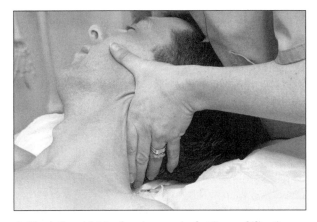

A physiotherapist performing cervical spine mobilization on a patient. (Paul Rapson/Photo Researchers, Inc.)

scientific evidence to support its use for this condition. Many people with neck pain use massage therapy for relief, but again, scientific support is lacking, and one study found fake laser acupuncture more effective than massage for neck pain. A treatment called prolotherapy, and the herb white willow, have shown promise for back pain and might also be useful for neck pain. In one study, an ambitious holistic treatment regimen for neck pain (including craniosacral osteopathy, Rosen bodywork, and Gestalt psychotherapy) failed to prove more effective than no treatment.

Other herbs and supplements sometimes recommended for neck pain, either on the basis of their use for related conditions or because of their known medical properties, include boswellia, butterbur, chondroitin, ginger, glucosamine, proteolytic enzymes, and turmeric.

Qigong is an ancient Chinese practice involving various breathing exercises and physical postures that are thought by its practitioners to enhance general health. In one study, qigong was no more effective than conventional physical therapy exercise techniques in the treatment of chronic, nonspecific neck pain. Biofeedback, hypnosis, and relaxation therapies may offer help for pain in general.

EBSCO CAM Review Board

FURTHER READING

Franca, D. L., et al. "Tension Neck Syndrome Treated by Acupuncture Combined with Physiotherapy." *Complementary Therapies in Medicine* 16 (2008): 268-277.

Haneline, M. T. "Chiropractic Manipulation and Acute Neck Pain." *Journal of Manipulative and Physiological Therapeutics* 28 (2005): 520-525.

Lansinger, B., et al. "Qigong and Exercise Therapy in Patients with Long-Term Neck Pain." *Spine* 32 (2007): 2415-2422.

Martinez-Segura, R., et al. "Immediate Effects on Neck Pain and Active Range of Motion After a Single Cervical High-Velocity Low-Amplitude Manipulation in Subjects Presenting with Mechanical Neck Pain." *Journal of Manipulative and Physiological Therapeutics* 29 (2006): 511-517.

Sarig-Bahat, H. "Evidence for Exercise Therapy in Mechanical Neck Disorders." *Manual Therapy* 8 (2003): 10-20.

Trinh, K., et al. "Acupuncture for Neck Disorders." *Spine* 32 (2007): 236-243.

See also: Acupressure; Acupuncture; Back pain; Bone and joint health; Bursitis; Carpal tunnel syndrome; Fibromyalgia: Homeopathic remedies; Injuries, minor; Massage therapy; Nonsteroidal anti-inflammatory drugs (NSAIDs); Osteoarthritis; Pain management; Progressive muscle relaxation; Soft tissue pain; Sports and fitness support: Enhancing recovery; Sports-related injuries: Homeopathic remedies; Temporomandibular joint syndrome (TMJ); Tendonitis; Yoga.

Neem

CATEGORY: Herbs and supplements

RELATED TERM: *Azadirachta indica*

DEFINITION: Natural plant product used to treat specific health conditions.

PRINCIPAL PROPOSED USES: None

OTHER PROPOSED USES: Fevers, respiratory diseases, skin diseases

OVERVIEW

The neem tree has been called the village pharmacy because its bark, leaves, sap, fruit, seeds, and twigs have so many diverse uses in the traditional medicine of India. This member of the mahogany family has been used medicinally for more than four thousand years and is held in such esteem that Indian poets called it *Sarva Roga Nivarini*, meaning "the One That Can Cure All Ailments." Mohandas Gandhi encouraged scientific investigation of the neem tree as part of his program to revitalize Indian traditions, which eventually led to more than two thousand research papers and intense commercial interest.

More than fifty patents have been filed on neem and neem-based products in the United States for control of insects in food and ornamental crops. However, the Indian government and many nongovernmental organizations have united to overthrow some patents of this type, which they regard as folk-wisdom piracy. One fear is that if neem is patented, indigenous people who already use it will lose the right to continue to do so. Another point is the fundamental question: Who owns the genetic diversity of plants? The nations where the plants originated or the transnational corporations that pay for the research into those plants? Although this area of international law is rapidly evolving, a patent on the spice turmeric has already been overturned, and a similar ruling involving neem may follow soon.

At least one hundred bioactive substances have been found in neem, including nimbidin, azadirachthins, and other triterpenoids and limonoids. Although the scientific evidence for all of neem's uses in health care remains preliminary, the intense interest in the plant will eventually lead to proper double-blind, placebo-controlled trials.

THERAPEUTIC DOSAGES

Because of the numerous parts of the neem tree used and the many different ways these parts can be prepared, the only possible recommendation for dosage is to follow the directions on the label of the neem product.

THERAPEUTIC USES

The uses of neem are remarkably diverse. In India, the sap is used for treating fevers, general debilitation, digestive disturbances, and skin diseases; the bark gum for respiratory diseases and other infections; the leaves for digestive problems, intestinal parasites, and viral infections; the fruit for debilitation, malaria, skin diseases, and intestinal parasites; and the seed and kernel oil for diabetes, fevers, fungal infections, bacterial infections, inflammatory diseases, and fertility prevention, and as an insecticide. However, there is no reliable research evidence to support any of these uses.

As with many plant products, test-tube studies indicate that, on direct contact, neem can kill or inhibit the growth of bacteria, fungi, and viruses. This does not mean, however, that neem acts as a systemic antibiotic if it is taken by mouth. Neem mouthwash and chewing gum might be helpful for preventing cavities because they can directly come in contact with cavity-causing bacteria, but this has not been proven. On the basis of extremely preliminary evidence, neem has also been advocated as a treatment for diabetes.

SAFETY ISSUES

Based on its extensive traditional use, neem seems to be quite safe. However, formal safety testing has involved only neem oil, the insecticide product made from the plant. While neem has been found adequately safe for use as an insecticide, animal studies suggest that long-term oral use of neem oil might produce toxic effects. In addition, other animal studies suggest that whole neem extract (which includes more substances than neem oil) may damage chromosomes, at least when taken in high doses or for an extended period of time. For all these reasons, as well as the lack of comprehensive safety investigation of neem products other than neem oil, it is recommended that young children, pregnant or nursing women, and individuals with severe liver or kidney disease avoid the use of neem.

EBSCO CAM Review Board

FURTHER READING

Juglal, S., R. Govinden, and B. Odhav. "Spice Oils for the Control of Co-occurring Mycotoxin-Producing Fungi." *Journal of Food Protection* 65 (2002): 683-687.

SaiRam, M., et al. "Anti-microbial Activity of a New Vaginal Contraceptive NIM-76 from Neem Oil (*Azadirachta indica*)." *Journal of Ethnopharmacology* 71 (2000): 377-382.

Vanka, A., et al. "The Effect of Indigenous Neem (*Adirachta indica*) Mouthwash on *Streptococcus mutans* and Lactobacilli Growth." *Indian Journal of Dental Research* 12 (2001): 133-144.

See also: Folk medicine; Herbal medicine.

Nettle

CATEGORY: Herbs and supplements
RELATED TERM: *Urtica dioica*
DEFINITION: Natural plant product used to treat specific health conditions.
PRINCIPAL PROPOSED USES: Allergies (nettle leaf), benign prostatic hyperplasia (nettle root)

OVERVIEW

Anyone who lives where nettle grows wild will eventually discover the powers of this dark green plant. Depending on the species, the fine hairs on its leaves and stem cause burning pain that lasts from hours to weeks. However, this well-protected herb has also been used as medicine. Nettle juice was used in Hippocrates' time to treat bites and stings, and European herbalists recommended nettle tea for lung disorders. Nettle tea was used by Native Americans as an aid in pregnancy, childbirth, and nursing.

THERAPEUTIC DOSAGES

Therapeutic dosages of nettle root extract vary according to preparation, and label instructions should be followed. Some nettle root products are standardized to their content of the substance scopoletin, but since this substance is not established as an active ingredient, the significance of this standardization remains unclear. For allergies, the studied dosage is 300 milligrams (mg) twice a day of freeze-dried nettle leaf.

THERAPEUTIC USES

Nettle root is now more commonly used medicinally than the above-ground portion of the herb. In Europe, nettle root is widely used for the treatment of benign prostatic hyperplasia (BPH), or prostate enlargement. Like saw palmetto, pygeum, and beta-sitosterol, nettle appears to reduce obstruction to urinary flow and decrease the need for nighttime urination. However, the evidence is not as strong for nettle as it is for these other treatments. Before self-treating prostate symptoms with nettle root, men should be sure to get a proper medical evaluation to rule out prostate cancer.

Nettle leaf has become a popular treatment for allergies (hay fever) based on one preliminary double-blind study. Nettle leaf is highly nutritious and, in cooked form, may be used as a general dietary supplement.

SCIENTIFIC EVIDENCE

The evidence is much better for nettle root and prostatic enlargement than for nettle leaf and allergies.

Nettle root. Nettle root as a treatment for benign prostatic hyperplasia has not been as well studied as saw palmetto, but the evidence is still substantial. In a double-blind, placebo-controlled study performed in Iran, 558 people were given either placebo or nettle root for six months. The results indicated that nettle root is significantly more effective than placebo on all major measures of BPH severity. Benefits were seen in three other double-blind studies as well, enrolling a total of more than 150 men.

There are theoretical reasons to believe that nettle root's effectiveness might be enhanced when it is combined with another herb used for prostate problems: pygeum. Nettle has also been studied in combination with saw palmetto, with mixed results. Nettle root contains numerous biologically active chemicals that may influence the prostate indirectly by interacting with sex hormones, or directly by altering the properties of prostate cells.

Nettle leaf. One preliminary double-blind, placebo-controlled study following sixty-nine people suggests that freeze-dried nettle leaf may at least slightly improve allergy symptoms. One small double-blind study suggests that direct application of stinging nettle leaf to a painful joint may improve symptoms.

SAFETY ISSUES

Because nettle leaf has a long history of food use, it is believed to be safe. Nettle root does not have as extensive a history to go by. Although detailed safety studies have not been reported, no significant adverse effects have been noted in Germany, where nettle root is widely used. In practice, it is nearly free of side effects. In one study of 4,087 people who took 600 to 1,200 mg of nettle root daily for six months, less than 1 percent reported mild gastrointestinal distress, and only 0.19 percent experienced allergic reactions (skin rash).

For theoretical reasons, there are some concerns that nettle may interact with diabetes, blood pressure, anti-inflammatory, and sedative medications, although there are no reports of any problems occurring. The safety of nettle root or leaf for pregnant or nursing mothers has not been established, and there are concerns based on animal studies and its traditional use for inducing abortions. However, nettle leaf tea is a traditional drink for pregnant and nursing women.

IMPORTANT INTERACTIONS

Nettle may conceivably interact with anti-inflammatory, antihypertensive, sedative, or blood-sugar-lowering medications (although this is not likely), so people taking these medications should be aware and cautious.

EBSCO CAM Review Board

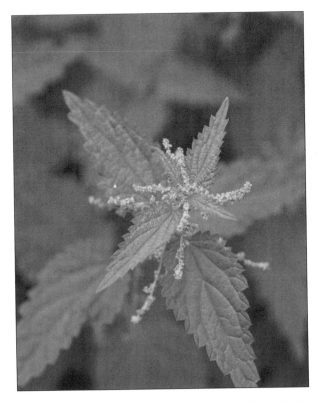

Nettle plant. (Voisin/Phanie/Photo Researchers, Inc.)

FURTHER READING

Konrad, L., et al. "Antiproliferative Effect on Human Prostate Cancer Cells by a Stinging Nettle Root (*Urtica dioica*) Extract." *Planta Medica* 66 (2000): 44-47.

Lopatkin, N., et al. "Long-term Efficacy and Safety of a Combination of Sabal and Urtica Extract for Lower Urinary Tract Symptoms." *World Journal of Urology* 23, no. 2 (2005): 139-146.

Marks, L. S., et al. "Effects of a Saw Palmetto Herbal Blend in Men with Symptomatic Benign Prostatic Hyperplasia." *Journal of Urology* 163 (2000): 1451-1456.

Randall, C., et al. "Randomized Controlled Trial of Nettle Sting for the Treatment of Base-of-thumb Pain." *Journal of the Royal Society of Medicine* 93 (2000): 305-309.

Safarinejad, M. R. "*Urtica dioica* for Treatment of Benign Prostatic Hyperplasia." *Journal of Herbal Pharmacotherapy* 5 (2006): 1-11.

Sokeland, J. "Combined Sabal and Urtica Extract Compared with Finasteride in Men with Benign Prostatic Hyperplasia: Analysis of Prostate Volume and Therapeutic Outcome." *BJU International* 86 (2000): 439-442.

See also: Benign prostatic hyperplasia; Beta-sitosterol; Herbal medicine; Pygeum; Saw palmetto.

Nicotinamide adenine dinucleotide

CATEGORY: Herbs and supplements

DEFINITION: Natural substance of the human body used as a supplement to treat specific health conditions.

PRINCIPAL PROPOSED USE: Jet lag

OTHER PROPOSED USES: Alzheimer's disease, chronic fatigue syndrome, depression, Parkinson's disease, sports performance enhancement

OVERVIEW

Nicotinamide adenine dinucleotide (NADH) is an important cofactor, or assistant, that helps enzymes in the work they do throughout the body. NADH particularly plays a role in the production of energy. It also participates in the production of L-dopa, which the body turns into the important neurotransmitter dopamine.

Based on these basic biochemical facts, NADH has been evaluated as a treatment for jet lag, Alzheimer's disease, Parkinson's disease, chronic fatigue syndrome, and depression, and as a sports supplement. However, only the first of these uses has any meaningful scientific evidence behind it, and even that is highly preliminary.

REQUIREMENTS AND SOURCES

Healthy bodies make all the NADH they need, using vitamin B_3 (also known as niacin or nicotinamide) as a starting point. The highest concentration of NADH in animals is found in muscle tissues, which means that meat might be a good source, were it not that most of the NADH in meat is destroyed during processing, cooking, and digestion. In reality, people do not get much NADH from their food.

THERAPEUTIC DOSAGES

The typical dosage for supplemental NADH ranges from 5 to 50 milligrams (mg) daily, often taken sublingually (under the tongue). Products said to be stabilized are available.

THERAPEUTIC USES

Two small double-blind, placebo-controlled trials suggest that NADH may be useful for enhancing mental function under conditions of inadequate sleep, such as jet lag.

Supplemental NADH has also been proposed as a treatment for Alzheimer's disease, chronic fatigue syndrome, depression, and Parkinson's disease. Additionally, it has been tried as a sports performance enhancer. However, although a few studies have been performed to evaluate these potential uses, none were designed in such a way as to produce scientifically meaningful results.

SCIENTIFIC EVIDENCE

In a double-blind, placebo-controlled trial, thirty-five individuals taking an overnight flight across four time zones were given either 20 mg of NADH or a placebo sublingually (under the tongue) on the morning of arrival. Participants were twice given tests of wakefulness and mental function: first at ninety minutes and then at five hours after landing. Individuals given NADH scored significantly better on these tests than those given a placebo.

The only other supporting evidence comes from an unpublished double-blind, placebo-controlled, cross-over study funded by the makers of an NADH product. In this study, twenty-five people were kept awake all night and their cognitive function was tested the following day. People given NADH performed significantly better on various measures of mental function than those given placebo. NADH did not, however, reduce daytime sleepiness or enhance mood.

SAFETY ISSUES

NADH appears to be quite safe when taken at a dosage of 5 mg daily or less. However, formal safety studies have not been completed, and safety in young children, pregnant or nursing women, and those with severe liver or kidney disease has not been established.

EBSCO CAM Review Board

FURTHER READING

Forsyth, L. M., et al. "Therapeutic Effects of Oral NADH on the Symptoms of Patients with Chronic Fatigue Syndrome." *Annals of Allergy, Asthma, and Immunology* 82 (1999): 185-191.

See also: Chronic fatigue syndrome; Fatigue; Herbal medicine; Jet lag.

Night vision, impaired

CATEGORY: Condition

RELATED TERMS: Night blindness, nyctalopia

DEFINITION: Treatment of the inability of the eyes to normally, and quickly, adapt to darkness or to recover from glare.

PRINCIPAL PROPOSED NATURAL TREATMENT: Bilberry

OTHER PROPOSED NATURAL TREATMENTS: Black currant, oligomeric proanthocyanidins, vitamin A, zinc

INTRODUCTION

The ability to see in poor light depends on the presence of a substance in the eye called rhodopsin, or visual purple. This substance is destroyed by bright light but rapidly regenerates in the dark. However, for some people, the adaptation to darkness or the recovery from glare takes an unusually long time. There is no medical treatment for this condition.

PRINCIPAL PROPOSED NATURAL TREATMENTS

The herb bilberry, a close relative of the American blueberry, is the most commonly mentioned natural treatment for impaired night vision. This use dates back to World War II, when pilots in Great Britain's Royal Air Force reported that a good dose of bilberry jam just before a mission improved their night vision, often dramatically. After the war, medical researchers investigated the constituents of bilberry and found a group of active chemicals called anthocyanosides. These naturally occurring antioxidants appear to

---

Vitamin A Deficiency and Impaired Vision

Vitamin A deficiency is common in developing countries but rarely seen in the United States. Approximately 250,000 to 500,000 malnourished children in the developing world become blind each year from a deficiency of vitamin A. In the United States, vitamin A deficiency is most often associated with strict dietary restrictions and excessive alcohol intake. Severe zinc deficiency, which is also associated with strict dietary limitations, often accompanies vitamin A deficiency. Zinc is required to make retinol-binding protein, which transports vitamin A through the body. Therefore, a deficiency in zinc limits the body's ability to move vitamin A stores from the liver to body tissues.

Night blindness is one of the first signs of vitamin A deficiency. In ancient Egypt, it was known that night blindness could be cured by eating liver, which was later found to be a rich source of the vitamin. Vitamin A deficiency contributes to blindness by making the cornea very dry, thereby damaging the retina and cornea.

---

have numerous potentially important actions within the eye.

However, neither anecdote nor basic scientific evidence of this type can prove a treatment effective. Only double-blind, placebo-controlled studies can do that. The evidence from studies of this type is more negative than positive, with all of the most recent studies finding no benefit.

For example, a double-blind crossover trial of fifteen persons found no short- or long-term improvements in night vision attributable to bilberry. Similarly negative results were seen in a double-blind, placebo-controlled crossover trial of eighteen persons and another trial of sixteen persons. Earlier studies had reported some benefit, but they were less rigorous in design. Thus, bilberry cannot be recommended as a treatment for improving night vision.

OTHER PROPOSED NATURAL TREATMENTS

Evidence from a small, double-blind, placebo-controlled study suggests that anthocyanosides from black currant might have some benefit for night vision. Oligomeric proanthocyanidins also have been recommended for improving night vision, although the evidence that they help is far too weak to rely upon. There is no question that deficiencies of vitamin A and zinc can also negatively affect night vision. However, there is no evidence to suggest that taking extra amounts of these nutrients will enhance vision.

EBSCO CAM Review Board

FURTHER READING

Gaby, A. R. "Nutritional Therapies for Ocular Disorders." *Alternative Medicine Review* 13 (2008): 191-204.

Levy, Y., and Y. Glovinsky. "The Effect of Anthocyanosides on Night Vision." *Eye* 12 (1998): 967-969.

Muth, E. R., J. M. Laurent, and P. Jasper. "The Effect of Bilberry Nutritional Supplementation on Night Visual Acuity and Contrast Sensitivity." *Alternative Medicine Review* 5 (2000): 164-173.

Nakaishi, H., et al. "Effects of Black Current Anthocyanoside Intake on Dark Adaptation and VDT Work-Induced Transient Refractive Alteration in Healthy Humans." *Alternative Medicine Review* 5 (2000): 553-562.

See also: Bilberry; Cataracts; Diabetes, complications of; Glaucoma; Macular degeneration; Retinitis pigmentosa.

Nitrofurantoin

CATEGORY: Drug interactions
DEFINITION: A drug used to prevent bladder infections.
INTERACTION: Magnesium
TRADE NAMES: Furadantin, Macrobid, Macrodantin

MAGNESIUM
Effect: Take at a Different Time of Day

Magnesium supplements might impair the absorption of nitrofurantoin, so one should not take magnesium during the two hours before or after using nitrofurantoin.

EBSCO CAM Review Board

FURTHER READING

Pronsky, Z. M., and J. P. Crowe. *Food Medication Interactions.* 16th ed. Birchrunville, Pa.: Food-Medication Interactions, 2010.

See also: Food and Drug Administration; Magnesium; Supplements: Introduction.

Nitroglycerin

CATEGORY: Drug interactions
DEFINITION: A commonly used drug treatment for quick relief of anginal pain.
INTERACTIONS: Arginine, folate, N-acetylcysteine, vitamin C, vitamin E
TRADE NAMES: Deponit, Minitran, Nitrek, Nitro-Bid, Nitro-Derm, Nitro-Dur, Nitro-Time, Nitrocine, Nitrodisc, Nitrogard, Nitroglyn, Nitrol, Nitrolingual, Nitrong, NitroQuick, Nitrostat, Transderm-Nitro
RELATED DRUGS: Isosorbide dinitrate, isosorbide mononitrate

N-ACETYLCYSTEINE (NAC)
Effect: Possible Benefits and Risks

NAC is a specially modified form of the dietary amino acid cysteine that has various proposed uses. Nitrates such as nitroglycerin lose some of their effectiveness over time. According to some studies, the supplement N-acetylcysteine might help these drugs work better. However, the combination of NAC and nitroglycerin appears to cause severe headaches.

Taking NAC with nitroglycerin may be beneficial in some cases. However, unpleasant side effects probably limit the use of this combination.

Angina is too serious a disease for self-treatment. Persons with angina should not take any supplement except on a physician's advice.

VITAMIN C
Effect: Supplementation Possibly Helpful

Vitamin C may help prevent the development of tolerance to nitrate medications such as nitroglycerin. According to a double-blind study of forty-eight persons, the use of vitamin C at a dose of 2,000 milligrams (mg) three times daily helped maintain the effectiveness of nitroglycerin. These findings are supported by other studies.

Angina is too serious a disease for self-treatment. Persons with angina should not take any supplement except on a physician's advice.

ARGININE

Effect: Supplementation Possibly Helpful

According to a small, double-blind, placebo-controlled crossover study, the use of arginine (700 mg four times daily) may help prevent tolerance to nitrate medications.

FOLATE

Effect: Supplementation Possibly Helpful

A small, double-blind trial suggests that folate supplements (at the high dose of 10 mg daily) may help prevent tolerance to nitrate medications.

VITAMIN E

Effect: Supplementation Possibly Helpful

A small, double-blind trial suggests that vitamin E at a dose of 200 mg three times daily may help prevent tolerance to nitrate medications.

EBSCO CAM Review Board

FURTHER READING

Bassenge, E., et al. "Dietary Supplement with Vitamin C Prevents Nitrate Tolerance." *Journal of Clinical Investigation* 31 (1998): 67-71.

Daniel, T. A., and J. J. Nawarskas. "Vitamin C in the Prevention of Nitrate Tolerance." *Annals of Pharmacotherapy* 4 (2000): 1193-1197.

Gori, T., et al. "Folic Acid Prevents Nitroglycerin-Induced Nitric Oxide Synthase Dysfunction and Nitrate Tolerance: A Human In Vivo Study." *Circulation* 104 (2001): 1119-1123.

McVeigh, G. E., et al. "Platelet Nitric Oxide and Superoxide Release During the Development of Nitrate Tolerance: Effect of Supplemental Ascorbate." *Circulation* 106 (2002): 208-213.

Parker, J. O., et al. "The Effect of Supplemental L-arginine on Tolerance Development During Continuous Transdermal Nitroglycerin Therapy." *Journal of the American College of Cardiology* 39 (2002): 1199-1203.

Watanabe, H., et al. "Randomized, Double-Blind, Placebo-Controlled Study of the Preventive Effect of Supplemental Oral Vitamin C on Attenuation of Development of Nitrate Tolerance." *Journal of the American College of Cardiology* 31 (1998): 1323-1329.

See also: Arginine; Folate; Food and Drug Administration; N-acetylcysteine; Supplements: Introduction; Vitamin C; Vitamin E.

Nitrous oxide

CATEGORY: Drug interactions
DEFINITION: Gas used as a local anesthetic in dentistry and in certain phases of cardiac bypass surgery.
INTERACTIONS: Folate, vitamin B_{12}

FOLATE AND VITAMIN B_{12}

Effect: Supplementation Possibly Helpful

Nitrous oxide can occasionally cause significant vitamin B_{12} deficiency, especially in people who are already borderline deficient in the vitamin (vegetarians, for example) or in such persons as dentists and anesthesiologists, who are frequently exposed to the gas. The effect on B_{12} impacts folate too.

Taking folate and B_{12} supplements at the U.S. Dietary Reference Intake (formerly known as the Recommended Dietary Allowance) levels should prevent any problems from developing.

EBSCO CAM Review Board

FURTHER READING

Ermens, A. A., et al. "Monitoring Cobalamin Inactivation During Nitrous Oxide Anesthesia by Determination of Homocysteine and Folate Plasma and Urine." *Clinical Pharmacology and Therapeutics* 49 (1991): 385-393.

Flippo, T. S., and W. D. Holder, Jr. "Neurologic Degeneration Associated with Nitrous Oxide Anesthesia in Patients with Vitamin B12 Deficiency." *Archives of Surgery* 128 (1993): 1391-1395.

See also: Folate; Food and Drug Administration; Supplements: Introduction; Vitamin B_{12}.

Nondairy milk

CATEGORY: Functional foods
DEFINITION: Milk produced from nonanimal sources, such as soy, rice, almond, multigrain, oat, and potato.
PRINCIPAL PROPOSED USE: Lactose intolerance
OTHER PROPOSED USES: None

OVERVIEW

Milk has changed, and for many people, that change is welcome news. According to an article published in

American Family Physician, up to 100 percent of Asians and American Indians, 80 percent of black and Latino people, and 15 percent of people of northern European descent have trouble digesting lactose.

Lactose, a milk sugar found in dairy products, is digested in the intestines by an enzyme called lactase. Many people do not produce enough lactase, and the result is a decreased ability to digest lactose known as lactose intolerance, which can result in bloating, gas, diarrhea, and stomach cramps. There are different degrees of lactose intolerance—some people may be able to handle moderate amounts of milk before feeling the effects of too little lactase, while others may only be able to handle a small amount or none at all. Overall, one in four Americans has some degree of lactose intolerance.

Not everyone who avoids cow's milk is lactose intolerant. In its whole state, milk has both saturated fat and cholesterol. Some people are concerned about the environmental impact and animal abuse associated with milk production. Others, such as Buddhists, have religious convictions or other personal reasons for avoiding cow's milk.

REQUIREMENTS AND SOURCES

Nondairy milks are abundant and now found in many supermarkets and other stores. Milk is made from soybeans, rice, nuts, oats, and potato (and combinations thereof) and is available in different flavors, with different fat contents (regular, reduced-fat, low-fat, or no-fat) and with various levels of nutrient fortification. Because of such a wide-ranging selection, one should read the ingredient and nutrition information for help selecting the best products for one's needs.

Soy milk. Soy milk is the most popular of the nondairy milk beverages. Each soy milk product on the market has its own texture, taste, and consistency, and in general, soy milk products are thicker and creamier than other nondairy milks.

Soybeans are the main ingredient in soy milk, followed by soy protein isolate—a concentrated soybean protein. Some soy milks contain tofu, but most soy milks are made from organic soybeans, although not all are free of genetically engineered beans. Soy milk is available in both liquid and powder forms.

Oat milk. Swedish farmers and scientists invented oat milk through a process called the Oste Process, which uses oat kernels and rapeseed (canola) oil to produce a neutral-tasting, highly stable beverage. The milk is also an excellent substitute for cow's milk in

---

Common Guidelines for Buying and Consuming Nondairy Milk

- Consider why you are buying the product: as a beverage, to use on cereal, or to use in recipes. You may need several different types.
- Choose products that meet your nutrient needs.
- Most nondairy beverages come in packages that generally last six months or longer unopened. Once opened, the milk must be refrigerated and used within seven to ten days.
- Not all brands taste the same. Experiment with several. Powdered forms are usually less expensive and allow you to vary the consistency.
- Nondairy beverages are not suitable for infants. Specially designed soy-based infant formulas are available.
- More than thirty brands of nondairy beverages are on the market. Among them are: Better Than Milk, Eden, Grainaissance, Harmony Farms, Lactaid, Mill Milk, Pacific Foods, Soyco Foods, Vitamite, White Wave, and Whyte's DariFree.

---

cooking and baking. Oat milk is low in fat and contains vitamin E, folic acid, amino acids, trace elements, and minerals. The extraction process allows much of the natural fiber to remain in the final product, which makes oat milk "oatmeal in a glass."

Rice, nut, and potato milks. Rice milk is lighter and sweeter than soy milk. Some people say it tastes closer to cow's milk than other nondairy choices. Almond milk is the most popular nut milk, although people who make their own often use walnuts, hazelnuts, or cashews, along with almonds. Potato milk is the newest addition to the nondairy case, and it is available in both liquid and powder form. Combination beverages often contain oats, barley, soybeans, and brown rice.

Nutrients. To get enough calcium and other nutrients from nondairy milk, one should buy fortified products. The nutrients most commonly added to nondairy milks are the same ones either added to or found in cow's milk: calcium, riboflavin, and vitamins C, D, and B_{12}. One should buy brands that contain 20 to 30 percent of the U.S. recommended daily allowance (RDA) for calcium, riboflavin, and vitamin B_{12}, which makes them nutritionally similar to cow's milk. Not all nondairy beverages are fortified, so one should check the labels.

USES AND APPLICATIONS

According to Robert Oser, a former chef at the world-famous Canyon Ranch Spa in Tucson, Arizona, and author of *Flavors of the Southwest*, nondairy milks not only are great in shakes and on cereal; they can be used for cooking and baking too. The results will depend on the fat content of the milk substitute used and on the brand. Substituting nondairy milk for cow's milk often can be done one-to-one in a recipe, but experimentation is often recommended. When making gravy, for example, one may need to add more corn starch or other thickeners than the recipe specifies.

Because rice and nut milks are sweeter and lighter than soy milk, they are good for desserts and curries, but less suitable for gravies and most entrees. Oat and potato milks are more neutral and complement soups and main dishes. Soy-based beverages and those containing a high amount of calcium carbonate can curdle at high temperatures, especially if the recipe uses acidic foods such as oranges or tomatoes.

Deborah Mitchell; reviewed by Brian Randall, M.D.

FURTHER READING

American Dietetic Association. "Calcium Consumption Versus Lactose Intolerance." Available at http://www.eatright.org.

_____. "Lactose Intolerance: A Matter of Degree." Available at http://www.eatright.org.

Go Dairy Free. http://www.godairyfree.org.

Goldberg, J. P., and S. C. Folta. "Milk: Can a 'Good' Food Be So Bad?" *Pediatrics* 110, no. 4 (2002): 826-832.

Swagerty, D. L., A. D. Walling, and R. M. Klein. "Lactose Intolerance." *American Family Physician* 65, no. 9 (2002). Available at http://www.aafp.org.

Vegetarian Resource Group. http://www.vrg.org.

See also: Calcium; Diarrhea; Diet-based therapies; Food allergies and sensitivities; Functional beverages; Functional foods: Introduction; Functional foods: Overview; Gas, intestinal; Soy; Vegan diet; Vegetarian diet.

Noni

CATEGORY: Herbs and supplements
RELATED TERMS: Indian mulberry, *Morinda citrifolia*
DEFINITION: Natural plant product used to treat specific health conditions.

PRINCIPAL PROPOSED USES: None
OTHER PROPOSED USES: Numerous

OVERVIEW

Morinda citrifolia, also known as noni or Indian mulberry, is a small evergreen shrub or tree of the plant family Rubiaceae. Native to the Pacific Islands, Polynesia, Asia, and Australia, it grows up to 10 feet high. The leaves are 8 or more inches long, dark green, oval shaped, and shiny, with deep veins. The flower heads are about an inch long and bear many small white flowers. These heads grow to become the mature fruit, 3 to 4 inches in diameter with a warty, pitted surface. Noni fruit starts out green, turns yellow with ripening, and has a foul odor, especially as it ripens to whiteness and falls to the ground.

Some cultures may eat noni fruit in times of scarcity (the unripened fruit is less noxious). Traditional Polynesian healers have apparently used the fruit for many conditions, such as bowel disorders (constipation and diarrhea), skin inflammation, infection, mouth sores, fever, contusions, and sprains, but it is said that only sick and desperate people will take it because of its unpleasant odor and bitter taste. However, the primary indigenous use of this plant appears to be of the leaves, as a topical treatment for wound healing.

In Chinese medicine, the root of *M. officinalis* is also a standard medication (known as *bai ji tian* or *pa chi tien*) used for the digestive system, kidneys, heart, and liver. Other traditional uses for the plant include making a red dye from the bark and a yellow dye from the root.

THERAPEUTIC DOSAGES

Commercial products that contain noni juice or a juice concentrate are widely available and heavily promoted. The odor has been eliminated, or the taste altered, for these preparations to make them more palatable. Tablets and capsules of the fruit and of the whole plant are also available.

The usual recommendation is the equivalent of 4 ounces of noni juice thirty minutes before breakfast. The typical recommendation is 2 tablespoons daily for liquid concentrates or 500 to 1,000 milligrams (mg) daily for powdered extracts.

According to noni promoters, it should be taken on an empty stomach and not together with coffee, tobacco, or alcohol. However, there is no scientific evidence for this recommendation.

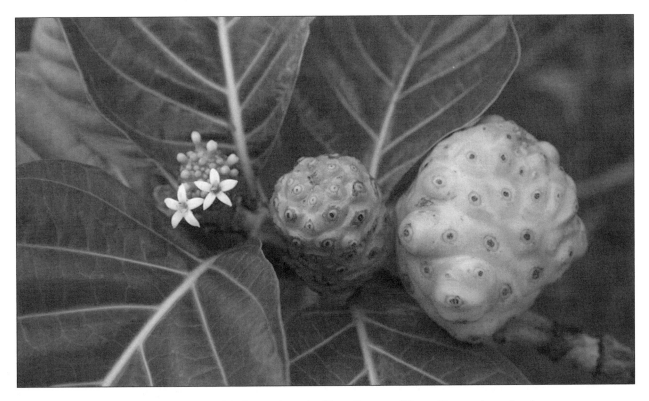

Flowers, immature fruit, and mature noni fruit on a branch. (Inga Spence/Photo Researchers, Inc.)

THERAPEUTIC USES

Noni has been heavily promoted for many uses, including abrasions, arthritis, atherosclerosis, bladder infections, boils, bowel disorders, burns, cancer, chronic fatigue syndrome, circulatory weakness, colds, cold sores, congestion, constipation, diabetes, drug addiction, eye inflammations, fever, fractures, gastric ulcers, gingivitis, headaches, heart disease, hypertension, improved digestion, immune weakness, indigestion, intestinal parasites, kidney disease, malaria, menstrual cramps, menstrual irregularities, mouth sores, respiratory disorders, ringworm, sinusitis, skin inflammation, sprains, stroke, thrush, and wounds. However, there is no evidence that it is effective.

Several animal studies have evaluated the effects of extracts derived from noni. The results suggest noni may have anticancer, immune-enhancing, and pain-relieving properties. However, most of these studies used unrealistically high doses that would be difficult to get from taking the juice itself. There have been no meaningful human trials of noni.

SAFETY ISSUES

Although use of noni is not commonly associated with side effects, comprehensive safety studies have not been performed. A small number of case reports hint that, in rare cases, use of noni might cause severe liver damage, potentially leading to a need for liver transplant. The risk is believed to be very low, however, if it exists at all. Nonetheless, people who have liver disease, who take medications that can harm the liver, or who consume alcohol to excess should not use noni. Maximum safe doses in young children and pregnant or nursing women remain unclear.

EBSCO CAM Review Board

FURTHER READING

Millonig, G., S. Stadlmann, and W. Vogel. "Herbal Hepatotoxicity: Acute Hepatitis Caused by a Noni Preparation (*Morinda citrifolia*)." *European Journal of Gastroenterology and Hepatology* 17, no. 4 (2005): 445-447.

Stadlbauer, V., et al. "Hepatotoxicity of NONI Juice: Report of Two Cases." *World Journal of Gastroenterology* 11 (2005): 4758-4760.

See also: Chinese medicine; Folk medicine; Herbal medicine.

Nonsteroidal anti-inflammatory drugs (NSAIDs)

CATEGORY: Drug interactions

DEFINITION: Drugs used to treat pain, fever, and inflammation.

INTERACTIONS: Arginine, chondroitin, citrate, cayenne, colostrum, dong quai, feverfew, folate, garlic, ginkgo, licorice, PC-SPES, policosanol, potassium citrate, reishi, St. John's wort, vinpocetine, vitamin C, vitamin E (possible mixed interaction), white willow

DRUGS IN THIS FAMILY: Aspirin, alternatively called acetylsalicylic acid or ASA (Adprin-B, Anacin, Arthritis Foundation Aspirin, Ascriptin, Aspergum, Asprimox, Bayer, BC, Bufferin, Buffex, Cama, Cope, Easprin, Ecotrin, Empirin, Equagesic, Fiorinal, Fiorital, Halfprin, Heartline, Genprin, Lanorinal, Magnaprin, Measurin, Micrainin, Momentum, Norwich, St. Joseph, Zorprin), celecoxib (Celebrex), choline salicylate (Arthropan), choline salicylate/magnesium salicylate (Tricosal, Trilisate), diclofenac potassium (Cataflam, Voltaren Rapide), diclofenac sodium (Arthrotec, Voltaren, Voltaren SR, Voltaren-XR), diclofenac sodium/misoprostol (Arthrotec), diflunisal (Dolobid), etodolac (Lodine, Lodine XL), fenoprofen calcium (Nalfon), flurbiprofen (Ansaid), ibuprofen (Advil, Arthritis Foundation Ibuprofen, Bayer Select Ibuprofen, Dynafed IB, Genpril, Haltran, IBU, Ibuprin, Ibuprohm, Menadol, Midol IB, Motrin, Nuprin, Saleto), indomethacin (Indochron E-R, Indocin, Indocin SR, Indomethacin, Indomethacin SR, Novo-Methacin), ketoprofen (Actron, Orudis, Orudis KT, Oruvail), ketorolac tromethamine (Toradol), magnesium salicylate (Doan's, Magan, Mobidin, Backache Maximum Strength Relief, Bayer Select Maximum Strength Backache, Momentum Muscular Backache Formula, Nuprin Backache, Mobigesic, Magsal), meclofenamate sodium (Mecolfen, Meclomen), mefenamic acid (Ponstan, Ponstel), nabumetone (Relafen), naproxen (EC-Naprosyn, Napron X, Naprosyn), naproxen sodium (Aleve, Anaprox, Anaprox DS, Naprelan), oxaprozin (Daypro), piroxicam (Feldene), salsalate or salicylic acid (Amigesic, Argesic-SA, Arthra-G, Disalcid, Marthritic, Mono-Gesic, Salflex, Salgesic, Salsitab), sodium salicylate (Pabalate), sodium thiosalicylate (Rexolate), sulfasalazine (Azulfidine EN-tabs, Salazopyrin, SAS-500), sulindac (Clinoril), tolmetin sodium (Tolectin, Tolectin DS)

ARGININE

Effect: Possible Harmful Interaction

Arginine is an amino acid found in many foods, including dairy products, meat, poultry, and fish. Supplemental arginine has been proposed as a treatment for various conditions, including heart problems.

Arginine has been found to stimulate the body's production of gastrin, a hormone that increases stomach acid. Because excessive acid can irritate the stomach, there are concerns that arginine could be harmful for persons taking drugs that can negatively affect the stomach (such as NSAIDs). It may be best not to mix arginine with NSAIDs unless approved by a doctor.

FEVERFEW

Effect: Possible Harmful Interaction

The herb feverfew (*Tanacetum parthenium*) is primarily used for the prevention and treatment of migraine headaches. NSAIDs are also used for migraines, so there is a chance that some persons might use both the herb and drug at once, a combination that may present risks.

The biggest concern with NSAIDs is that they can cause stomach ulcers, which may progress to bleeding or perforation without pain or other warning symptoms. This stomach damage is caused by drug interference with the body's protective prostaglandins. Newer NSAIDs called COX-2 inhibitors may be less likely to produce this side effect. Feverfew also affects prostaglandins, so combining it with an NSAID might increase the risk of stomach problems.

GARLIC, GINKGO

Effect: Possible Harmful Interaction

Among many other proposed uses, the herb garlic (*Allium sativum*) is taken to lower cholesterol. One of the possible side effects of garlic is a decreased ability of the blood to clot, leading to an increased bleeding tendency. Therefore, one should not combine garlic and aspirin or other NSAIDs except under medical supervision.

Among many other uses, the herb ginkgo is used to treat Alzheimer's disease and ordinary age-related memory loss. Some evidence suggests that ginkgo might also decrease the ability of the blood to clot, probably through effects on platelets. However, one double-blind study found that ginkgo does not increase the anticoagulant effects of aspirin; another study found that while it did not interact with the antiplatelet drug clopidogrel, the herb did interact slightly with the related drug cilostazol. Taken together, this evidence still suggests that one should not take ginkgo while using aspirin or other NSAIDs, except under medical supervision.

POLICOSANOL (SUGARCANE SOURCE)
Effect: Possible Harmful Interaction

A sugarcane-derived form of the supplement policosanol is used to reduce cholesterol levels. It also interferes with platelet clumping, creating potential benefit and a risk of interactions with blood-thinning drugs.

A thirty-day, double-blind, placebo-controlled trial of twenty-seven people with high cholesterol levels found that policosanol at 10 milligrams (mg) a day markedly reduced the ability of blood platelets to

Combining NSAIDs with Dietary and Herbal Supplements and Prescription Drugs

Harmful, even life-threatening results can occur after taking a combination of supplements; using these products with medications (whether prescription or over-the-counter, including nonsteroidal anti-inflammatory drugs, or NSAIDs); or substituting them in place of medicines prescribed by a doctor. Health consumers should be alert to any advisories about these products. Coumadin (a prescription medicine), *Ginkgo biloba* (an herbal supplement), aspirin (an over-the-counter NSAID), and vitamin E (a dietary supplement) can each thin the blood. Taking any of these products alone or together can increase the potential for internal bleeding or stroke.

clump together. Another double-blind, placebo-controlled study of thirty-seven healthy volunteers found evidence that the blood-thinning effect of policosanol increased as the dose was increased: the larger the policosanol dose, the greater the effect.

Another double-blind placebo-controlled study of forty-three healthy volunteers compared the effects of policosanol (20 mg daily), aspirin (100 mg daily), and policosanol and aspirin combined at these same doses. The results again showed that policosanol substantially reduced the ability of blood platelets to stick together, and that the combined therapy exhibited additive effects.

Based on these findings, one should avoid combining aspirin or other NSAIDs with sugarcane policosanol except under medical supervision. Beeswax policosanol, discussed below, is substantially different from sugarcane policosanol.

PC-SPES
Effect: Possible Harmful Interaction

PC-SPES is an herbal combination that has shown promise for the treatment of prostate cancer. One case report suggests that PC-SPES might increase risk of bleeding complications if combined with blood-thinning medications. Subsequent evidence has indicated that PC-SPES contains the strong prescription blood thinner warfarin, making this interaction inevitable.

POTASSIUM CITRATE
Effect: Possible Harmful Interaction

Potassium citrate and other forms of citrate (such as calcium citrate and magnesium citrate) may be used to prevent kidney stones. These agents work by making the urine less acidic. This effect on the urine may lead to decreased blood levels and therapeutic effects of several drugs, including aspirin and other salicylates (choline salicylate, magnesium salicylate, salsalate, sodium salicylate, and sodium thiosalicylate). One should avoid these citrate compounds during therapy with aspirin or salicylates, except under medical supervision.

REISHI
Effect: Possible Harmful Interaction

One study suggests that reishi impairs platelet clumping. This creates the potential for an interaction with any blood-thinning medication.

DONG QUAI, ST. JOHN'S WORT

Effect: Possible Harmful Interaction

The herb dong quai (*Angelica sinensis*) is often recommended for menstrual disorders such as dysmenorrhea, premenstrual syndrome, and irregular menstruation. St. John's wort (*Hypericum perforatum*) is primarily used to treat mild to moderate depression.

Certain NSAIDs, including most notably piroxicam, can cause increased sensitivity to the sun, amplifying the risk of sunburn or skin rash. Because St. John's wort and dong quai may also cause this problem, taking these herbal supplements during NSAID therapy might add to this risk. One should use sunscreen or wear protective clothing during sun exposure if also taking one of these herbs while using an NSAID.

VINPOCETINE

Effect: Possible Harmful Interaction

The substance vinpocetine is sold as a dietary supplement for the treatment of age-related memory loss and impaired mental function. Vinpocetine is thought to inhibit blood platelets from forming clots. For this reason, it should not be combined with medications or natural substances that impair the blood's ability to clot normally, as this may lead to excessive bleeding. One study found only a minimal interaction between the blood-thinning drug warfarin and vinpocetine, but one should use caution anyway.

VITAMIN E

Effect: Possible Mixed Interaction

Vitamin E appears to add to aspirin's blood-thinning effects. One study suggests that the combination of aspirin and even relatively small amounts of vitamin E (50 mg daily) may lead to a significantly increased risk of bleeding. In another study of 28,519 men, vitamin E supplementation at a low dose of about 50 IU (international units) daily was associated with an increase in fatal hemorrhagic strokes, the kind of stroke caused by bleeding within the brain. However, there was a reduced risk of the more common ischemic stroke, caused by obstruction of a blood vessel in the brain, and the two effects were found essentially to cancel each other out.

Weak evidence from one animal study hints that vitamin E might reduce stomach inflammation caused by NSAIDs. One should seek medical advice before combining vitamin E and aspirin.

WHITE WILLOW

Effect: Possible Harmful Interaction

The herb white willow (*Salix alba*), also known as willow bark, is used to treat pain and fever. White willow contains a substance that is converted by the body into a salicylate similar to aspirin. It is therefore possible that taking NSAIDs and white willow could lead to increased risk of side effects, just as would occur if one combined NSAIDs with aspirin.

HERBS AND SUPPLEMENTS

Effect: Possible Harmful Interaction

Based on their known effects or constituents, the herbs dong quai, garlic, ginger (*Zingiber officinale*), horse chestnut (*Aesculus hippocastanum*), and red clover (*Trifolium pratense*), and the substances fish oil, mesoglycan, and OPCs (oligomeric proanthocyanidins), might present an increased risk of bleeding if combined with aspirin.

CITRATE

Effect: Possible Harmful Interaction

Potassium citrate, sodium citrate, and potassium-magnesium citrate are sometimes used to prevent kidney stones. These supplements reduce urinary acidity and can, therefore, lead to decreased blood levels and decreased effectiveness of NSAIDs.

CAYENNE

Effect: Supplementation Possibly Helpful

Cayenne (*Capsicum annuum* or *C. frutescens*) and other hot peppers used in chili and various dishes contain as their "hot" ingredient capsaicin, a substance that is thought to be stomach-protective. For years, people have believed that spicy foods were a cause of stomach ulcers. However, preliminary evidence suggests that cayenne peppers might actually help protect the stomach against ulcers caused by aspirin and possibly other NSAIDs.

In a study involving eighteen healthy volunteers, one group received chili powder, water, and aspirin; the control group received only water and aspirin. Chili powder was found to significantly protect the stomach against damage from aspirin, a known stomach irritant. It was suggested that this protective effect might result from capsaicin-induced stimulation of blood flow in the lining of the stomach.

Further support for this theory comes from a study in rats, which found that capsaicin protected the stomach against damage caused by aspirin, ethanol (consumable alcohol), and acid. Increasing the dose of capsaicin brought even greater benefit, as did increasing the time between giving capsaicin and giving the other agents. An earlier study in rats found that capsaicin conferred similar protection against aspirin damage.

Some researchers have used these data to advocate chili or capsaicin as treatment for peptic ulcer disease. However, one should check with a doctor before trying to self-treat this serious condition.

COLOSTRUM

Effect: Supplementation Possibly Helpful

Colostrum is the fluid that women's breasts produce during the first day or two after giving birth. The fluid gives newborns a rich mixture of antibodies and growth factors that help them get a good start on nutrition. According to one study involving rats, taking colostrum from cows (bovine colostrum) as a supplement might help protect against the ulcers caused by NSAIDs.

FOLATE

Effect: Supplementation Possibly Helpful

Folate (also known as folic acid) is a B vitamin that plays an important role in many vital aspects of health, including preventing neural-tube birth defects and possibly reducing the risk of heart disease. Because inadequate intake of folate is widespread, persons taking any medication that depletes or impairs folate even slightly may need supplementation.

There is some evidence that NSAIDs might produce this effect. In test-tube studies, many NSAIDs have been found to interfere with folate activity. In addition, a study of twenty-five people with arthritis receiving the drug sulfasalazine found evidence of folate deficiency. In another report, a woman taking 650 mg of aspirin every four hours for three days experienced a significant fall in blood levels of folate. Based on this preliminary evidence, folate supplementation may be warranted for persons taking drugs in the NSAID family.

LICORICE

Effect: Supplementation Possibly Helpful

Licorice root (*Glycyrrhiza glabra* or *G. uralensis*), a member of the pea family, has been used since ancient times as both food and medicine. Preliminary evidence suggests that a specific form of licorice called DGL (deglycyrrhizinated licorice) might help protect the stomach against damage caused by the use of aspirin and possibly other NSAIDs. (DGL is a modified version of licorice that is safer to use.)

In a double-blind study of nine healthy volunteers, participants were given aspirin alone (325 mg) or aspirin (325 mg) plus DGL (175 mg). Stomach damage (as measured by blood loss) was found to be about 20 percent less when DGL was given with aspirin. As part of the same study, DGL also was found to reduce stomach damage caused by aspirin in rats, though the benefit was small. It is possible that larger doses of DGL might provide greater protection.

VITAMIN C

Effect: Supplementation Possibly Helpful

Test-tube studies suggest that aspirin promotes the loss of vitamin C through the urine, which could lead to tissue depletion of the vitamin. In addition, low vitamin C levels have been noted in persons with rheumatoid arthritis, and this has been attributed to aspirin therapy taken for this condition. Vitamin C supplementation may be advisable in persons who regularly take aspirin.

POLICOSANOL (BEESWAX FORM)

Effect: Possible Helpful Interaction

The supplement policosanol is a mixture of numerous related substances, and its exact composition varies with its source. Policosanol made from sugar cane appears to reduce cholesterol levels. Policosanol from beeswax may help protect the stomach from damage caused by NSAIDs. However, it is not clear if beeswax policosanol amplifies the "blood thinning" effect of anti-inflammatory drugs in the same manner as sugarcane policosanol.

CHONDROITIN

Effect: Possible Harmful Interaction

Based on chondroitin's chemical similarity to the anticoagulant drug heparin, it has been suggested that chondroitin also might have anticoagulant effects. There are no case reports of any problems related to this, and studies suggest that chondroitin has at most a mild anticoagulant effect. Nonetheless, chondroitin should not be combined with NSAIDs except under physician supervision.

EBSCO CAM Review Board

FURTHER READING

Aruna, D., and M. U. Naidu. "Pharmacodynamic Inter-
action Studies of *Ginkgo biloba* with Cilostazol and
Clopidogrel in Healthy Human Subjects." *British
Journal of Clinical Pharmacology* 63 (2007): 333-338.

Ernst, Edzard, Max H. Pittler, and Barbara Wider,
eds. *Complementary Therapies for Pain Management:
An Evidence-Based Approach.* New York: Mosby/Else-
vier, 2007.

Górski, Andrzej, Hubert Krotkiewski, and Michał
Zimecki, eds. *Inflammation.* Boston: Kluwer Academic, 2001.

Wolf, H. R. "Does *Ginkgo biloba* Special Extract EGb 761
Provide Additional Effects on Coagulation and
Bleeding When Added to Acetylsalicylic Acid 500mg
Daily?" *Drugs in Research and Development* 7 (2006):
163-172.

See also: Arginine; Cayenne; Colostrum; Food and
Drug Administration; Ginkgo; Herbal medicine; Lic-
orice; Pain management; Policosanol; Supplements:
Introduction; Vinpocetine; Vitamin E.

Nopal

CATEGORY: Herbs and supplements
RELATED TERMS: *Opuntia*, prickly pear cactus
DEFINITION: Natural plant product used to treat spe-
cific health conditions.
PRINCIPAL PROPOSED USES: Diabetes, hangover
from use of alcohol
OTHER PROPOSED USES: High cholesterol, prostate
enlargement

OVERVIEW

The nopal, or prickly pear cactus, is one of the
major national symbols of Mexico and appears on
the Mexican flag. This cactus has a long history of
use as food and medicine. Its fleshy, leaflike stems
(cladodes), especially when young, are eaten as
vegetables. The fruit is eaten raw, fermented into a
beer, or turned into a cheeselike food. Medicinally,
nopal fruit, stems, and flowers have been used to
treat diabetes, stomach problems, fatigue, shortness
of breath, easy bruising, prostate enlargement, and
liver disease. Nopal is also a significant source of protein, vitamins, and minerals.

THERAPEUTIC DOSAGES

Neither the optimum dosage nor the most active
species of nopal cactus has been established. The one
double-blind study that has been conducted used a
special extract made from the skin of the fruit of
Opuntia ficus indica.

THERAPEUTIC USES

Although the results of animal studies and highly
preliminary trials in humans are somewhat contradictory, taken together they suggest that nopal fruit and
stems might have some benefit for diabetes. However,
only properly designed and sufficiently large double-
blind, placebo-controlled trials can reveal for sure
whether nopal is effective, and none have been reported for this use of nopal.

The only properly designed study of nopal involved
use of the cactus for treating hangover symptoms. In
this double-blind, placebo-controlled study of sixty-
four people, use of an extract made from the skin of
nopal fruit significantly reduced hangover symptoms
compared with a placebo. The greatest improvements
were seen in symptoms of nausea, loss of appetite, and
dry mouth. Overall, the rate of severe hangover symptoms was 50 percent lower in the treatment group
compared with the placebo group. The researchers
involved in this study hypothesized that hangovers are
caused by inflammation and that the herb reduced inflammation.

There is weak evidence that nopal fruit, leaves, or
stems might be helpful for improving cholesterol profile. Other studies suggest that nopal stems and fruit
might have anti-inflammatory, pain-relieving, and
stomach-protective effects. Finally, test-tube studies
suggest that the flower of the nopal cactus might be
helpful for prostate enlargement (BPH).

SAFETY ISSUES

As a widely eaten food, nopal is presumed safe.
However, safety in young children, pregnant or
nursing women, and individuals with severe liver or
kidney disease has not been established.

EBSCO CAM Review Board

FURTHER READING

Linares, E., C. Thimonier, and M. Degre. "The Effect
of NeOpuntia on Blood Lipid Parameters: Risk
Factors for the Metabolic Syndrome (Syndrome
X)." *Advances in Therapy* 24 (2007): 1115-1125.

Wiese, J., et al. "Effect of *Opuntia ficus indica* on Symptoms of the Alcohol Hangover." *Archives of Internal Medicine* 164 (2004): 1334-1340.

See also: Diabetes; Herbal medicine.

Nosebleeds

CATEGORY: Condition
RELATED TERM: Epistaxis
DEFINITION: Treatment of bleeding of the nose.
PRINCIPAL PROPOSED NATURAL TREATMENT: Citrus bioflavonoids
OTHER PROPOSED NATURAL TREATMENTS: Bilberry, bromelain, oligomeric proanthocyanidins, proteolytic enzymes, shepherd's purse, vitamin C

INTRODUCTION

A nosebleed can arise from many causes, including dry winter air, colds, injuries, or the common if unsavory habit of picking one's nose. In many cases, no cause can be identified with certainty.

Sometimes nosebleeds arise more frequently because of faulty or weak collagen, a strengthening protein present in blood vessel walls and the surrounding connective tissue. Collagen problems may lead to nosebleeds in people who take corticosteroids and those with a condition called fragile capillaries. Corticosteroids, including nasal steroids used for allergies, can thin the collagen in the mucous membranes lining the nose. In fragile capillaries, weak or defective collagen in blood vessel walls may contribute to bleeding. People with such collagen problems may have problems with bleeding gums, heavy menstrual periods, and bruising in addition to nosebleeds.

Rarely, the cause of nosebleeds and other bleeding lies in the blood itself. Anything that reduces blood clotting may lead to nosebleeds. Drugs such as warfarin (Coumadin) or heparin and the regular use of aspirin decrease the blood's tendency to clot. (Persons taking such medications who begin to experience nosebleeds should consult their doctor.) Even natural substances such as ginkgo, policosanol, high-dose vitamin E, and garlic may increase the tendency to bleed.

Conventional treatments for nosebleeds include various maneuvers for stopping acute bleeding, followed by the diagnosis and treatment of any underlying problems. Sometimes a physician can prevent future nosebleeds by cauterizing the responsible blood vessel.

PRINCIPAL PROPOSED NATURAL TREATMENTS

One supplement that may help prevent nosebleeds is citrus bioflavonoids. Bioflavonoids (or flavonoids) are plant substances that bring color to many fruits and vegetables. Citrus fruits are a rich source of bioflavonoids, including disomin, hesperidin, rutin, and naringen.

A double-blind, placebo-controlled study of ninety-six people with fragile capillaries found that a combination of the bioflavonoids diosmin and hesperidin decreased symptoms of capillary fragility, such as nosebleeds and bruising. In this six-week trial, participants (41 percent of whom had problems with nosebleeds) took two tablets daily of the bioflavonoid combination or placebo. Those who received bioflavonoids had significantly greater improvements in both their symptoms and their capillary strength, compared to those taking placebo. However, the researchers did not state how much the nosebleeds improved.

OTHER PROPOSED NATURAL TREATMENTS

Oligomeric proanthocyanidins (OPCs) are bioflavonoid-like compounds found in large amounts in grape seed and grape extract products. Test-tube studies have found that OPCs protect collagen, partly by inhibiting an enzyme that breaks it down. One rather poorly designed double-blind study of thirty-seven people, most of whom had fragile capillaries, found that OPCs were more effective than placebo in decreasing capillary fragility; however, the study authors left many questions unanswered in their report, making it hard to determine how seriously to take their results, and they did not address nosebleeds specifically.

Related chemicals called anthocyanosides are present in high concentrations in the herb bilberry. Like OPCs, anthocyanosides may strengthen capillaries through their effects on collagen. Proteolytic enzymes (such as bromelain) are also thought to help stabilize capillaries. However, no studies have directly addressed the potential value of either of these treatments for nosebleeds.

Vitamin C is vital for the development of normal collagen. People with scurvy (severe vitamin C deficiency) may bleed easily from the nose and may develop spontaneous bruises and other bleeding symptoms.

However, there is no evidence that vitamin C supplementation helps to decrease nosebleeds in the absence of true scurvy, a condition that is rare today.

The herb shepherd's purse (*Capsella bursae pastoris*) has been traditionally used as a topical application to control nosebleeds, although scientific evidence of its effectiveness is lacking. The herb should not be used during pregnancy, because it is thought to stimulate uterine contractions.

EBSCO CAM Review Board

FURTHER READING

Galley, P., and M. Thiollet. "A Double-Blind, Placebo-Controlled Trial of a New Veno-active Flavonoid Fraction (S 5682) in the Treatment of Symptomatic Capillary Fragility." *International Angiology* 12 (1993): 69-72.

Javed, F., A. Golagani, and H. Sharp. "Potential Effects of Herbal Medicines and Nutritional Supplements on Coagulation in ENT Practice." *Journal of Laryngology and Otology* 122 (2008): 116-119.

Shakeel, M., et al. "Complementary and Alternative Medicine in Epistaxis: A Point Worth Considering During the Patient's History." *European Journal of Emergency Medicine* 17 (2010): 17-19.

See also: Citrus bioflavonoids; Sinusitis; Wounds, minor.

O

Oak bark

CATEGORY: Herbs and supplements
RELATED TERM: *Quercus* and species
DEFINITION: Natural plant product used to treat specific health conditions.
PRINCIPAL PROPOSED USE: Diarrhea
OTHER PROPOSED USES: Canker sores, eczema, hemorrhoids, sore throat

OVERVIEW

The oak tree, respected for millennia as a source of strong, dense wood, also has a considerable tradition of medicinal use. The astringent, tannin-rich bark of the oak tree has been recommended for such diverse conditions as internal hemorrhage, diarrhea, dysentery, cancer, and pneumonia.

THERAPEUTIC DOSAGES

A typical oral dose of oak bark is 1 gram three times daily. For application as a treatment for eczema, an oak bark tea is made by boiling 1 to 2 tablespoons of the bark for twenty minutes in 2 cups of water, and this is applied to the rash three to five times daily. Oak tinctures and extracts should be used according to label instructions.

THERAPEUTIC USES

Currently, Germany's Commission E recommends oak bark internally for treatment of diarrhea and topically for sore throat, mouth sores, hemorrhoids, and eczema. However, there is no meaningful scientific evidence that oak bark offers any therapeutic benefit in these or any other conditions. Only double-blind, placebo-controlled studies can prove a treatment effective, and none have been performed on oak bark.

Oak bark contains numerous substances in the tannin family, especially ellagitannin, along with potentially active substances in the saponin family. Tannins are thought to have an astringent effect, meaning that they reduce tissue swelling and stop bleeding, and they are traditionally thought to be useful for diarrhea. However, oak bark has never been studied as a treatment for diarrhea. Saponins are often said to act as expectorants, enhancing the ability to cough up phlegm. Again, however, there is no direct evidence that oak bark is useful for coughs or related conditions.

Evidence too weak to be relied upon hints that oak bark may have value for kidney stones, possibly reducing pain and slowing stone growth. In addition, test-tube studies indicate that oak bark solutions applied topically might have activity against various microorganisms, including *Staphylococcus* bacteria, and might also exert cancer-preventive effects. However, it is a long way from such studies to actual evidence of clinical benefit.

SAFETY ISSUES

Although comprehensive safety testing has not been performed, use of oak bark is

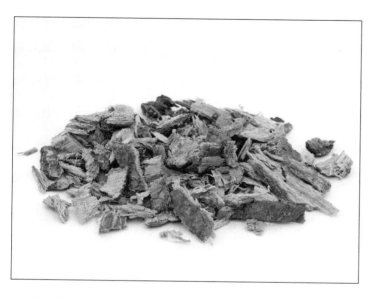

Dried oak bark is used to make a tea (infusion) that is thought to have astringent properties. (Geoff Kidd/Photo Researchers, Inc.)

not generally associated with any side effects other than the occasional digestive upset or allergic reaction. Safety in young children, pregnant or nursing women, and people with severe liver or kidney disease has not been established.

EBSCO CAM Review Board

FURTHER READING

Cerda, B., F. A. Tomas-Barberan, and J. C. Espin. "Metabolism of Antioxidant and Chemopreventive Ellagitannins from Strawberries, Raspberries, Walnuts, and Oak-Aged Wine in Humans: Identification of Biomarkers and Individual Variability." *Journal of Agricultural and Food Chemistry* 53 (2005): 227-235.

Gulluce, M., et al. "Antimicrobial Effects of *Quercus ilex* L. Extract." *Phytotherapy Research* 18 (2004): 208-211.

Voravuthikunchai, S., et al. "Effective Medicinal Plants Against Enterohaemorrhagic *Escherichia coli* O157:H7." *Journal of Ethnopharmacology* 94 (2004): 49-54.

Voravuthikunchai, S. P., and L. Kitpipit. "Activity of Medicinal Plant Extracts Against Hospital Isolates of Methicillin-Resistant *Staphylococcus aureus*." *Clinical Microbiology and Infections* 11 (2005): 510-512.

See also: Diarrhea; Herbal medicine.

Oat straw

CATEGORY: Herbs and supplements

RELATED TERMS: Avena sativa, green oats, oat straw, wild oat extract

DEFINITION: Natural plant product used to treat specific health conditions.

PRINCIPAL PROPOSED USES: None

OTHER PROPOSED USES: Benign prostatic hypertrophy, enhancing female sexual function, enhancing male sexual function, smoking cessation

OVERVIEW

When an oat plant matures, it produces a fruit that becomes the grain called oats, a heart-healthy, high-fiber food. This article does not address this form of oat. Rather, described here are those products made from the green, unripe oat straw, sold under the names *Avena sativa*, green oats, and wild oat extract.

Traditionally, oat straw was considered a mild nervine, an herb thought to calm and heal nervous symptoms. On this basis, it was used to treat insomnia, stress, anxiety, and nervousness. In addition, oat straw tea was used for arthritis, and an alcohol extract of oat straw for the treatment of narcotic and cigarette addiction. However, there is no evidence that it is effective when used for any of these purposes.

THERAPEUTIC DOSAGES

Oat straw extract should be taken according to the manufacturer's directions. Alcohol tincture of oat straw is typically used at a dose of ½ to 1 teaspoon three times per day.

THERAPEUTIC USES

Oat straw is widely marketed for enhancing male sexual function, and a combination of oat straw and saw palmetto is said to help sexual dysfunction in women. The same combination is supposedly helpful for enlargement of the prostate. However, the only evidence for these claims comes from unpublished studies conducted by the manufacturer of oat straw products. Because these studies are not available in full, it is not possible to judge their validity.

For example, one double-blind, placebo-controlled trial of seventy-five men and women reportedly found that use of an oat straw product enhanced sexual experience for men but not for women. It is not clear whether the results were statistically significant or exactly how the researchers arrived at their conclusions. Another study discussed on the same Web page supposedly found that oat straw combined with saw palmetto produced similar benefits for women, but it is not clear whether this trial was double-blind.

It has been claimed that oat straw works by increasing the amount of free testosterone in the blood. Many oat straw Web sites state that, with advancing age, testosterone in the body tends to become bound up and inactivated, that this leads to numerous problems including failing sexual function, and that oat straw reverses this process. However, none of the parts of this argument are fully substantiated. The argument is speculation piled on speculation.

Oat straw has also been advocated as a stop-smoking treatment. However, despite promising results in one rather informal study, reported in a letter to the journal *Nature* in 1971, the balance of the evidence suggests that alcohol tincture of wild oats is not helpful for quitting smoking.

SAFETY ISSUES

There are no known or suspected health risks with oat straw. However, comprehensive safety studies have not been reported.

EBSCO CAM Review Board

FURTHER READING

Anand, C. L. "Effect of *Avena sativa* on Cigarette Smoking." *Nature* 233 (1971): 496.

Bye, C., et al. "Lack of Effect of *Avena sativa* on Cigarette Smoking." *Nature* 252 (1974): 580-581.

Gabrynowicz, J. W. "Letter: Treatment of Nicotine Addiction with *Avena sativa*." *Medical Journal of Australia* 2 (1974): 306-307.

See also: Herbal medicine; Saw palmetto; Sexual dysfunction in men; Sexual dysfunction in women; Smoking addiction.

Obesity and excess weight

CATEGORY: Condition

RELATED TERMS: Overweight, weight control, weight loss aids

DEFINITION: Treatment to aid in the loss of excess body weight.

PRINCIPAL PROPOSED NATURAL TREATMENTS: Chromium, fiber, pyruvate

OTHER PROPOSED NATURAL TREATMENTS: Acupuncture, Ayurveda, calcium, *Coleus forskohlii*, combination herb/supplement therapies, conjugated linoleic acid, dehydroepiandrosterone, diacylglycerol, ephedrine (alone or with caffeine), evening primrose oil, 5-hydroxytryptophan, green tea, glucomannan, *Hoodia gordonii*, hydroxycitric acid (*Garcinia cambogia*), hypnotherapy, L-carnitine, low-carbohydrate diet, low-glycemic-index diet, medium-chain triglycerides, spirulina, vitamin C, vitamin D

INTRODUCTION

Losing weight can be a lifelong challenge. Researchers who study obesity consider it a chronic health condition that must be managed much like high blood pressure or high cholesterol. This means that there is no easy cure.

Losing just 5 to 10 percent of one's total weight can lower blood pressure, improve cholesterol profile, prevent diabetes, improve blood sugar control if one already has diabetes, and reduce the risk of developing osteoarthritis of the knee. A combination of improved diet and regular exercise might be the best way to lose weight and keep it off.

Although early weight-loss drugs, such as amphetamines and Fen-Phen (fenfluramine and phentermine), have had a poor safety record, sibutramine (Meridia) appears to be safe and modestly effective for weight loss. Newer drugs will likely offer greater benefits.

It is commonly stated that the high-fructose corn syrup that is added to many foods is a major cause of obesity. However, while there is little doubt that, in general, excess intake of calories promotes obesity, the specific relationship of this substance to weight gain remains questionable.

PRINCIPAL PROPOSED NATURAL TREATMENTS

Chromium. Chromium is a mineral the body needs in only small amounts, but it is important to human nutrition. Although it has principally been studied for improving blood sugar control in people with diabetes, chromium has also been tried for reducing total weight and body fat percentage, with some success. Both of these potential benefits involve chromium's effects on insulin. Before an explanation of how chromium may help, some background information on how the body controls its blood sugar levels will be provided here.

The body needs a constant level of glucose (sugar) in the blood. When a person digests a carbohydrate meal, glucose levels rise. Protein meals have the same effect, although to a lesser extent. The body responds by secreting insulin. Insulin causes the cells of the body to absorb glucose out of the blood, thereby reducing circulating blood sugar.

Once cells have taken in glucose, they can burn it for energy or convert it to a storage form. Liver and muscle cells can store a limited amount of glucose as glycogen. Fat cells can convert unlimited amounts of glucose into energy stored as fat.

The process also goes the opposite way. When the body has used up the food from its last meal, blood glucose levels drop. Just as the body does not respond well to glucose levels that are too high, low glucose levels also cause problems. The body, in response, applies its control mechanisms to raise blood sugar levels. It does so by reducing its output of insulin and also by raising levels of another hormone called glucagon. The net effect is that energy storage depots are mobilized. Glycogen is converted back into glucose. In addition, fat cells release their contents into the bloodstream to supply an alternative energy source. In summary, high insulin levels build fat, whereas low insulin levels break down fat.

Based on this push-pull effect, to lose weight, one should keep insulin levels low. Dieting is the most obvious method of reducing insulin. When a person does not take in enough calories to supply the body's daily needs, insulin levels fall and the body breaks down fat cells. Exercising is another method to reduce insulin; by increasing the body's energy requirements, exercise causes insulin levels to fall and fat cells to break down.

It is difficult to consistently use more energy than one takes in. Hunger takes over, and a person wants to eat. If there were some way to trigger fat breakdown without going hungry, it would make weight loss much easier.

There is another important connection between insulin and weight to consider. Persons who weigh too much often develop insulin resistance. In this condition, certain cells of the body become less sensitive to insulin. The body senses this and, thus, increases insulin production until it overcomes the resistance. It is possible that fat cells respond to these increased levels of insulin by storing even more fat.

Chromium is thought to improve the body's responsiveness to insulin. Combining this belief with the insulin-weight connections, some researchers have proposed that chromium may assist in decreasing weight or improving body composition (the ratio of fatty tissue to lean tissue).

The main argument is the following: Chromium increases insulin sensitivity. This causes levels of insulin to fall. With reduced amounts of insulin in the blood, fat cells are less inclined to store fat, so weight loss may become easier. In addition, there is some evidence that chromium partially blocks insulin's effects on fat cells, interfering with its fat-building effect. This could also promote weight loss. Another small study suggests that chromium may work by influencing the brain and its role in appetite and food cravings.

There are several flaws in these arguments, though. For example, even very small amounts of insulin in the blood effectively suppress fat breakdown. Another

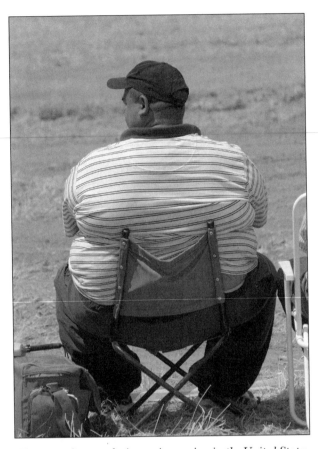

The rates of severe obesity are increasing in the United States. (© Armand Upton/Dreamstime.com)

problem is that during insulin resistance, fat cells also appear to become resistant to insulin. Insulin resistance, in other words, might be a natural method of regulating weight gain. Chromium supplements might have the undesired effect of increasing the ability of fat cells to respond to insulin, helping them to better store fat.

However, theory takes one only so far. It is more important to review the results of studies in which people were given chromium supplements to reduce their weight.

About ten well-designed, double-blind, placebo-controlled trials have evaluated chromium's potential benefit for weight loss. In the largest study, 219 people were given either placebo, 200 micrograms (mcg) of chromium picolinate daily, or 400 mcg of chromium picolinate daily. Participants were not advised to follow any particular diet. For seventy-two days, people taking chromium experienced significantly greater weight loss (more than 2.5 pounds versus about 0.25 pound) than those not taking chromium. Persons taking chromium actually gained lean body mass, so the difference in loss of fatty tissue was greater: more than 4 pounds versus less than 0.50 pound. However, a high dropout rate makes the results of this study somewhat unreliable.

In a smaller double-blind study by the same researcher, 130 moderately overweight persons attempting to lose weight were given either placebo or 400 mcg of chromium daily. Although hints of benefit were seen, they were too slight to be statistically significant. Several other small, double-blind, placebo-controlled studies also failed to find evidence of the benefit of chromium picolinate as an aid to weight loss. One study failed to find benefit with a combination of chromium and conjugated linoleic acid.

When larger studies find positive results and smaller studies do not, it often indicates that the treatment under study is only weakly effective. This may be the case with chromium as a weight-loss treatment.

Pyruvate. Pyruvate supplies the body with pyruvic acid, a natural compound that plays important roles in the manufacture and use of energy. Theoretically, taking pyruvate might increase the body's metabolism, particularly of fat.

Several small studies enrolling about 150 people have found evidence that pyruvate or DHAP (a combination of pyruvate and the related substance dihydroxyacetone) can aid weight loss or improve body composition, or both. For example, in a six-week, double-blind, placebo-controlled trial, fifty-one people were given either pyruvate (6 grams [g] daily), placebo, or no treatment. All participated in an exercise program. In the treated group, significant decreases in fat mass (2.1 kilograms [kg]) and percentage body fat (2.6 percent) were seen, along with a significant increase in muscle mass (1.5 kg). No significant changes were seen in the placebo or nontreatment groups.

Another placebo-controlled study (blinding not stated) used a much higher dose of pyruvate (22 to 44 g daily, depending on total calorie intake). In this trial, thirty-four slightly overweight people were put on a mildly weight-reducing diet for four weeks. Subsequently, one-half were given a liquid dietary supplement containing pyruvate. In six weeks, people in the pyruvate group lost a small amount of weight (about 1.5 pounds), while those in the placebo group did not lose weight. Most of the weight loss came from fat.

Another placebo-controlled study evaluated the effects of DHAP when people who had previously lost weight increased their calorie intake. Seventeen severely overweight women were put on a restricted diet as inpatients for three weeks, during which time they lost approximately 17 pounds. They were then given a high-calorie diet. Approximately one-half of the women also received 15 g of pyruvate and 75 g of dihydroxyacetone daily. The results found that after three weeks of this weight-gaining diet, persons receiving the supplements gained only about 4 pounds, compared to about 6 pounds in the placebo group. Close evaluation showed that pyruvate specifically blocked the regain of fat weight. Larger studies (one hundred participants or more) are needed, however, to establish the benefits of pyruvate for weight loss.

Fiber. Dietary fiber is important to many intestinal tract functions, including digestion and waste excretion. It also appears to have a mild cholesterol-lowering effect and might help reduce the risk of some kinds of cancer (although the evidence is a bit contradictory).

Fiber might also be useful for losing weight. It is thought to work in a simple way by filling the stomach and causing a feeling of fullness, while providing little to no calories. Fiber might also interfere with the absorption of fat.

There are two kinds of fiber: soluble fiber, which swells up and holds water, and insoluble fiber, which does not. Soluble fiber is found in psyllium seed (sold as a laxative), apples, and oat bran. Most other plant-based foods contain insoluble fiber. Fiber supplements may contain a variety of soluble or insoluble fibers from grain, citrus, vegetable, and even shellfish sources.

Several double-blind, placebo-controlled studies have evaluated fiber supplements as an aid to weight loss. The results have been somewhat inconsistent, but in general it appears that some forms of fiber may slightly enhance weight loss.

In one of the largest studies, ninety-seven mildly overweight women on a strict low-calorie diet were given either placebo or an insoluble fiber (type not stated) three times daily for eleven weeks. Women given fiber lost almost 11 pounds compared to about 7 pounds in the placebo group. Participants using the fiber reported less hunger.

Researchers were not finished with the study participants. For an additional sixteen weeks, the diet was changed to one that supplied more calories. As expected, participants regained some weight during this period. Nonetheless, by the end of the sixteen weeks, persons taking fiber were still 8 pounds lighter than at the beginning of the study, while those taking placebo were only 6 pounds lighter.

Another study evaluated whether the benefits of dietary fiber endure in six months of dieting. This double-blind trial of fifty-two overweight people found that the use of insoluble dietary fiber (in a product made from beet, barley, and citrus) almost doubled the degree of weight loss compared with placebo. Once more, participants using the fiber supplement reported less hunger.

Two other double-blind, placebo-controlled studies evaluated a similar insoluble fiber product. The first enrolled sixty moderately overweight women and put them on a 1,400-calorie diet along with placebo or fiber for two months. The other study was similar but enrolled only forty-five women and followed them for three months. The results of both studies again showed improved weight loss and reduced feelings of hunger in the treated groups. However, a twenty-four-week study of fifty-three moderately overweight persons found no difference in effect between placebo and 4 g of insoluble fiber daily. Another study failed to find benefit with either of two soluble fiber supplements (methylcellulose or pectin plus beta glucan) in terms of weight, hunger, or satiety.

Glucomannan, a source of soluble dietary fiber from the tubers of *Amorphophallus konjac*, has also been tried for weight loss, with positive results in adults. In a double-blind, placebo-controlled trial of twenty overweight persons, researchers found that the use of glucomannan significantly improved weight loss in an eight-week period. Benefits were also seen in a double-blind, placebo-controlled trial of twenty-eight overweight persons who had just had a heart attack. However, another trial studied the effectiveness of glucomannan as a weight-loss agent in sixty overweight children and found no benefit.

An eight-week, double-blind, placebo-controlled trial of fifty-nine overweight people evaluated the effects of chitosan, a mostly insoluble fiber from crustaceans, taken at a dose of 1.5 g before each of the two biggest meals of the day. No special diets were assigned. The results showed that, on average, participants in the placebo group gained more than 3 pounds during the study, while those taking chitosan lost more than 2 pounds. However, a subsequent twenty-four-week, double-blind, placebo-controlled study of 250 people using the same dosage of chitosan failed to find benefit. Negative results were also seen in an eight-week, double-blind, placebo-controlled trial of fifty-one women given 1,200 mg twice daily and in a twenty-eight-day double-blind trial of thirty overweight people using 1 g twice daily. Although benefits have shown up in other studies, the balance of evidence indicates that chitosan probably does not work. Furthermore, chitosan supplements may at times contain toxic levels of arsenic.

A few trials have evaluated the effects only on hunger and satiety rather than on weight loss. One study found that the soluble fiber pectin (from apples) reduces hunger sensations. Another found that the soluble fiber guar gum slows stomach emptying and increases the sensation of fullness. However, a later study evaluated the effects of guar gum in twenty-five women undergoing a weight-loss program and found no influence on hunger. In another study, consuming fiber from barley led to an increase in calorie consumption.

The optimum dose of fiber and the proper time to take it have not been determined. In the first three studies noted, insoluble fiber supplements were given twenty to thirty minutes before each meal at a dose of about 2.3 g, along with a large glass of water.

Fiber supplements should be taken with water to keep the fiber from blocking the digestive tract. Even when they are used properly, mild gastrointestinal side effects such as gas and bloating may occur. As a positive side effect, fiber supplements may reduce high levels of cholesterol and blood pressure.

OTHER PROPOSED TREATMENTS

5-hydroxytryptophan. The supplement 5-hydroxy-tryptophan (5-HTP) is thought to affect serotonin levels. Because serotonin is thought to play a role in weight regulation, 5-HTP has been investigated as a possible weight-loss aid. A total of four small, double-blind, placebo-controlled clinical trials have been reported.

The first of these, a double-blind crossover study, found that the use of 5-HTP (at a daily dose of 8 mg per kilogram of body weight) reduced caloric intake even though the nineteen participants made no conscious effort to eat less. Participants given placebo consumed about 2,300 calories per day, while those taking 5-HTP ate only 1,800 calories daily. The use of 5-HTP appeared to lead to a significantly enhanced sense of satiety after eating. In five weeks, women taking 5-HTP effortlessly lost more than 3 pounds.

A follow-up study by the same research group enrolled twenty overweight women who were trying to lose weight. Participants received either 5-HTP (900 mg per day) or placebo for two consecutive six-week periods. In the first period, there was no dietary restriction, while in the second period, participants were encouraged to follow a defined diet that was expected to lead to weight loss.

Participants receiving placebo did not lose weight during either period. However, those receiving 5-HTP lost about 2 percent of their initial body weight during the no-diet period and an additional 3 percent while on the diet. Thus, a woman with an initial weight of 170 pounds lost about 3.5 pounds after six weeks of using 5-HTP without dieting and another 5 pounds while dieting. Once again, participants taking 5-HTP experienced quicker satiety. Similar benefits were seen in a double-blind study of fourteen overweight women given 900 mg of 5-HTP daily.

Finally, a double-blind, placebo-controlled study of twenty overweight persons with adult-onset (type 2) diabetes found that the use of 5-HTP (750 mg per day) without intentional dieting resulted in about a 4.5-pound weight loss in two weeks. The use of 5-HTP reduced carbohydrate intake by 75 percent and fat intake to a lesser extent.

All of these studies, however, were performed by a single research group. In science, results are not considered valid until they are independently replicated by different researchers. In addition, all these studies were small in size. For these reasons, further research is necessary before 5-HTP can be considered a proven weight-loss agent.

Garcinia cambogia. Hydroxycitric acid (HCA), a derivative of citric acid, is found primarily in a small, sweet, purple fruit called *Garcinia cambogia*, the Malabar tamarind. Although animal and test-tube studies and one human trial suggest that HCA might encourage weight loss, other studies have found no benefit. In an eight-week, double-blind, placebo-controlled trial of sixty overweight people, the use of HCA at a dose of 440 mg three times daily produced significant weight loss compared with placebo.

In contrast, a twelve-week, double-blind, placebo-controlled trial of 135 overweight persons, who were given either placebo or 500 mg of HCA three times daily, found no effect on body weight or fat mass. However, this study has been criticized for using a high-fiber diet, which is thought to impair HCA absorption.

Other small placebo-controlled studies found HCA had no effect on metabolism, appetite, or weight. It is not clear whether *G. cambogia* is an effective treatment for weight loss.

Caffeine and ephedrine. Caffeine and ephedrine (found in ephedra, an herb also known as ma huang) are central nervous system stimulants. Considerable evidence suggests ephedrine-caffeine combinations can modestly assist in weight loss.

For example, in a double-blind, placebo-controlled trial, 180 overweight people were placed on a weight-loss diet and given either ephedrine-caffeine (20 mg/200 mg), ephedrine alone (20 mg), caffeine alone (200 mg), or placebo three times daily for twenty-four weeks. The results showed that the ephedrine-caffeine treatment significantly enhanced weight loss, resulting in a loss of more than 36 pounds compared to only 29 pounds in the placebo group. Neither ephedrine nor caffeine alone produced any benefit. Contrary to some reports, participants did not develop tolerance to the treatment. For the entire six months of the trial, the treatment group maintained the same relative weight loss advantage over the placebo group. While this study found benefit only with caffeine-ephedrine and not with ephedrine alone, other studies have found that ephedrine alone also offers some weight-loss benefits.

It is not known how ephedrine-caffeine works. However, caffeine has actions that cause fat breakdown and enhance metabolism. Ephedrine suppresses appetite and increases energy expenditure. The combination appears to produce synergistic effects, with appetite suppression probably the most important overall factor.

Ephedrine presents serious medical risks and should be used only under physician supervision. In the United States, the sale of ephedrine-containing products is banned.

Medium-chain triglycerides. Some evidence suggests that consumption of medium-chain triglycerides (MCTs) might enhance the body's tendency to burn fat. This has led to investigations of MCTs as a weight-loss aid. However, the results of clinical trials have been fairly unimpressive.

In a four-week, double-blind, placebo-controlled trial, sixty-six women were put on a diet very low in carbohydrates to induce a state called ketosis. One-half of the women received a liquid supplement containing ordinary fats; the other one-half received a similar supplement in which the ordinary fats were replaced by MCTs.

The results indicated that the MCT supplement significantly increased the rate of "fat burning" during the first two weeks of the trial and also reduced the loss of muscle mass. However, these benefits declined during the last two weeks of the trial, which suggests that the effects of MCTs are temporary. Studies that involved substituting MCTs for ordinary fats in a low-calorie diet have shown minimal relative benefits at best.

A related supplement called structured medium- and long-chain triacylglycerols (SMLCT) has been created to provide the same potential benefits as MCTs, but in a form that can be used as cooking oil. In a preliminary double-blind trial, SMLCT showed some promise as a "fat burner."

Other approaches to weight loss. A special type of fat known as diacylglycerol has shown promise as a weight-loss aid. For example, in a twenty-four-week, double-blind, placebo-controlled study, 131 overweight men and women were placed on a weight-loss diet including supplementary foods containing either diacylglycerols or ordinary fats. The results showed that participants who were using diacylglycerols lost more weight than participants who were using ordinary fats. Diacylglycerols appear to be safe.

In four preliminary controlled trials, a patented, proprietary blend of fats added to yogurt has shown potential weight-loss benefit. Also, Korean pine nut oil (PinnoThinac), which is high in free fatty acids, was shown in one study (that compared the pine nut oil to olive oil) to reduce the appetite of forty-two overweight women.

Beans partially interfere with the body's ability to digest carbohydrates, which is why they cause flatulence. Based on this process, products containing the French white bean *Phaseolus vulgaris* have been widely marketed as weight-loss aids. However, published studies have generally failed to find these carbohydrate blockers effective for this purpose. According to one manufacturer, more concentrated

extracts of *P. vulgaris*, taken in higher doses, actually can work. The evidence for this claim, until 2007, rested entirely on unpublished studies not independently verified.

A relevant trial was at last published in 2007. In this double-blind, placebo-controlled study, sixty slightly overweight people were given either placebo or a phaseolus extract once daily, thirty minutes before a main meal rich in carbohydrates. The results of the thirty-day study indicated that phaseolus treatment led to a significantly greater reduction of body weight and improvement of lean/fat ratio compared with placebo.

Some evidence suggests that the supplements creatine and colostrum may each slightly improve body composition (fat-to-muscle ratio) compared with placebo among persons undergoing an exercise program. It has been suggested too that calcium supplements, or high-calcium diets, may slightly enhance weight loss, but evidence is more negative than positive. However, because bones may grow thin during rapid weight loss, it may make sense to take calcium supplements when intentionally losing weight. (When weight loss is induced by exercise rather than diet, bone loss does not seem to occur.)

A six-month double-blind study found that the supplement dehydroepiandrosterone (DHEA) at a dose of 50 mg daily may help decrease abdominal fat and improve insulin sensitivity (thereby potentially helping to prevent diabetes) in the elderly. However, another study failed to find DHEA at 40 mg twice daily helpful for weight loss in severely overweight adolescents. A supplement related to DHEA, 3-acetyl-7-oxo-dehydroepiandrosterone (also called 7-oxy or 7-keto-DHEA), has shown some promise for enhancing weight loss.

Results of two small, double-blind, placebo-controlled studies suggest that vitamin C supplements might aid in weight loss. A related study found that marginal vitamin C deficiency might interfere with deliberate attempts to lose weight. Also, one small, double-blind study indicates that a concentrated extract of the herb *Coleus forskohlii* might increase the rate of fat burning.

A double-blind, placebo-controlled trial that enrolled 158 moderately overweight persons tested a mixture of chromium, cayenne, inulin (a nondigestible carbohydrate), and phenylalanine (an amino acid), and other herbs and nutrients. All participants lost weight in the four-week trial. Those using the supplement lost a bit more weight, but the difference was not mathematically significant. However, some positive news came from close examination of the results. Among those taking the supplement, a significantly higher percentage of the weight loss came from fat instead of muscle.

One study found benefit with a combination treatment containing niacin-bound chromium combined with *Gymnema sylvestre* and HCA. Another study reported weight-loss effects with a combination of HCA, pantothenic acid, chamomile, lavender, damask rose, and the Hawaiian herb *Cananga odorata*. A very small study hints that soy isoflavones might help reduce buildup of abdominal fat.

Weight-loss benefits were seen in a double-blind trial of 150 overweight people given either placebo or one of two doses of a combination therapy containing chitosan, chromium, and HCA. Benefits were also seen in a forty-five-day double-blind, placebo-controlled trial of forty-four overweight people that tested a combination product containing yerba mate, guarana, and damiana. Minimal benefits were seen in a twelve-week double-blind study evaluating a combination of asparagus, green tea, black tea, guarana, maté, kidney beans, *Garcinia cambogia*, and high-chromium yeast.

A double-blind, placebo-controlled study evaluated the effects of a mixture containing *Citrus aurantium* (bitter orange), caffeine, and St. John's wort. *C. aurantium* contains various stimulant chemicals related to nasal spray decongestants. The results suggest that this combination might assist weight loss, but the study was so small (twenty-three participants divided into three groups) that the results mean little.

Ayurvedic herbs have shown some promise for weight loss. In a three-month, double-blind, placebo-controlled study, seventy overweight people were divided into four groups: placebo, *Triphala guggul* (a mixture of five Ayurvedic ingredients) plus *Gokshuradi guggul* (a mixture of eight Ayurvedic ingredients), *T. guggul* plus *Sinhanad guggul* (a mixture of six Ayurvedic herbs), or *T. guggul* plus *Chandraprabha vati* (a mixture of thirty-six Ayurvedic ingredients). Reportedly, all three Ayurvedic ingredients produced significant weight loss and improvements in cholesterol compared with placebo; furthermore, the improvements produced by the respective treatments were close to identical.

One study failed to find benefit with a proprietary mixture of astragalus, gallic acid, ginger, red sage, rhubarb, and turmeric. Studies attempting to determine whether evening primrose oil can aid in weight loss have yielded mixed results. Another study failed to find benefit with the edible cactus *Caralluma fimbriata*.

Conjugated linoleic acid (CLA) is a mixture of different isomers, or chemical forms, of linoleic acid. CLA has been proposed as a fat-burning substance, improving lean-to-fat-mass ratios and reducing total fat mass, but on balance, the benefit appears to be slight. Also, some studies have raised concerns that the use of CLA by overweight people could raise insulin resistance and therefore increase the risk of diabetes. In addition, the use of CLA might impair endothelial function and levels of C-reactive protein and, thereby, increase cardiovascular risk.

One study found that the topical application of glycyrrhetinic acid, a constituent of licorice, can reduce fat thickness in the thigh. A mixture of the herbs *Magnolia officinalis* and *Phellodendron amurense* is said to help reduce stress-induced overeating, but the only supporting evidence for this claim is a study too small to provide meaningful results. The herb *Hoodia gordonii*, often known simply as hoodia, has been marketed as a weight-loss treatment. However, the evidence that it works is limited to one small unpublished trial funded by the manufacturer.

Hypnosis is popular as an aid to weight loss. However, a careful analysis of published studies suggests that the benefits are slight at best. Although acupuncture is widely used for weight loss, the evidence from published studies is incomplete and inconsistent.

One double-blind study failed to find capsaicin (the "hot" in cayenne pepper) helpful for preventing weight regain after weight loss, but it did seem to cause some increase in fat metabolism. A rather theoretical study found that two ingredients in green tea may interact to increase metabolism, and on this basis green tea became a popular weight control supplement. However, other evidence indicates that if green tea increases metabolism, the effect is extremely small. One study conducted in Thailand reported weight-loss benefits with green tea; however, a Dutch study failed to find green tea helpful for preventing weight regain after weight loss. In another study, the use of green tea failed to produce significant weight loss in overweight women with polycystic ovary syndrome.

Green tea extract enriched with catechins (an active ingredient in green tea) has done better, enhancing weight loss in one substantial but somewhat flawed trial. Oolong tea enriched with green tea catechins found some apparent weight-loss benefit. However, a study in overweight Japanese children did not support the effectiveness of green tea catechins for weight reduction. Similar results were obtained in another placebo-controlled trial involving seventy-eight overweight women after twelve weeks of treatment.

Other supplements that have been studied but not found effective include spirulina, L-carnitine, and oligomeric proanthocyanidin complexes from grape seed. An enormous number of other supplements are marketed for weight loss, but they are sold without meaningful supporting evidence. For example, certain supplements are said to be lipotropic, meaning that they help the body metabolize fat or slow down the rate at which it is stored. Vitamins B_5 and B_6, biotin, choline, inositol, lecithin, and lipoic acid are often placed in this category. However, there is no real evidence that they will help one lose weight.

A number of amino acids, including phenylalanine, tyrosine, methionine, and glutamine, are said to reduce hunger. Because the herb kava appears to be helpful for anxiety, it has been proposed as a treatment for mood-related overeating. The antidepressant herb St. John's wort has been recommended with much the same reasoning.

Seaweeds such as kelp, bladderwrack, and sargassi are often added to diet formulas, under the assumption that they will affect the thyroid gland through their iodine content. (An underactive thyroid can cause weight gain.) However, the effect of iodine on thyroid function depends on whether a person is iodine deficient. Excess iodine can actually suppress the action of the thyroid. The herb guggul (*Commiphora mukul*) is often claimed to enhance thyroid function, and for this reason it is often sold as a weight-loss agent. However, there is little evidence that it actually affects the thyroid, and a small double-blind trial found it no more effective than placebo for weight loss.

Numerous herbs and supplements with potential or known effects on insulin or blood sugar levels are widely added to weight-loss formulas, again without any evidence that they are effective. These herbs and supplements include alfalfa, *Anemarrhena asphodeloides*, arginine, *Azadirachta indica* (neem), bilberry leaf, bitter melon (*Momordica charantia*), *Catharanthus roseus*, Coc-

cinia indica, Cucumis sativus, Cucurbita ficifolia, Cuminum cyminum (cumin), *Euphorbia prostrata*, garlic, glucomannan, *Guaiacum coulteri*, *Guazuma ulmifolia*, guggul, holy basil (*Ocimum sanctum*), *Lepechinia caulescens*, *Musa sapientum* L. (banana), nopal cactus (*Opuntia streptacantha*), onion, *Psacalium peltatum*, pterocarpus, *Rhizophora mangle*, *Salacia oblonga*, salt bush, *Spinacea oleracea*, *Tournefortia hirsutissima*, *Turnera diffusa*, and vanadium.

Herbs with laxative or diuretic properties or reputations are also popular in weight-loss formulas, although they are unlikely to produce anything beyond a slight temporary effect. These include barberry, buchu, cascara sagrada bark, cassia powder, cleavers, cornsilk, couchgrass, dandelion root, fig, goldenrod, hydrangea root, juniper berry, peppermint, prune, senna leaf, tamarind, turkey rhubarb root, and uva ursi.

Herbs that are supposed to strengthen the body in general are found in many diet formulas, including ashwagandha, *Cordyceps*, *Eleutherococcus*, fo-ti, ginseng, maitake, reishi, schisandra, and suma.

Other herbs and supplements sometimes recommended for weight loss for reasons that are unclear include buckthorn, cayenne, chickweed, coenzyme Q_{10}, cranberry, fennel, flaxseed, ginger, ginkgo, gotu kola, grape seed extract, hawthorn, licorice, milk thistle, parsley, passionflower, plantain, white willow, yellow dock, yucca, and zinc.

Numerous dietary methods have been proposed for aiding weight loss. The Mediterranean diet, which is relatively high in fiber and monounsaturated fats (such as olive oil), has attracted attention as an effective method for weight management. Two of the most popular alternative diets for weight loss are low-carbohydrate diets and low-glycemic-index (low-GI) diets. On average, it appears that all dietary weight-loss approaches are about equally helpful, provided one sticks to the "rules." However, it is possible that a low-GI diet and the Mediterranean diet are more beneficial than a low-fat diet in people with type 2 diabetes and prediabetes.

One study found that reducing one's consumption of high-sugar beverages has a minor effect, if any. Also, it has often been suggested that a vegetarian diet enhances weight loss, but this has not been proven.

EBSCO CAM Review Board

FURTHER READING

Burke, L. E., et al. "Effects of a Vegetarian Diet and Treatment Preference on Biochemical and Dietary

Variables in Overweight and Obese Adults." *American Journal of Clinical Nutrition* 86 (2007): 588-596.

Ebbeling, C. B., H. A. Feldman, et al. "Effects of Decreasing Sugar-Sweetened Beverage Consumption on Body Weight in Adolescents." *Pediatrics* 117 (2006): 673-680.

Ebbeling, C. B., M. M. Leidig, et al. "Effects of a Low-Glycemic Load vs. Low-Fat Diet in Obese Young Adults." *Journal of the American Medical Association* 297 (2007): 2092-2102.

Gardner, C. D., et al. "Comparison of the Atkins, Zone, Ornish, and LEARN Diets for Change in Weight and Related Risk Factors Among Overweight Premenopausal Women." *Journal of the American Medical Association* 297 (2007): 969-977.

Hsu, C. H., et al. "Effect of Green Tea Extract on Obese Women." *Clinical Nutrition* 27 (2008): 363-370.

Jull, A. B., et al. "Chitosan for Overweight or Obesity." *Cochrane Database of Systematic Reviews* (2008): CD003892. Available through *EBSCO DynaMed Systematic Literature Surveillance* at http://www.ebscohost.com/dynamed.

Melanson, K. J., et al. "Effects of High-Fructose Corn Syrup and Sucrose Consumption on Circulating Glucose, Insulin, Leptin, and Ghrelin, and on Appetite in Normal-Weight Women." *Nutrition* 23 (2007): 103-112.

Shai, I., et al. "Weight Loss with a Low-Carbohydrate, Mediterranean, or Low-Fat Diet." *New England Journal of Medicine* 359 (2008): 229-241.

Winzenberg, T., et al. "Calcium Supplements in Healthy Children Do Not Affect Weight Gain, Height, or Body Composition." *Obesity* 15 (2007): 1789-1798.

Yazaki, Y., et al. "A Pilot Study of Chromium Picolinate for Weight Loss." *Journal of Alternative and Complementary Medicine* 16 (2010): 291-299.

See also: Chitosan; Chromium; Ephedra; Glucomannan; Pyruvate.

Obsessive-compulsive disorder (OCD)

CATEGORY: Condition

DEFINITION: Treatment of recurrent and persistent thoughts or images known as obsessions and resultant repetitive behaviors known as compulsions.

PRINCIPAL PROPOSED NATURAL TREATMENTS: None

OTHER PROPOSED NATURAL TREATMENTS: 5-hydroxytryptophan, inositol, relaxation therapy, repetitive transcranial magnetic stimulation, St. John's wort, yoga

INTRODUCTION

Obsessive-compulsive disorder (OCD) is a psychological condition that involves recurrent and persistent thoughts or images known as obsessions that are experienced as intrusive and that cause distress. These obsessions are not simply excessive worries about real-life problems; they take on an unrealistic quality. In order to combat their obsessions, people with OCD engage in repetitive behaviors known as compulsions, and they often do so following rigid and self-imposed rules.

The cause of OCD is not known. Antidepressant drugs that affect serotonin levels, such as selective serotonin reuptake inhibitors (SSRIs), often relieve symptoms significantly, but the reasons for this effect are not clear. Psychotherapeutic and behavioral methods may also help to treat OCD.

PROPOSED NATURAL TREATMENTS

The supplement inositol is thought to increase the body's sensitivity to serotonin. On this basis, inositol has been studied for use in a number of psychological conditions, including OCD.

In a small double-blind trial, the use of inositol at a dose of 18 grams (g) daily for six weeks significantly improved symptoms of OCD compared with placebo. However, some evidence suggests that inositol does not increase the effectiveness of standard drugs for OCD.

One study found that people with OCD have lower than normal levels of vitamin B_{12}. This suggests, but absolutely does not prove, that vitamin B_{12} supplements might be helpful for the condition.

The herb St. John's wort has antidepressant properties and is thought to affect serotonin levels. On this basis, it has been tried for OCD, but there is no reliable evidence that it is effective for the disorder. On a similar basis, the supplement 5-hydroxytryptophan has been suggested as a treatment for OCD, but again there is no meaningful evidence that the supplement works.

A form of magnet therapy called repetitive transcranial magnetic stimulation (rTMS) has shown promise for the treatment of depression. However, a double-blind, placebo-controlled study of eighteen people with OCD found no evidence of benefit through the use of rTMS.

In a small randomized trial, a yoga meditation technique called kundalini was more effective for OCD than a relaxation therapy involving mindfulness meditation after three months. However, another small study found mindfulness meditation more helpful than no intervention for OCD symptoms.

HERBS AND SUPPLEMENTS TO USE WITH CAUTION

Various herbs and supplements may interact with drugs used to treat OCD, so persons with OCD who are considering the use of herbs and supplements should first consult a doctor to discuss safe treatment options.

EBSCO CAM Review Board

FURTHER READING

Alonso, P., et al. "Right Prefrontal Repetitive Transcranial Magnetic Stimulation in Obsessive-compulsive Disorder." *American Journal of Psychiatry* 158 (2001): 1143-1145.

Fux, M., J. Benjamin, and R. H. Belmaker. "Inositol Versus Placebo Augmentation of Serotonin Reuptake Inhibitors in the Treatment of Obsessive-compulsive Disorder." *International Journal of Neuropsychopharmacology* 2 (1999): 193-195.

Hanstede, M., Y. Gidron, and I. Nyklicek. "The Effects of a Mindfulness Intervention on Obsessive-Compulsive Symptoms in a Non-clinical Student Population." *Journal of Nervous and Mental Disease* 196 (2008): 776-779.

Seedat, S., and D. J. Stein. "Inositol Augmentation of Serotonin Reuptake Inhibitors in Treatment-Refractory Obsessive-Compulsive Disorder." *International Clinical Psychopharmacology* 14 (1999): 353-356.

Shannahoff-Khalsa, D. S., et al. "Randomized Controlled Trial of Yogic Meditation Techniques for Patients with Obsessive-Compulsive Disorder." *CNS Spectrums* 4 (1999): 34-47.

Taylor, L. H., and K. A. Kobak. "An Open-Label Trial of St. John's Wort (*Hypericum perforatum*) in Obsessive-Compulsive Disorder." *Journal of Clinical Psychiatry* 61 (2000): 575-578.

See also: Anxiety and panic attacks; Attention deficit disorder; Autism spectrum disorder; Bipolar disorder; Depression, mild to moderate; Eating disorders; Mental health; Relaxation therapies; Seasonal affective disorder; SSRIs.

Office of Cancer Complementary and Alternative Medicine

CATEGORY: Organizations and legislation
DEFINITION: The consumer hub for U.S. government information on complementary and alternative medicine for persons with cancer and those who treat them.
DATE: Founded in 1998

MISSION AND OBJECTIVES

The Office of Cancer Complementary and Alternative Medicine (OCCAM) works to improve the quality of cancer care through the support and advancement of research in evidence-based complementary and alternative medical (CAM) practices. OCCAM also provides quality information about CAM for health care professionals, researchers, and the public. The focus of the office is to coordinate CAM activities in diagnosing, preventing, and treating cancer through managing cancer-related symptoms and cancer treatment side effects. OCCAM's focus on cancer distinguishes it from the related National Center for Complementary and Alternative Medicine, part of the National Institutes of Health (NIH).

HISTORY

Before establishing a separate division for CAM, the National Cancer Institute (NCI) of the NIH was interested in using CAM to treat cancer. In the 1940s, the NCI looked at studies to treat cancer with various CAM therapies. One treatment alternative reviewed by the NCI was the chemical compound laetrile, a purified amygdalin found in the pits of fruits and nuts, lima beans, sorghum, and clover. The Gerson regimen, named for German physician Max Gerson, also was considered. This regimen used a diet of raw and fresh organic fruits, vegetables, and juices, and coffee enemas, supplements, and detoxification, to help the body heal itself of cancer. The NCI also examined the Hoxley treatment, which employed herbs and salves to treat cancer; the NCI found no evidence that this treatment was effective.

NCI's interest in CAM for cancer treatment continued during the next several decades, leading to the development of the Best Case Series in 1991. This program provided a way for CAM practitioners to use scientific approaches with rigorous research to evaluate these therapies in the treatment of cancer.

In 1998, OCCAM was founded under the leadership of Jeffrey D. White, a board-certified cancer oncologist and researcher who joined the NCI in 1990. The Best Case Series was moved from the Cancer Therapy Evaluation program at NCI to the then-new OCCAM. The following year, the CAM Cancer Research Interest Group and Invited Speaker Series was established at OCCAM.

In 2006, OCCAM published the first NCI annual report on CAM. The following year, the office moved to the Division of Cancer Treatment and Diagnosis at the NCI. In 2008, OCCAM published "Survey of Cancer Researchers Regarding Complementary and Alternative Medicine" in the *Journal of the Society of Integrative Oncology*. That same year, the NCI provided more than $121 million for CAM research in more than four hundred projects.

BEST CASE SERIES PROGRAM

One notable program coordinated through OCCAM is the NCI Best Case Series (BCS) program. Established in 1991, BCS evaluates CAM research data through independent reviews of records and review of the test results of persons with cancer who were treated with CAM therapies. With valid data supporting CAM cancer therapies, the NIH can then determine funding for further research in CAM effectiveness.

CAM practitioners are encouraged to submit their research on persons treated for tumor regression to the BCS program. To be accepted for review, the practitioner must meet specific criteria, including having a patient with a definitive diagnosis of cancer, having detailed records of cancer response, and having a chronicled treatment history.

Marylane Wade Koch, M.S.N., R.N.

FURTHER READING

Cassileth, B. "Gerson Regimen." *Oncology* (Williston Park) 24, no. 2 (2010): 201.

National Cancer Institute. "Thinking About Complementary and Alternative Medicine: A Guide for People with Cancer." Available at http://www.cancer.gov/cancertopics/cam/thinking-about-cam. A booklet that explains CAM and what choices are available to people with cancer.

Office of Cancer Complementary and Alternative Medicine. http://www.cancer.gov/cam. This site provides health professionals, persons with cancer, and the general public information about complementary and alternative medicine in treating cancer.

Rees, Alan M., ed. *The Complementary and Alternative Medicine Information Source Book.* Phoenix, Ariz.: Oryx Press, 2001. Defines CAM terms and the background of CAM and includes a listing of resources.

Rosenbaum, Earnest H., and Isadora Rosenbaum. *Everyone's Guide to Cancer Supportive Care: A Comprehensive Handbook for Patients and Their Families.* 4th ed. Kansas City, Mo.: Andrews McMeel, 2005. Comprehensive guide with more than fifty chapters. Includes Web resources on CAM.

Smith, W. B., et al. "Survey of Cancer Researchers Regarding Complementary and Alternative Medicine." *Journal of the Society of Integrative Oncology* 6, no. 1 (2008): 2-12. Survey results published by the NCI to assess the interest and concern of 329 research respondents in CAM.

See also: Dietary Supplement Health and Education Act of 1994; Food and Drug Administration; Health freedom movement; National Center for Complementary and Alternative Medicine; National Health Federation; Office of Dietary Supplements; Regulation of CAM.

Office of Dietary Supplements

CATEGORY: Organizations and legislation
DEFINITION: A U.S. government office formed to enhance knowledge of dietary supplements to ensure medical understanding and consumer safety.
DATE: Founded in 1995

INTRODUCTION

The U.S. Office of Dietary Supplements (ODS) was established in 1995, as mandated by the Dietary Supplement Health and Education Act of 1994. ODS was formed to better understand the science behind dietary supplements, to identify useful and harmful

Office of Dietary Supplements: Strategic Plan 2010–2014

The Office of Dietary Supplements (ODS) has outlined several goals as part of its 2010-2014 Strategic Plan. Goal 4—Make the Most Up-To-Date Scientific Knowledge About Dietary Supplements Publicly Available—is presented here, in part.

Information about dietary supplements is available from a wide variety of sources, including government and commercial providers; articles published in scientific journals, books, and magazines; and sellers of these products. Even web-savvy health consumers and health practitioners find it difficult to navigate these resources, critically evaluate their contents, and extract the information needed to assess supplement efficacy, safety, and quality.

A need exists for one authoritative source to collect, evaluate, and summarize science-based, reliable information on dietary supplements and to present this information in various forms to diverse audiences in a range of venues. ODS, as that authoritative source, plans to accelerate its efforts to synthesize this information and bring it to the attention of federal agencies, health care providers, investigators, and consumers.

supplements, and to disseminate reliable information to the medical community and the public. As part of the National Institutes of Health (NIH), the office collaborates with other government organizations, including the National Center for Complementary and Alternative Medicine (NCCAM) and the U.S. Food and Drug Administration (FDA), to raise public awareness of the benefits and risks of dietary supplements. ODS, NCCAM, and the FDA evaluate the methods of action of thousands of supplements and develop tools to understand their use within given populations.

DIETARY SUPPLEMENTS

As the name suggests, dietary supplements are any tablets, pills, capsules, or liquids that are taken orally to enhance a person's diet. There are approximately thirty thousand dietary supplements available in the United States. Between 50 and 75 percent of American adults, and possibly one-third of all children in the

United States, use some type of supplement, including vitamins, minerals, and weight-reduction supplements, for health promotion and disease prevention.

FDA regulation of dietary supplements, which are often complex mixtures, is less strict than it is for prescription and nonprescription pharmaceuticals, leading to an enhanced role for ODS. Manufacturers of supplements do not need to follow standard guidelines, nor do they need to back up medical claims, such as claims that a product lowers the risk of a certain disease, with scientific research. As a result, the manufacture of dietary supplements is not standardized, and some products fail to meet their health claims. To increase the authority of the ODS and to ensure public safety, the FDA, in 2009, issued an evaluation of health claims of both conventional foods and dietary supplements.

HIGHLIGHTS AND ACCOMPLISHMENTS

Since its inception, ODS has helped to fund dietary supplement research grants and projects that examine usage rates and that evaluate, for example, the science behind supplements; has developed reference databases (which cite approximately 750,000 world references); has sponsored conferences and workshops; has led campaigns to educate the public on the potential risks of supplements; and has helped establish good manufacturing practices (GMPs) to ensure the quality of dietary supplements. These efforts are supported by six Dietary Supplement Research Centers located at different universities in the United States. Ongoing research programs include studies on glucosamine and chondroitin for knee osteoarthritis, on saw palmetto as a urinary aid for males, and on the potential cardiovascular benefits of omega-3 fatty acids.

Through ODS-sponsored research, many dietary supplements have proven essential to maintaining health: Calcium is now known as effective in reducing the risk of osteoporosis; certain vitamins and antioxidant supplements have been found to help reduce the effects of macular degeneration; and iron supplements during pregnancy are now known to be essential in preventing maternal anemia and reducing the rate of premature births. Other supplements have been found to be potentially harmful. Beta-carotene, which was promoted as reducing the risk of developing cancer, was later found to increase lung cancer rates in people who smoke cigarettes. Ephedra and ephedrine-containing supplements for weight reduction are now banned in the United States because of the side effects from taking the supplements, side effects that include high blood pressure and heart damage.

Renée Euchner, B.S.N.

FURTHER READING

Betz, J. M., et al. "The NIH Analytical Methods and Reference Materials Program for Dietary Supplements." *Analytical and Bioanalytical Chemistry* 389 (2007): 19-25.

Costello R. B., and P. Coates. "In the Midst of Confusion Lies Opportunity: Fostering Quality Science in Dietary Supplement Research." *Journal of the American College of Nutrition* 20 (2001): 21-25.

Dwyer, J. T., D. B. Allison, and P. M. Coates. "Dietary Supplements in Weight Reduction." *Journal of the American Dietary Association* 105, no. 5, suppl. (2005): 80-86.

Dwyer, J. T., et al. "Measuring Vitamins and Minerals in Dietary Supplements for Nutrition Studies in the USA." *Analytical and Bioanalytical Chemistry* 389 (2007): 37-46.

Haggans, C., et al. "Computer Access to Research on Dietary Supplements: A Database of Federally Funded Dietary Supplement Research." *Journal of Nutrition* 135 (2005): 1796-1799.

Office of Dietary Supplements. National Institutes of Health. http://www.ods.od.nih.gov.

Timbo, B. B., et al. "Dietary Supplements in a National Survey: Prevalence of Use and Reports of Adverse Events." *Journal of the American Dietary Association* 106 (2006): 1966-1974.

See also: Dietary Supplement Health and Education Act of 1994; Food and Drug Administration; Health freedom movement; National Center for Complementary and Alternative Medicine; National Health Federation; Regulation of CAM; Supplements: Introduction.

Ohsawa, George

Also known as: Yukikazu Sakurazawa
CATEGORY: Biography
IDENTIFICATION: Japanese philosopher who introduced the macrobiotic diet and philosophy to Europe

BORN: October 18, 1893; Kyoto, Japan
DIED: April 23, 1966; Tokyo, Japan

OVERVIEW

George Ohsawa was a Japanese philosopher, teacher, and writer said to have brought the macrobiotic diet and associated philosophy to Europe from Japan. His practices were largely based on the long-standing Asian principle of yin and yang, a certain type of equilibrium or balance believed to bring health and well-being to those who follow the related principles.

Ohsawa was born to a poor family and thus had no money for higher education. Despite this, he is said to have been an excellent student, and he reportedly educated himself in many subjects in his early life. Around 1913, he began studying in Tokyo with Manabu Nishibata, who was a direct disciple of Japanese physician Sagen Ishizuka, potentially the originator of formal macrobiotics (*shokuiku*). Ohsawa's studies at this time were reportedly focused on the examination of *shokuiku*. In some of his publications, Ohsawa claimed that he cured himself of tuberculosis at about the age of eighteen years using traditional dietary principles that originated in Japan and China.

Ohsawa wrote many books (in various languages) about the macrobiotic diet and related principles. He wrote that observance of macrobiotics could improve not only human physical health but also emotional health. In one of his books, he indicated that macrobiotics could shed light on a number of social problems and even causes of war, a time-appropriate claim given that he was writing during a period when atomic war was looming. According to Japanese records, Ohsawa was a peace activist.

Ohsawa also was said to have practiced an ancient Japanese method called *sanpaku*, whereby a person's health and overall well-being can be predicted based on the coloring of the white areas around the iris of the eyes. Using this ancient method, he reportedly predicted the premature deaths of certain American public figures, including U.S. President John F. Kennedy and actor-entertainer Marilyn Monroe.

A number of Ohsawa's disciples were instrumental in further spreading the macrobiotic diet and its philosophy to the Western world, including parts of Europe, South America, and North America. In particular, a student of Ohsawa named Herman Aihara founded a study center and foundation in San Francisco named in Ohsawa's honor—the George Ohsawa

Macrobiotic Foundation—which remains in operation, dedicated to providing education and products relevant to macrobiotics and Ohsawa's teachings.

Brandy Weidow, M.S.

FURTHER READING

Brown, Simon. *Macrobiotics for Life.* Berkeley, Calif.: North Atlantic Books, 2009.

"Macrobiotics." In *Complementary and Alternative Medicine Sourcebook*, edited by Amy L. Sutton. Detroit: Omnigraphics, 2010.

Ohsawa, George. *Macrobiotics: An Invitation to Health and Happiness.* Chico, Calif.: George Ohsawa Macrobiotic Foundation, 1978.

_____. *The Unique Principle: The Philosophy of Macrobiotics.* Chico, Calif.: George Ohsawa Macrobiotic Foundation, 1973.

_____. *Zen Macrobiotics: The Art of Rejuvenation and Longevity.* 4th ed. Chico, Calif.: George Ohsawa Macrobiotic Foundation, 1995.

See also: Diet-based therapies; Hufeland, Christoph Wilhelm; Ishizuka, Sagen; Macrobiotic diet.

Oligomeric proanthocyanidins

CATEGORY: Herbs and supplements

RELATED TERMS: Grape seed extract, pine bark extract, procyanidolic oligomers (PCOs), pycnogenol

DEFINITION: Natural plant product used to treat specific health conditions.

PRINCIPAL PROPOSED USES: Easy bruising, edema following injury or surgery, travelers' thrombosis, varicose veins, weight loss

OTHER PROPOSED USES: Aging skin, allergies, asthma, atherosclerosis prevention, attention deficit disorder, cancer prevention, diabetes (blood sugar control), diabetic neuropathy and retinopathy, hemorrhoids, hypertension, impaired night vision, impotence, liver cirrhosis, lupus, menopause, periodontal disease, premenstrual syndrome

OVERVIEW

One of the best-selling herbal products of the early 1990s was an extract of the bark of French maritime pine. This substance consists of a family of chemicals known scientifically as oligomeric proanthocyanidin complexes (OPCs) or procyanidolic oligomers (PCOs). Similar (but not identical) substances are also found in grape seed. The research record is complicated by the fact that certain identically named proprietary products have consisted at different times of various proportions of these related substances. OPCs are marketed for a wide variety of uses. However, there is no solid evidence that they are effective for any medical condition.

REQUIREMENTS AND SOURCES

OPCs are not a single chemical but a group of closely related compounds. Several food sources contain similar chemicals: red wine, cranberries, blueberries, bilberries, tea (green and black), black currant, onions, legumes, parsley, and the herb hawthorn. However, most OPC supplements are made from either grape seed or the bark of the maritime pine. These two OPC sources lead to products that are not necessarily identical in function, although there do seem to be many similarities. In the discussion of scientific studies below, the source of the OPCs used are indicated wherever possible. In some cases, however, identifying the exact product is difficult, as both grape seed and pine bark OPCs, or their combination, have at various times been sold under the same name.

THERAPEUTIC DOSAGES

For the treatment of specific medical conditions, studies have used doses of 150 to 300 milligrams (mg) daily. For use as a general antioxidant, 50 mg of OPCs daily is often recommended; however, there is no evidence that this dose provides any health benefits.

THERAPEUTIC USES

The best-documented use of OPCs is to treat chronic venous insufficiency, a condition closely related to varicose veins. In both of these conditions, blood pools in the legs, causing aching, pain, heaviness, swelling, fatigue, and unsightly visible veins. Fairly good preliminary evidence suggests that OPCs from pine bark or grape seed can relieve the leg pain and swelling of chronic venous insufficiency. However, no studies have evaluated whether regular use of OPCs can make visible varicose veins disappear or prevent new ones from developing. Other small, double-blind trials suggest that OPCs may help reduce swelling caused by injuries or surgery.

Evidence from one small, double-blind trial suggests that OPCs from bilberry and grape seed may reduce the general fluid retention and swelling that can occur in premenstrual syndrome (PMS). One large study found some evidence that the use of OPCs from pine bark might help prevent the leg blood clots that can develop on a long airplane flight.

Some studies suggest OPCs from pine bark, alone or with arginine, may be helpful for erectile dysfunction (impotence). For example, in a double-blind, placebo-controlled trial, 124 men (aged thirty to fifty) with moderate erectile dysfunction were randomized to take Prelox (a formulation of pine bark extract and arginine) or a placebo for six months. The men who took Prelox experienced improvement in their condition over those who took a placebo.

In a double-bind, placebo-controlled study of sixty-one children with attention deficit disorder (ADD), use of OPCs from pine bark (at a dose of 1 gram per kilogram per day) appeared to improve some measurements of disease severity.

Two small, double-blind pilot studies suggest that OPCs from pine bark might help reduce asthma symptoms. OPCs are also often recommended for allergies, but an eight-week double-blind trial of forty-nine individuals found no benefit with grape seed extract. On a slightly more positive note, a preliminary trial involving thirty-nine people with seasonal allergies found that those who took OPCs at least five weeks before the start of the season experienced more symptom relief compared with the control group. And those that took OPCs for a longer period of time (for example, seven to eight weeks before the season) seemed to have better results.

OPCs might marginally improve blood sugar control in people with diabetes, according to a double-blind study of seventy-seven people with type 2 diabetes. Some evidence suggests that OPCs protect and strengthen collagen and elastin. Theoretically, this could mean that OPCs are helpful for aging skin, and they are widely sold for this purpose, but there is no direct evidence that the herbs work.

Hemorrhoids are varicose veins in and around the anus. Since OPCs are used to treat varicose veins, it is thought that this substance would also be helpful for people who have hemorrhoids. A randomized trial involving eighty-four people with hemorrhoids found that both the oral and topical forms of Pycnogenol (pine bark extract) eased symptoms, including bleeding.

One study suggests that while OPCs alone may not reduce levels of cholesterol, some benefits may occur when they are taken in combination with chromium. OPCs are strong antioxidants. Vitamin E defends against fat-soluble oxidants, and vitamin C neutralizes water-soluble ones, but OPCs are active against both types. Based on the (unproven) belief that antioxidants offer many health benefits, regular use of OPCs has been proposed as a measure to prevent cancer, diabetic neuropathy and diabetic retinopathy, and heart disease.

OPCs have been tried as a treatment for impaired night vision, lupus (systemic lupus erythematosus), easy bruising, high blood pressure, and liver cirrhosis. However, more research needs to be performed to discover whether it actually provides any benefits in these conditions. A double-blind, placebo-controlled study of questionable validity reported that use of OPCs from pine bark produced benefits in all symptoms of menopause.

One study failed to find OPCs significantly helpful for weight loss. Another failed to find OPCs helpful for reducing the side effects of radiation therapy for breast cancer.

SCIENTIFIC EVIDENCE

Venous insufficiency (varicose veins). There is fairly good preliminary evidence for the use of OPCs to treat people with symptoms of venous insufficiency. A double-blind, placebo-controlled study of seventy-one subjects found that grape seed OPCs, taken at a dose of 100 mg three times daily, significantly improved major symptoms, including heaviness, swelling, and leg discomfort. Over a period of one month, 75 percent of the participants treated with OPCs improved substantially. This result does not seem quite so impressive when one notes that significant improvement

Selected Alternative Names for Oligomeric Proanthocyanidins

Condensed tannins, French marine pine bark extract, French maritime pine bark extract, leucoanthocyanidins, maritime bark extract, OPCs, pine bark, pine bark extract, *Pinus pinaster, Pinus maritima,* procyanidin oligomers, procyanodolic oligomers, Pycnogenol, pygenol also was seen in 41 percent of the placebo group; nonetheless, OPCs still did significantly better than a placebo.

A two-month double-blind, placebo-controlled trial of forty people with chronic venous insufficiency found that 100 mg of pine bark OPCs three times daily significantly reduced edema, pain, and the sensation of leg heaviness. A similar study of twenty individuals also found OPCs from pine bark effective.

A placebo-controlled study (blinding not stated) that enrolled 364 people with varicose veins found that treatment with grape seed OPCs produced statistically significant improvements compared with baseline. There was a lesser response in the placebo group, but whether this difference was statistically significant was not stated.

OPCs have also been compared against other natural treatments for venous insufficiency. A double-blind study of fifty people with varicose veins of the legs found that doses of 150 mg per day of grape seed OPCs were more effective in reducing symptoms and signs than the bioflavonoid diosmin. Similarly, a double-blind study of thirty-nine people found pine bark OPCs more effective than the herb horse chestnut.

Edema after surgery or injury. Breast cancer surgery often leads to swelling of the arm. A double-blind, placebo-controlled study of sixty-three postoperative breast cancer patients found that 600 mg of grape seed OPCs daily for six months reduced edema, pain, and peculiar sensations known as paresthesias. Also, in a double-blind, placebo-controlled study of thirty-two people who had received facial surgery, edema disappeared much faster in the group treated with grape seed OPCs.

Another ten-day, double-blind, placebo-controlled study enrolling fifty participants found that grape seed OPCs improved the rate at which edema disappeared following sports injuries.

Blood clots after plane flights. It is commonly thought, though not proven, that the immobility endured during a long plane flight can lead to the development of potentially dangerous blood clots in the legs known as deep venous thrombosis (DVTs). Travelers at high risk are often recommended to take aspirin to thin their blood prior to flying.

One crossover study of twenty-two smokers found that 100 mg of OPCs had a blood-thinning effect equivalent to 500 mg of aspirin. On the basis of this, a large double-blind study was performed to evaluate whether OPCs from pine bark could help reduce risk of blood clots on long airplane flights. The study followed 198 people thought to be at high risk for blood clots. Some participants were given 200 mg of OPCs two to three hours prior to the flight, 200 mg six hours later, and 100 mg the next day; others received a placebo on the same schedule. The average flight length was about eight hours. The results indicated that use of OPCs significantly reduced risk of blood clots. There were five cases of DVTs or superficial thrombosis in the placebo group, compared with none in the OPC group, a difference that was statistically significant.

Another substantial double-blind study (204 participants) found benefit with a product that contains OPCs combined with nattokinase. Nattokinase, also known as natto, is an extract of fermented soy thought to have some blood-clot-dissolving properties.

Periodontal disease. Inflammation of the gums (gingivitis) and plaque formation lead to periodontal disease, one of the most common causes of tooth loss. A fourteen-day double-blind, placebo-controlled trial of forty people evaluated the potential benefits of a chewing gum product containing 5 mg of OPCs from pine bark. Use of the OPC gum resulted in significant improvements in gum health and reductions in plaque formation; no similar benefits were seen in the placebo group.

Atherosclerosis. Although there are no reliable human studies, animal evidence suggests that OPCs can slow or reverse atherosclerosis. This suggests (but definitely does not prove) that OPCs might be helpful for preventing heart disease.

SAFETY ISSUES

OPCs have been extensively tested for safety and are generally considered to be essentially nontoxic. Side effects are rare, but when they do occur they are limited to occasional allergic reactions and mild digestive distress.

However, one study unexpectedly found that a combination of OPCs and vitamin C might slightly increase blood pressure in people with high blood pressure. Neither treatment alone had this effect. These results may have been a statistical fluke, but nonetheless people with hypertension should use the combination of vitamin C and OPCs only with caution. One study, though, found that Pycnogenol (pine bark extract) may help improve kidney function in people with metabolic syndrome who take high blood pressure medicine. Maximum safe dosages for young children, pregnant or nursing women, and those with severe liver or kidney disease have not been established.

IMPORTANT INTERACTIONS

OPCs may have some anticoagulant properties when taken in high doses, so individuals on blood-thinner drugs, such as warfarin (Coumadin), heparin, clopidogrel (Plavix), ticlopidine (Ticlid), pentoxifylline (Trental), or aspirin should use them only under medical supervision.

EBSCO CAM Review Board

FURTHER READING

Belcaro, G., et al. "Pycnogenol Treatment of Acute Hemorrhoidal Episodes." *Phytotherapy Research* 24, no. 3 (2010): 438-444.

Cisár, P., et al. "Effect of Pine Bark Extract (Pycnogenol) on Symptoms of Knee Osteoarthritis." *Phytotherapy Research* 22, no. 8 (2008): 1087-1092.

Kar, P., et al. "Effects of Grape Seed Extract in Type 2 Diabetic Subjects at High Cardiovascular Risk: A Double-Blind Randomized Placebo-Controlled Trial Examining Metabolic Markers, Vascular Tone, Inflammation, Oxidative Stress, and Insulin Sensitivity." *Diabetic Medicine* 26, no. 5 (2009): 526-531.

Ledda, A., et al. "Investigation of a Complex Plant Extract for Mild to Moderate Erectile Dysfunction in a Randomized, Double-Blind, Placebo-Controlled, Parallel-Arm Study. *BJU International* 106, no. 7 (2010): 1030-1033.

Ryan, J., et al. "An Examination of the Effects of the Antioxidant Pycnogenol on Cognitive Performance, Serum Lipid Profile, Endocrinological and Oxidative Stress Biomarkers in an Elderly Population." *Journal of Psychopharmacology* 22, no. 5 (2008): 553-562.

Steigerwalt, R., et al. "Pycnogenol Improves Microcirculation, Retinal Edema, and Visual Acuity in Early Diabetic Retinopathy." *Journal of Ocular Pharmacology and Therapeutics* 2009;25(6):537-540.

Wilson, D., et al. "A Randomized, Double-Blind, Placebo-Controlled Exploratory Study to Evaluate the Potential of Pycnogenol for Improving Allergic Rhinitis Symptoms." *Phytotherapy Research* 24, no. 8 (2010): 1115-1119.

See also: Grape seed; Herbal medicine; Varicose veins; Venous insufficiency: Homeopathic remedies.

Olive leaf

CATEGORY: Herbs and supplements
RELATED TERM: *Olea europaea*
DEFINITION: Natural plant product used to treat specific health conditions.
PRINCIPAL PROPOSED USES: None
OTHER PROPOSED USES: Antibiotic, diabetes, gout, high blood pressure

OVERVIEW

Olive leaf contains a substance called oleuropein, which breaks down in the body to another substance called enolinate.

THERAPEUTIC DOSAGES

Because olive leaf extracts vary widely, label instructions regarding dosing should be followed.

THERAPEUTIC USES

Web sites that promote olive leaf extracts state that enolinate kills harmful bacteria, viruses, and fungi in the body but, at the same time, nurtures microbes that are good for health. This remarkable claim, however, has no meaningful scientific justification.

SCIENTIFIC EVIDENCE

It is true that oleuropein, enolinate, and other olive leaf constituents or their breakdown products can kill microbes in test-tube studies. However, it is a long way from test-tube studies to evidence of efficacy in humans. Only double-blind, placebo-controlled studies can prove a treatment effective, and the only study of this type reported for olive leaf was too flawed to prove anything. This small, poorly designed trial supposedly found that olive leaf extract reduces blood pressure. However, the study was too small and too poorly designed to produce meaningful results. The only other support for the widespread claim that olive leaf reduces blood pressure comes from test-tube and animal studies that are too preliminary to rely upon. Other animal studies weakly suggest that olive leaf might help control blood sugar levels in diabetes and reduce symptoms of gout.

SAFETY ISSUES

Olive leaf has not undergone comprehensive safety testing. However, based on the limited evidence available, it does not appear to commonly cause much more in the way of immediate side effects than occasional digestive distress. Safety in young children, pregnant or nursing women, and people with severe liver or kidney disease has not been established.

EBSCO CAM Review Board

FURTHER READING

Aziz, N. H., et al. "Comparative Antibacterial and Antifungal Effects of Some Phenolic Compounds." *MicroBios* 93 (1998): 43-54.

Bisignano, G., et al. "On the In-Vitro Antimicrobial Activity of Oleuropein and Hydroxytyrosol." *Journal of Pharmacy and Pharmacology* 51 (1999): 971-974.

Lee-Huang, S., et al. "Anti-HIV Activity of Olive Leaf Extract (OLE) and Modulation of Host Cell Gene Expression by HIV-1 Infection and OLE Treatment." *Biochemical and Biophysical Research Communications* 307 (2003): 1029-1037.

See also: Antibiotics, general; Herbal medicine.

Optimal health

CATEGORY: Therapies and techniques
RELATED TERMS: Holistic health, whole-body wellness
DEFINITION: Experiencing life to its fullest potential through a balanced mental, physical, emotional, spiritual, and social state of being.
PRINCIPLE PROPOSED USES: Alzheimer's disease, acquired immune deficiency syndrome, anxiety, arthritis, cancer, dementia, depression, diabetes, fibromyalgia, heart disease, hypertension, insomnia, leukemia, liver disease, lupus, lymphoma, Parkinson's disease, rheumatism, spinal cord injury, stress reduction
OTHER PROPOSED USES: Addiction, anemia, anorexia, attention deficit disorder, autism, bipolar disorder, bulimia, cerebral palsy, chronic pain reduction, memory enhancement, muscular dystrophy, muscular sclerosis, paralysis, stroke

OVERVIEW

In the 1970s, a new movement called optimal health began to focus on attaining a condition of the greatest possible mental, physical, and spiritual wellness, rather than focus only on the treatment of dis-

ease after its appearance. As people came to better understand their ability to positively impact their own health, they became more proactive in their lifestyle choices. Greater emphasis was placed on body, mind, and spirit as an integrative whole, with the necessity for developing each to its fullest potential to achieve a healthy and whole person.

MECHANISM OF ACTION

Optimal health concentrates on fortifying physical, mental, and spiritual well-being to the greatest extent attainable, so that a person may live the best life possible. To assist the body in achieving its premier state of performance, a person focuses on exercise, diet, nutrition, detoxification, cleansing, supplements, yoga, massage, and sleep therapies. To facilitate maximum intellectual acuity, a person employs reading, writing, puzzles, games, classes, support groups, and social interaction. To become more in tune with the divine, to be more spiritual, a person practices meditation, hypnosis, fasting, psychic cleansing, aura healing, metaphysical retreats, soul rebirthing, and vision quests.

USES AND APPLICATIONS

Nutrition is a major factor of any optimal-health plan, and many specialized diets are used. Most feature little or no red meat and little or no poultry and fish, with an emphasis on whole grains, fruits, and vegetables. All processed foods, which contain chemicals and preservatives, are avoided. Some diets advise strict vegetarian regimes, while others, like the vegan dietary model, allow no meat or dairy products. Rice, beans, legumes, fresh fruits, vegetables, and whole grains, all cooked in olive oil, are essential in achieving optimal health. Drinking large amounts of either bottled or purified water is also necessary to flush harmful toxins from the body and to keep it adequately hydrated.

A minimum of eight hours of sleep each night is mandatory to keep the body functioning at its peak, so supplements such as melatonin and valerian root are often useful as sleep aids for insomnia. An exercise regime, especially aerobic exercise like walking, cycling, or swimming, is indispensable for maintaining the body's strength and stamina. Yoga and massage are likewise highly effective at reducing stress and furthering mobility.

Fasting and cleansing therapies, using detoxification and enemas (principally coffee enemas), are useful in eliminating the build-up of chemicals and free radicals in the body's digestive system. Various supplements, such as green tea extract, calcium, fish oil, and vitamins C, B, D, and E, are important in supplanting the body's cardiovascular and immune systems.

Intellectual challenge and stimulation, particularly involving social activity, are fundamental for mental sharpness and psychological well-being. Isolation should be avoided at all costs; friends, family, and a social support network are crucial elements of optimal health. Meditation, expanded consciousness, and transcendental thinking encourage spiritual growth and foster purposeful living.

SCIENTIFIC EVIDENCE

There have been no double-blind, placebo-controlled studies of optimal health, because research would not be feasible. However, hundreds of studies have verified that a vegetarian or vegan diet can slow or even reverse heart disease; regular aerobic exercise and fish oil also are extremely beneficial for cardiovascular health. Voluminous research shows the importance of eight hours of sleep nightly, eight glasses of water daily, and healthy social relationships. Double-blind studies have revealed no beneficial results of coffee enemas; however, green tea has repeatedly been shown to contain powerful immune-system-boosting antioxidants.

CHOOSING A PRACTITIONER

In looking for an optimal-health practitioner, one should choose a licensed medical physician, preferably a doctor specializing in integrative medicine. An integrative medicine specialist will possess advanced knowledge and training in administering and balancing the best of Western and Eastern medicines. The American Medical Association is the preeminent source for physician referrals.

SAFETY ISSUES

Women who are pregnant or persons taking prescription medications should take no supplements without first receiving approval from a licensed medical physician, because dangerous interactions between supplements and prescription drugs may occur, resulting in negative side effects or allergic reactions. All fasting and cleansing dietary plans should be examined cautiously to be certain that they include sufficient nutritional sustenance while purifying the body of toxins. Weight-loss plans, particularly, must be monitored closely to avoid potentially adverse ramifications, especially to the cardiovascular system.

Mary E. Markland, M.A.

FURTHER READING

Bushell, William, Erin Olivo, and Neil Theise. *Longevity, Regeneration, and Optimal Health: Integrating Eastern and Western Perspectives.* Hoboken, N.J.: New York Academy of Sciences, 2009.

Eden, Donna, and David Feinstein. *Energy Medicine: Balancing Your Body's Energies for Optimal Health, Joy, and Vitality.* 2d ed. New York: Jeremy P. Tarcher/Penguin, 2008.

Johnson, Duke. *The Optimal Health Revolution: How Inflammation Is the Root Cause of the Biggest Killers and How the Cutting-Edge Science of Nutrigenomics Can Transform Your Long-Term Health.* Dallas: BenBella Books, 2009.

Rau, Thomas, and Susan Wyler. *The Swiss Secret to Optimal Health: Dr. Rau's Diet for Whole Body Healing.* New York: Berkley Publishing Group, 2009.

Weil, Andrew. *Eight Weeks to Optimum Health: A Proven Program for Taking Full Advantage of Your Body's Natural Healing Power.* 2d ed. New York: Alfred A. Knopf, 2006.

See also: Detoxification; Diet-based therapies; Exercise; Health freedom movement; Integrative medicine; Massage therapy; Mental health; Popular Health movement; Supplements: Introduction; Vegan diet; Vegetarian diet; Wellness, general; Wellness therapies; Whole medicine; Yoga.

Oral contraceptives

CATEGORY: Drug interactions
RELATED TERMS: Birth control pills, contraceptives
DEFINITION: Drugs used to prevent pregnancy.
INTERACTIONS: Androstenedione, dong quai, folate, grapefruit juice, indole-3-carbinol, milk thistle, resveratrol, rosemary, St. John's wort, soy
TRADE NAMES: Alesse, Brevicon, Demulen, Desogen, Estrostep, Genora, Jenest, Levlen, Levlite, Levora, Loestrin, Lo/Ovral, Micronor, Mircette, Modicon, Nelova, Nordette, Norethin, Norinyl, Nor-Q.D., Ortho-Cept, Ortho Cyclen, Ortho-Novum, Ortho

Tri-Cyclen, Ovcon, Ovral, Ovrette, Tri-Levlen, Tri-Norinyl, Triphasil, Zovia

FOLATE

Effect: Supplementation Possibly Helpful

Although the evidence is not consistent, women who are taking oral contraceptives (OCs) may need extra folate. Because folate deficiency is fairly common, even among women who are not taking OCs, and because the body should not lack an essential nutrient, taking a folate supplement on general principle is a good idea.

OTHER NUTRIENTS

Effect: Supplementation Possibly Helpful

Evidence from several studies suggests that OCs might interfere with the absorption or metabolism of magnesium, vitamin B_2, vitamin C, and zinc. With the exception of the trials involving magnesium,

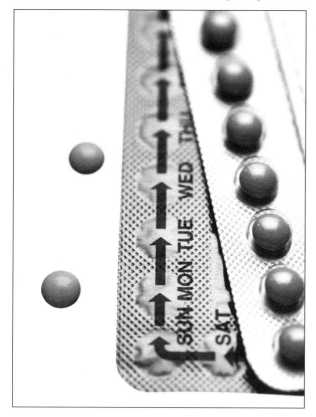

Oral contraceptive pills. (Kevin Curtis/Photo Researchers, Inc.)

these studies used older, high-dose OCs. Modern, low-dose OCs may not affect nutrients to the same extent.

ST. JOHN'S WORT

Effect: Decreased Effectiveness of Drug

Reliable case reports, as well as controlled clinical trials, indicate that St. John's wort interferes with the effectiveness of oral contraceptives and may have led to unwanted pregnancies.

INDOLE-3-CARBINOL

Effect: Possible Reduced Effectiveness of Drug

Indole-3-carbinol (I3C) is a substance found in broccoli that is thought to have cancer-preventive effects. One of its mechanisms of action is thought to involve facilitating the inactivation of estrogen, as well as blocking its effects on cells. The net result could be decreased effectiveness of oral contraceptives.

DONG QUAI, ST. JOHN'S WORT

Effect: Possible Harmful Interaction

OCs have been reported to cause increased sensitivity to the sun, amplifying the risk of sunburn or skin rash. Because dong quai and St. John's wort may also cause this problem, taking these herbal supplements while taking OCs might add to this risk. It may be a good idea to wear sunscreen or protective clothing during sun exposure if one takes one of these herbs while using OCs.

ROSEMARY

Effect: Possible Harmful Interaction

Weak evidence hints that the herb rosemary may enhance the liver's ability to deactivate estrogen in the body. This could potentially interfere with the activity of medications that contain estrogen.

GRAPEFRUIT JUICE

Effect: Possible Harmful Interaction

Grapefruit juice slows the body's normal breakdown of several drugs, including estrogen, allowing it to build up to potentially excessive levels in the blood. A recent study indicates this effect can last for three days or more following the last glass of juice. If one takes estrogen, the safest approach is to avoid grapefruit juice altogether.

RESVERATROL

Effect: Possible Harmful Interaction

The supplement resveratrol has a chemical structure similar to that of the synthetic estrogen diethylstilbestrol and produces estrogenic-like effects. For this reason, it should not be combined with prescription estrogen products.

MILK THISTLE

Effect: Possible Decreased Action of Drug

One report has noted that an ingredient of milk thistle, silibinin, can inhibit a bacterial enzyme called beta-glucuronidase. This enzyme helps oral contraceptives work. Taking milk thistle could, therefore, reduce the effectiveness of OCs.

ANDROSTENEDIONE

Effect: Theoretical Harmful Interaction

Androstenedione has become popular as a sports supplement, on the theory that it increases testosterone levels, as well as sports performance. However, there is no evidence that it is effective. In addition, androstenedione appears more likely to elevate estrogen than testosterone levels. This could increase risks of developing estrogen-related diseases, including breast and uterine cancers. Women taking estrogen should not take androstenedione.

SOY

Effect: Probably No Interaction

Fears have been expressed by some experts that soy or soy isoflavones might interfere with the action of oral contraceptives. However, one study of thity-six women suggests that such concerns are groundless.

EBSCO CAM Review Board

FURTHER READING

Bradlow, H. L., et al. "Multifunctional Aspects of the Action of Indole-3-Carbinol as an Antitumor Agent." *Annals of the New York Academy of Sciences* 889 (1999): 204-13.

Jobst, K. A., et al. "Safety of St. John's Wort (*Hypericum perforatum*)." *The Lancet* 355 (2000): 575.

Martini, M. C., et al. "Effects of Soy Intake on Sex Hormone Metabolism in Premenopausal Women." *Nutrition and Cancer* 34 (1999): 133-139.

Meng, Q., et al. "Indole-3-Carbinol Is a Negative Regulator of Estrogen Receptor-Alpha Signaling in Human Tumor Cells." *Journal of Nutrition* 130 (2000): 2927-2931.

Michnovicz, J. J. "Increased Estrogen 2-Hydroxylation in Obese Women Using Oral Indole-3-Carbinol." *International Journal of Obesity and Related Metabolic Disorders* 22 (1998): 227-229.

Pfrunder, A., et al. "Interaction of St. John's Wort with Low-Dose Oral Contraceptive Therapy." *British Journal of Clinical Pharmacology* 56 (2003): 683-690.

Takanaga, H., et al. "Relationship Between Time After Intake of Grapefruit Juice and the Effect on Pharmacokinetics and Pharmacodynamics of Nisoldipine in Healthy Subjects." *Clinical Pharmacology and Therapeutics* 67 (2000): 201-214.

See also: Food and Drug Administration; Supplements: Introduction.

Oral hypoglycemics

CATEGORY: Drug interactions

DEFINITION: Medications used for controlling blood sugar in persons with type 2 diabetes.

INTERACTIONS: Coenzyme Q_{10}, dong quai, *Ginkgo biloba*, herbs and supplements, ipriflavone, magnesium, potassium citrate, St. John's wort, vitamin B_{12}

DRUGS IN THIS FAMILY: Acarbose (Prandase, Precose), acetohexamide (Dymelor), chlorpropamide (Diabinese), glimepiride (Amaryl), glipizide (Glucotrol, Glucotrol XL), glyburide or glibenclamide (DiaBeta, Glynase, Micronase), metformin (Glucophage), miglitol (Glyset), phenformin, pioglitazone (Actos), rosiglitazone (Avandia), repaglinide (Prandin), tolazamide (Tolinase), tolbutamide (Orinase), troglitazone (Rezulin)

VITAMIN B$_{12}$

Effect: Supplementation Possibly Helpful

The biguanide oral hypoglycemic drugs metformin and phenformin can cause malabsorption of vitamin B_{12}. In turn, this can lead to vitamin B_{12} deficiency. Taking vitamin B_{12} supplements should easily solve this problem.

COENZYME Q$_{10}$ (CoQ$_{10}$)

Effect: Possible Benefits and Risks

Studies suggest that the oral hypoglycemic drugs

glyburide, phenformin, and tolazamide may inhibit the normal production of the substance CoQ_{10}. While there is no direct evidence that taking extra CoQ_{10} will provide any specific benefit, supplementing with CoQ_{10} on general principle might make sense.

In addition, there is some evidence that the use of CoQ_{10} could improve blood sugar control for persons with diabetes. However, one might also need to reduce one's medication dosage.

IPRIFLAVONE

Effect: Might Require Reduction in Medication Dosage

There is some evidence that the supplement ipriflavone might increase blood levels of oral hypoglycemic drugs. This could lead to a risk of blood sugar levels falling too low. Persons taking oral hypoglycemic medications should not take ipriflavone without first consulting a physician.

MAGNESIUM

Effect: Might Require Reduction in Medication Dosage

Magnesium supplements might increase the absorption of chlorpropamide (and, by inference, other oral hypoglycemics), possibly requiring a dosage reduction.

HERBS AND SUPPLEMENTS

Effect: Might Require Reduction in Medication Dosage

Meaningful preliminary evidence suggests that the use of the following herbs and supplements could potentially improve blood sugar control and thus require a reduction in daily doses of oral hypoglycemic medication: aloe, chromium, fenugreek, ginseng, gymnema, and vanadium.

Weaker evidence suggests that the following herbs and supplements could potentially have the same effect under certain circumstances: *Anemarrhena asphodeloides*, arginine, *Azadirachta indica*, bilberry leaf, biotin, bitter melon, carnitine, *Catharanthus roseus*, *Coccinia indica*, CoQ_{10}, conjugated linoleic acid, *Cucumis sativus*, *Cucurbita ficifolia*, *Cuminum cyminum* (cumin), *Euphorbia prostrata*, garlic, glucomannan, *Guaiacum coulteri*, *Guazuma ulmifolia*, guggul, holy basil, *Lepechinia caulescens*, lipoic acid, *Medicago sativa* (alfalfa), *Musa sapientum* L. (banana), niacinamide, nopal cactus, onion, *Phaseolus vulgaris*, *Psacalium peltatum*, Pterocarpus, *Rhizophora mangle*, salt bush, *Spinacea oleracea*, *Tournefortia hirsutissima*, *Turnera diffusa*, and vitamin E.

POTASSIUM CITRATE

Effect: Possible Harmful Interaction

Potassium citrate and other forms of citrate (such as calcium citrate and magnesium citrate) may be used to prevent kidney stones. These agents work by making the urine less acidic. This effect on the urine may lead to decreased blood levels and therapeutic effects of chlorpropamide and possibly other oral hypoglycemic drugs. For this reason, it may be advisable to avoid these citrate compounds during treatment with oral hypoglycemic drugs.

Ginkgo biloba

Effect: Possible Harmful Interactions

It has been suggested that ginkgo might cause problems for persons with type 2 diabetes, both by altering blood levels of medications and by directly affecting the blood-sugar-regulating system of the body. However, the most recent and best-designed studies have failed to find any such actions. Until this situation is clarified, people with diabetes should use ginkgo only under physician supervision.

DONG QUAI, ST. JOHN'S WORT

Effect: Possible Harmful Interaction

Some oral hypoglycemic drugs have been reported to cause increased sensitivity to the sun, amplifying the risk of sunburn or skin rash. Because St. John's wort and dong quai may also cause this problem, taking these herbal supplements during treatment with oral hypoglycemic drugs might add to this risk. It may be a good idea to wear sunscreen or protective clothing during sun exposure if one takes any of these herbs while using an oral hypoglycemic medication.

EBSCO CAM Review Board

FURTHER READING

Hodgson, J. M., et al. "Coenzyme Q(10) Improves Blood Pressure and Glycaemic Control: A Controlled Trial in Subjects with Type 2 Diabetes." *European Journal of Clinical Nutrition* 56 (2002): 1137-1142.

Kudolo, G. B., et al. "Short-Term Ingestion of *Ginkgo biloba* Extract Does Not Alter Whole Body Insulin Sensitivity in Non-diabetic, Pre-diabetic, or Type 2 Diabetic Subjects." *Clinical Nutrition* 25 (2006): 123-134.

Pronsky, Z. M., and J. P. Crowe. *Food Medication Interactions.* 16th ed. Birchrunville, Pa.: Food-Medication Interactions, 2010.

Ting, R. Z., et al. "Risk Factors of Vitamin B12 Deficiency in Patients Receiving Metformin." *Archives of Internal Medicine* 166 (2006): 1975-1979.

See also: Diabetes; Diabetes: Homeopathic remedies; Food and Drug Administration; Insulin; Supplements: Introduction.

Oregano oil

CATEGORY: Herbs and supplements
RELATED TERM: *Origanum vulgare*
DEFINITION: Natural plant product used to treat specific health conditions.
PRINCIPAL PROPOSED USE: Yeast hypersensitivity syndrome
OTHER PROPOSED USES: Colds and flu, human immunodeficiency virus support, intestinal parasites

OVERVIEW

The common food spice oregano grows wild in the mountains of Mediterranean countries. In ancient Greece, oregano or its essential oil was used for the treatment of wounds, snake bites, spider bites, and respiratory problems. Respiratory uses dominated the medicinal history of oregano in medieval Europe, but in the nineteenth century, physicians in the Eclectic School (a medical movement that emphasized herbal treatment) used oregano for promoting menstruation.

THERAPEUTIC DOSAGES

A typical dose of oregano oil is 100 milligrams (mg) three times daily of a product standardized to contain 55 to 65 percent of the presumed active ingredient carvacrol.

THERAPEUTIC USES

In the 1990s, the concept of the yeast hypersensitivity syndrome (often called systemic candidiasis, or candida) became popular in alternative medicine circles. This theory states, in brief, that many people develop excessive levels of the yeast *Candida albicans* and subsequently experience symptoms of allergy to the yeast in their bodies. The symptoms of this purported syndrome include common conditions such as fatigue and headache. A succession of anticandidal treatments

have been offered. Oregano oil is one of the more recent of these products.

SCIENTIFIC EVIDENCE

It is true that oregano oil is toxic to many different types of microorganisms, including fungi and parasites. However, the same is the case with hundreds of essential oils of herbs, not to mention vinegar, alcohol, and bleach. It is a long way from killing microorganisms in a test tube or on the surface of a block of cheese to medicinal effects in the body. Only double-blind, placebo-controlled studies in humans can prove a treatment effective, and none have been performed on oregano oil. Nonetheless oregano oil is widely marketed as a treatment for candida.

There is a related theory that many people suffer from undiagnosed intestinal parasites; oregano oil is marketed for treatment of this purported problem as well. Oregano oil is also advocated for dozens of other illnesses, ranging from asthma and human immunodeficiency virus infection to rheumatoid arthritis, though without any reliable justification.

Web sites selling oregano oil additionally point out that it has antioxidant properties. While true, this does not, by itself, indicate any health benefits. Most major studies of antioxidants have failed to identify the specific benefits that were once seen as likely to result from supplementation with these substances.

SAFETY ISSUES

There are no specific safety risks known to be associated with use of oregano oil products. However, in

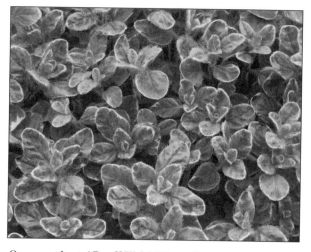

Oregano plant. (Geoff Kidd/Photo Researchers, Inc.)

general, essential oils of herbs can be toxic when taken even in relatively small quantities. Allergic reactions are also possible. Safety in young children, pregnant or nursing women, and people with severe liver or kidney disease has not been established.

EBSCO CAM Review Board

FURTHER READING

Friedman, M., P. R. Henika, and R. E. Mandrell. "Bactericidal Activities of Plant Essential Oils and Some of Their Isolated Constituents Against *Campylobacter jejuni, Escherichia coli, Listeria monocytogenes,* and *Salmonella enterica." Journal of Food Protection* 65 (2002): 1545-1560.

Juglal, S., R. Govinden, and B. Odhav. "Spice Oils for the Control of Co-occurring Mycotoxin-Producing Fungi." *Journal of Food Protection* 65 (2002): 683-687.

Lahlou, M. "Potential of *Origanum compactum* as a Cercaricide in Morocco." *Annals of Tropical Medicine and Parasitology* 96 (2002): 587-593.

Lambert, R. J., et al. "A Study of the Minimum Inhibitory Concentration and Mode of Action of Oregano Essential Oil, Thymol, and Carvacrol." *Journal of Applied Microbiology* 91 (2001): 453-462.

Mejlholm, O., and P. Dalgaard. "Antimicrobial Effect of Essential Oils on the Seafood Spoilage Microorganism *Photobacterium phosphoreum* in Liquid Media and Fish Products." *Letters in Applied Microbiology* 34 (2002): 27-31.

Nielsen, P. V., and R. Rios. "Inhibition of Fungal Growth on Bread by Volatile Components from Spices and Herbs, and the Possible Application in Active Packaging, with Special Emphasis on Mustard Essential Oil." *International Journal of Food Microbiology* 60 (2000): 219-229.

Sokovic, M., et al. "Antifungal Activities of Selected Aromatic Plants Growing Wild in Greece." *Nahrung/Food* 46 (2002): 317-320.

See also: Antioxidants; Candida/yeast hypersensitivity syndrome; Herbal medicine.

Oregon grape

CATEGORY: Herbs and supplements

RELATED TERMS: *Berberis aquifolium, Mahonia aquifolium*

DEFINITION: Natural plant product used to treat specific health conditions.

PRINCIPAL PROPOSED USE: Psoriasis

OTHER PROPOSED USES: Acne, athlete's foot and other fungal infections, eczema

OVERVIEW

The roots and bark of the shrub *Mahonia aquifolium* (commonly known as Oregon grape) have traditionally been used both orally and topically to treat skin problems. They were also used for other conditions such as gastritis, fever, hemorrhage, jaundice, gall bladder disease, and cancer. In addition, mahonia was used as a bitter tonic to improve appetite.

According to some experts, *M. aquifolium* is identical to the plant named *Berberis aquifolium,* but others point to small distinctions. *B. vulgaris,* commonly called barberry, is a close relative of these herbs but is not identical.

THERAPEUTIC DOSAGES

Topical ointments or creams containing 10 percent Oregon grape extract are generally applied three times daily to the affected areas.

THERAPEUTIC USES

Oregon grape is primarily used today as a topical treatment for psoriasis. Growing evidence suggests that it may help reduce symptoms, although it does not seem to be as effective for this purpose as standard medications.

Oregon grape has been proposed as a treatment for other skin diseases, such as fungal infections (such as athlete's foot), eczema, and acne. However, the evidence is either extremely preliminary or inconclusive. For example, a double-blind, placebo-controlled study of eighty-eight people with eczema tested a cream containing extracts of *M. aquifolium, Viola tricolor,* and *Centella asiatica.* The results failed to show benefit overall.

Many studies have been performed on purified berberine, a major chemical constituent of Oregon grape and other herbs such as goldenseal, but it is not clear whether their results apply to the whole herb. In addition, impossibly high dosages of the herb would be required to duplicate the amount of berberine used in many of these studies.

SCIENTIFIC EVIDENCE

Evidence from two double-blind, placebo-controlled studies and one comparative trial suggest that cream made from the herb Oregon grape may help reduce symptoms of psoriasis, although it does not seem to be as effective as standard medications.

In a double-blind study published in 2006, two hundred people were given either a cream containing 10 percent Oregon grape extract or a placebo twice a day for three months. The results indicate that the people using Oregon grape experienced greater benefits than those in the placebo group, and the difference was statistically significant. The treatment was well tolerated, though in a few people it caused a rash or a burning sensation.

Benefits were also seen in a double-blind, placebo-controlled study of eighty-two people with psoriasis. However, the study design had a significant flaw: The treatment salve was darker in color than the placebo, possibly allowing participants to guess which was which.

Another study found that dithranol, a conventional drug used to treat psoriasis symptoms, was more effective than Oregon grape. Regrettably, the authors fail to state whether this study was double-blind. Forty-nine participants applied one treatment to their left side and the other to their right side for four weeks. Skin biopsies were then analyzed and compared with samples taken at the beginning of the study. The physicians evaluating changes in skin tissue were unaware which treatments had been used on the samples. Greater improvements were seen in the dithranol group.

A large open study in which 443 participants with psoriasis used Oregon grape topically for twelve weeks found the herb to be helpful for 73.7 percent of the group. Without a placebo group, it is not possible to know whether Oregon grape was truly responsible for the improvement seen, but the trial does help to establish the herb's safety and tolerability. Laboratory research suggests Oregon grape has some effects at the cellular level that might be helpful in psoriasis, such as slowing the rate of abnormal cell growth and reducing inflammation.

SAFETY ISSUES

Oregon grape appears to be safe when used as directed. In the large open study described above, only 5 of the 443 participants reported side effects of burning, redness, and itching. However, because Oregon grape contains berberine, which has been reported to cause uterine contractions and to increase levels of bilirubin, oral consumption of Oregon grape should be avoided by pregnant women. Safety in young children, nursing women, or people with severe liver or kidney disease has not been established. There is an additional concern regarding the berberine content of Oregon grape. One study found that berberine impairs metabolism of the drug cyclosporine, thereby raising its levels. This could potentially cause toxicity.

EBSCO CAM Review Board

FURTHER READING

Bernstein, S., et al. "Treatment of Mild to Moderate Psoriasis with Relieva, a *Mahonia aquifolium* Extract." *American Journal of Therapeutics* 13 (2006): 121-126.

Klovekorn, W., A. Tepe, and U. Danesch. "A Randomized, Double-Blind, Vehicle-Controlled, Half-side Comparison with a Herbal Ointment Containing *Mahonia aquifolium*, *Viola tricolor*, and *Centella asiatica* for the Treatment of Mild-to-moderate Atopic Dermatitis." *International Journal of Clinical Pharmacology and Therapeutics* 45 (2007): 583-591.

Wu, X., et al. "Effects of Berberine on the Blood Concentration of Cyclosporin A in Renal Transplanted Recipients: Clinical and Pharmacokinetic Study." *European Journal of Clinical Pharmacology* 61, no. 8 (2005): 567-572.

See also: Barberry; Herbal medicine; Psoriasis.

Ornithine alpha-ketoglutarate

CATEGORY: Herbs and supplements
DEFINITION: Natural substance of the human body used as a supplement to treat specific health conditions.
PRINCIPAL PROPOSED USE: Recovery from severe injury
OTHER PROPOSED USES: Liver cirrhosis, sports supplement

OVERVIEW

Ornithine alpha-ketoglutarate (OKG) is manufactured from two amino acids, ornithine and glutamine. These amino acids are considered conditionally essential, meaning that ordinarily, a person does not need to consume them in food because the body can manufacture them from other nutrients. However, during periods of severe stress, such as recovery from major trauma or severe illness, the body may not be able to manufacture them in sufficient quantities and may require an external source.

Ornithine and glutamine are thought to have anabolic effects, meaning that they stimulate the body to build muscle and other tissues. These amino acids also appear to have anti-catabolic effects. This is a closely related but slightly different property; ornithine and glutamine appear to block the effect of hormones that break down muscle and other tissues (catabolic hormones).

Evidence suggests that use of OKG (and related amino acids) may offer benefits for hospitalized patients recovering from serious illness or injury. Based on these findings (and a leap of logic), OKG has been extensively marketed as a sports supplement for helping to build muscle. However, the fact that OKG helps seriously ill people build muscle does not mean that it will have the same effect in athletes, and there is no direct evidence to indicate that it does.

REQUIREMENTS AND SOURCES

The amino acids that make up OKG are found in high-protein foods such as meat, fish, and dairy products. Supplements are available in tablet or pill form.

THERAPEUTIC DOSAGES

A typical dose of OKG is 5 to 25 grams (g) daily. It may be necessary to increase dosage slowly to avoid digestive upset.

THERAPEUTIC USES

OKG may play a role in the treatment of individuals recovering from severe physical trauma. When the body experiences severe trauma–such as injury, major surgery, or burns–it goes into what is called a catabolic state. In this temporary condition, the body tends to tear itself down rather than build itself up. The catabolic hormone cortisone plays a major role in inducing catabolism. In the catabolic state, the body fails to utilize protein found in the diet, and high levels of protein breakdown products appear in the urine. Calcium levels in urine also rise, as bones begin to weaken.

The opposite of a catabolic state is an anabolic state, in which the body tends to build itself up. Studies of hospitalized patients recovering from severe illnesses or injuries suggest that OKG blocks the catabolic effects of cortisone and also directly stimulates anabolic activity. It is not clear how OKG accomplishes this. It may directly affect the enzymes involved in hormone metabolism. Another possibility is that

OKG may increase levels of growth hormone (an anabolic hormone), at least when it is taken in high enough doses (12 mg a day or more). It has also been suggested that OKG increases insulin release, which would have anabolic effects; however, this has been disputed.

Based on these findings, OKG has become popular as a bodybuilding supplement. However, there are no reported double-blind studies of OKG alone as a sports supplement. One study evaluated a combined arginine and ornithine supplement and found some evidence of benefit. OKG and the related substance ornithine-l-aspartate have shown some promise for hepatic encephalopathy, a life-threatening complication of liver cirrhosis.

SAFETY ISSUES

Because it is simply ornithine and glutamine, OKG is presumably safe. However, high doses (over 5 to10 g) can cause diarrhea and stomach cramps. The maximum safe dosages for young children, women who are pregnant or nursing, and those with serious liver or kidney disease have not been established.

EBSCO CAM Review Board

FURTHER READING

Coudray-Lucas, C., et al. "Ornithine Alpha-ketoglutarate Improves Wound Healing in Severe Burn Patients: A Prospective Randomized Double-Blind Trial Versus Isonitrogenous Controls." *Critical Care Medicine* 28 (2000): 1772-1776.

Jiang, Q., et al. "L-ornithine-l-aspartate in the Management of Hepatic Encephalopathy: A Meta-analysis." *Journal of Gastroenterology and Hepatology* 24, no. 1 (2009): 9-14.

Kircheis, G., et al. "Clinical Efficacy of L-ornithine-L-aspartate in the Management of Hepatic Encephalopathy." *Metabolic Brain Disorders* 17 (2002): 453-462.

Neu, J., V. DeMarco, and N. Li. "Glutamine: Clinical Applications and Mechanisms of Action." *Current Opinion in Clinical Nutrition and Metabolic Care* 5 (2002): 69-75.

Reynolds, T. M. "The Future of Nutrition and Wound Healing." *Journal of Tissue Viability* 11, no. 1 (2001): 5-13.

See also: Burns, minor; Herbal medicine; Injuries, minor; Sports and fitness support: Enhancing recovery; Wounds, minor.

Orthomolecular medicine

CATEGORY: Therapies and techniques

RELATED TERMS: Megavitamin therapy, nutritional medicine

DEFINITION: The prevention and treatment of disease by eliminating from the body those substances that contribute to malnutrition, such as sugar, salt, and animal fat, and by optimizing the amounts of such substances as vitamins and minerals.

PRINCIPAL PROPOSED USES: Cancer, common cold, heart disease, schizophrenia, wounds and injuries

OTHER PROPOSED USES: Alcoholism, asthma, chronic fatigue, digestive disorders, osteoarthritis

OVERVIEW

In 1968, Linus Pauling, a preeminent American chemist and two-time Nobel laureate, introduced the term "orthomolecular" to signify human health as "the right molecules in the right amount" in the body. He had earlier discovered the first disease described as "molecular" when he showed that sickle cell anemia is caused by a defect in the hemoglobin molecule. He later explored the role of molecular deficiencies in mental illness and, following the advice of biochemist Irwin Stone, began taking large amounts (megadoses) of vitamin C (ascorbic acid), which reduced the numbers and the severity of his bouts with the common cold.

Pauling then investigated the scientific literature and found studies that indicated that a high ingestion of vitamin C protected people against colds. Because medical and nutritional authorities had largely ignored these studies, Pauling compiled his findings and published the book *Vitamin C and the Common Cold* (1970) to alert consumers, doctors, and nutritionists about the results of his literature review.

Pauling's book initiated the so-called vitamin C controversy, which pitted Pauling and a growing number of supporters against members of the medical and nutritional establishment, who generally criticized his claims. In the early 1970s, Pauling and others founded the Institute of Orthomolecular Medicine (later renamed the Linus Pauling Institute of Science and Medicine) near Stanford University. The institute was designed, among other things, to do research on how the deficiencies and surpluses of certain bodily substances affect human health. This research led to the publication of the book *Cancer and Vitamin C* (1979), which Pauling coauthored with the oncologist Ewan Cameron. Pauling then published *How to Live Longer and Feel Better* (1986), his final book. After Pauling's death in 1994, his institute was moved to Oregon State University, where Pauling had obtained his undergraduate degree. The institute's research mission remained orthomolecular medicine and nutrition, a goal shared with many orthomolecular doctors all over the world.

MECHANISM OF ACTION

Millions of years of evolution in *Homo sapiens* has led the human body to develop an armamentarium of substances that facilitate the health necessary for survival. According to orthomolecular physicians, however, modern diets often lack the proper amounts of essential vitamins, minerals, proteins, and other nutrients, and contain harmful amounts of such substances as sugar, salt, and animal fats. A person can maintain good health by eliminating substances that contribute to malnutrition and by optimizing the amounts of such substances as vitamins and minerals.

USES AND APPLICATIONS

After interviewing a person seeking care and after analyzing that person's blood, urine, and hair, the orthomolecular doctor attempts, through diet, supplements, and lifestyle modification, to restore a proper balance of chemical constituents in the body. The physician may prescribe megadoses of vitamin C, vitamin E,

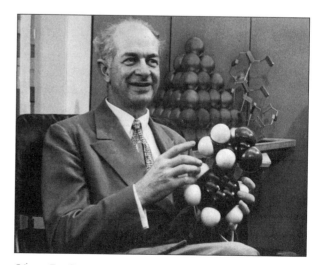

Linus Pauling introduced the term "orthomolecular" to signify human health as "the right molecules in the right amount" in the body. (Hulton Archive/Getty Images)

and niacin and restrict the ingestion of such processed foods as refined sugar, white flour, and animal fats.

SCIENTIFIC EVIDENCE

Because of the overwhelming data gathered by researchers in numerous double-blind studies of humans and nonhuman animals, general agreement exists among physicians and nutritionists that certain vitamins, minerals, proteins, carbohydrates, and fats are essential for good health. Controversies have developed, however, about what constitutes truly advantageous amounts of these substances. For example, Pauling believed that the Food and Nutrition Board of the U.S. Food and Drug Administration set the recommended dietary allowances of many of these substances much too low. As scientific evidence to bolster his claim, Pauling cited his own work, "Evolution and the Need for Ascorbic Acid," in which he analyzes the diets of primates, showing that they ingested two to three grams of ascorbic acid per day. Furthermore, animals who manufacture their own vitamin C do so in mega- rather than micro-amounts.

In rebuttal of the claims of Pauling and orthomolecular doctors who support his views, other researchers performed laboratory and clinical studies that showed, for example, that megavitamin therapy had no value for people suffering from mental illness. Most famously, two Mayo Clinic studies (1979 and 1985) concluded that vitamin C was an ineffective treatment for persons with cancer. Scientific studies continued during the succeeding decades on the effectiveness of megadoses of vitamins and other nutrients for various illnesses, with some studies supporting the benefits but many indicating no or even negative consequences. Even as many people continue to use dietary supplements, many conventional health practitioners reject most of the doctrines of the orthomolecular proponents.

CHOOSING A PRACTITIONER

Although orthomolecular medicine is widely considered an alternative medicine, it generally involves cooperation with conventional doctors and is thus more complementary than alternative in nature. For example, when Pauling and his wife were suffering from cancer, both used megavitamin therapy as a complement to surgery.

The International Society of Orthomolecular Medicine and many national societies provide lists of orthomolecular practitioners. Orthomolecular Health Medicine, founded in 1994, has a referral service.

SAFETY ISSUES

Proponents of orthomolecular medicine insist that megadoses of vitamins and other nutrients are perfectly safe, but critics insist that relying solely on nutritional rather than pharmacological treatment, when necessary, is dangerous. Researchers who support criticism of orthomolecular medicine have gathered evidence that confirms the hazards of megadoses of such fat-soluble vitamins as A and E. Megadoses of other vitamins have been associated with increased risk of heart disease, kidney stones, hypertension, and other diseases.

Robert J. Paradowski, Ph.D.

Linus Pauling on Orthomolecular Medicine

Linus Pauling briefly defines the terms "ortho" and "orthomolecular medicine" in a 1983 interview, excerpted here.

Ortho means "right"—the right molecules in the right amounts. Orthomolecular medicine is the use of the right molecules or orthomolecular substances that are normally present in the human body in the amounts that lead to the best of health and the greatest decrease in disease. It is the most effective prevention in the treatment of disease.

Source: Linus Pauling, interview by Deborah Kesten, *Healthline*, April 1983.

FURTHER READING

Bender, David A. *Nutritional Biochemistry of the Vitamins.* 2d ed. New York: Cambridge University Press, 2003. In this reference work intended for physicians, nutritionists, and clinicians, Bender has gathered an immense amount of information on the biochemical, medical, and physiological effects of vitamins. His data tend to support the traditional view of vitamins as micronutrients. Figures and tables, bibliography, and index.

Gratzer, Walter B. *Terrors of the Table: The Curious History of Nutrition.* New York: Oxford University Press, 2005. Gratzer treats mainstream scientists as the heroes and Pauling and his orthomolecular supporters as the villains. Further reading, references, and index.

Hoffer, Abram, and Andrew W. Saul. *Orthomolecular Medicine for Everyone: Megavitamin Therapeutics for Families and Physicians.* Laguna Beach, Calif.: National Health, 2008. Written by two orthomolecular practitioners, this book surveys the field, advocating megavitamin therapy as safe, effective, and inexpensive.

Linus Pauling Online, Oregon State University. http://pauling.library.oregonstate.edu.

Pauling, Linus. *How to Live Longer and Feel Better.* Corvallis: Oregon State University Press, 2006. This new edition of a book originally published in 1986 makes available again what has been called "the strongest presentation ever written on the need for supplemental vitamins."

_____. *Vitamin C and the Common Cold.* San Francisco: Freeman, 1970. This best-selling and prizewinning book contains a chapter on orthomolecular medicine and helpful appendixes, references, and an index.

Williams, Roger J., and Dwight K. Kalita, eds. *A Physician's Handbook on Orthomolecular Medicine.* New ed. New Canaan, Conn.: Keats, 1979. The editors have collected articles by orthomolecular doctors and researchers from around the world, though some reviewers, representing conventional medicine, found the claims of many contributors unsupported by scientific evidence.

See also: Supplements: Introduction; Vitamins and minerals; Wellness, general.

Osha

CATEGORY: Herbs and supplements
RELATED TERMS: Colorado cough root, *Ligusticum porteri*
DEFINITION: Natural plant product used to treat specific health conditions.
PRINCIPAL PROPOSED USES: Cough, indigestion, respiratory infections

OVERVIEW

Native to high altitudes in the Southwest and Rocky Mountain states, the root of the osha plant (*Ligusticum porteri*) is a traditional Native American remedy for respiratory infections and digestive problems. A related plant, *L. wallichii*, has a long history of use in Chinese medicine, and most of the scientific studies on osha were actually performed on this species.

THERAPEUTIC DOSAGES

Osha products vary in their concentration and should be taken according to directions on the label.

THERAPEUTIC USES

Osha is frequently recommended for use at the first sign of a respiratory infection. Like a sauna, it will typically induce sweating, and according to folk wisdom this may help avert the development of a full-blown cold. Osha is also taken during respiratory infections as a cough suppressant and expectorant, hence the common name Colorado cough root. However, there have not been any double-blind, placebo-controlled studies to verify these proposed uses.

Chinese research suggests that *L. wallichii* can relax smooth muscle tissue (perhaps thereby moderating the cough reflex) and inhibit the growth of various bacteria. Whether these findings apply to osha as well is unknown. Like other bitter herbs, osha is said to improve symptoms of indigestion and increase appetite.

SAFETY ISSUES

Osha is believed to be safe, although the scientific record is far from complete. Traditionally, it is not recommended for use in pregnancy. Safety in young children, nursing women, and those with severe liver or kidney disease also has not been established. One potential risk with osha is contamination with hemlock parsley, a deadly plant with a similar appearance.

EBSCO CAM Review Board

FURTHER READING

Bensky, D., A. Gamble, and T. J. Kaptchuk. *Chinese Herbal Medicine: Materia Medica.* Seattle: Eastland Press; 1986.

Moore, M. *Medicinal Plants of the Mountain West: A Guide to the Identification, Preparation, and Uses of Traditional Medicinal Plants Found in the Mountains, Foothills, and Upland Areas of the American West.* Santa Fe: Museum of New Mexico Press, 1979.

See also: Chinese medicine; Cough; Dyspepsia; Herbal medicine.

Osteoarthritis

CATEGORY: Condition
RELATED TERMS: Arthritis, degenerative joint disease
DEFINITION: Treatment of damage to joint cartilage.
PRINCIPAL PROPOSED NATURAL TREATMENTS:

- *Reducing symptoms and slowing progression:* Chondroitin sulfate, glucosamine
- *Reducing symptoms only:* Acupuncture, avocado-soybean unsaponifiables, cetylated fatty acids, s-adenosylmethionine

OTHER PROPOSED NATURAL TREATMENTS:

- *Herbs and supplements:* Ayurveda, boswellia, bromelain, cat's claw, Chinese herbal medicine, comfrey (topical), devil's claw, ginger, green-lipped mussel, krill oil, methyl sulfonyl methane, multimineral supplement, niacinamide, proteolytic enzymes, rose hips, velvet antler, white willow, zinc
- *Therapies:* Balneotherapy, bee venom, magnet therapy, prolotherapy, relaxation therapies, Tai Chi, yoga

PROBABLY INEFFECTIVE TREATMENTS: Mesoglycan, vitamin E

INTRODUCTION

In osteoarthritis, the cartilage in joints has become damaged, disrupting the smooth gliding motion of the joint surfaces. The result is pain, swelling, and deformity. The pain of osteoarthritis typically increases with joint use and improves at rest. Although X rays can find evidence of arthritis, the level of pain and stiffness experienced by people does not match the extent of injury noticed on X rays.

Many theories exist about the causes of osteoarthritis, but no one really knows what causes the disease. Osteoarthritis is often described as wear-and-tear arthritis, but evidence suggests that this simple explanation is not correct. For example, osteoarthritis frequently develops in many joints at the same time, often symmetrically on both sides of the body, even when there is no reason to believe that equal amounts of wear and tear are present. Another intriguing finding is that osteoarthritis of the knee is commonly (and mysteriously) associated with osteoarthritis of the hand. These factors, and others, have led to the suggestion that osteoarthritis may actually be a body-wide disease of the cartilage.

During one's lifetime, cartilage is constantly being turned over by a balance of forces that both break down and rebuild it. One prevailing theory suggests that osteoarthritis may represent a situation in which the degrading forces become chaotic. Some of the proposed natural treatments for osteoarthritis described here may inhibit enzymes that damage cartilage.

When the cartilage damage in osteoarthritis begins, the body responds by building new cartilage. For several years, this compensating effort can keep the joint functioning well. Some natural treatments appear to work by assisting the body in repairing cartilage. Eventually, however, building forces cannot keep up with destructive ones, and what develops is end-stage osteoarthritis. This is the familiar picture of pain and impaired joint function.

The conventional medical treatment for osteoarthritis consists mainly of anti-inflammatory drugs, such as naproxen and Celebrex. The main problem with anti-inflammatory drugs is that they can cause ulcers. Another possible problem is that they may actually speed the progression of osteoarthritis by interfering with cartilage repair and by promoting cartilage destruction. In contrast, two of the treatments described here might actually slow the course of the disease, although this has not been proven.

PRINCIPAL PROPOSED NATURAL TREATMENTS

Several natural treatments for osteoarthritis have a meaningful, though not definitive, body of supporting evidence indicating that they can reduce pain and improve function. In addition, there is some evidence that glucosamine and chondroitin might offer the additional benefit of helping to prevent progressive joint damage.

Glucosamine. Inconsistent evidence hints that glucosamine can reduce symptoms of mild to moderate arthritis; a small amount of evidence indicates that regular use can slow down the gradual worsening of arthritis that normally occurs with time.

Glucosamine appears to stimulate cartilage cells in the joints to make proteoglycans and collagen, two proteins essential for the proper function of joints. Glucosamine may also help prevent collagen from breaking down.

Glucosamine is widely accepted as a treatment for osteoarthritis. However, the supporting evidence that it works is somewhat inconsistent, with several of the most recent studies failing to find benefit. Two types of studies have been performed: those that compared glucosamine with placebo and those that compared it with standard medications.

In the placebo-controlled category, one of the best trials was a three-year double-blind study of 212 people with osteoarthritis of the knee. Participants receiving glucosamine showed reduced symptoms compared to those receiving placebo. Benefits were also seen in other double-blind, placebo-controlled studies, enrolling more than eight hundred people and ranging in length from four weeks to three years. Even more double-blind studies enrolling more than four hundred people compared glucosamine with ibuprofen and found glucosamine just as effective as the drug.

Most recent studies, however, have not shown benefit. In four studies involving almost five hundred people, the use of glucosamine failed to improve symptoms to any greater extent than placebo. In a study involving 222 participants with hip osteoarthritis, two years of treatment with glucosamine was no better than placebo at improving pain or function. Another study involving 147 women with osteoarthritis found glucosamine to be no more effective than home exercises over an eighteen-month period. A third study evaluated the effects of stopping glucosamine after it was taken by participants for six months. In this double-blind trial of 137 people with osteoarthritis of the knee, participants who stopped using glucosamine (and unknowingly took placebo instead) did no worse than people who stayed on glucosamine. In a fourth, large (1,583-participant) study, neither glucosamine (as glucosamine hydrochloride) nor glucosamine plus chondroitin was more effective than placebo. Another study also failed to find benefit with glucosamine plus chondroitin. Finally, in a systematic review including randomized trials involving 3,803 persons with osteoarthritis of the hip or knee, researchers found that neither glucosamine alone, chondroitin alone, nor the combination of glucosamine and chondroitin relieved pain. It appears that most of the positive studies were funded by manufacturers of glucosamine products. Most of the studies performed by neutral researchers failed to find benefit.

Many popular glucosamine products combine this supplement with methylsulfonylmethane (MSM). One study published in India reported that both MSM and glucosamine improved arthritis symptoms compared with placebo but that the combination of MSM and glucosamine was even more effective than either supplement separately.

Two studies reported that glucosamine can slow the progression of osteoarthritis. However, as with the positive studies of glucosamine for reducing

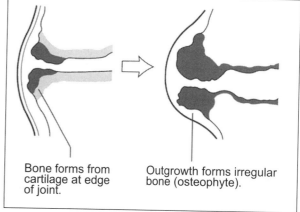

Bone forms from cartilage at edge of joint.

Outgrowth forms irregular bone (osteophyte).

Osteoarthritis results when irregular bone growth occurs at the edge of a joint, causing impaired movement of the joint and pressure on nerves in the area.

symptoms, both of these studies were funded by a major glucosamine manufacturer.

A three-year, double-blind, placebo-controlled study of 212 persons found indications that glucosamine may protect joints from further damage. Over the course of the study, persons given glucosamine showed some actual improvement in pain and mobility, while those given placebo worsened steadily. Furthermore, X rays showed that glucosamine treatment prevented progressive damage to the knee joint. A separate three-year study enrolling 202 people found similar results.

A follow-up analysis five years after the conclusion of the foregoing two studies found suggestive evidence that the use of glucosamine reduced the need for knee replacement surgery. However, the aforementioned study involving 222 persons with osteoarthritis of the hip failed to show any significant change on X ray findings following two years of glucosamine treatment compared with placebo.

Chondroitin sulfate. The supplement chondroitin is often combined with glucosamine. Several studies also have evaluated chondroitin used alone, with some positive results, both for improving symptoms and for slowing the progression of the disease. On balance, however, the evidence for chondroitin's effectiveness for osteoarthritis remains inconsistent.

According to some double-blind, placebo-controlled studies, chondroitin may relieve symptoms of osteoarthritis. One study enrolled eighty-five people with osteoarthritis of the knee and followed them for six months. Participants received either 400 milligrams (mg) of chondroitin sulfate twice daily or a placebo. At the end of the trial, doctors rated the improvement as good or very good in 69 percent of those taking chondroitin sulfate but in only 32 percent of those taking placebo.

Another way of comparing the results is to look at maximum walking speed among participants. Whereas persons in the chondroitin group were able to improve their walking speed gradually over the course of the trial, walking speed did not improve in the placebo group. Additionally, there were improvements in other measures of osteoarthritis, such as pain level, with benefits seen as early as one month. This suggests that chondroitin was able to stop the arthritis from gradually getting worse. Good results were seen in a twelve-month double-blind trial that compared chondroitin with placebo in 104 persons with arthritis of the knee, and in a twelve-month trial of 42 participants.

Another study evaluated the intermittent or "on and off" use of chondroitin. In this study, 120 people received either placebo or 800 mg of chondroitin sulfate daily for two separate, three-month periods in one year. The results showed that even when it was taken intermittently, the use of chondroitin improved symptoms. Benefits were also seen in two short-term trials involving about 240 persons.

Generally positive results were also seen in other studies, including one that found chondroitin about as effective as the anti-inflammatory drug diclofenac. However, a large (1,583-participant) and well-designed study failed to find either chondroitin or glucosamine plus chondroitin more effective than placebo. When this study is pooled together with the two other best-designed trials, no overall benefit is seen. It has been suggested that chondroitin, like glucosamine, may show benefit primarily in studies funded by manufacturers of the product being tested.

Some evidence suggests that, like glucosamine, chondroitin might slow the progression of arthritis. An important feature of the foregoing study of forty-two persons was that the persons taking a placebo showed progressive joint damage over the year, but among those taking chondroitin sulfate, no worsening of the joints was seen. In other words, chondroitin sulfate seemed to protect from further damage the joints of those with osteoarthritis.

A longer and larger double-blind, placebo-controlled trial also found evidence that chondroitin sulfate can slow the progression of osteoarthritis. The study enrolled 119 people and lasted three years. Thirty-four of the participants received 1,200 mg of chondroitin sulfate per day; the rest received placebo. Over the course of the study, researchers took X rays to determine how many joints had progressed to a severe stage.

During the three years of the study, only 8.8 percent of those who took chondroitin sulfate developed severely damaged joints, whereas almost 30 percent of those who took placebo progressed to this extent. Similar long-term benefits were seen in two other studies, enrolling more than two hundred people.

Additional evidence comes from animal studies. Researchers measured the effects of chondroitin sulfate (administered both orally and via injection directly into the muscle) in rabbits, in which cartilage damage had been induced in one knee by the injection of an enzyme. After eighty-four days of treatment, the damaged knees in the animals that had been given chondroitin sulfate had significantly more cartilage left than the knees of the untreated animals. Taking chondroitin sulfate by mouth was as effective as taking it through an injection.

Looking at the sum of the evidence, it does appear that chondroitin sulfate may actually protect joints

---

What Is Cartilage?

Cartilage, the hard but slippery coating on the end of each bone, is 65 to 80 percent water. The remaining three components—collagen, proteoglycans, and chondrocytes—are described here.

- *Collagen.* A family of fibrous proteins, collagens are the building blocks of skin, tendon, bone, and other connective tissues.
- *Proteoglycans.* Made up of proteins and sugars, strands of proteoglycans interweave with collagens and form a mesh-like tissue. This allows cartilage to flex and absorb physical shock.
- *Chondrocytes.* Found throughout cartilage, chondrocytes are cells that produce cartilage and help it stay healthy as it grows. Sometimes, however, chondrocytes release substances called enzymes that destroy collagen and other proteins. Researchers are trying to learn more about chondrocytes.

from damage in osteoarthritis. However, the scientific record suffers from a paucity of truly independent researchers.

S-adenosylmethionine. A substantial body of scientific evidence indicates that S-adenosylmethionine (SAMe) can relieve symptoms of arthritis. Numerous double-blind studies involving more than one thousand participants suggest that SAMe is approximately as effective for this purpose as standard anti-inflammatory drugs. However, there is no meaningful evidence that SAMe slows the progression of the disease.

One of the best double-blind studies enrolled 732 persons and followed them for four weeks. Over this period, 235 of the participants received 1,200 mg of SAMe per day, while a similar number took either placebo or 750 mg daily of the standard drug naproxen. The majority of the participants had experienced moderate symptoms of osteoarthritis of either the knee or the hip for an average of six years.

The results indicate that SAMe provided as much pain-relieving effect as naproxen and that both treatments were significantly better than placebo. However, differences did exist between the two treatments. Naproxen worked more quickly, producing readily apparent benefits at the two-week follow-up, whereas the full effect of SAMe was not apparent until four weeks. By the end of the study, both treatments were producing the same level of benefit.

In a double-blind study that compared SAMe with the newer anti-inflammatory drug Celebrex, the drug worked faster than the supplement, but in time both were providing equal benefits.

Evidence regarding slowing the progression of arthritis is limited to studies involving animals rather than people.

Avocado-soybean unsaponifiables. Special extracts of avocado and soybeans called avocado-soybean unsaponifiables (ASUs) have been investigated as a treatment for osteoarthritis with promising results in studies enrolling several hundred people.

For example, in a double-blind trial, 260 persons with arthritis of the knee were given either placebo or ASU at 300 or 600 mg daily. The results over three months showed that the use of ASU significantly improved arthritis symptoms compared with placebo. There was no significant difference seen between the two doses tested. It does not appear that ASU can slow the progression of osteoarthritis.

Cetylated fatty acids. A type of naturally occurring fatty acid called cetylated fatty acids have shown growing promise for osteoarthritis. They are used both as topical creams and as oral supplements. Three double-blind placebo-controlled studies have found cetylated fatty acids helpful for osteoarthritis. Two involved a topical product and one used an oral formulation.

In one of the studies using a cream, forty people with osteoarthritis of the knee applied either cetylated fatty acid or placebo to the affected joint. The results over thirty days showed greater improvements in range of motion and functional ability among people using the real cream than among those using the placebo cream. In another thirty-day study, also enrolling forty people with knee arthritis, the use of cetylated fatty acid cream improved postural stability, presumably because of decreased pain levels. In addition, a sixty-eight-day, double-blind, placebo-controlled study of sixty-four people with knee arthritis tested an oral cetylated fatty acid supplement (the supplement also contained lesser amounts of lecithin and fish oil). Participants in the treatment group experienced improvements in swelling, mobility, and pain level compared to those in the placebo group. Inexplicably, the study report does not discuss whether or not side effects occurred. While this is a promising body of research, it is far from definitive.

Advertising claims for cetylated fatty acids go far beyond the existing evidence. For example, a number of Web sites claim that cetylated fatty acids are more effective than glucosamine or chondroitin. However, no comparison studies have been performed upon which such a claim could be rationally based.

Acupuncture. Acupuncture has shown inconsistent benefit as a treatment for osteoarthritis. A 2006 meta-analysis (systematic statistical review) of studies on acupuncture for osteoarthritis found eight trials that were similar enough to be considered together. These studies enrolled 2,362 people. The authors of the meta-analysis concluded that acupuncture should be regarded as an effective treatment for osteoarthritis.

However, one study comprised almost one-half of all the people considered in this meta-analysis, and it failed to find real acupuncture more effective than sham acupuncture. In this study, published in 2006, 1,007 people with knee osteoarthritis were given either real acupuncture, fake acupuncture, or standard therapy over six weeks. Though both real acupuncture and fake acupuncture were more effective than no acupuncture, there was no significant difference in benefits between the two acupuncture groups. In general, larger studies are more reliable than small ones. For this reason, it is always somewhat questionable when meta-analysis combines one large negative study and a number of smaller positive ones to come up with a positive outcome.

Another review, published in 2007, concluded that real acupuncture produces distinct benefits in osteoarthritis compared to no treatment but that fake acupuncture is effective for osteoarthritis too. When comparing real acupuncture to fake acupuncture, the difference in outcome (while it might possibly be statistically significant) is so trivial as to make no difference in real life. In other words, virtually all of the benefit of acupuncture for osteoarthritis is a placebo effect.

OTHER PROPOSED NATURAL TREATMENTS

A six-week, double-blind, placebo-controlled study of 247 persons with osteoarthritis of the knee evaluated a combination herbal product containing ginger and the Asian spice galanga (*Alpinia galanga*). The results showed that participants in the ginger and galanga group improved to a significantly greater extent than those receiving placebo. However, despite news reports claiming that this study proves ginger effective for osteoarthritis, this study only provides information on the effectiveness of the herbal combination. The two double-blind studies performed on ginger alone were small and produced contradictory results. Furthermore, another study found that massage combined with the topical application of essential oils made from ginger and orange was no better than massage plus olive oil in persons with osteoarthritis of the knee.

A three-week double-blind study of 220 people with osteoarthritis of the knee found that the use of a cream containing the herb comfrey reduced symptoms significantly more than a placebo cream.

The herb white willow contains the aspirin-like substance salicin. A two-week, double-blind, placebo-controlled trial of seventy-eight persons with arthritis found evidence that willow extracts can relieve osteoarthritis pain. However, another double-blind study enrolling 127 people with osteoarthritis found white willow less effective than a standard anti-inflammatory drug and no more effective than placebo. The likely explanation for these contradictory results is that white willow at usual doses provides relatively modest benefits.

The supplement MSM, as described in a foregoing study, has shown promise for osteoarthritis when taken with glucosamine. Benefits were also seen in a twelve-week, double-blind, placebo-controlled trial of fifty people with osteoarthritis, utilizing MSM at a dose of 3 grams twice daily. However, in a comprehensive review of six studies involving 681 persons with osteoarthritis of the knee, researchers concluded it is not possible to convincingly determine whether or not MSM is beneficial.

Other treatments with incomplete supporting evidence from double-blind trials include Ayurvedic herbal combination therapy, boswellia, cat's claw, a proprietary complex of minerals with or without cat's claw, devil's claw, proteolytic enzymes, rose hips, soy protein, and vitamin B_3.

Traditional Chinese herbal medicine has also shown some promise for osteoarthritis. However, one study that compared a commonly used Chinese herbal product (Duhuo Jisheng Wan) to the drug diclofenac found that the herb worked more slowly than the drug, yet produced about an equal rate of side effects.

Growing but definitive evidence suggests that the natural substance hyaluronic acid may help reduce osteoarthritis symptoms when it is injected into an affected joint. However, there is absolutely no reason to believe that oral hyaluronic acid should help, and one study failed to show any significant benefit.

Incomplete and inconsistent evidence from human and animal studies only weakly suggests that green-lipped mussel might alleviate osteoarthritis symptoms. A badly designed human study hints that krill oil might be helpful as well. One double-blind study involving dogs found some evidence of benefit with elk velvet antler.

Numerous other herbs and supplements sometimes recommended for osteoarthritis include beta-carotene, boron, cartilage, chamomile, copper, dandelion, D-phenylalanine, feverfew, molybdenum, selenium, turmeric, and yucca. However, there is little to no evidence that these treatments are effective.

Other studies provide limited evidence that certain supplements proposed for osteoarthritis do not work. For example, a two-year double-blind study of 136 people with knee arthritis found vitamin E ineffective for either reducing symptoms or slowing the progression of the disease. In addition, a six-month, double-blind, placebo-controlled trial of seventy-seven people with osteoarthritis failed to find any symptomatic benefit with vitamin E. Similarly, in a large (almost four-hundred-participant), five-year, double-blind, placebo-controlled study, the use of injected mesoglycan failed to slow the progression of osteoarthritis. A fairly small study failed to find the enzyme bromelain helpful for reducing symptoms.

Prolotherapy is a special form of injection therapy that is popular among some alternative practitioners. A double-blind, placebo-controlled study evaluated the effects of three prolotherapy injections (using a 10 percent dextrose solution) at two-month intervals in sixty-eight people with osteoarthritis of the knee. At six-month follow-up, participants who had received prolotherapy showed significant improvements in pain at rest and while walking, reduction in swelling, fewer episodes of "buckling," and better range of flexion, compared to those who had received placebo treatment. The same research group performed a similar double-blind trial of twenty-seven persons with osteoarthritis in the hands. The results at six-month follow-up showed that range of motion and pain with movement improved significantly in the treated group compared with the placebo group.

Several double-blind, placebo-controlled studies suggest that pulsed electromagnetic field therapy, a special form of magnet therapy, can improve symptoms of osteoarthritis. One small study provides extremely weak supporting evidence for the more ordinary form of magnet therapy: static magnets. A subsequent, much larger study of static magnets failed to find real magnets more effective than placebo magnets, but a manufacturing error may have obscured genuine benefits (some people in the placebo group were accidentally given active magnets). In another placebo-controlled trial, the use of a magnetic knee wrap for twelve weeks was associated with a significant increase in quadriceps (thigh muscle) strength in persons with knee osteoarthritis.

Limited evidence supports the use of bee venom injections for osteoarthritis. Hot water therapy (balneotherapy), relaxation therapies, and various forms of exercise, including hatha yoga and Tai Chi, have also all shown some promise. However, for none of these therapies is the supporting evidence convincing.

HERBS AND SUPPLEMENTS TO USE WITH CAUTION

Various herbs and supplements may interact adversely with drugs used to treat osteoarthritis, so one should be cautious when considering the use of herbs and supplements.

EBSCO CAM Review Board

FURTHER READING

Arjmandi, B. H., et al. "Soy Protein May Alleviate Osteoarthritis Symptoms." *Phytomedicine* 11 (2005): 567-575.

Brien, S., et al. "Systematic Review of the Nutritional Supplements Dimethyl Sulfoxide (DMSO) and Methylsulfonylmethane (MSM) in the Treatment of Osteoarthritis." *Osteoarthritis and Cartilage* 16 (2008): 1277-1288.

Brismee, J. M., et al. "Group and Home-Based Tai Chi in Elderly Subjects with Knee Osteoarthritis." *Clinical Rehabilitation* 21 (2007): 99-111.

Chen, C. Y., et al. "Effect of Magnetic Knee Wrap on Quadriceps Strength in Patients with Symptomatic Knee Osteoarthritis." *Archives of Physical Medicine and Rehabilitation* 89 (2008): 2258-2264.

Clegg, D. O., et al. "Glucosamine, Chondroitin Sulfate, and the Two in Combination for Painful Knee Osteoarthritis." *New England Journal of Medicine* 354 (2006): 795-808.

Deutsch, L. "Evaluation of the Effect of Neptune Krill Oil on Chronic Inflammation and Arthritic Symptoms." *Journal of the American College of Nutrition* 26 (2007): 39-48.

Kawasaki, T., et al. "Additive Effects of Glucosamine or Risedronate for the Treatment of Osteoarthritis of the Knee Combined with Home Exercise." *Journal of Bone and Mineral Metabolism* 26 (2008): 279-287.

Lee, M. S., M. H. Pittler, and E. Ernst. "Tai Chi for Osteoarthritis." *Clinical Rheumatology* 27 (2008): 211-218.

Manheimer, E., et al. "Meta-analysis: Acupuncture for Osteoarthritis of the Knee." *Annals of Internal Medicine* 146 (2007): 868-877.

Reichenbach, S., et al. "Meta-analysis: Chondroitin for Osteoarthritis of the Knee or Hip." *Annals of Internal Medicine* 146 (2007): 580-590.

Tishler, M., et al. "The Effect of Balneotherapy on Osteoarthritis: Is an Intermittent Regimen Effective?" *European Journal of Internal Medicine* 15 (2004): 93-96.

Wandel, S., et al. "Effects of Glucosamine, Chondroitin, or Placebo in Patients with Osteoarthritis of Hip or Knee." *British Medical Journal* 341 (2010): c4675.

See also: Acupuncture; Bone and joint health; Chondroitin; Exercise; Glucosamine; Nonsteroidal anti-inflammatory drugs (NSAIDs); Osteoarthritis: Homeopathic remedies; Pain management; Rheumatoid arthritis; SAMe; Tai Chi.

Osteoarthritis: Homeopathic remedies

CATEGORY: Homeopathy

DEFINITION: The use of highly diluted remedies to treat damage to joint cartilage.

STUDIED HOMEOPATHIC REMEDIES: *Calcarea carbonica*; *C. fluorica*; *Kali carbonicum*; *Rhus tox*; topical homeopathic remedy containing *Symphytum officinale*, *Rhus toxicodendron*, and *Ledum palustre*

SCIENTIFIC EVALUATIONS OF HOMEOPATHIC REMEDIES

One double-blind study compared the effectiveness of the homeopathic remedy *Rhus tox* 6x with the anti-inflammatory drug fenoprofen and with placebo. However, the results were not promising. At the conclusion of the study, fenoprofen was found to provide significantly greater pain relief than *Rhus tox*, and the homeopathic remedy proved no more effective than placebo.

A much larger double-blind study compared a homeopathic gel containing the remedies *Symphytum officinale*, *Rhus toxicodendron*, and *Ledum palustre* with a gel made from the anti-inflammatory drug piroxicam. Of the 184 people with knee arthritis who were enrolled in this study, 172 were followed for the full four weeks. The results showed that the two treatments were equally effective.

However, these results are not as promising as they might at first appear. Oral piroxicam is a well-established therapy for osteoarthritis, but the effectiveness of piroxicam gel is far from clear. Thus, it is possible that this study simply proved that the two gels were equally ineffective. Furthermore, the homeopathic remedies contained in the gel were more like herbal treatments than homeopathic treatments because they were not extremely diluted.

TRADITIONAL HOMEOPATHIC TREATMENTS

Classical homeopathy offers possible homeopathic treatments for osteoarthritis. These therapies are chosen based on various specific details of the person seeking treatment. If the arthritis pain and stiffness is worse in the morning, is relieved by heat but aggravated by cold, and improves with movement, then the affected person may fit the symptom picture for *Rhus toxicodendron*.

Calcarea carbonica is used for arthritis made worse by coldness or dampness, especially when it is the knees that are especially painful. People prescribed this remedy are often overweight and out of shape. *C. fluorica* is often recommended for arthritis related to past injuries. *Kali carbonicum* may be used when arthritis has led to permanently swollen or deformed joints.

EBSCO CAM Review Board

FURTHER READING

Breuer, G. S., et al. "Perceived Efficacy among Patients of Various Methods of Complementary Alternative Medicine for Rheumatologic Diseases." *Clinical and Experimental Rheumatology* 23 (2005): 693-696.

Shipley, M., et al. "Controlled Trial of Homeopathic Treatment of Osteoarthritis." *The Lancet* 1 (1983): 97-98.

Van Haselen RA, Fisher PA. "A Randomized Controlled Trial Comparing Topical Piroxicam Gel with a Homeopathic Gel in Osteoarthritis of the Knee." *Rheumatology* 39 (2000): 714-719.

See also: Aging; Bone and joint health; Homeopathy; Osteoarthritis; Rheumatoid arthritis: Homeopathic remedies.

Osteopathic manipulation

CATEGORY: Therapies and techniques

RELATED TERMS: Cranial osteopathy, craniosacral therapy, Jones counterstrain, mobilization, muscle energy technique, myofascial release, osteopathic medicine, osteopathy, strain-counterstrain

DEFINITION: Treatment through manipulation of soft tissues and joints outside the spine.

PRINCIPAL PROPOSED USES: Back pain, enhancing recovery from surgery or serious illness, fibromyalgia, general health, musculoskeletal pain, neck pain

OTHER PROPOSED USES: Asthma, general health, sinus infections, tendonitis

OVERVIEW

Osteopathy originated as a nineteenth-century alternative medical approach focusing on physical manipulation. Today, osteopathic physicians study and practice the same types of medical and surgical techniques as conventional medical doctors. Some of osteopathy's original techniques still persist, however. Taken together, these techniques are called osteopathic manipulation (OM). OM is less well known to the public than chiropractic spinal manipulation, but it has shown promise for many of the same conditions, such as back pain and tension headaches.

History of osteopathic manipulation. Osteopathic medicine was founded in 1874 by Andrew Taylor Still, an American physician. Physicians educated in this method were called doctors of osteopathy, or D.O.'s. Subsequently, however, schools of osteopathic medicine became integrated with conventional medical schools, and today the license of D.O. is legally equivalent to that of medical doctor (M.D.).

Forms of osteopathic manipulation. Osteopathic and chiropractic techniques overlap, but they are not identical. As a general rule, chiropractors focus most of their attention on the spine, while osteopathic practitioners devote more of the their efforts to the manipulation of soft tissues and joints outside the spine. Another general difference is that chiropractic spinal manipulation tends to make use of rapid short movements (spinal manipulation, which is a high-velocity, low-amplitude technique), while OM typically concentrates on gentle, larger movements (mobilization, which is a low-velocity, high-amplitude technique). Neither of these distinctions is absolute, and many chiropractic and osteopathic methods do not fit neatly into these categories.

There are several specific osteopathic techniques in wide use, many of which are named after their founders. Some of the more popular are muscle energy technique, Jones counterstrain (also known as strain-counterstrain), myofascial release, and cranialsacral therapy (formally known as osteopathy in the cranial field).

Muscle energy technique. The muscle energy technique involves bending a joint just up to the point where muscular resistance to movement begins (the barrier), and then holding the joint there while the patient gently resists. The pressure is maintained for a few seconds and then released. After a brief pause to allow the affected muscles to relax, the practitioner then moves the joint a little farther into the barrier, which will usually have shifted slightly toward improved mobility during the interval.

Strain-counterstrain technique. The strain-counterstrain technique (Jones counterstrain) involves finding tender points and then manipulating the joint connected to them to find a position where the tenderness decreases toward zero. Once this precise angle is

found, it is held for ninety seconds and then released. Like muscle-energy work, strain-counterstrain progressively increases range of motion and, it is hoped, decreases muscle spasm and pain.

Myofascial release. Myofascial release focuses on the fascial tissues that surround muscles. The practitioner first positions the painful area either at the edge of the barrier to movement or, alternatively, at the opposite extreme (the area of greatest comfort). Next, while the patient breathes slowly and easily, the practitioner palpates the fascial tissues, looking for a subtle sensation that indicates the tissues are ready to "unwind." After receiving this indication, the practitioner then helps the tissue to follow a pattern of spontaneous movement. This process is repeated over several sessions until a full release is achieved. Myofascial release is said to be especially useful in pain conditions that have persisted for months or years.

Cranialsacral therapy. Cranialsacral therapy, more properly called cranial osteopathy (or cranial), is a specialized technique based on the scientifically unconfirmed belief that the tissues surrounding the brain and spinal cord undergo a rhythmic pulsation. This "cranial rhythm" is said to cause subtle movements of the bones of the skull. A practitioner of cranialsacral therapy gently manipulates these bones in time with the rhythm (as determined by the practitioner's awareness) to repair "cranial lesions." This therapy is said to be helpful for numerous conditions ranging from headaches and sinus allergies to multiple sclerosis and asthma. However, many researchers have serious doubts that the cranial rhythm even exists.

USES AND APPLICATIONS

Osteopathic manipulation is primarily used to treat musculoskeletal pain conditions, such as back pain, shoulder pain, and tension headaches. OM is often said to be specifically effective for conditions that have persisted for some time, as opposed to chiropractic spinal manipulation, which, according to this view, is most effective for treatment of injuries that have occurred recently. However, there is no meaningful scientific support for this belief. Some advocates of OM believe that it has numerous additional benefits, including the enhancement of overall health and well-being.

SCIENTIFIC EVIDENCE

There is little evidence that osteopathic manipulation is helpful for the treatment of any medical condition. There are several possible reasons for this, but one is fundamental: Even with the best of intentions, it is difficult to properly ascertain the effectiveness of a hands-on therapy like OM.

Only one form of study can truly prove that a treatment is effective: the double-blind, placebo-controlled trial. However, it is not possible to fit OM into a study design of this type.

Because of these problems, all studies of OM fall short of optimum design. Many have compared OM with no treatment. However, studies of that type cannot provide reliable evidence about the efficacy of a treatment: If a benefit is seen, there is no way to determine whether it was a result of OM specifically or just attention generally. (Attention alone will almost always produce some reported benefit.)

More meaningful trials used fake osteopathy for the control group. Such studies are single-blind because the practitioner is aware of applying phony treatment. However, this design can introduce potential bias in the form of subtle unconscious communication between practitioner and patient.

"Osteopathy to Cure Disease"

The founder of osteopathy, Andrew Taylor Still, discusses the healing method of osteopathic manipulation in his book Philosophy of Osteopathy *(1899). His brief discussion is excerpted here.*

The osteopath seeks first physiological perfection of form, by normally adjusting the osseous framework, so that all arteries may deliver blood to nourish and construct all parts. Also that the veins may carry away all impurities dependent upon them for renovation. Also that the nerves of all classes may be free and unobstructed while applying the powers of life and motion to all divisions, and the whole system of nature's laboratory. A full and complete supply of arterial blood must be generated and delivered to all parts, organs and glands, by the channels called the arteries. And when it has done its work, then without delay the veins must return all to heart and lungs for renewal. We must know some delay of fluids has been established on which nature begins the work of renewal by increased action of electricity, even to the solvent action of fever heat, by which watery substances evaporate and relieve the lymphatic system of stagnant, watery secretions. Thus fever is a natural and powerful remedy.

Still other studies have simply involved giving people OM and seeing if they improve. These trials are particularly meaningless; it has long since been proven that both participants and examining physicians will think, at minimum, that they observe improvement in people given a treatment, whether or not the treatment does anything on its own; such studies are not reported here. Given these caveats, the following is a summary of what science knows about the effects of OM.

Possible effects of OM. Most studies of OM have involved its potential use for various pain conditions. In a study of 183 people with neck pain, the use of osteopathic methods provided greater benefits than standard physical therapy or general medical care. Participants receiving OM showed faster recovery and experienced fewer days off work. OM appeared to be less expensive overall than the other two approaches; however, researchers strictly limited the allowed OM sessions, making direct cost comparisons questionable. Another study evaluated a rather ambitious combined therapy for the treatment of chronic pain caused by whiplash injury (craniosacral therapy with Rosen bodywork and Gestalt psychotherapy). The results failed to find this assembly of treatments more effective than no treatment.

In a fourteen-week, single-blind study of twenty-nine elderly persons with shoulder pain, real OM proved more effective than placebo OM. Although participants in both groups improved, those in the treated group showed relatively greater increase in range of motion in the shoulder. In a larger study of 150 adults with shoulder complaints, researchers found that adding manipulative therapy to usual care improved shoulder and neck pain at twelve weeks.

In a small randomized, placebo-controlled trial, researchers used oscillating-energy manual therapy, an osteopathic technique based on the principle of craniosacral therapy, to treat twenty-three persons with chronic tendonitis of the elbow (tennis elbow or lateral epicondylitis). Persons in the treatment group showed significant improvement in grip strength, pain intensity, function, and activity limitation because of pain. These results, however, are limited by the small size of the study and the fact that the therapist delivering the treatment could not be "blinded."

In another study, twenty-four women with fibromyalgia were divided into five groups: standard care, standard care plus OM, standard care plus an educational approach, standard care plus moist heat, and standard care plus moist heat and OM. The results indicate that OM plus standard care is better than standard care alone and that OM is more effective than less specific treatments, such as moist heat or general education. However, because this was not a blinded study (participants knew which group they were in), the results cannot be taken as reliable.

A study of twenty-eight people with tension headaches compared one session of OM with two forms of sham treatment. The study found evidence that real treatment provided a greater improvement in headache pain.

Although OM has shown some promise for the treatment of back pain, one of the best-designed trials failed to find it a superior alternative to conventional medical care. In this twelve-week study of 178 people, OM proved no more effective than standard treatment for back pain. Another study, this one enrolling 199 people and following them for six months, failed to find OM more effective than fake OM. This study also included a no-treatment group; both real and fake OM were more effective than no treatment. A much smaller study reportedly found that muscle energy technique enhances recovery from back pain, but this study does not appear to have used a meaningful placebo treatment.

Some studies have evaluated the potential benefits of OM for speeding healing in people recovering from surgery or serious illness. The best of these studies compared OM with light touch in fifty-eight elderly people hospitalized for pneumonia. The results indicate that the use of osteopathy aided recovery.

In a much less meaningful study, OM was compared to no treatment in people recovering from knee or hip surgery. While the people receiving OM recovered more quickly, these results mean very little, because any form of attention should be expected to produce greater apparent benefits than no attention. A similarly weak study suggests that OM might also be helpful for people hospitalized with pancreatitis. A small study found some evidence that OM might be helpful for childhood asthma.

CHOOSING A PRACTITIONER

Although there are many licensed doctors of osteopathy, most practice conventional medicine and do not specialize in OM. Some do, and many have been certified by the American Osteopathic Board of Neuromusculoskeletal Medicine. In addition, many

physical therapists and massage therapists use some osteopathic techniques, with variable amounts of training.

SAFETY ISSUES

Most forms of OM, because of their gentle nature, are believed to be quite safe. However, mild short-term pain may occur immediately following treatment. In addition, some osteopathic practitioners use the high-velocity thrusts common to chiropractic and might, therefore, introduce some slight safety risks.

EBSCO CAM Review Board

FURTHER READING

Bergman, G. J., et al. "Manipulative Therapy in Addition to Usual Care for Patients with Shoulder Complaints." *Journal of Manipulative and Physiological Therapeutics* 33 (2010): 96-101.

Gamber, R. G., et al. "Osteopathic Manipulative Treatment in Conjunction with Medication Relieves Pain Associated with Fibromyalgia Syndrome." *Journal of the American Osteopathic Association* 102 (2002): 321-325.

Guiney, P. A., et al. "Effects of Osteopathic Manipulative Treatment on Pediatric Patients with Asthma." *Journal of the American Osteopathic Association* 105 (2005): 7-12.

Licciardone, J. C., et al. "Osteopathic Manipulative Treatment for Chronic Low Back Pain." *Spine* 28 (2003): 1355-1362.

Ventegodt, S., et al. "A Combination of Gestalt Therapy, Rosen Body Work, and Cranio Sacral Therapy Did Not Help in Chronic Whiplash-Associated Disorders." *Scientific World Journal* 4 (2005): 1055-1068.

Wilson, E., et al. "Muscle Energy Technique in Patients with Acute Low Back Pain." *Journal of Orthopaedic and Sports Physical Therapy* 33 (2003): 502-512.

See also: Back pain; Bone and joint health; Chiropractic; Craniosacral therapy; Manipulative and body-based therapies; Massage therapy; Pain management; Rolfing.

Osteoporosis

CATEGORY: Condition
RELATED TERM: Bone loss
DEFINITION: Treatment of bone loss caused by aging, smoking, lack of exercise, and other factors.

PRINCIPAL PROPOSED NATURAL TREATMENTS: Calcium and vitamin D, genistein and other isoflavones, ipriflavone, strontium, vitamin K

OTHER PROPOSED NATURAL TREATMENTS: Black cohosh, black tea, boron, dehydroepiandrosterone, *Epimedium brevicornum*, estriol, fish oil, gamma-linolenic acid, reducing high homocysteine with folate and vitamin B$_{12}$, magnesium, manganese, phosphorus, progesterone, royal jelly, silicon, Tai Chi, trace minerals

HERBS AND SUPPLEMENTS TO USE WITH CAUTION: Vitamin A

INTRODUCTION

Many factors are known or suspected to accelerate the rate of bone loss. These factors include smoking, alcohol, low calcium intake, lack of exercise, various medications, and several illnesses. Excessive consumption of vitamin A may also increase the risk of osteoporosis, and rapid weight loss may increase the risk in postmenopausal women. Raw-food vegetarians are also likely to have significant bone thinning.

In general, women are far more prone to osteoporosis than men. For this reason, the following discussion focuses almost entirely on women.

Hormone replacement therapy prevents or reverses osteoporosis in women. However, long-term use of hormone replacement therapy has been found to be unsafe, so conventional medical treatment for osteoporosis in women centers mainly on drugs in the bisphosphonate family, including Fosamax (taken with calcium and vitamin D).

Exercise, especially weight-bearing exercise, almost certainly helps strengthen bone (although the evidence for this is weaker than one might expect). Minimal evidence suggests that the Chinese exercise Tai Chi may also provide some benefit.

PRINCIPAL PROPOSED NATURAL TREATMENTS

There is good evidence that people with osteoporosis, or who are at risk for it, should take calcium and vitamin D supplements regardless of what other treatments they may be using. Substances called isoflavones found in soy and other plants may be helpful for osteoporosis (and for general menopausal symptoms). Vitamin K and a newer supplement called strontium ranelate have also shown promise. A semisynthetic isoflavone called ipriflavone has shown considerable promise for osteoporosis, but safety concerns have decreased its popularity.

Calcium and vitamin D. Calcium is necessary to build and maintain bone. Humans need vitamin D too, as the body cannot absorb calcium without it. Many people do not get enough calcium in their daily diet. Although the body can manufacture vitamin D when exposed to the sun, supplemental vitamin D may be necessary because of the common use of sunscreen.

According to most studies, calcium supplements (especially as calcium citrate, and taken with vitamin D) appear to be modestly helpful in slowing bone loss in postmenopausal women. Contrary to some reports, milk does appear to be a useful source of calcium for this purpose. Any improvements in bone density rapidly disappear once the supplements are stopped. People who ensure that they continue calcium use may do better than those who forget from time to time. Vitamin D without calcium, however, does not appear to offer more than minimal bone-protective benefits for the elderly.

The effect of calcium and vitamin D supplementation in any form is relatively minor and may not be strong enough to reduce the rate of osteoporotic fractures. A large study of more than three thousand postmenopausal women age sixty-five to seventy-one years found that three years of daily supplementation with calcium and vitamin D was not associated with a significant reduction in the incidence of fractures. The use of calcium supplements early in life might prevent problems later, especially when children also engage in physical exercise; however, study results are somewhat contradictory.

One study found benefits for elderly men using a calcium- and vitamin D-fortified milk product. However, there are some concerns that excessive calcium intake could raise the risk of prostate cancer in men.

Vitamin D and calcium taken together may also have a modestly protective effect against the severe bone loss caused by corticosteroid drugs such as prednisone. Certain other supplements may enhance the effects of calcium and vitamin D. One study found that adding various trace minerals (zinc at 15 milligrams [mg], copper at 2.5 mg, and manganese at 5 mg) produced further improvement. However, copper by itself may not be helpful.

There is some evidence that essential fatty acids may also enhance the effectiveness of calcium. In one study, sixty-five postmenopausal women were given calcium with either placebo or a combination of omega-6 fatty acids (from evening primrose oil) and omega-3 fatty acids (from fish oil) for eighteen months. At the end of the study period, the group receiving essential fatty acids had higher bone density and fewer fractures than the placebo group. In contrast to this, however, a similar twelve-month double-blind trial of forty-two postmenopausal women found no benefit from essential fatty acids. The explanation for the discrepancy may lie in the differences among the women studied. The first study involved women living in nursing homes, while the second studied healthier women living on their own. The second group of women may have been better nourished and already receiving sufficient essential fatty acids in their diet. Vitamin K may also enhance the effect of calcium.

Vitamin D may offer another benefit for osteoporosis in the elderly: Most, though not all, studies have found that vitamin D supplementation improves balance in the elderly (especially women) and reduces the risk of falling. Because the most common adverse consequence of osteoporosis is a fracture caused by a fall, this could offer a meaningful benefit. Also, there is weak, preliminary evidence that calcium supplementation in healthy, postmenopausal women may slightly increase the risk of cardiovascular events, such as myocardial infarction.

Genistein and other isoflavones. Soy contains substances called isoflavones that produce effects in the body somewhat similar to the effects of estrogen. (For this reason, they are called phytoestrogens.) Although study results are not entirely consistent, growing evidence suggests that genistein and other isoflavones can (like estrogen) help prevent bone loss.

For example, in a one-year, double-blind, placebo-controlled study, ninety women age forty-seven to fifty-seven were given genistein at a dose of 54 mg per day or standard hormone replacement therapy (HRT) or placebo. The results showed that genistein prevented bone loss in the back and hip to approximately the same extent as HRT. No adverse effects on the uterus or breast were seen. A subsequent two-year double-blind study of 389 postmenopausal women with mild bone loss found that 54 mg of genistein plus calcium and vitamin D improved bone density to a greater extent than did calcium and vitamin D alone. However, a fairly high percentage of participants given genistein experienced substantial digestive distress.

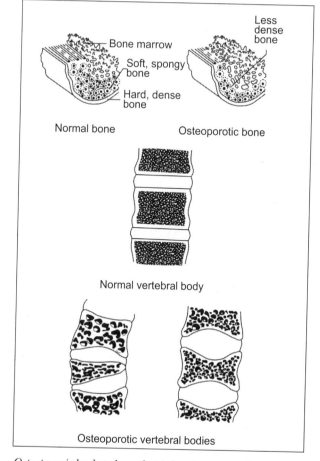

Osteoporosis leads to bone that is less dense, more brittle, more easily broken, and degenerative.

In a one-year, double-blind, placebo-controlled study of 203 postmenopausal Chinese women, the use of soy isoflavones at a dose of 80 mg daily had mildly positive protective effects on bone mass in the hip. This supplement contained 46.4 percent daidzein, 38.8 percent glycetein, and 14.7 percent genistein.

Another study evaluated an isoflavone supplement made from red clover (containing 6 mg biochanin A, 16 mg formononetin, 1 mg genistein, and 0.5 mg daidzein daily). In this one-year, double-blind, placebo-controlled study of 205 people, the use of red clover isoflavones significantly reduced loss of bone in the lumbar spine. Benefits were also seen in a one-year, double-blind, placebo-controlled study using an extract made from the soy product tofu.

However, it is not clear that the consumption of foods rich in isoflavones offers the same benefits. For

Osteoporosis and Genistein

Genistein is a phytoestrogen, a naturally occurring substance with estrogen-like properties. There are two main types of phytoestrogens: isoflavones and lignans. Soy is the most common food source of isoflavones, and, in turn, genistein is the most abundant isoflavone in soy. Red clover is also a good source of genistein.

Based on its estrogen-like properties, genistein has been studied as a substitute for hormone replacement therapy. It has shown some promise for treating symptoms that occur early in menopause, such as hot flashes, and for problems that occur later, such as osteoporosis.

A study published in 2007 confirms earlier research regarding genistein's benefits for osteoporosis. In this double-blind trial, 389 postmenopausal women with mildly reduced bone density were first put on a low-soy diet for four weeks to make sure they did not have any genistein in their system. Participants were then given either placebo or 54 milligrams of genistein daily for twenty-four months. In addition, all participants were given calcium and vitamin D.

The primary end point evaluated by the researchers was bone density in the hip and spine. The results were quite positive. At the end of the study, bone density had increased in participants given genistein, while it decreased in those given placebo; furthermore, this difference was statistically significant. As an additional plus, genistein did not produce the typical, and harmful, estrogen-like effects on the uterus. However, genistein did cause significant gastrointestinal side effects in almost 20 percent of those taking it.

These findings are definitely promising. However, the study does have some limits. The participants all had mild bone loss, technically osteopenia. It is not clear whether genistein would work for the more severe bone loss of true osteoporosis. Furthermore, the study was not designed to determine whether genistein could reduce the rate of fractures caused by osteoporosis, which is the most important issue. Osteoporotic fractures are related not only to bone density but also to the structure of bone, and it is not clear whether genistein is helpful in this regard. Finally, it is not clear how genistein compares to the modern nonhormone treatments for osteoporosis, especially drugs in the bisphosphonate family.

Steven Bratman, M.D.

example, in placebo-controlled study involving 237 healthy women in the early stages of menopause, the consumption of isoflavone-enriched foods (providing an average of 110 mg isoflavone daily) for one year had no effect on bone density or metabolism.

The effect of isoflavones on bone may be more complex than that of estrogen. Bone is always undergoing two opposite processes at once: bone breakdown and bone formation. Estrogen acts on the first of these processes by inhibiting bone breakdown. Isoflavones may affect both sides of the equation at once: inhibiting bone breakdown, while at the same time enhancing new bone formation.

In about one of three people, intestinal bacteria convert some soy isoflavones into a substance called equol. Isoflavones may have a greater bone-protecting effect in such equol producers.

Strontium. Growing evidence indicates that the mineral strontium (as strontium ranelate) is effective as an aid in the treatment of osteoporosis. The best and largest study on strontium was a double-blind, placebo-controlled study of 1,649 postmenopausal women with osteoporosis. In this three-year study, a dose of strontium ranelate at 2 grams (g) daily significantly increased bone density in the spine and hip and significantly decreased the rate of vertebral fractures.

While some treatments for osteoporosis act to increase bone formation and others act to decrease bone breakdown, some evidence suggests that strontium ranelate has a dual effect, providing both these benefits at once. There is one major caveat, however. All major controlled clinical trials of strontium ranelate have involved some of the same researchers. Entirely independent confirmation is needed. It is not clear to what extent the "ranelate" portion of strontium ranelate is necessary for this benefit, or whether other strontium salts would work too. (The strontium used in these studies is not the same as the radioactive strontium that was such a concern during the decades of above-ground atomic testing in the mid-twentieth century.)

Vitamin K. Increasing, but inconsistent, evidence indicates that vitamin K may help prevent osteoporosis. It may work by reducing bone breakdown, rather than by enhancing bone formation.

Perhaps the best evidence for a beneficial effect comes from a three-year, double-blind, placebo-controlled trial of 181 women. Participants, all postmenopausal women between the ages of fifty and sixty years, were divided into three groups: placebo, calcium plus vitamin D plus magnesium, or calcium plus vitamin D plus magnesium plus vitamin K (at a dose of 1 g daily). Researchers monitored bone loss by using a standard dual-energy X-ray absorptiometry bone density scan. The results showed that the study participants using vitamin K with the other nutrients did not lose as much bone as those in the other two groups. However, another placebo-controlled trial involving 452 older men and women with normal levels of calcium and vitamin D failed to demonstrate any beneficial effects of 500 micrograms per day of vitamin K supplementation on bone health over a three-year period.

Ipriflavone. Ipriflavone is a semisynthetic variation of soy isoflavones. Ipriflavone appears to help prevent osteoporosis by interfering with bone breakdown. Estrogen works in much the same way, but ipriflavone does not appear to produce estrogenic effects anywhere else in the body other than in bone. For this reason, it probably does not increase the risk of breast or uterine cancer. However, it also does not reduce the hot flashes, night sweats, mood changes, or vaginal dryness of menopause. In addition, it may cause health risks of its own.

Numerous double-blind, placebo-controlled studies involving more than seventeen hundred participants have examined the effects of ipriflavone on various forms of osteoporosis. Overall, it appears that ipriflavone can stop the progression of osteoporosis and perhaps reverse it to some extent. For example, a two-year double-blind study followed 198 postmenopausal women who had evidence of bone loss. At the end of the study, there was a gain in bone density of 1 percent in the ipriflavone group compared to a loss of 0.7 percent in the placebo group.

Conversely, the largest and longest study of ipriflavone found no benefit. In this three-year trial of 474 postmenopausal women, no differences in extent of osteoporosis were seen between ipriflavone and placebo groups. However, for reasons that are not clear, the researchers in this study gave women only 500 mg of calcium daily. All other major studies of ipriflavone gave participants 1,000 mg of calcium daily. It is possible that ipriflavone requires the higher dose of calcium to work properly.

Ipriflavone may also be helpful for preventing osteoporosis in women who are taking Lupron or corticosteroids, medications that accelerate bone loss. (However, the combined use of ipriflavone and drugs that suppress the immune system, such as corticosteroids, presents risks.)

There is some evidence that combining ipriflavone with estrogen may improve benefits against osteoporosis. However, it is not known whether such combinations increase or decrease the other benefits and adverse effects of estrogen-replacement therapy. Finally, for reasons that are not clear, ipriflavone appears to be able to reduce pain in osteoporosis-related fractures.

OTHER PROPOSED NATURAL TREATMENTS

It is often said that magnesium supplements are helpful for strong bones, but there is only minimal evidence to support this claim. It has been suggested (though with little meaningful supporting evidence) that the typical American diet causes the body to become acidic, and that this in turn leads to bone loss. One study tested potassium citrate as a treatment for bone loss, in the belief that this supplement would counteract this hypothesized diet-related acidity. The results in this one-year study of 161 postmenopausal women indicated that potassium citrate reduced bone loss to a greater extent than did the placebo (potassium chloride). This study had numerous problems in design, analysis, and reporting, so it does not necessarily show anything about dietary "acidity." It may, however, indicate that the citrate part of potassium citrate has some bone-protective effects. If this is true, it could in turn explain why calcium citrate has, in some studies, proven more effective for treating or preventing osteoporosis than other forms of calcium.

Observational studies hint that higher levels of homocysteine might increase the risk of osteoporosis. Vitamins B_{12}, B_6, and folate are known to reduce homocysteine levels. On this basis, supplementation with these vitamins has been proposed for preventing or mitigating the effects of osteoporosis. One double-blind study found weak evidence that supplemental folate and vitamin B_{12} (known to reduce homocysteine) might reduce risk of osteoporotic fractures in people who had had a stroke. However, two other studies failed to find that the use of mixed B-vitamins had any positive effect on bone density or chemical markers of bone turnover.

Some evidence suggests that the hormone dehy-droepiandrosterone (DHEA) may be helpful for preventing or treating osteoporosis, especially in postmenopausal women older than age seventy years. Also, one study found weak evidence that DHEA might be helpful for preventing the osteoporosis that sometimes develops in women with anorexia nervosa.

Chinese studies suggest that the herb *Epimedium brevicornum* has phytoestrogenic effects and, on this basis, may be helpful for preventing bone loss. (*E. brevicornum* is related, but not identical, to *E. sagittatum*, otherwise known as horny goat weed.)

Preliminary evidence suggests that black tea may help protect against osteoporosis. Similarly weak evidence hints that the herb black cohosh might help prevent osteoporosis. Although it has long been stated that high phosphorus intake from the consumption of soft drinks might lead to osteoporosis, there is no solid evidence for this claim. Elevated intake of phosphorus may help prevent osteoporosis. The reason is that bone contains both calcium and phosphate.

According to one preliminary study, but not another, boron may be helpful for preventing osteoporosis. However, there are some concerns that boron supplements may raise levels of the body's own estrogen, especially in women on estrogen-replacement therapy, and therefore might present an increased risk of cancer. To increase boron intake, one should eat more fruits and vegetables.

One study widely advertised as showing that silicon is helpful for osteoporosis actually failed to show much of anything. Extremely weak evidence hints at possible benefit for osteoporosis through the use of royal jelly.

Although it has long been believed that consuming too much protein (especially animal-based protein) increases the risk of osteoporosis, the balance of available evidence suggests the reverse: If anything, high intake of protein appears to help strengthen bone. One study found that calcium supplements may do a better job of strengthening bones in people with relatively high protein intake than in those with lower intake.

It has been suggested both that water fluoridation helps prevent osteoporosis and also that it causes the condition; on balance, however, the evidence suggests that it does neither. Another study failed to find arginine supplements helpful for enhancing bone density.

Progesterone. Many books promote the idea that natural progesterone prevents or even reduces osteoporosis. In this case, the term "natural" means the same progesterone found in the body. It is still made synthetically, but it is called natural progesterone to distinguish it from its chemical cousins known as progestins. Generally, prescription "progesterone" is actually a progestin.

The progesterone-osteoporosis story began with test-tube and other preliminary studies suggesting that progesterone or progestins can stimulate the activity of cells that build bone. Subsequently, a poorly designed and uncontrolled study (actually, a series of case histories from one physician's practice) purportedly demonstrated that progesterone cream can slow or even reverse osteoporosis.

However, a one-year double-blind trial of 102 women using either progesterone cream (providing 20 mg progesterone daily) or placebo cream, along with calcium and multivitamins, found no evidence of any improvements in bone density attributable to progesterone. Furthermore, in a three-year study of 875 women, combination treatment with estrogen and oral progesterone was no more effective for osteoporosis than estrogen alone.

Estriol. Some alternative medicine practitioners have popularized the use of a special form of estrogen called estriol, claiming that, unlike standard estrogen, it does not increase the risk of cancer. However, this claim is unfounded.

Controlled trials performed in Japan have found that estriol helps prevent bone loss in menopausal women, although one small study found no benefit. However, like other forms of estrogen, oral estriol stimulates the growth of uterine tissue. This leads to a risk of uterine cancer.

In a placebo-controlled study of 1,110 women, greater uterine tissue stimulation was seen among women given estriol orally (1 to 2 mg daily) than among those given placebo. Another large study found that oral estriol increased the risk of uterine cancer. In another study of 48 women given estriol at a dose of 1 mg twice daily, uterine tissue stimulation was seen in the majority of cases.

In contrast, a twelve-month double-blind trial of oral estriol (2 mg daily) in sixty-eight Japanese women found no effect on the uterus. It may be that the high levels of soy in the Japanese diet altered the results. Additionally, test-tube studies suggest that estriol is just as likely to cause breast cancer as any other form of estrogen. Women who use estriol should consider it like any other form of estrogen.

HERBS AND SUPPLEMENTS TO USE WITH CAUTION

While the evidence is not yet strong, some research suggests that excessive intake of vitamin A may increase the risk of osteoporosis. Also, herbs and supplements may interact adversely with drugs used to treat osteoporosis, so persons should be cautious when considering the use of herbs and supplements.

EBSCO CAM Review Board

FURTHER READING

Atkinson, C., et al. "The Effects of Phytoestrogen Isoflavones on Bone Density in Women." *American Journal of Clinical Nutrition* 79 (2004): 326-333.

Avenell, A., et al. "Oral Vitamin D3 and Calcium for Secondary Prevention of Low-Trauma Fractures in Elderly People." *The Lancet* 365 (2005): 1621-1628.

Barger-Lux, M. J., et al. "Calcium Supplementation Does Not Augment Bone Gain in Young Women Consuming Diets Moderately Low in Calcium." *Journal of Nutrition* 135 (2005): 2362-2366.

Bischoff-Ferrari, H. A., and B. Dawson-Hughes. "Where Do We Stand on Vitamin D?" *Bone* 41, suppl. 1 (2007): S13-S-19.

Bolland, M. J., et al. "Vascular Events in Healthy Older Women Receiving Calcium Supplementation." *British Medical Journal* 336 (2008): 262-266.

Bolton-Smith, C., et al. "Two-Year Randomized Controlled Trial of Vitamin K1 (Phylloquinone) and Vitamin D3 plus Calcium on the Bone Health of Older Women." *Journal of Bone and Mineral Research* 22 (2007): 509-519.

Booth, S. L., et al. "Effect of Vitamin K Supplementation on Bone Loss in Elderly Men and Women." *Journal of Clinical Endocrinology and Metabolism* 93 (2008): 1217-1223.

Brink, E., et al. "Long-term Consumption of Isoflavone-Enriched Foods Does Not Affect Bone Mineral Density, Bone Metabolism, or Hormonal Status in Early Postmenopausal Women." *American Journal of Clinical Nutrition* 87 (2008): 761-770.

Carpenter, T. O., et al. "A Randomized Controlled Study of Effects of Dietary Magnesium Oxide Supplementation on Bone Mineral Content in Healthy Girls." *Journal of Clinical Endocrinology and Metabolism* 91 (2006): 4866-4872.

Cockayne, S., et al. "Vitamin K and the Prevention of Fractures." *Archives of Internal Medicine* 166 (2006): 1256-1261.

Courteix, D., et al. "Cumulative Effects of Calcium Supplementation and Physical Activity on Bone Accretion in Premenarchal Children." *International Journal of Sports Medicine* 26 (2005): 332-338.

Daly, R. M., S. Bass, and C. Nowson. "Long-Term Effects of Calcium-Vitamin-D(3)-Fortified Milk on Bone Geometry and Strength in Older Men." *Bone* 39 (2006): 946-953.

Dodiuk-Gad, R. P., et al. "Sustained Effect of Short-Term Calcium Supplementation on Bone Mass in Adolescent Girls with Low Calcium Intake." *American Journal of Clinical Nutrition* 81 (2005): 168-174.

Fontana, L., et al. "Low Bone Mass in Subjects on a Long-Term Raw Vegetarian Diet." *Archives of Internal Medicine* 165 (2005): 684-689.

Harwood, R. H., et al. "A Randomised, Controlled Comparison of Different Calcium and Vitamin D Supplementation Regimens in Elderly Women After Hip Fracture." *Age and Ageing* 33 (2004): 45-51.

Herrmann, M., et al. "The Effect of B-Vitamins on Biochemical Bone Turnover Markers and Bone Mineral Density in Osteoporotic Patients." *Clinical Chemistry and Laboratory Medicine* 45 (2007): 1785-1792.

Jankowski, C. M., et al. "Effects of Dehydroepiandrosterone Replacement Therapy on Bone Mineral Density in Older Adults." *Journal of Clinical Endocrinology and Metabolism* 91 (2006): 2986-2993.

Kelley, G. A., and K. S. Kelley. "Exercise and Bone Mineral Density at the Femoral Neck in Postmenopausal Women." *American Journal of Obstetrics and Gynecology* 194 (2006): 760-767.

Lanou, A. J., et al. "Calcium, Dairy Products, and Bone Health in Children and Young Adults: A Re-evaluation of the Evidence." *Pediatrics* 115 (2005): 736-743.

Martyn-St. James, M., and S. Carroll. "High-Intensity Resistance Training and Postmenopausal Bone Loss." *Osteoporosis International* 17 (2006): 1225-1240.

Reid, I. R., et al. "Randomized Controlled Trial of Calcium in Healthy Older Women." *American Journal of Medicine* 119 (2006): 777-785.

Von Mühlen, D., et al. "Effect of Dehydroepiandrosterone Supplementation on Bone Mineral Density, Bone Markers, and Body Composition in Older Adults." *Osteoporosis International* 19 (2008): 699-707.

Wayne, P. M., et al. "The Effects of Tai Chi on Bone Mineral Density in Postmenopausal Women." *Archives of Physical Medicine and Rehabilitation* 88 (2007): 673-680.

See also: Aging; Bone and joint health; Breast-feeding support; Calcium; Elder health; Estrogen; Exercise; Ipriflavone; Menopause; Progesterone; Soy; Strontium; Vitamin D; Vitamin K; Women's health.

Oxerutins

CATEGORY: Herbs and supplements
RELATED TERMS: Hydroxyethylrutosides, troxerutin
DEFINITION: Natural plant substance used to treat specific health conditions.
PRINCIPAL PROPOSED USES: Hemorrhoids, venous insufficiency
OTHER PROPOSED USES: Lower-leg edema in people with diabetes, lymphedema, postsurgical edema, vertigo

OVERVIEW

Oxerutins are a group of chemicals derived from a naturally occurring bioflavonoid called rutin. This supplement has been widely used in Europe since the mid-1960s as a treatment for conditions in which blood or lymph vessels leak fluid. Considerable evidence suggests that oxerutins are effective. However, it is difficult to find this supplement in North America.

REQUIREMENTS AND SOURCES

Although they are closely related to a natural flavonoid, oxerutins are not found in food. They can be taken only in supplement form.

THERAPEUTIC DOSAGES

For varicose veins/venous insufficiency, oxerutins are usually taken in dosages ranging from 900 to 1,200 milligrams (mg) daily. A typical schedule is 1,000 mg daily, taken in two separate doses of 500 mg. For treating lymphedema and postsurgical edema, a typical dosage is a good deal higher: 3,000 mg daily.

One particular oxerutin called troxerutin may be taken alone (in similar dosages) as a treatment for varicose veins. There is no evidence that rutin itself is effective.

THERAPEUTIC USES

"Varicose" means enlarged or distended. A varicose vein is abnormally enlarged, allowing blood to pool and stagnate instead of moving it efficiently toward the heart. Surface veins of the leg are those most vulnerable to becoming varicose. Venous insufficiency is a closely related condition affecting larger veins deep within the leg. In either case, blood pools within the vein and exerts pressure against the vein walls and capillaries, resulting in pain, aching, swelling, and feelings of heaviness and fatigue. In addition, varicose veins present a cosmetic problem: bulging, often ropy, blue or purple lines visible on the skin of the lower legs. Strong evidence shows that oxerutins can be helpful for venous insufficiency/varicose veins, improving aching, swelling, and fatigue in the legs. Mixed evidence suggests that oxerutins might also be helpful for the leg ulcers that can develop in venous insufficiency. There is no evidence that oxerutins can improve the cosmetic appearance of varicose veins. Oxerutins have also been found effective for treating varicose veins when they occur during pregnancy. Hemorrhoids are a special type of varicose vein, and oxerutins may be helpful for treating them as well, although there have been some negative studies.

Some evidence suggests that oxerutins may be helpful for lymphedema (chronic arm swelling caused by damage to the lymph drainage system) following surgery for breast cancer, as well as for edema in the immediate postsurgical period. Preliminary evidence, including small double-blind trials, suggests that oxerutins might also be helpful for reducing lower extremity swelling in people with diabetes. In these trials, oxerutin therapy did not affect blood sugar control.

One small double-blind study suggests oxerutins may be helpful for reducing vertigo and other symptoms of Meniere's disease. This use is based on a theory that Meniere's disease is caused by excessive fluid leaking from capillaries in the inner ear.

SCIENTIFIC EVIDENCE

Varicose veins/venous insufficiency. About twenty double-blind, placebo-controlled studies, enrolling a total of more than two thousand participants, have examined oxerutins' effectiveness for treating varicose veins and venous insufficiency. Virtually all found oxerutins significantly more effective than placebo, giving substantial relief from swelling, aching, leg

Oxerutins for Hemorrhoids

Oxerutins have been used in the treatment of hemorrhoids, which are swollen and inflamed veins around the anus or in the lower rectum. The rectum is the last part of the large intestine leading to the anus.

External hemorrhoids are located under the skin around the anus. Internal hemorrhoids develop in the lower rectum and may protrude, or prolapse, through the anus. Most prolapsed hemorrhoids shrink back inside the rectum on their own. Severely prolapsed hemorrhoids may protrude permanently and require treatment.

Swelling in the anal or rectal veins causes hemorrhoids. Several factors may cause this swelling, including chronic constipation or diarrhea, straining during bowel movements, sitting on the toilet for long periods of time, and a lack of fiber in the diet.

Another cause of hemorrhoids is the weakening of the connective tissue in the rectum and anus that occurs with age. Pregnancy can cause hemorrhoids by increasing pressure in the abdomen, which may enlarge the veins in the lower rectum and anus. For most women, hemorrhoids caused by pregnancy disappear after childbirth.

pains, and other uncomfortable symptoms, while causing no significant side effects.

For example, one large double-blind, placebo-controlled study published in 1983 enrolled 660 people with symptoms of venous insufficiency. Three out of four participants were randomly assigned to receive oxerutins (1,000 mg daily), while one out of four was given a placebo. After four weeks of treatment, those who took oxerutins reported less heaviness, aching, cramps, and restless leg or pins-and-needles symptoms than those who took placebo. According to the researchers' calculations, oxerutins had produced significantly better results than placebo. This report has been criticized, however, for omitting key information (such as whether any participants also wore support stockings) and for failing to present data in a usable form.

A more recent, better-designed study supported these positive findings. This twelve-week double-blind, placebo-controlled study enrolled 133 women with moderate chronic venous insufficiency. Half received 1,000 mg of oxerutins daily, and the rest took a matching placebo. All participants were also fitted with standard compression stockings and wore them for the duration of the study. The researchers measured subjective symptoms, such as aches and pains, as well as objective measures of edema in the leg.

Those who took oxerutins had significantly less lower-leg edema than those in the placebo group. Furthermore, these results lasted through a six-week follow-up period, even though participants were no longer taking oxerutins. Compression stockings, on the other hand, produced no lasting benefit after participants stopped wearing them. They gave symptomatic relief while they were worn, but they did not improve capillary circulation in a lasting way, as oxerutins apparently did. Regarding aching, sensations of heaviness, and other uncomfortable symptoms, however, there was little difference between the two groups. The authors theorized that the compression stockings gave both groups so much symptomatic relief that it was difficult to demonstrate a separate subjective benefit of oxerutin therapy. Many other double-blind, placebo-controlled studies have also found benefits with oxerutins for varicose veins and venous insufficiency.

As mentioned above, there is some evidence that troxerutin–one of the compounds in the standardized mixture sold as oxerutins–may be effective when taken alone. One study found it more effective than a placebo, but another (very small) study found it less effective than the standard oxerutin mixture.

Pregnant women are at especially high risk for varicose veins and venous insufficiency. A 1975 study examined sixty-nine pregnant women with varicose leg veins and found that oxerutins (900 mg daily) were significantly more effective than a placebo against pain and swelling. A more recent study also found positive results, but because it was neither placebo-controlled nor double-blind, its results mean little (other than to suggest that oxerutins are safe in pregnancy).

Skin ulcers sometimes form on the legs of people with varicose veins or venous insufficiency when capillary circulation has become too impaired to keep the skin healthy. A French study published in 1987 found that oxerutins combined with compression stockings were significantly more helpful for leg ulcers than the stockings alone. Other positive results have been reported as well. However, some experiments found oxerutins to have no benefit in treating or preventing leg ulcers. Until more research is done, the most that can be said is that oxerutins might be helpful for leg ulcers, especially if combined with compression stockings.

Hemorrhoids. Some evidence suggests that oxerutins might be helpful for hemorrhoids, as well. A double-blind study enrolling ninety-seven pregnant women found oxerutins (1,000 mg daily) significantly better than a placebo in reducing the pain, bleeding, and inflammation of hemorrhoids.

Lymphedema. Women who have undergone surgery for breast cancer may experience a lasting and troublesome side effect: swelling in the arm caused by damage to the lymph system. Along with the veins, the lymph system is responsible for returning fluid to the heart, but when the system is damaged, fluid can accumulate. Three double-blind, placebo-controlled studies enrolling more than one hundred people have examined the effectiveness of oxerutins in this condition.

In one trial, oxerutins worked significantly better than a placebo at reducing swelling, discomfort, immobility, and other measures of lymphedema over a six-month treatment period, with better results appearing each month–suggesting that, for women with this condition, the full effect of oxerutins might take months to be realized. Two smaller studies also found oxerutins to be more effective than placebo, but the researchers were not sure that the improvement was large enough to make a real difference. In all of these studies, the dosage used was 3 grams (g) daily, about three times the typical dosage for venous insufficiency.

Post-surgical edema. Swelling often occurs in the recovery period following surgery. In one double-blind trial, researchers gave oxerutins or placebo for five days to forty people recovering from minor surgery or other minor injuries, and they found oxerutins significantly helpful in reducing swelling and discomfort.

SAFETY ISSUES

Oxerutins appear to be safe and well tolerated. In most studies, oxerutins have produced no more side effects than placebo. For example, in a study of 104 elderly people with venous insufficiency, twenty-six participants taking oxerutins reported adverse events, compared with twenty-five in the placebo group. The most commonly observed side effects were gastrointestinal symptoms, headaches, and dizziness.

Oxerutins have been given to pregnant women in some studies, with no apparent harmful effects. However, their safety for pregnant or nursing women cannot be regarded as absolutely proven. In addition, the safety of oxerutins has not been established for people with severe liver or kidney disease.

EBSCO CAM Review Board

FURTHER READING

Incandela, L., et al. "HR (Paroven, Venoruton; 0-(beta-hydroxyethyl)-rutosides) in Venous Hypertensive Microangiopathy." *Journal of Cardiovascular Pharmacology and Therapeutics* 7 (2002): S7-S10.

_____. "Treatment of Diabetic Microangiopathy and Edema with HR (Paroven, Venoruton; 0-(beta-hydroxyethyl)-rutosides)." *Journal of Cardiovascular Pharmacology and Therapeutics* 7 (2002): S11-S15.

Petruzzellis, V., et al. "Oxerutins (Venoruton): Efficacy in Chronic Venous Insufficiency." *Angiology* 53 (2002): 257-263.

See also: Edema; Herbal medicine; Hemorrhoids; Varicose veins.

P

PABA

CATEGORY: Herbs and supplements
RELATED TERM: Para-aminobenzoic acid
DEFINITION: Natural food product used to treat specific health conditions.
PRINCIPAL PROPOSED USE: Peyronie's disease
OTHER PROPOSED USES: Male infertility, scleroderma, vitiligo

OVERVIEW

Para-aminobenzoic acid (PABA) is best known as the active ingredient in sunblock. This use of PABA is not really medicinal: Like a pair of sunglasses, PABA physically blocks ultraviolet rays when it is applied to the skin. There are, however, some proposed medicinal uses of oral PABA supplements. PABA is sometimes suggested as a treatment for various diseases of the skin and connective tissue, as well as for male infertility. However, most of the clinical data on PABA comes from very old studies, some from the early 1940s.

REQUIREMENTS AND SOURCES

PABA is not believed to be an essential nutrient. Nonetheless, it is found in foods, mainly in grains and meat. Small amounts of PABA are usually present in B-vitamin supplements as well as in some multiple vitamins.

THERAPEUTIC DOSAGES

A typical therapeutic dosage of PABA is 300 to 400 milligrams (mg) daily. Some studies have used much higher dosages. However, serious side effects have been found in dosages above 8 grams (g) daily. People should not take more than 400 mg daily except on medical advice.

THERAPEUTIC USES

PABA has been suggested as a treatment for Peyronie's disease, a condition in which the penis becomes bent owing to the accumulation of fibrous plaques. However, there has been only one reported double-blind placebo-controlled study properly examining this use. This trial enrolled 103 men with Peyronie's disease and followed them for one year. The results showed that use of PABA at a dose of 3 g taken four times daily significantly slowed the progression of Peyronie's disease; it did not, however, reduce preexisting plaque.

PABA has also been suggested as a treatment for scleroderma, a disease that creates fibrous tissue in the skin and internal organs. A four-month double-blind, placebo-controlled study of 146 people with long-standing, stable scleroderma did not support this, failing to find any evidence of benefit. However, half the participants in this trial dropped out before the end, making the results unreliable.

Based on one small World War II-era study, PABA has been suggested for treating male infertility as well as vitiligo, a condition in which patches of skin lose their pigment, resulting in pale blotches. However, this study did not have a control group, so its results are not meaningful. Ironically, a recent study suggests that high dosages of PABA can cause vitiligo.

SAFETY ISSUES

PABA is probably safe when taken at a dosage up to 400 mg daily. Possible side effects at this dosage are minor, including skin rash and loss of appetite. Higher doses are a different story, however. There has been one reported case of severe liver toxicity in a woman taking 12 g daily of PABA. The woman's liver recovered completely after she discontinued her use of this supplement. Also, a recent study suggests that 8 g daily of PABA can cause vitiligo, the patchy skin disease. There are questions that need to be answered about the safety of high-dose PABA therapy.

Persons should not take more than 400 mg daily except under medical supervision. Safety in young children, pregnant or nursing women, and those with serious liver or kidney disease has not been determined.

IMPORTANT INTERACTIONS

PABA may interfere with certain medications, including sulfa antibiotics such as Bactrim or Septra, so persons taking these medications should not take PABA supplements except on medical advice.

EBSCO CAM Review Board

FURTHER READING

Vinnicombe, H. G., and J. P. Derrick. "Dihydropteroate Synthase from *Streptococcus pneumoniae*: Characterization of Substrate Binding Order and Sulfonamide Inhibition." *Biochemical and Biophysical Research Communication* 258 (1999): 752-757.

Weidner, W., et al. "Potassium Paraaminobenzoate (POTABA) in the Treatment of Peyronie's Disease." *European Urology* 47 (2005): 530-536.

See also: Antibiotics, general; Burns, minor; Herbal medicine; Peyronie's disease; Scleroderma; Sunburn; Vitiligo.

Pain management

CATEGORY: Therapies and techniques
DEFINITION: Complementary and alternative therapies and techniques to aid in the relief and management of pain.

OVERVIEW

For people with mild to moderate chronic pain, medication may offer relief. However, many people find they can gain long-term control over their pain through complementary methods, such as heat or cold application, music, relaxation, exercise, meditation, acupuncture, and a positive attitude.

"For the vast majority of people who have chronic pain, there just are not any pharmacologic or physical interventions that can totally eliminate the pain," says University of Washington (Seattle) pain management expert Dennis C. Turk.

"Pain is a chronic condition, just like hypertension or diabetes," Turk explains. "When you have a chronic condition, you need to do more things for yourself. It

is going to last a long time. It is best to help yourself and learn to self-manage and control your pain."

OPTIONS

In addition to traditional pain relievers, nondrug methods of pain relief may help a person gain that control. Some techniques–such as imagery and the use of hot and cold–relax the muscles, help one sleep, and distract one from symptoms. Other techniques, such as music, films, and recorded comedy routines, can take one's mind off physical complaints, as does losing oneself in a good book.

While some remedies require little expertise or help from others, some may require instruction from a professional. Ronald Glick, the director of the University of Pittsburgh Pain Evaluation and Treatment Center, recommends that patients seek advice from a chronic pain specialist who can coordinate all aspects of management, including physical therapies and psychological techniques. While these pain relief techniques help many people with chronic pain, they are not cures for pain.

Heat and cold. "The most important thing about heat and cold is that it gives a sense of control," Turk says. "They are things you can do yourself to help relieve the pain, which can immediately reduce the emotional stress."

– *Direct application.* "Heat and cold can be quite helpful for people with musculoskeletal conditions," says Turk. "Something as simple as a bag of frozen peas wrapped in a towel can be a useful self-management technique that relieves muscle tension in the back, neck, and shoulders." Most people are familiar with holding an ice pack on a twisted ankle or lying on a heating pad for a sore back. However, hot and cold treatments can be used in other ways. Moist heat can be applied with a warm towel or through a soak in a bath tub. An elastic bandage can hold an ice pack in place. A paper cup filled with water and kept in the freezer becomes a tool for localized cold massage, while iced wash cloths can cover a larger area.

– *Timing.* One should apply heat or cold therapy for periods not to exceed fifteen minutes and should allow the area to return to normal body temperature before reapplying the therapy. Some people obtain added relief by alternating heat and ice. Others use heat before exercising and use ice after.

Skin protection. One should always place a towel between the cold or heat and the skin and should not lie directly on a heating pad.

Relaxation. "Relaxation response" is a term coined by Herbert Benson of the Mind-Body Medical Institute in Boston. It is an array of beneficial physiologic effects associated with focused relaxation, some of which may mitigate the perception of pain. For best results, one should make relaxation a part of one's daily routine.

There are a number of ways to invoke the relaxation response, and many audiotapes are available to help. One popular approach is to assume a comfortable position, take several deep breaths, and then focus on breathing, or on a word or a sound, while passively avoiding intruding thoughts.

Muscle relaxation exercises. Progressive muscle relaxation is a technique that may be effective for both muscle spasm pain and stress reduction. "Relaxation skills are useful in reducing muscle tension and can help reduce frustration and some of the stress," says Jennifer Markham of the University of Pittsburgh Pain Clinic. Progressive muscle relaxation involves focusing attention on each muscle group until it feels heavy and relaxed. One usually begins in the feet and gradually progresses upward.

Imagery exercises. Imagery, which often accompanies the management of pain through relaxation, allows

Cognitive Behavioral Therapy for Pain

Pain is a normal, protective reaction to an injury or illness. It is the body's signal that it is time to take care of a problem. Chronic pain is pain that continues for weeks, months, or years. It may be related to such chronic illnesses as arthritis, disorders of the nerves, or cancer pain. It may begin with an injury or short illness but continue even when the physical damage is no longer evident.

For many persons, chronic pain management includes tackling only the physical symptoms of pain, but many cognitive, behavioral, and emotional aspects can hamper or help healing. How you think and feel about your health or illness will impact your recovery and how much the pain will interfere with your everyday life.

Negative thought patterns like "I'll never get better" or "This pain stops me from doing everything" may influence the decisions you make about your health care. If you feel there is little to no chance of successful treatment, you may be less likely to seek beneficial treatment or may continue with unsuccessful treatments. However, if you believe success is possible, you are more likely to participate in seeking and completing recovery treatments.

Stress also can be a major part of a pain cycle. Managing any chronic condition is stressful enough on its own. Aside from the stress of the illness itself, financial concerns and strained relationships secondary to the illness can add to stress. This regular stress stimulates physical responses in the body, which can increase pain and delay healing.

Identifying these factors, learning more positive thought patterns, and developing better communication techniques can be important in managing chronic pain.

Cognitive behavioral therapy (CBT) is a specialized form of therapy designed to help one take these steps.

A common assumption is that people with chronic pain are only imagining their pain. However, part of CBT is to help acknowledge that the pain is real and to develop healthy thought patterns to manage it. The therapy will be based on your specific need, but it often involves creating realistic beliefs about pain, treatment options, and outcomes. Your therapist will help you to develop positive thinking and self-talk, reduce behaviors that continue an illness-way-of-life, increase positive behaviors that get you toward your goal, improve communication skills with family and medical team, and develop pain-management skills.

The overall goal is to replace ways of living that do not work with methods that do. The changes will help you gain more control over your life, instead of living solely through what pain you have.

CBT may be done in a one-on-one or group setting, depending on your needs. Your therapy may also include other persons, such as a spouse or other family members. Most often, the treatment is short-term, lasts between six to twenty sessions, and requires practice and homework to be most effective.

Chronic pain is often caused or exacerbated by a combination of issues, some of which can be immediately addressed, while others may take longer to resolve. CBT, in the meantime, can play a role in helping you manage pain and improve your quality of life. It will help you develop the skills to reshape your thinking, so that you can improve your treatment effects and decrease new cycles of pain.

Pamela Jones, M.A.; reviewed by Rosalyn Carson-DeWitt, M.D.

one to visualize what it would be like to "let the pain go." If one knows what is causing the pain–for instance, a pinched nerve in the spine–the idea is to picture the encroaching vertebral space opening and freeing the trapped nerve. By calling on a variety of senses, one can go to a favorite place, such as the beach or the mountains. Music, nature sounds, and instructional tapes make it easier for beginners to escape to a mental paradise.

"Relaxation techniques redirect your thinking from physical pain and onto something else," says Penney Cowan, founder and executive director of the American Chronic Pain Association. "Imagining the beach, the sun on your face, and the warmth of the sand helps divert your mind from how much your head is hurting."

Biofeedback. Biofeedback offers a measurable response to relaxation and imagery techniques. Through the use of sensors connected to a computer, one receives visual or auditory cues that indicate an increase or decrease in muscle tension, heart rate, and skin temperature. Using this feedback, one trains oneself to control body functions not normally thought about. Biofeedback may be useful in chronic pain or other conditions associated with muscle spasm or tension, such as some headaches.

Exercise. Although one may not feel like getting off the couch because of the pain, exercising within the confines of one's physical limitations can decrease pain. The reasons for this are complex, but one prominent theory is that exercise releases endorphins, which are natural pain-relieving chemicals in the brain. "Exercise is absolutely critical," says Turk. "The type of exercise will depend on the condition, but as a general rule of thumb, the more active you remain and the more you use your muscles, the better off you're going to be."

A physical therapist can tailor an initial exercise plan based on a person's capacity to exercise and then gradually make recommendations for increasing how much to do and for how long. Pain experts recommend pacing activities. Overdoing it on good days can cause more pain later. Experts recommend reducing exercise during a flare-up of pain, but it is important to resume an exercise routine as soon as possible.

Acupuncture. Acupuncture is a form of Chinese medicine. It involves insertion of very thin needles into the skin at different and specific points on the body. It has been shown to be effective for the treatment of chronic back pain. It requires several treatments, usually between two and five, before a response can be seen. Results of acupuncture also largely depend on the skills of the acupuncturist.

Meditation. The benefits of meditation go beyond relaxation response. Daily meditation may be an excellent tool in fighting chronic pain. There are a variety of different meditation techniques, and one should choose a mediation style that is comfortable. Meditation is not a religious practice and can be done easily in the privacy of one's home.

Hypnotherapy. Hypnosis has nothing to do with popular images of stage performance. It was first utilized as a therapeutic modality more than one hundred years ago, and it is a technique that can be useful in chronic pain management. Hypnotherapy is performed by a trained and licensed therapist. The exact way that hypnosis works is not fully understood. It is known, however, to induce a state of focused awareness, which can alleviate many forms of pain.

Attitude and communication. How one thinks about one's aches and discomforts, one's level of anxiety and depression, one's expectations, and one's ability to cope determines how much pain one feels. Cognitive-behavior modification techniques help change unhealthy attitudes and habits that can develop when pain is chronic.

A person should concentrate on his or her abilities and find pleasure in the things he or she can do rather than dwelling on activities that have become difficult because of pain. One should communicate with family members. "Psychology helps people begin to understand they do have some control, even if they don't have a magic wand to make the pain go away," says Markham. "When they realize they have some control [over their pain], it gives them hope."

Debra Wood, R.N., and Steven Bratman, M.D.;
reviewed by Brian Randall, M.D.

FURTHER READING

Gatlin, C. G., and L. Schulmeister. "When Medication Is Not Enough: Nonpharmacologic Management of Pain." *Clinical Journal of Oncology Nursing* 11 (2007): 699-704.

Lee, H., K. Schmidt, and E. Ernst. "Acupuncture for the Relief of Cancer-Related Pain." *European Journal of Pain* 9 (2005): 437.

Rydholm, M., and P. Strang. "Acupuncture for Patients in Hospital-Based Home Care Suffering from Xerostomia." *Journal of Palliative Care* 15 (1999): 20.

Wright, L. D. "Meditation: A New Role for an Old Friend." *American Journal of Hospice and Palliative Care* 23 (2006): 323-327.

See also: Acupressure; Acupuncture; Back pain; Biofeedback; Breast pain, cyclic; Childbirth support: Homeopathic remedies; Guided imagery; Head injury: Homeopathic remedies; Herbal medicine; Hypnotherapy; Injuries, minor; Manipulative and body-based practices; Meditation; Music therapy; Neck pain; Nonsteroidal anti-inflammatory drugs (NSAIDs); Relaxation therapies; Soft tissue pain; Sports and fitness support: Enhancing recovery; Sports-related injuries: Homeopathic remedies; Surgery support; Wounds, minor.

Palmer, Daniel David

CATEGORY: Biography

IDENTIFICATION: Canadian-born magnetic healer who founded the field of chiropractic medicine

BORN: March 7, 1845; Toronto, Ontario, Canada

DIED: October 20, 1913; Los Angeles, California

OVERVIEW

Daniel David (D. D.) Palmer was a magnetic healer who founded the chiropractic field in the 1890s. He had moved to the United States when he was twenty years of age, and during his early years he worked as a teacher, beekeeper, and grocery store owner. He had no formal medical training but had long been interested in magnetic healing, spirituality, and other health philosophies.

While working as a magnetic healer in Iowa, Palmer was said to have restored a man's compromised hearing. Palmer noticed a lump in the man's back and speculated that it was responsible for the man's hearing problem. He reportedly treated the man with self-developed chiropractic methods, restoring the man's hearing. Palmer postulated that "a subluxated (misaligned) vertebra [was] the cause of 95 percent of all diseases" and that "the other 5 percent [were] caused by displaced joints other than those of the vertebral column." He claimed that chiropractic-based methods served to restore normal

---

Radiating from the Spine

The developer of chiropractic, Daniel David Palmer, discusses the significance of the nervous system in regulating not only health but also illness and disease. This excerpt is from his book The Science of Chiropractic *(1906).*

Between vertebrae are nerves which perform the various functions of the body. When the intervertebral cartilage becomes condensed, less elastic, and thinner, the vertebrae are drawn closer together, occluding the foramina, slightly impinging nerves, causing a lack of functional force; vigor is impaired, and in proportion old age advances. If we keep our vertebrae separated, movable and free, age stiffness will be eliminated.

We have been taught to observe effects; the real cause, closed joints, have not been noticed by the medical world. . . .

The brain sends its messages through the spinal cord to all parts of the body. The spinal marrow passes down thru the spinal canal, and contains nerves which control the nervous system and tactile impressions. The nerves branch out from the spinal cord in all directions, absolutely controlling every part of the anatomy. So potent is this control that all action, whether normal or abnormal, is absolutely dependent upon the condition of the nerve radiating from the spine. A wrench of the vertebral column invariably leads to some disturbance of that portion to which the nerves proceed and end.

---

nerve flow by realigning a person's spinal vertebrae or other joints; this alignment would restore the person's health. He also claimed that chiropractic medicine could overcome "intellectual abnormalities," stating that "Chiropractors correct abnormalities of the intellect as well as those of the body."

Palmer eventually founded the Palmer School of Chiropractic in 1897. However, in 1906, he was prosecuted in Iowa for practicing medicine without a license (he had never attended medical school) and was briefly jailed for this offense. Soon after, Palmer's son, B. J. Palmer, bought and took over administration of the school, although B. J. went on to sell the school some years later. D. D. Palmer went on to establish other chiropractic schools in California, Oregon, and Oklahoma in subsequent years.

D. D. Palmer regarded chiropractic as partly religious in nature. At one time, he stated that he had "received chiropractic from the other world." Some reports suggest he credited his previous spiritual leader and teacher, possibly receiving "inspiration" from him posthumously. Palmer may have stated at one point that, as the founder of chiropractic, he was like persons who have founded religions. Because of such statements, Palmer has had many critics.

Palmer died in 1913; according to official records, he died of typhoid fever. The school that D. D. Palmer founded in Iowa has survived to date.

Brandy Weidow, M.S.

FURTHER READING

Ernst, E. "Chiropractic: A Critical Evaluation." *Journal of Pain and Symptom Management* 35, no. 5 (2008): 544-562.

Frigard, L. Ted. "Still Versus Palmer: A Remembrance of the Famous Debate." *Dynamic Chiropractic* 21, issue 3 (January 27, 2003).

See also: Chiropractic; Pain management; Pseudoscience.

Pancreatitis

CATEGORY: Condition
RELATED TERMS: Acute pancreatitis, chronic pancreatitis
DEFINITION: Treatment of inflammation of the pancreas.
PRINCIPAL PROPOSED NATURAL TREATMENT: Digestive enzymes
OTHER PROPOSED NATURAL TREATMENTS: Antioxidants (beta-carotene, grape seed extract, lipoic acid, methionine, milk thistle, selenium, vitamin C, vitamin E), multivitamin-multimineral supplements
NATURAL TREATMENT TO AVOID: Probiotics

INTRODUCTION

The pancreas is an organ that creates enzymes necessary to properly digest starch, protein, and fat. In addition, cells responsible for creating insulin are found in the pancreas. Pancreatitis is a condition in which the pancreas is inflamed. When pancreatitis is prolonged, pancreatic function declines, leading to malabsorption of nutrients and, possibly, to diabetes.

Pancreatitis occurs in three forms: acute (short-term) pancreatitis, recurrent acute pancreatitis, and chronic pancreatitis. Acute pancreatitis is a painful condition, but with treatment it ordinarily resolves in three to seven days. Causes include alcohol abuse, gallstones, extremely high blood levels of triglycerides, direct trauma to the pancreas, abdominal surgery and procedures, kidney failure, infection, and certain medications. The treatment of acute pancreatitis consists primarily of resting the pancreas by discontinuing all eating and drinking. Intravenous fluids are used to maintain fluid balance.

Recurrent acute pancreatitis involves multiple bouts of acute pancreatitis, sometimes in the context of a more mild, chronic condition. Each bout is treated as described in the foregoing paragraph.

Chronic pancreatitis is a more gradual process that leads to partial or complete pancreatic failure. Its most common cause is alcohol abuse, although the condition may also occur for other reasons or for no known reason. Chronic pancreatitis causes many symptoms, including most prominently abdominal pain, weight loss, diarrhea because of undigested fat, and mild diabetes. Treatment primarily involves the use of digestive enzymes (and, if necessary, insulin), dietary changes, and pain medication. If a person's alcohol abuse contributed to the chronic pancreatitis, he or she should stop drinking.

PRINCIPAL PROPOSED NATURAL TREATMENTS

Digestive enzymes, the mainstay of treatment for chronic pancreatitis, can be considered natural products. The digestive enzymes prescribed by physicians for pancreatitis are not necessarily more powerful than their dietary supplement equivalent, and some experimentation with different products might lead to the best results. Excessive consumption of digestive enzymes can cause harm, however, and for this reason a doctor's supervision is strongly recommended.

OTHER PROPOSED NATURAL TREATMENTS

Chronic pancreatitis leads to malabsorption of fat, which can lead to deficiencies of fat-soluble vitamins, such as vitamin A and vitamin E. In addition, chronic pancreatitis might impair absorption of vitamin B_{12} and possibly other nutrients. While it is not clear that these deficiencies are severe enough to cause harm, it makes sense for people with pancreatitis to consider taking a multivitamin-multimineral supplement as nutritional "insurance."

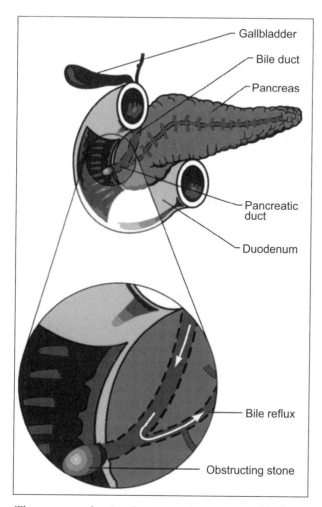

Gallbladder

Bile duct

Pancreas

Pancreatic
duct

Duodenum

Bile reflux

Obstructing stone

The pancreas, showing the pancreatic duct; when this duct is blocked, bile may reflux, leading to "autodigestion" of the pancreas.

Antioxidants are substances that help the body neutralize free radicals. Free radicals are dangerous, naturally occurring substances that are thought to play a role in pancreatitis and many other conditions. A small, double-blind, placebo-controlled trial of people with pancreatitis (chronic as well as recurring acute) examined the effectiveness of an antioxidant supplement providing 9,000 international units (IU) of beta-carotene, 540 milligrams (mg) of vitamin C, 270 IU of vitamin E, 600 micrograms (mcg) of selenium, and 2,000 mg of methionine daily. The results showed improvement in both symptoms and laboratory signs of disease severity. Similar results were found in a randomized trial of 127 men with chronic pancreatitis; six

months of antioxidant treatment led to significant reduction in pain compared with placebo. Other natural supplements with antioxidant properties sometimes recommended for chronic pancreatitis include grape seed extract (a source of oligomeric proanthocyanidins), lipoic acid, and milk thistle.

In a detailed review of four studies, researchers concluded that the use probiotics did not benefit persons with severe acute pancreatitis. Furthermore, according to one study, the use of probiotics led to an increased risk of mortality in persons with severe acute pancreatitis and should, therefore, be avoided.

EBSCO CAM Review Board

FURTHER READING

Besselink, M. G., et al. "Probiotic Prophylaxis in Predicted Severe Acute Pancreatitis." *The Lancet* 371 (2008): 651-659.

Bhardwaj, P., et al. "A Randomized Controlled Trial of Antioxidant Supplementation for Pain Relief in Patients with Chronic Pancreatitis." *Gastroenterology* 136 (2009): 149-159.

Marotta, F., et al. "Fat-Soluble Vitamin Concentration in Chronic Alcohol-Induced Pancreatitis: Relationship with Steatorrhea." *Digestive Diseases and Sciences* 39 (1994): 993-998.

Sun, S., et al. "Probiotics in Patients with Severe Acute Pancreatitis." *Langenbeck's Archives of Surgery* 394 (2009): 171-177.

See also: Antioxidants; Cholesterol, high; Gallstones; Gastrointestinal health; Insulin; Kidney stones.

Pantothenic acid and pantethine

CATEGORY: Herbs and supplements
RELATED TERMS: Pantothenate, vitamin B_5
DEFINITION: Natural food substances used as supplements to treat specific health conditions.
PRINCIPAL PROPOSED USES: High cholesterol, high triglycerides
OTHER PROPOSED USES: Performance enhancement, rheumatoid arthritis, stress

OVERVIEW

The body uses pantothenic acid (better known as vitamin B_5) to make proteins and other important chemicals needed to metabolize fats and carbohydrates. Pantothenic acid is also used in the manufacture of hormones, red blood cells, and acetylcholine, an important neurotransmitter (signal carrier between nerve cells).

As a supplement, pantothenic acid has been proposed as a treatment for rheumatoid arthritis, enhancing sports performance, and fighting stress in general. In the body, pantothenic acid is converted to a related chemical known as pantethine. For reasons that are not clear, pantethine supplements (but not pantothenic acid supplements) appear to reduce blood levels of triglycerides and possibly also to improve the cholesterol profile.

REQUIREMENTS AND SOURCES

The Greek word *pantothenic* means "everywhere," and pantothenic acid is indeed found in a wide range of foods. For this reason, pantothenic acid deficiency is rare. The official U.S. and Canadian recommendations for daily intake of pantothenic acid are as follows: 1.7 milligrams (mg) for infants up to six months of age, 1.8 mg for infants from seven to twelve months old, 2 mg for children from one to three years old, 3 mg for children from four to eight years old, 4 mg for children nine to thirteen years old, 5 mg for those aged fourteen and older, 6 mg for pregnant women, and 7 mg for nursing women.

Brewer's yeast, torula (nutritional) yeast, and calf liver are excellent sources of pantothenic acid. Peanuts, mushrooms, soybeans, split peas, pecans, oatmeal, buckwheat, sunflower seeds, lentils, rye flour, cashews, and other whole grains and nuts are good sources as well, as are red chili peppers and avocados. Pantethine is not found in foods in appreciable amounts.

THERAPEUTIC DOSAGES

For lowering triglycerides, the typical recommended dosage of pantethine is 300 mg three times daily. Dosages of pantothenic acid as high as 660 mg three times daily are sometimes recommended for people with rheumatoid arthritis.

THERAPEUTIC USES

Inconsistent evidence from small double-blind trials suggests that pantethine might lower blood levels of triglycerides and, to a lesser extent, of cholesterol. High triglycerides, like high cholesterol, increase risk of heart disease and strokes. Some people have only modestly elevated cholesterol but very high triglycerides, so pantethine may be especially useful for them.

Weak evidence hints that pantothenic acid might be helpful for rheumatoid arthritis. Pantothenic acid is also recommended as an athletic performance enhancer, but there is no evidence that it works. It is also sometimes referred to as an antistress nutrient because it plays a role in the function of the adrenal glands, but whether it really helps the body withstand stress is not known.

SCIENTIFIC EVIDENCE

High triglycerides/high cholesterol. Three small double-blind, placebo-controlled studies suggest that pantethine can reduce total blood triglycerides and perhaps improve cholesterol levels as well. For example, a double-blind placebo-controlled study followed twenty-nine people with high cholesterol and triglycerides for eight weeks. The dosage used was 300 mg three times daily, for a total daily dose of 900 mg. In this study, subjects taking pantethine experienced a 30 percent reduction in blood triglycerides, a 13.5 percent reduction in low-density lipoproteins (LDL, or

What Is Cholesterol?

Cholesterol is a waxy, fat-like substance that is found in all cells of the body. The body needs some cholesterol to make hormones, vitamin D, and substances that help a person to digest foods. The body makes all the cholesterol it needs. However, cholesterol is also found in some foods.

Cholesterol travels through the bloodstream in small packages called lipoproteins. These packages are made of fat (lipid) on the inside and proteins on the outside. Two kinds of lipoproteins carry cholesterol throughout the body: low-density lipoproteins (LDL) and high-density lipoproteins (HDL). Having healthy levels of both types of lipoproteins is important.

LDL cholesterol is sometimes called bad cholesterol. A high LDL level leads to a buildup of cholesterol in a person's arteries. (Arteries are blood vessels that carry blood from the heart to other parts of the body.) HDL cholesterol is sometimes called good cholesterol because it carries cholesterol from other parts of the body to the liver. The liver removes the cholesterol from the body.

bad cholesterol), and a 10 percent rise in high-density lipoproteins (HDL, or good cholesterol). However, other small studies have found no benefit. These contradictory results do not necessarily mean that pantethine is ineffective, as chance plays a considerable role in the outcome of small studies. Rather, they suggest that larger studies need to be performed to establish (or disprove) panthethine's potential efficacy.

Several open studies have specifically studied the use of pantethine to improve cholesterol and triglyceride levels in people with diabetes and found it effective without causing harmful effects. These findings are supported by experiments in rabbits, which show that pantethine may prevent the buildup of plaque in major arteries. However, it is not known how pantethine acts in the body to reduce triglycerides.

Rheumatoid arthritis. There is weak evidence for using pantothenic acid to treat rheumatoid arthritis. One observational study found sixty-six people with rheumatoid arthritis had less pantothenic acid in their blood than twenty-nine healthy people. The more severe the arthritis, the lower the blood levels of pantothenic acid. However, this result does not prove that pantothenic acid supplements can effectively reduce any of the symptoms of rheumatoid arthritis.

To follow up on this finding, researchers then conducted a small placebo-controlled trial involving eighteen subjects to see whether pantothenic acid would help. This study found that 2 grams (g) daily of pantothenic acid (in the form of calcium pantothenate) reduced morning stiffness, pain, and disability significantly better than a placebo. However, a study this small does not mean much on its own.

SAFETY ISSUES

No significant side effects have been reported for pantothenic acid or pantethine, used by themselves or with other medications. As noted above, pantethine has been used in people with diabetes, without apparent adverse effects. However, maximum safe dosages for young children, pregnant or nursing women, or people with serious liver or kidney disease have not been established.

EBSCO CAM Review Board

FURTHER READING

Coronel, G., et al. "Treatment of Hyperlipidemia in Diabetic Patients on Dialysis with a Physiological Substance." *American Journal of Nephrology* 11 (1991): 32-36.

See also: Cholesterol, high; Herbal medicine; Rheumatoid arthritis; Triglycerides, high.

Parasites, intestinal

CATEGORY: Condition
RELATED TERMS: Giardia, pinworms, worms
DEFINITION: Treatment of diseases caused by parasites in the intestines.
PRINCIPAL PROPOSED NATURAL TREATMENTS: None
OTHER PROPOSED NATURAL TREATMENTS: Anise, berberine (found in barberry, goldenseal, goldenthread, and Oregon grape), black walnut fruit, cloves, curled mint, essential oils, garlic, gentian, grapefruit seed extract, lapacho, neem, olive leaf, oregano, papaya, propolis, pumpkin seed, sweet Annie, tansy, *Terminalia arjuna*, thyme, wormseed, wormwood

INTRODUCTION

The human intestines play host to an enormous variety of bacteria and fungi. Most of these are harmless or even helpful. However, other microscopic organisms can also take up residence in the intestines. Such organisms are called intestinal parasites. Common parasites include amoebas (especially *Entamoeba histolytica*), *Cryptosporidium*, giardia (*Giardia lamblia*), hookworm (*Ancylostoma duodenale* and *Necator americanus*), pinworm (*Enterobius vermicularis*), roundworm (*Ascaris lumbricoides*), and tapeworm (*Taenia* species).

Intestinal parasites can cause a wide variety of symptoms, including gas, bloating, diarrhea, abdominal cramping, bloody stools, itching in the anus, and weight loss. Some parasites are no more than a nuisance, while others can cause serious disease and even death.

Conventional treatment for parasites begins with careful identification of the particular parasite involved, followed by the use of medications capable of destroying the infestation. Careful attention to hygiene while traveling in developing countries can help prevent future infections with parasites.

PROPOSED NATURAL TREATMENTS

Intestinal parasites are hardy organisms not easily killed. Traditional remedies used for parasites are generally fairly toxic. Until recently, conventional treatments for parasites were also quite toxic. However,

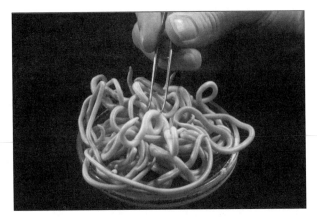

Nematode worms are the largest of the human intestinal parasites. (CNRI/Photo Researchers, Inc.)

now that safe drugs have been developed, it can be said as a general rule that conventional therapies for parasites are less toxic and almost certainly more effective than natural remedies.

Despite this, many natural products are marketed for the treatment of parasites. The profusion of such offerings is due primarily to a particular current of thought among some alternative practitioners that states that parasites are the underlying cause of many illnesses. Most such natural products are made of herbs that kill parasites in the test tube. However, it is a long way from a test-tube study to meaningful effects in humans, and there is no reliable meaningful evidence that any of these natural therapies are useful in a practical sense. Some herbs commonly mentioned for the treatment of parasitic infections include anise, black walnut fruit, cloves, curled mint, essential oils, garlic, gentian, grapefruit seed extract, lapacho, neem, olive leaf, oregano, propolis, pumpkin seed, sweet Annie, tansy, *Terminalia arjuna*, thyme, wormseed, and wormwood.

The substance berberine has shown some promise for the treatment of parasites, and it was, for a time, evaluated as a potential new antiparasitic drug. Berberine is found in barberry, goldenseal, goldenthread, Oregon grape, and other herbs, and for this reason these herbs are commonly mentioned as useful for the treatment of parasitic infections. However, the only studies relevant to these herbs used purified chemical berberine. To obtain the same amount of berberine in the form of an herb, one would have to consume massive (and possibly toxic) quantities.

One placebo-controlled study conducted in Africa concluded that the use of dried papaya seeds could reduce levels of intestinal parasites generally. However, this study had significant problems in design and reporting. Also, the form of papaya used in this trial was not equivalent to the digestive enzyme papain.

EBSCO CAM Review Board

FURTHER READING

Kaneda, Y. "In Vitro Effects of Berberine Sulphate on the Growth and Structure of *Entamoeba histolytica*, *Giardia lamblia*, and *Trichomonas vaginalis*." *Annals of Tropical Medicine and Parasitology* 85 (1991): 417-425.

Okeniyi, J. A., et al. "Effectiveness of Dried Carica Papaya Seeds Against Human Intestinal Parasitosis." *Journal of Medicinal Food* 10 (2007): 194-196.

Soffar, S. A., et al. "Evaluation of the Effect of a Plant Alkaloid (Berberine Derived from *Berberis aristata*) on *Trichomonas vaginalis* In Vitro." *Journal of the Egyptian Society of Parasitology* 31 (2001): 893-904.

See also: Diarrhea; Dyspepsia; Gastrointestinal health; Ulcers.

Parkinson's disease

CATEGORY: Condition

RELATED TERMS: Paralysis agitans, parkinsonism

DEFINITION: Treatment of the chronic condition caused by the death of nerve cells in certain parts of the brain.

PRINCIPAL PROPOSED NATURAL TREATMENTS: Coenzyme Q_{10}, cytidinediphosphocholine (also called citicholine)

OTHER PROPOSED NATURAL TREATMENTS: Acupuncture, Alexander technique, creatine, D-phenylalanine, 5-hydroxytryptophan, glutathione, L-methionine, magnet therapy, nicotinamide adenine dinucleotide, phosphatidylserine, policosanol, S-adenosylmethionine, vitamin C, vitamin E

HERBS AND SUPPLEMENTS TO USE ONLY WITH CAUTION: Amino acids (such as branched-chain amino acids, methionine, and phenylalanine), 5-hydroxytryptophan, iron, kava, S-adenosylmethionine, vitamin B_6

INTRODUCTION

Parkinson's disease is a chronic disorder typically affecting people older than age fifty-five years. The condition is caused by the death of nerve cells in certain parts of the brain, leading to characteristic problems with movement. These problems include a "pill rolling" tremor in the hands (so called because it appears that the person is rolling a small object between thumb and forefinger), difficulty initiating walking, a shuffling gait, decreased facial expressiveness, and trouble speaking. Thinking ability may become impaired in later stages of the disease, and depression is common.

Although the underlying cause of Parkinson's disease is unknown, many researchers believe that free radicals may play a role in destroying some of the nerve cells. The nerve cells that are affected in Parkinson's disease work by supplying the neurotransmitter dopamine to another part of the brain. Most treatments for Parkinson's disease work by artificially increasing the brain's dopamine levels. Simply taking dopamine pills will not work, however, because the substance cannot travel from the bloodstream into the brain. Instead, most people with Parkinson's disease take levodopa (L-dopa), which can pass into the brain and be converted there into dopamine. Many people take levodopa with carbidopa, a drug that increases the amount of levodopa available to make dopamine.

Initially, levodopa produces dramatic improvement in symptoms; however, over time, levodopa becomes less effective and more likely to produce side effects. Other drugs may be useful too, including bromocriptine, trihexyphenidyl, entacapone, tolcapone, selegiline, and pergolide. There are also surgical treatments that can decrease symptoms, such as pallidotomy and deep brain stimulation.

PRINCIPAL PROPOSED NATURAL TREATMENTS

Cytidinediphosphocholine.   Cytidinediphosphocholine (CDP-choline) is a substance that occurs naturally in the human body. It is closely related to choline, a nutrient commonly put in the B vitamin family. For reasons that are not completely clear, CDP-choline seems to increase the amount of dopamine in the brain. On this basis, it has been tried for Parkinson's disease. Support for the use of CDP-choline also comes from studies in which the supplement was administered by injection.

In a four-week, single-blind study of seventy-four people with Parkinson's disease, researchers tested whether oral CDP-choline might help levodopa be more effective. Researchers divided participants into two groups: One group received their usual levodopa dose, the other received one-half their usual dose without knowing what dosage they were getting. All the participants took 400 milligrams (mg) of oral CDP-choline three times daily. Even though 50 percent of the participants were taking only one-half their usual dose of levodopa, both groups scored equally well on standardized tests designed to evaluate the severity of Parkinson's disease symptoms.

In general, CDP-choline appears to be safe. The study of oral CDP-choline for Parkinson's disease reported only a few brief, nonspecific side effects such as nausea, dizziness, and fatigue. In a study of 2,817 elderly people who took oral CDP-choline for up to sixty days for problems other than Parkinson's disease, side effects were few and mild and reported in only about 5 percent of participants. Two-thirds of

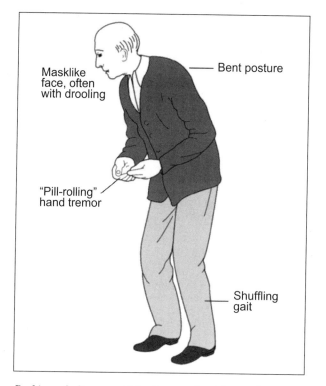

Parkinson's disease, which often attacks older people, is characterized by debilitating symptoms that become more severe as the disease progresses.

these side effects were gastrointestinal (nausea, stomach pain, and diarrhea), and none required stopping CDP-choline. The dose in this study was 550 to 650 mg per day, about one-half the dose used for Parkinson's disease.

Coenzyme Q_{10}. The supplement coenzyme Q_{10} (CoQ_{10}) has been widely advertised as effective for treating Parkinson's disease. However, there is only minimal evidence that it works, and there is some evidence that it does not.

A study published in 2002 raised hopes that CoQ_{10} might help slow the progression of Parkinson's disease. In this sixteen-month, double-blind, placebo-controlled trial, eighty people with Parkinson's disease were given either CoQ_{10} (at a dose of 300, 600, or 1,200 mg daily) or placebo. Participants in this trial had early stages of the disease and did not yet need medication. The results appeared to suggest that the supplement, especially at the highest dose, might have slowed disease progression. However, for a variety of statistical reasons, the results were quite inconclusive.

A subsequent double-blind, placebo-controlled study of twenty-eight people with Parkinson's disease (that was well-controlled by medications) indicated that 360 mg of CoQ_{10} daily could produce a mild improvement in some symptoms. Based on these results, a more substantial study was undertaken, enrolling 131 people with Parkinson's disease (again, well-controlled by medications). It did not work. While benefits were seen in both the placebo group and the CoQ_{10} group, the supplement failed to prove more effective than placebo.

OTHER PROPOSED NATURAL TREATMENTS

Several other natural products have been studied for preventing or treating Parkinson's disease, with mixed results.

S-adenosylmethionine. Whether a symptom of the disease or a response to disability, depression affects many people with Parkinson's disease, and the long-term use of levodopa may contribute to this problem. Research suggests that levodopa can deplete the brain of a substance called S-adenosylmethionine (SAMe). As SAMe has been found in a number of small studies to have antidepressant effects, it is possible that depleting it might trigger depression.

Researchers conducted a trial to determine if taking SAMe supplements could decrease depression

in twenty-one people with Parkinson's disease who were taking levodopa. In this double-blind study, each participant received either a combination of oral and injected SAMe or a placebo daily for thirty days, followed by the alternative treatment for another thirty days. Although other symptoms of Parkinson's did not change, depression improved after two weeks in 72 percent of those taking SAMe, while only 30 percent noted improvement with placebo. It is not known if oral SAMe alone would have similar effects.

Although SAMe might appear to be an excellent accompaniment to levodopa, there is another side to the issue. During treatment with levodopa, SAMe participates in breaking down levodopa and gets used up in the process. It is possible that taking extra SAMe could lead to the decreased effectiveness of levodopa. In the foregoing short-term study, SAMe did not interfere with levodopa's effects, but longer-term use might do so. For persons who have Parkinson's disease, it is safest to use SAMe only under the supervision of a physician.

Phosphatidylserine. Phosphatidylserine is a major component of cell membranes. Several studies have found phosphatidylserine supplementation effective for improving mental function in people with Alzheimer's disease. One trial examined its use in sixty-two people, all of whom had both Parkinson's disease and Alzheimer's-type dementia. The results appeared to indicate some benefit, but because of the incompleteness of the report on this trial, it is difficult to draw conclusions.

Vitamin E. Because of indications that free radicals play a role in causing Parkinson's disease, treatment with high doses of vitamin E has been tried to determine if it slows the progression of Parkinson's disease. However, a large study yielded disappointing results. In this trial, eight hundred persons newly diagnosed with Parkinson's disease took 2,000 international units of tocopherol (synthetic vitamin E) or placebo daily for an average of fourteen months. Vitamin E had no effect in delaying symptoms of the disease, and it failed to reduce the side effects of levodopa.

Vitamin C. One problem with levodopa treatment for Parkinson's disease is the on-off effect, in which a person taking levodopa will move more freely for some hours, followed by sudden "freezing up." Vitamin C has been tried as a remedy for the on-off effect in a small double-blind study, but the results were so minimal that the researchers did not feel justified in recommending it.

Other treatments. The herb *Mucuna pruriens* contains L-dopa. One small study reportedly found evidence that the use of the herb as an L-dopa source offers advantages over purified L-dopa given as a medication itself.

Other proposed natural treatments for Parkinson's disease have minimal or conflicting evidence supporting them. These treatments include nicotinamide adenine dinucleotide, glutathione, policosanol, and the amino acids D-phenylalanine and L-methionine. Caution is advised with the latter three, as they might affect the function of levodopa.

A two-year study failed to find more than minimal benefits at most with creatine, and weak evidence hints that the supplement 5-hydroxytryptophan (5-HTP) might be helpful for depression in people with Parkinson's disease. However, 5-HTP should not be combined with the drug carbidopa.

A double-blind, placebo-controlled trial of ninety-nine people found that repetitive transcranial magnetic stimulation (rTMS) delivered in eight weekly treatments can improve Parkinson's symptoms. A two-month, double-blind, placebo-controlled trial of eighteen people found that rTMS improved Parkinson's symptoms. Similar benefits were seen in three other small controlled studies. Also, when combining the results of ten randomized trials in persons with Parkinson's, researchers noted a significant benefit for rTMS (using higher frequencies).

A postural training method called the Alexander technique has shown some promise. A small placebo-controlled study found that the use of bright lights, best known as a treatment for seasonal affective disorder, may also help relieve various symptoms of Parkinson's disease, possibly by reducing levels of melatonin in the brain.

In two studies, acupuncture failed to provide much benefit for Parkinson's disease. In two comprehensive reviews of multiple clinical trials, independent sets of researchers concluded that there was no well-established evidence for acupuncture's effectiveness in Parkinson's.

HERBS AND SUPPLEMENTS TO USE WITH CAUTION

Persons with Parkinson's disease should avoid taking the herb kava. Preliminary reports suggest that kava may counter the effects of dopamine and pos-

sibly reduce the effectiveness of medications for Parkinson's.

Other substances may also interact with Parkinson's drugs. Iron supplements can interfere with the absorption of levodopa and carbidopa and should not be taken within two hours of either medication. Amino acid supplements, such as branched-chain amino acids, can temporarily decrease levodopa's effectiveness, as may methionine and phenylalanine, two amino acids studied for treatment of Parkinson's disease.

Vitamin B_6 in doses higher than 5 mg per day also might impair the effectiveness of levodopa and should be avoided. However, if one takes levodopa-carbidopa combinations, this restriction may not necessarily apply. One should consult a physician about an appropriate dose of vitamin B_6.

Certain herbal formulas used in traditional Chinese herbal medicine to treat upset stomach might reduce the effectiveness of levodopa. The supplement 5-HTP has a potentially dangerous interaction with carbidopa. Using the two substances together may increase the chance of developing symptoms resembling those of the disease scleroderma.

One report suggests that by amplifying the action of levodopa, policosanol might increase side effects called dyskinesias. Finally, weak evidence hints that prolonged (over many years) intake of high levels of iron and manganese might increase the risk of developing Parkinson's disease.

EBSCO CAM Review Board

FURTHER READING

Bender, A., et al. "Creatine Supplementation in Parkinson Disease." *Neurology* 67 (2006): 1262-1264.

Elahi, B., and R. Chen. "Effect of Transcranial Magnetic Stimulation on Parkinson Motor Function." *Movement Disorders* 24 (2009): 357-363.

Katzenschlager, R., et al. "*Mucuna pruriens* in Parkinson's Disease." *Journal of Neurology, Neurosurgery, and Psychiatry* 75 (2004): 1672-1677.

Lam, Y. C., et al. "Efficacy and Safety of Acupuncture for Idiopathic Parkinson's Disease." *Journal of Alternative and Complementary Medicine* 14 (2008): 663-671.

Paus, S., et al. "Bright Light Therapy in Parkinson's Disease." *Movement Disorders* 22 (2007): 1495-1498.

Storch, A., et al. "Randomized, Double-Blind, Placebo-Controlled Trial on Symptomatic Effects of Coenzyme Q(10) in Parkinson Disease." *Archives of Neurology* 64 (2007): 938-944.

See also: Coenzyme Q$_{10}$; Levodopa/carbidopa; Phosphatidylserine; SAMe; Vitamin C; Vitamin E.

Parsley

CATEGORY: Herbs and supplements

RELATED TERMS: *Petroselinum crispum, P. hartense, P. sativum*

DEFINITION: Natural plant product used to treat specific health conditions.

PRINCIPAL PROPOSED USES: None

OTHER PROPOSED USES: Abortifacient, amenorrhea, colic, flatulence, indigestion, kidney stones

OVERVIEW

Parsley is a culinary herb used in many types of cooking and as a nearly universal adornment to restaurant food. Originally a native plant of the Mediterranean region, parsley is grown today throughout the world. It is a nutritious food, providing dietary calcium, iron, carotenes, ascorbic acid, and vitamin A.

Parsley's traditional use for inducing menstruation may be explained by evidence that apiol and myristicin, two substances contained in parsley, stimulate contractions of the uterus. Indeed, extracted apiol has been tried for the purpose of causing abortions. A tea made from the seeds of parsley is also a traditional remedy for colic, indigestion, and intestinal gas.

THERAPEUTIC DOSAGES

The usual dose of parsley leaf or root is 6 grams (g) of dried plant per day, consumed in three doses of 2 g each, steeped in 150 ml of water. Extract of parsley leaf and root are made at a ratio of 1 g of plant to 1 milliliter (ml) of liquid and used at a dose of 2 ml three times daily. Tea made from parsley seeds is used at a lower dosage of 2 to 3 g per day, using 1 g of seed per cup of tea.

THERAPEUTIC USES

Germany's Commission E suggests the use of parsley leaf or root to relieve irritation of the urinary tract (such as may occur in bladder infections) and to aid in passing kidney stones. Although there is no evidence that parsley is helpful for these conditions, parsley is believed to have a diuretic effect because of it its constituents apiol and myristicin. As diuretics

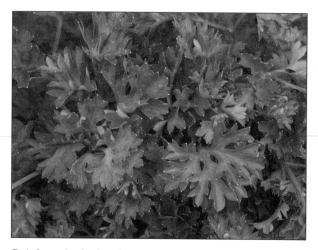

Dried parsley leaf and root are used for medicinal purposes. (Bonnie Sue Rauch/Photo Researchers, Inc.)

would increase the flow of urine, this might help the body wash out bacteria as well as stones. However, no studies have evaluated whether parsley is actually beneficial for either health problem.

A test-tube study evaluated parsley extract as a topical antibiotic, finding that the extract had a weak effect against *Staphylococcus* bacteria. However, it did not appear to be strong enough to be practically useful for this purpose.

SAFETY ISSUES

As a widely eaten food, parsley is generally regarded as safe. However, excessive quantities of parsley should be avoided during pregnancy, based on the evidence that myristicin and apiol can stimulate the uterus. Myristicin may also cross the placenta and increase the heart rate of the fetus.

Parsley is known as a plant that can cause photosensitivity, which is an increased tendency to sunburn; this result, however, occurs from prolonged physical contact with the leaves, not from oral consumption of parsley. Maximum safe intake of parsley in young children, pregnant or nursing women, and people with severe liver or kidney disease has not been established.

IMPORTANT INTERACTIONS

Those persons taking lithium should use parsley only under a doctor's supervision.

EBSCO CAM Review Board

FURTHER READING

Blumenthal, M. *Herbal Medicine Expanded Commission E Monograph.* Newton, Mass.: Integrative Medicine Communications, 2000.

Kreydiyyeh, S. I., and J. Usta. "Diuretic Effect and Mechanism of Action of Parsley." *Journal of Ethnopharmacology* 79 (2002): 353-357.

See also: Diuretics, loop; Diuretics, potassium-sparing; Diuretics, thiazide; Herbal medicine.

Passionflower

CATEGORY: Herbs and supplements
RELATED TERM: *Passiflora incarnata*
DEFINITION: Natural plant product used to treat specific health conditions.
PRINCIPAL PROPOSED USES: Anxiety, drug addiction
OTHER PROPOSED USES: Insomnia, nervous stomach

OVERVIEW

The passionflower vine is a native of the Western hemisphere, named for symbolic connections drawn between its appearance and the crucifixion of Jesus. Native North Americans used passionflower primarily as a mild sedative. It quickly caught on as a folk remedy in Europe and was thereafter adopted by professional herbalists as a sedative and digestive aid.

THERAPEUTIC DOSAGES

The proper dosage of passionflower is 1 cup three times daily of a tea made by steeping 1 teaspoon of dried leaves for ten to fifteen minutes. Passionflower tinctures and powdered extracts should be taken according to the label instructions.

THERAPEUTIC USES

In 1985, Germany's Commission E officially approved passionflower as a treatment for nervous unrest. The herb is considered to be a mildly effective treatment for anxiety and insomnia, less potent than kava and valerian, but nonetheless useful. Like melissa (lemon balm), chamomile, and valerian, passionflower is also used for nervous stomach. However, there is only weak supporting scientific evidence that passionflower works for these purposes. Preliminary trials suggest that passionflower might be helpful for anxiety and chemical dependency. Animal studies suggest that passionflower extracts can reduce agitation and prolong sleep. The active ingredients in passionflower are not known.

SCIENTIFIC EVIDENCE

Anxiety. A four-week double-blind study of thirty-six individuals with anxiety (specifically, generalized anxiety disorder) compared passionflower to the standard drug oxazepam. Oxazepam worked more quickly, but by the end of the four-week trial, both treatments proved equally effective. Furthermore, passionflower showed a comparative advantage in terms of side effects: Use of oxazepam was associated with more job-related problems (such as daytime drowsiness). In a placebo-controlled trial involving sixty surgical patients, passionflower significantly reduced anxiety up to ninety minutes prior to surgery.

Chemical dependency. A fourteen-day double-blind trial enrolled sixty-five men addicted to opiate drugs and compared the effectiveness of passionflower and the drug clonidine together against clonidine alone. Clonidine is a drug widely used to assist narcotic withdrawal. It effectively reduces physical symptoms such as increased blood pressure. However, clonidine does not help emotional symptoms, such as drug craving, anxiety, irritability, agitation, and depression. These symptoms can be quite severe and often cause enrollees in drug treatment programs to end participation. In this fourteen-day study, the use of passionflower along with clonidine significantly eased the emotional aspects of withdrawal compared with clonidine alone.

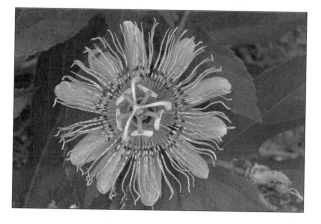

Passionflower has been studied as a treatment for anxiety. (John Serrao/Photo Researchers, Inc.)

SAFETY ISSUES

Passionflower is on the U.S. Food and Drug Administration's Generally Recognized as Safe (GRAS) list. The alkaloids harman and harmaline found in passionflower have been found to act somewhat like the drugs known as MAO inhibitors and also to stimulate the uterus, but whether whole passionflower has these effects remains unknown. Passionflower might increase the action of sedative medications. Finally, there are five case reports from Norway of individuals becoming temporarily mentally impaired from a combination herbal product containing passionflower. It is not clear whether the other ingredients may have played a role. Safety has not been established for pregnant or nursing mothers, very young children, or those with severe liver or kidney disease.

IMPORTANT INTERACTIONS

Passionflower may exaggerate the effect of sedative medications, so those taking these medications should use passionflower only under a physician's advice.

EBSCO CAM Review Board

FURTHER READING

Akhondzadeh, S., et al. "Passionflower in the Treatment of Generalized Anxiety: A Pilot Double-Blind Randomized Controlled Trial with Oxazepam." *Journal of Clinical Pharmacology and Therapeutics* 26 (2001): 363-367.

_____. "Passionflower in the Treatment of Opiates Withdrawal." *Journal of Clinical Pharmacology and Therapeutics* 26 (2001): 369-373.

Dhawan, K., et al. "Anxiolytic Activity of Aerial and Underground Parts of *Passiflora incarnata*." *Fitoterapia* 72 (2001): 922-926.

Movafegh, A., et al. "Preoperative Oral *Passiflora incarnata* Reduces Anxiety in Ambulatory Surgery Patients." *Anesthesia and Analgesia* 106 (2008): 1728-1732.

See also: Anxiety and panic attacks; Chamomile; Clonidine; Herbal medicine; Kava; Valerian.

PC-SPES

CATEGORY: Herbs and supplements
RELATED TERMS: *Dendranthema morifolium, Ganoderma lucidium* (reishi mushroom), *Glycyrrhiza glabra* (licorice), *Isatis indigotica, Panax pseuodoginseng, Rabdosia rubescens, Scutellaria baicalensis, Serenoa repens* (saw palmetto)

DEFINITION: Natural plant product used to treat specific health conditions.
PRINCIPAL PROPOSED USE: Prostate cancer

OVERVIEW

PC-SPES was, ostensibly, a formulation of eight natural products (seven herbs and one mushroom): *Isatis indigotica, Glycyrrhiza glabra* (licorice), *Panax* pseudoginseng, *Ganoderma lucidium* (reishi mushroom), *Scutellaria baicalensis, Dendranthema morifolium, Robdosia rubescens*, and *Serenoa repens* (saw palmetto). The name PC-SPES is derived from the common abbreviation for prostate cancer (PC) and the Latin word *spes*, meaning "hope." After its commercial launch in 1996, PC-SPES received considerable interest from the general public and reputable medical researchers as a treatment for prostate cancer. However, this claim turned out to be a fraud.

PC-SPES was not truly a purely herbal product; samples dating to 1996 were found to contain a form of pharmaceutical estrogen, diethylstilbestrol (DES), indomethacin (an anti-inflammatory medication in the ibuprofen family), and warfarin (a strong blood thinner). Samples subsequent to 1999 contained less DES, but they also showed less effectiveness in treating prostate cancer.

There is little doubt that DES is active against prostate cancer, but it presents a variety of risks, including blood clots in the legs. The other two pharmaceutical contaminants might actually reduce this risk (which may be why they were covertly added), but they present various risks of their own.

THERAPEUTIC DOSAGES

The standard dosage of PC-SPES was six to nine 320-milligram (mg) capsules per day, taken on an empty stomach at least two hours before or after meals.

THERAPEUTIC USES

The only proposed use of PC-SPES was the treatment of prostate cancer. The formulation was tried at various stages of the disease, and preliminary research indicated that it had potential, particularly for treating prostate cancer that is no longer responsive to hormone therapies. Benefits were reported in the two main types of prostate cancer: hormone-sensitive and hormone-insensitive cancer. However, when the covert addition of pharmaceuticals was discovered, interest in this so-called herbal combination ended.

Scientific Evidence

All the results reported in the following paragraphs are consistent with the known effects of hormones related to estrogen and may be due to the DES present in PC-SPES rather than to the herbal constituents.

Test-tube studies of cancer cells found that PC-SPES decreases cell growth; promotes tumor cell death, and reduces PSA (prostate-specific antigen) levels in both hormone-sensitive and hormone-insensitive prostate cancers; and exerts estrogenic effects. In a rat study, PC-SPES treatment reduced the occurrence of prostate cancer tumors, inhibited their growth, and slowed the rate of cancer spread (metastasis) to the lungs. In one uncontrolled human study, PC-SPES produced a significant decrease in PSA levels for most of the thirty-three volunteers tested. Similar results were seen in another study of sixty-nine individuals by the same author and in a study of seventy people conducted by another researcher. Benefits were seen in other uncontrolled trials, as well.

Safety Issues

Because of the presence of unlisted pharmaceuticals, PC-SPES should not be used. Side effects of PC-SPES closely resemble those of estrogen when taken by men for the treatment of prostate cancer; it may cause breast or nipple tenderness or swelling, loss of body hair, hot flashes, and loss of libido. Some individuals have also reported leg cramps, nausea and vomiting, and blood clots in the legs. Side effects of PC-SPES increase with dosage. Also, there is one case report of PC-SPES taken at twice the recommended dose causing internal bleeding, presumably because of the presence of warfarin (Coumadin), a strong blood thinner.

EBSCO CAM Review Board

Further Reading

De la Taille, A., et al. "Herbal Therapy PC-SPES: In Vitro Effects and Evaluation of Its Efficacy in Sixty-nine Patients with Prostate Cancer." *Journal of Urology* 164 (2000): 1229-1234.

Moyad, M. A., K. J. Pienta, and J. E. Montie. "Use of PC-SPES, a Commercially Available Supplement for Prostate Cancer, in a Patient with Hormone-Nave Disease." *Urology* 54 (1999): 319-324.

Oh, W. K., et al. "Activity of the Herbal Combination, PC-SPES, in the Treatment of Patients with Androgen-Independent Prostate Cancer." *Urology* 57 (2001): 122-126.

Pfeifer, B. L., et al. "PC-SPES, a Dietary Supplement for the Treatment of Hormone-Refractory Prostate Cancer." *BJU International* 85 (2000): 481-485.

Small, E. J., et al. "Prospective Trial of the Herbal Supplement PC-SPES in Patients with Progressive Prostate Cancer." *Journal of Clinical Oncology* 18 (2000): 3595-3603.

Weinrobe, M. C., and B. Montgomery. "Acquired Bleeding Diathesis in a Patient Taking PC-SPES." *New England Journal of Medicine* 345 (2001): 1213-1214.

See also: Cancer treatment support; Ginseng; Herbal medicine; Licorice; Men's health; Prostatitis; Reishi; Saw palmetto.

Pelargonium sidoides

Category: Herbs and supplements
Related terms: Kalwerbossie, rabassam, South African geranium, umckaloabo
Definition: Natural plant product used to treat specific health conditions.
Principal proposed uses: Acute bronchitis, sore throat
Other proposed uses: Colds and flu, sinusitis, tonsillitis

Overview

Pelargonium sidoides is a plant in the geranium family that grows in South Africa. It has heart-shaped leaves and narrow flowers of deep, saturated red. It has a long history of traditional use in southern Africa for treatment of respiratory problems. The root is the part used medicinally.

Therapeutic Dosages

A typical adult dose of the tested standardized root extract is 30 drops three times daily. For children aged six to eleven, this dose is typically reduced to 20 drops three times daily. However, other products besides the tested formulation may vary in strength. Therefore, label instructions should be followed regarding dosing.

THERAPEUTIC USES

An alcohol extract made from *P. sidoides* has become popular in Germany as a treatment for various respiratory problems, including acute bronchitis, the common cold, sinusitis, pharyngitis (sore throat), and tonsillitis. Fairly large studies have been performed to substantiate some of these uses. For example, in one double-blind, placebo-controlled study, 468 adults with recent onset of acute bronchitis were given either placebo or a standard alcohol extract of *P. sidoides* three times daily for a week. The results showed a significantly greater improvement in symptoms in the treatment group compared with the placebo group. On average, participants who received the real treatment were able to return to work two days earlier than those given a placebo. Benefits were also seen in two other double-blind, placebo-controlled studies enrolling a total of almost 350 people with acute bronchitis. When researchers pooled the results of four well-designed, placebo-controlled trials, they found that a standardized extract of *Pelargonium* performed significantly better than a placebo at reducing the symptoms of bronchitis by the seventh day of treatment. Given this evidence, *Pelargonium* appears to be effective for acute bronchitis.

Another double-blind, placebo-controlled study enrolled 143 children aged six to ten with a nondangerous form of strep throat (technically, non-group A beta hemolytic strep tonsillopharyngitis). On average, the total duration of the illness was reduced by two days in the treatment group compared with the placebo group. Only a medical test can distinguish between the relatively nondangerous form of strep throat studied in this trial (non-group A strep) and strep throat of the potentially very dangerous A form (group A strep). For this reason, physician supervision is essential.

Finally, a double-blind study of 133 adults who had just come down with the common cold found that use of a standardized *Pelargonium* extract at a dose of 30 milliliters (ml) three times daily significantly reduced the severity and duration of symptoms compared with a placebo. It is not known how *P. sidoides* might work, but its action is hypothesized to involve both direct antibacterial effects and immune function modification.

What Is a Botanical?

A botanical is a plant, such as *Pelargonium sidoides*, or plant part valued for its medicinal or therapeutic properties, flavor, or scent. Herbs are a subset of botanicals. Products made from botanicals that are used to maintain or improve health may be called herbal products, botanical products, or phytomedicines. Botanicals are sold in many forms: as fresh or dried products; as liquid or solid extracts; as tablets, capsules, or powders; in tea bags; and in other forms.

An extract such as *Pelargonium sidoides* is made by soaking the botanical in a liquid that removes specific types of chemicals. The liquid can be used as is or evaporated to make a dry extract for use in capsules or tablets.

SAFETY ISSUES

In clinical trials enrolling a total of over twenty-five hundred adults and children, use of the tested, standardized extract produced few side effects, other than the usual occasional allergic reactions or digestive upset. However, comprehensive safety testing has not been completed. There is no reliable evidence regarding safety in children under the age of six, pregnant or nursing women, and people with severe liver or kidney disease.

EBSCO CAM Review Board

FURTHER READING

Bereznoy, V. V., et al. "Efficacy of Extract of *Pelargonium sidoides* in Children with Acute Non-group A Beta-hemolytic *Streptococcus* Tonsillopharyngitis." *Alternative Therapies in Health and Medicine* 9 (2003): 68-79.

Chuchalin, A. G., B. Berman, and W. Lehmacher. "Treatment of Acute Bronchitis in Adults with a *Pelargonium sidoides* Preparation (EPs 7630)." *Explore (NY)* 1 (2006): 437-445.

Kayser, O., et al. "Immunomodulatory Principles of *Pelargonium sidoides*." *Phytotherapy Research* 15 (2001): 122-126.

Kolodziej, H., et al. "Pharmacological Profile of Extracts of *Pelargonium sidoides* and Their Constituents." *Phytomedicine* 10 (2003): 18-24.

Lizogub, V. G., R. S. Riley, and M. Heger. "Efficacy of a *Pelargonium sidoides* Preparation in Patients with the Common Cold." *Explore (NY)* 3 (2007): 573-584.

Matthys, H., and M. Heger. "Treatment of Acute Bronchitis with a Liquid Herbal Drug Preparation from *Pelargonium sidoides* (EPs 7630)." *Current Medical Research Opinions* 23 (2007): 323-331.

See also: Colds and flu; Bronchitis; Herbal medicine; Strep throat.

Penicillamine

CATEGORY: Drug interactions
DEFINITION: Drug used to treat rheumatoid arthritis and Wilson's disease, an inherited disorder affecting copper metabolism and causing cirrhosis and brain and eye problems.
INTERACTIONS: Copper, iron, vitamin B_6, zinc
TRADE NAMES: Cuprimine, Depen

COPPER

Effect: Avoid in Cases of Wilson's Disease

When used to treat Wilson's disease, penicillamine works by removing copper from the body. One should avoid taking copper supplements while also using penicillamine for this condition.

VITAMIN B_6

Effect: Possible Need for Supplementation

Penicillamine might increase the need for vitamin B_6. Taking 25 to 50 milligrams (mg) of supplemental vitamin B_6 daily is often recommended.

ZINC

Effect: Supplementation Possibly Helpful, but Take at a Different Time of Day

Long-term use of penicillamine can cause zinc deficiency. However, zinc can impair penicillamine absorption, so persons should not take zinc supplements during the two hours before or after taking penicillamine.

IRON

Effect: Take at a Different Time of Day

Penicillamine attaches to the mineral iron, which impairs the absorption of both substances. Persons who need iron supplements should not take them during the two hours before or after taking penicillamine.

EBSCO CAM Review Board

FURTHER READING

Campbell, N. R., and B. B. Hasinoff. "Iron Supplements: A Common Cause of Drug Interactions." *British Journal of Clinical Pharmacology* 31, no. 3 (1991): 251-255.

Pronsky, Z. M., and J. P. Crowe. *Food Medication Interactions.* 16th ed. Birchrunville, Pa.: Food-Medication Interactions, 2010.

See also: Copper; Food and Drug Administration; Iron; Supplements: Introduction; Vitamin B_6; Zinc.

Pennyroyal

CATEGORY: Herbs and supplements
RELATED TERMS: *Hedeoma pulegioides, Mentha pulegium*
DEFINITION: Natural plant product used to treat specific health conditions.
PRINCIPAL PROPOSED USES: None recommended

OVERVIEW

The name pennyroyal refers to two related plants: *Mentha pulegium* (European pennyroyal) and *Hedeoma pulegioides* (American pennyroyal). Pennyroyal is a member of the mint family. Applied topically, pennyroyal has been used since the time of ancient Greece to repel fleas and other insects. Pennyroyal has been taken internally in Europe and North America for a variety of conditions, including colds and influenza, coughs, kidney problems, headache, and upset stomach, as well as to induce abortion. Traditional herbalists do not appear to have noticed an essential fact about pennyroyal: It is toxic to the liver. In modern times, people have died as a consequence of using this herb according to traditional indications.

The essential oil of pennyroyal contains a substance called pulegone. In the body, pulegone is converted to the toxic chemical menthofuran. Low levels of menthofuran may not produce any untoward effects. At a certain point, however, depending on the individual, menthofuran poisons the nervous system, causing symptoms such as dizziness, vertigo, hallucinations, seizures, and possibly unconsciousness. Liver damage, possibly leading to liver failure, occurs subsequently.

Because of these safety risks and the fact that pennyroyal has not been proven effective for a single medical use, this herb should be avoided entirely. It is

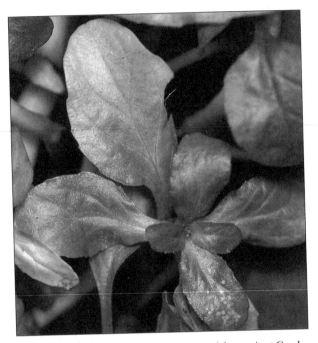

Pennyroyal has been used since the time of the ancient Greeks, but it can have severe side effects. (Jeanne White/Photo Researchers, Inc.)

not even recommended for use topically as an insect repellant, because it is possible that enough pulegone could be absorbed to cause harm.

EBSCO CAM Review Board

FURTHER READING

Anderson, I. B., et al. "Pennyroyal Toxicity: Measurement of Toxic Metabolite Levels in Two Cases and Review of the Literature." *Annals of Internal Medicine* 124 (1996): 726-734.

See also: Herbal medicine.

Pentoxifylline

CATEGORY: Drug interactions
DEFINITION: A drug that makes the blood less "sticky" and is used to increase blood circulation.
INTERACTIONS: Chondroitin, garlic, ginkgo, herbs and supplements, PC-SPES, policosanol, reishi, vinpocetine, white willow
TRADE NAME: Trental

CHONDROITIN

Effect: Possible Harmful Interaction

Based on chondroitin's chemical similarity to the anticoagulant drug heparin, it has been suggested that chondroitin might have anticoagulant effects as well. There are no case reports of any problems relating to this, and studies suggest that chondroitin has at most a mild anticoagulant effect. Nonetheless, chondroitin should not be combined with pentoxifylline except under physician supervision.

GARLIC, GINKGO

Effect: Possible Harmful Interaction

The herb garlic (*Allium sativum*) is taken to lower cholesterol, among many other proposed uses. One of the possible side effects of garlic is an increased tendency to bleed. Therefore, one should not combine garlic and pentoxifylline except under medical supervision. The herb ginkgo (*Ginkgo biloba*) has been used to treat Alzheimer's disease and ordinary age-related memory loss, among many other uses. Ginkgo appears to reduce the ability of platelets (blood-clotting cells) to stick together. Several case reports suggest that this blood-thinning effect of ginkgo may be associated with an increased risk of serious abnormal bleeding episodes in persons taking the herb.

Because of these risks, one should not combine ginkgo and pentoxifylline without physician supervision.

PC-SPES

Effect: Possible Harmful Interaction

PC-SPES is an herbal combination that once showed promise for the treatment of prostate cancer. One case report suggests that PC-SPES might increase risk of bleeding complications if combined with blood-thinning medications. Subsequent evidence has indicated that PC-SPES contains the strong prescription blood-thinner warfarin (Coumadin), making this interaction inevitable.

POLICOSANOL

Effect: Possible Harmful Interaction

The supplement policosanal is used to reduce cholesterol levels. It also interferes with platelet clumping, creating a risk of interactions with blood-thinning drugs.

For example, a thirty-day, double-blind, placebo-controlled trial of twenty-seven persons with high cholesterol levels found that policosanol at 10 milligrams (mg) daily markedly reduced the ability of blood platelets to clump together. Another double-blind placebo-controlled study of thirty-seven healthy volunteers found evidence that the blood-thinning effect of policosanol increased as the dose was increased: the larger the policosanol dose, the greater the effect. However, another double-blind placebo-controlled study of forty-three healthy volunteers compared the effects of policosanol (20 mg daily), the blood-thinner aspirin (100 mg daily), and policosanol and aspirin combined at these same doses. The results again showed that policosanol substantially reduced the ability of blood platelets to stick together and that the combined therapy exhibited additive effects. Based on these findings, one should not combine pentoxifylline and policosanol except under medical supervision.

REISHI

Effect: Possible Harmful Interaction

One study suggests that reishi impairs platelet clumping. This creates the potential for an interaction with any blood-thinning medication.

VINPOCETINE

Effect: Possible Harmful Interaction

The substance vinpocetine is sold as a dietary supplement for the treatment of age-related memory loss and impaired mental function. Vinpocetine is thought to inhibit blood platelets from forming clots. For this reason, it should not be combined with medications or natural substances that impair the blood's ability to clot normally, as this may lead to excessive bleeding. One study found only a minimal interaction between the blood-thinning drug warfarin (Coumadin) and vinpocetine, so one should use caution.

WHITE WILLOW

Effect: Possible Harmful Interaction

The herb white willow (*Salix alba*), also known as willow bark, is used to treat pain and fever. White willow contains a substance that is converted by the body into a salicylate similar to the blood thinner aspirin. For this reason, white willow might add to the effects of pentoxifylline, possibly thinning the blood too much. It may be advisable to avoid white willow while taking pentoxifylline, except under medical supervision.

HERBS AND SUPPLEMENTS

Effect: Possible Harmful Interaction

Herbs and supplements that impair the blood's ability to coagulate (clot) might add to the effects of pentoxifylline, possibly increasing the risk of excessive bleeding. This includes most prominently vitamin E.

Numerous other substances could conceivably present this risk, including mesoglycan, bromelain (from the fruit and stem of pineapple, *Ananas comosus*), chamomile (*Matricaria recutita*), *Coleus forskohlii*, danshen (*Salvia miltorrhiza*), dong quai (*Angelica sinensis*), feverfew (*Tanacetum parthenium*), fish oil, ginger (*Zingiber officinale*), horse chestnut (*Aesculus hippocastanum*), OPC's (oligomeric proanthocyanidins), papaya (*Carica papaya*), and red clover (*Trifolium pratense*).

EBSCO CAM Review Board

FURTHER READING

Rosenblatt, M., and J. Mindel. "Spontaneous Hyphema Associated with Ingestion of *Ginkgo biloba* Extract." *New England Journal of Medicine* 336 (1997): 1108.

Rowin, J., and S. L. Lewis. "Spontaneous Bilateral Subdural Hematomas with Chronic *Ginkgo biloba* Ingestion." *Neurology* 46 (1996): 1775-1776.

Vale, S. "Subarachnoid Hemorrhage Associated with *Ginkgo biloba*." *The Lancet* 35 (1998): 36.

Weinrobe, M. C., and B. Montgomery. "Acquired Bleeding Diathesis in a Patient Taking PC-SPES." *New England Journal of Medicine* 345 (2001): 1213-1214.

See also: Chondroitin; Food and Drug Administration; Garlic; Ginkgo; PC-SPES; Policosanol; Reishi; Supplements: Introduction; Vinpocetine; White Willow.

Peppermint

CATEGORY: Herbs and supplements
RELATED TERM: *Mentha piperita*
DEFINITION: Natural plant product used to treat specific health conditions.
PRINCIPAL PROPOSED USES: Dyspepsia, irritable bowel syndrome, other forms of spasms in the digestive tract
OTHER PROPOSED USES
• *Inhaled:* Nausea, respiratory congestion

- **Topical:** Breast-feeding support, tension headache
- **Oral:** Gallstones

OVERVIEW

Peppermint is a relative of numerous wild mint plants, deliberately bred in the late seventeenth century in England to become the delightful-tasting plant so well known today. It is widely used as a beverage tea and as a flavoring or scent in a wide variety of products.

Peppermint tea also has a long history of medicinal use, primarily as a digestive aid and for the symptomatic treatment of cough, colds, and fever. Peppermint oil is used for chest congestion (Vicks VapoRub), as a local anesthetic (Solarcaine, Ben-Gay), and most recently in the treatment of irritable bowel disease, also known as spastic colon.

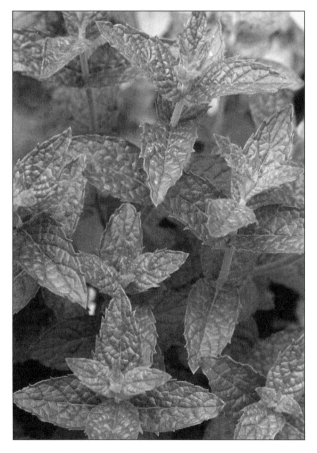

Peppermint tea and oil have both been used medicinally. (Adrian Thomas/Photo Researchers, Inc.)

THERAPEUTIC DOSAGES

The proper dosage of peppermint oil when treating irritable bowel syndrome is 0.2 to 0.4 milliliter (ml) three times a day of an enteric-coated capsule. The capsule has to be enteric-coated to prevent stomach distress. When used in herbal combinations to treat stomach problems, peppermint oil is taken at lower doses, and it is not enteric-coated.

THERAPEUTIC USES

Peppermint oil has shown promise for a variety of conditions that involve spasm of the intestinal tract. Most studies have involved irritable bowel syndrome (IBS), for which peppermint oil has shown considerable promise. Peppermint oil may also be helpful for reducing the pain caused by medical examinations of the colon and stomach, as well for decreasing the intestinal gas pain that frequently follows surgery. Peppermint oil may also be helpful for dyspepsia (a condition that is similar to IBS but involves the stomach instead of the intestines). Weak evidence, far too preliminary to rely upon, hints that peppermint oil might help dissolve gallstones.

Peppermint oil is also used in another way: as aromatherapy. This means that it is inhaled, often by adding it to a humidifier. Weak evidence hints that inhaled peppermint oil might be helpful for relief of mucus congestion of the lungs and sinuses. Even weaker evidence hints that inhaled peppermint oil might relieve postsurgical nausea. Similarly weak evidence hints that peppermint oil, applied to the forehead, might relieve tension headaches. Finally, a study performed in Iran reported that applying peppermint water (essentially, lukewarm peppermint tea) directly to the nipples helped prevent dryness and cracking caused by breast-feeding.

SCIENTIFIC EVIDENCE

Irritable bowel syndrome (IBS). There have been numerous studies of peppermint oil for IBS. In one of the larger studies, 110 people with IBS were given either enteric-coated peppermint oil (187 milligrams, or mg) or a placebo three to four times daily, fifteen to thirty minutes before meals, for four weeks. The results showed significant improvements in abdominal pain, bloating, stool frequency, and flatulence. In a similar study, people who took peppermint oil capsules for eight weeks also had less abdominal pain and discomfort compared with the placebo group.

Not all of these studies have shown that peppermint oil is beneficial, though. It has been suggested that these inconsistencies were caused by the accidental inclusion of people who had conditions unrelated to IBS that cause similar symptoms. Presumably, peppermint oil may be less effective for these problems. A study published in 2007 pretested participants for lactose intolerance and celiac disease, the two conditions most easily mistaken for IBS. A total of fifty-seven people with IBS symptoms and no evidence of the other two problems were enrolled in the study. Over a period of four weeks, participants were given either a placebo or peppermint oil. At the end of the study period, 75 percent of the patients in the peppermint oil group showed a marked reduction of IBS symptoms (defined, for this purpose, as a reduction of IBS symptom scores by more than 50 percent). In comparison, only 38 percent of the participants given a placebo showed an improvement of this magnitude, and this difference was statistically significant.

Other forms of spasm in the digestive tract. A barium enema involves introducing a solution containing the metal barium into the lower intestines. It commonly causes intestinal pain and spasm. A double-blind study of 141 individuals found that adding peppermint oil to the barium reduced the severity of intestinal spasm that occurred. Benefits were also seen in a large study conducted by different researchers. Another study found that peppermint oil reduced spasm in the stomach during a procedure called upper endoscopy. One study found that use of peppermint oil after C-section surgery reduced discomfort caused by intestinal gas.

Dyspepsia (minor indigestion). Peppermint oil is often used in combination with other essential oils to treat minor indigestion. For example, a double-blind, placebo-controlled study including thirty-nine individuals found that an enteric-coated peppermint-caraway oil combination taken three times daily for four weeks significantly reduced dyspepsia pain compared with placebo. Of the treatment group, 63.2 percent was free of pain after four weeks, compared with 25 percent of the placebo group.

Results from a double-blind, comparative study including 118 individuals suggest that the combination of peppermint and caraway oil is comparably effective to the no-longer-available drug cisapride. After four weeks, the herbal combination reduced dyspepsia

---

Peppermint Oil for Irritable Bowel Syndrome

Peppermint oil has shown promise as a treatment for irritable bowel syndrome (IBS). Peppermint contains menthol, a substance that relaxes the muscles of the small intestine. A number of studies have found that a special formulation of peppermint oil (enteric-coated, which is designed to open up only once the capsule has passed out of the stomach) can relieve symptoms. However, other studies of peppermint oil for IBS have failed to find benefit; the evidence has been sufficiently contradictory to keep the effectiveness of peppermint oil an open question.

It has been suggested that the inconsistencies seen in previous studies were caused by the accidental inclusion of people who had conditions that are unrelated to IBS but cause similar symptoms. Presumably, peppermint oil may be less effective for these conditions.

A study published in 2007 attempted to correct this problem by pretesting participants for the two conditions most easily mistaken for IBS: lactose intolerance and celiac disease. Fifty-seven people with IBS symptoms and evidence that they were free of the other two conditions were enrolled in the study. Over a period of four weeks, participants were given either placebo or peppermint oil.

At the end of the study period, 75 percent of the participants in the peppermint oil group showed a marked improvement in IBS symptoms. ("Marked improvement" was defined as a reduction of IBS symptom scores by more than 50 percent). In comparison, only 38 percent of the participants given placebo showed an improvement of this magnitude. The difference between these outcomes was statistically significant.

Steven Bratman, M.D.

---

pain by 69.7 percent, whereas the conventional treatment reduced pain by 70.2 percent.

A preparation of peppermint, caraway, fennel, and wormwood oils was compared with the drug metoclopramide in another double-blind study enrolling sixty individuals. After seven days, 43.3 percent of the treatment group was pain free compared with 13.3 percent of the metoclopramide group. Metoclopramide works by reducing gastric emptying time (in other words, speeding the passage of food from the stomach into the intestines). Interestingly, some evidence suggests that peppermint oil may have the same effect.

SAFETY ISSUES

At the normal dosage, enteric-coated peppermint oil is believed to be reasonably safe in healthy adults. However, case reports and one study in rats hint that peppermint might reduce male fertility. The species *Mentha spicata* may be more problematic in this regard than the more common *M. piperita*. Excessive doses of peppermint oil can be toxic, causing kidney failure and even death. Very high intake of peppermint oil can also cause nausea, loss of appetite, heart problems, loss of balance, and other nervous system problems. Safety in young children, pregnant or nursing women, and those with severe liver or kidney disease has not been established. In particular, peppermint can cause jaundice in newborn babies, so it should not be used for colic.

Use of peppermint oil may increase levels of the drug cyclosporine in the body. Persons taking cyclosporine who wish to take peppermint oil should notify their physician in advance, so that their blood levels of cyclosporine can be monitored and their dose adjusted if necessary. Conversely, those persons already taking both peppermint oil and cyclosporine should not stop taking the peppermint without informing their physicians. Ceasing to take peppermint may cause cyclosporine levels to fall.

IMPORTANT INTERACTIONS

Those taking cyclosporine should not use peppermint oil (or stop using it) except in consultation with a physician.

EBSCO CAM Review Board

FURTHER READING

Cappello, G., et al. "Peppermint Oil (Mintoil) in the Treatment of Irritable Bowel Syndrome." *Digestive Liver Disease* 39, no. 6 (2007): 530-536.

Ford, A. C., et al. "Effect of Fibre, Antispasmodics, and Peppermint Oil in the Treatment of Irritable Bowel Syndrome." *British Medical Journal* 337 (2008) a2313.

Inamori, M., et al. "Early Effects of Peppermint Oil on Gastric Emptying: A Crossover Study Using a Continuous Real-Time (13)c · Breath Test (BreathID System)." *Journal of Gastroenterology* 42 (2007): 539-542.

Merat, S., et al. "The Effect of Enteric-Coated, Delayed-Release Peppermint Oil on Irritable Bowel Syndrome." *Digestive Diseases and Sciences* 55, no. 5 (2010): 1385-1390.

Sayyah, Melli M., et al. "Effect of Peppermint Water on Prevention of Nipple Cracks in Lactating Primiparous Women." *International Breastfeeding Journal* 2 (2007): 7.

See also: Caraway; Cyclosporine; Diarrhea; Dyspepsia; Gastrointestinal health; Herbal medicine; Irritable bowel syndrome (IBS); Wormwood.

Peptic ulcer disease: Homeopathic treatment

CATEGORY: Therapies and techniques
RELATED TERMS: *Helicobacter pylori*, homeopathic remedies, miasm
DEFINITION: Treatment of peptic ulcer disease with homeopathic remedies.

OVERVIEW

Peptic ulcer disease (PUD) manifests as open sores in the lining of the esophagus, stomach, or duodenum (upper intestine). The most common symptom is abdominal pain. Persons with PUD may also vomit blood or experience bloody (dark, tarry) stools. Appetite changes are common, as is weight loss.

Homeopathic practitioners use a variety of remedies (homeopathic medications) to treat PUD. Randomized-controlled trials have shown the effectiveness of homeopathic treatment for a number of gastrointestinal conditions, but no such studies have examined the efficacy of homeopathic treatment for peptic ulcers.

CAUSAL FACTORS

A number of immediate causes of PUD have been determined. First, the bacterium *Helicobacter pylori* is found in the stomach and intestines of most people with peptic ulcers. *H. pylori* reduces the resistance of the protective lining of the esophagus, stomach, and upper intestine to digestive acid, and sores result. In many people, however, the bacterium does not cause problems. *H. pylori* appears to be a necessary but not sufficient variable in understanding the origins of many cases of PUD. Medications, including overuse

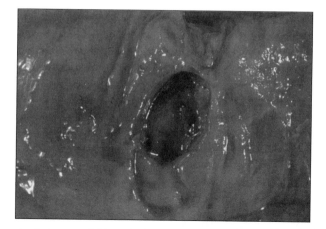

At the center of this excised portion of the human stomach is a bleeding peptic ulcer. (Dr. E. Walker/Photo Researchers, Inc.)

of nonsteroidal anti-inflammatory drugs such as aspirin, ibuprofen, and other pain relief drugs, are a second cause of PUD. In addition, persons with the disease often have a family history of PUD.

Homeopaths recognize these causes of peptic ulcers. Homeopathic theory also seeks to elucidate the underlying reasons why some people have a susceptibility to ulcer development, while others do not. As noted, many people infected by *H. pylori* do not develop peptic ulcers. Samuel Hahnemann, who founded homeopathy in the eighteenth century, theorized that people have inherited disease tendencies, which he called miasms. Ancestors experienced diseases that affect the genetic inheritance of their descendants. The descendants do not necessarily inherit the actual disease; instead, they have tendencies toward certain types of symptoms when the body is weakened by stress or poor environmental conditions, or both. Persons who develop peptic ulcers, for example, might have inherited what Hahnemann called the syphilitic miasm. Persons with this miasm tend to develop ulcerations of various types and tissue abnormalities that can lead to hemorrhages, among other symptoms. Peptic ulcers are only one of a number of specific conditions they might develop.

Current understanding of genetic mutations supports Hahnemann's general theory. Diseases can cause genetic mutations that are passed to descendants. Not all homeopaths believe miasmatic theory, but they do agree that peptic ulcers will develop when

the body's defenses are weakened by stress and environmental influences and when such a person is unable to reestablish homeostasis.

TREATMENTS AND REMEDIES

Homeopathy is a holistic healing modality. It is concerned with treating the whole person. Most persons with PUD will be experiencing symptoms or have other diseases; the classical homeopath will seek to find a remedy that covers all of the person's symptoms. For example, a person might have severe headaches and PUD. The homeopath will choose (from the many existing remedies) the remedy that covers as many symptoms as possible. Treatment is thus individuated.

Miasmic theory might help a homeopath determine the best remedy, which is thought to stimulate the body to heal itself and to return it to homeostasis. Homeopathic remedies come from many sources, including plants, minerals, and animal substances. Four remedies are commonly used for peptic ulcers. Also listed here are the specific symptoms and modalities that might indicate these remedies.

Argentum nitricum is used to treat ulceration of the intestines or stomach that is accompanied by the vomiting of blood. *Kali bichromatum* is used to treat intestinal ulceration accompanied by chronic diarrhea. Lachesis is used to treat gastric ulceration in persons who feel worse when they wake up in the morning. Pulsatilla is used to treat gastric ulceration in persons who cannot tolerate eating much fat and who feel better in the open air.

RESEARCH STUDIES

Though homeopaths regularly treat peptic ulcers and claim clinical success, the effectiveness of homeopathy in treating PUD has not been established by randomized-controlled trials (RCTs). RCTs have demonstrated the efficacy of homeopathy for a number of conditions. Though many of the studies have methodological flaws, the quality scores of the studies are similar to those found for biomedical treatments of disease. RCTs have indicated that homeopathy can successfully address a variety of gastrointestinal problems, including diarrhea, gallbladder disease, and irritable bowel syndrome.

A small pilot study of sixty persons with dyspepsia (only four of whom had been diagnosed with PUD) found that the control group (which received standard gastrointestinal treatment) and the homeopathy and acupuncture groups all showed improvement after six months, then reached a plateau. Statistical analysis showed no significant differences in outcomes between groups. RCTs specifically examining the effectiveness of homeopathic remedies in treating peptic ulcers are needed. Homeopathic studies are easily double-blinded, but the individuated nature of treatment requires that the remedies used vary according to the symptoms of the person with PUD.

Roxanne Friedenfels, Ph.D.

FURTHER READING

Holcombe, C. "*Helicobacter pylori*: The African Enigma." *Gut* 33 (1992): 429-431. Review of evidence showing high rates, in Africa, of *H. pylori* infection but low incidence of gastric ulcers.

Koretz, Ronald, and Michael Rotblatt. "Complementary and Alternative Medicine in Gastroenterology: The Good, the Bad, and the Ugly. " *Clinical Gastroenterology and Hepatology* 2 (2004): 957-967. Peer-reviewed article summarizing CAM treatments of gastrointestinal conditions. Also looks at RCTs of homeopathy.

Paterson, Charlotte, et al. "Treating Dyspepsia with Acupuncture and Homeopathy: Reflections on a Pilot Study by Researchers, Practitioners, and Participants." *Complementary Therapies in Medicine* 11 (2003): 78-84. Peer-reviewed pilot study showing similar efficacy of conventional treatment, acupuncture, and homeopathy after six months of treatment.

Ullman, Dana. *Discovering Homeopathy*. Berkeley, Calif.: North Atlantic Books, 1991. A homeopathic practitioner gives an overview of homeopathic history, theory, and treatment of acute and chronic disease.

See also: Dyspepsia; Gastroesophageal reflux disease; Gastrointestinal health; Homeopathy; Ulcers.

Perilla frutescens

CATEGORY: Herbs and supplements
RELATED TERMS: Chinese basil, rosmarinic acid
DEFINITION: Natural plant product used to treat specific health conditions.
PRINCIPAL PROPOSED USE: Allergic rhinitis (hay fever)
OTHER PROPOSED USES: Depression, rheumatoid arthritis

OVERVIEW

A member of the mint family, perilla is used in a variety of Asian foods to add both flavor and color. It is also grown ornamentally in gardens. The stem of the plant is used in Chinese medicine for treatment of morning sickness. The leaves are said to be helpful for asthma, colds and flu, and other lung problems.

THERAPEUTIC DOSAGES

A typical dosage of perilla should supply 50 to 200 milligrams (mg) of rosmarinic acid daily. Perilla also contains luteolin, a substance that may also have anti-allergic actions. For this reason, perilla products are often enriched with luteolin as well, typically providing 5 to 10 mg daily.

THERAPEUTIC USES

Extracts of perilla have undergone study as a treatment for allergic rhinitis (hay fever). Perilla contains high levels of the substance rosmarinic acid (also found in the herb rosemary and many other plants). Rosmarinic acid appears to have anti-inflammatory and antiallergic actions. In a three-week double-blind, placebo-controlled study of twenty-nine people with seasonal allergic rhinitis, participants were given one of three treatments: a placebo, *Perilla frutescens* extract enriched to contain 50 mg of rosmarinic acid, or an extract enhanced to contain 200 mg of rosmarinic acid. The results showed that both perilla products reduced symptoms to a greater extent than a placebo.

Animal studies hint that perilla might also be useful for a different type of allergy: the severe, rapid reaction known as anaphylaxis, commonly associated with shellfish, peanut, and bee sting allergies. Weak evidence suggests that rosmarinic acid, perilla, or both may have anticancer effects and might also have benefits for rheumatoid arthritis and other autoimmune diseases, as well as for depression.

SAFETY ISSUES

In the small clinical trials and animal studies conducted thus far, the use of perilla or rosmarinic acid (or both) has not been associated with significant adverse effects. Because of the wide use of perilla in Asian cooking and of the prevalence of rosmarinic acid in many spices, these substances are assumed to have a relatively high level of safety. However, comprehensive safety testing has not been reported. Safety in young children, pregnant or nursing women, and people with severe liver or kidney disease has not been established.

EBSCO CAM Review Board

FURTHER READING

Makino, T., et al. "Anti-allergic Effect of *Perilla frutescens* and Its Active Constituents." *Phytotherapy Research* 17 (2003): 240-243.

Osakabe, N., H. Takano, et al. "Anti-inflammatory and Anti-allergic Effect of Rosmarinic Acid (RA): Inhibition of Seasonal Allergic Rhinoconjunctivitis (SAR) and Its Mechanism." *Biofactors* 21 (2005): 127-131.

Osakabe, N., A. Yasuda, et al. "Rosmarinic Acid Inhibits Epidermal Inflammatory Responses: Anticarcinogenic Effect of *Perilla frutescens* Extract in the Murine Two-Stage Skin Model." *Carcinogenesis* 25 (2004): 549-557.

Renzulli, C., et al. "Effects of Rosmarinic Acid Against Aflatoxin B1 and Ochratoxin-A-Induced Cell Damage in a Human Hepatoma Cell Line (Hep G2)." *Journal of Applied Toxicology* 24 (2004): 289-296.

Takano, H., et al. "Extract of *Perilla frutescens* Enriched for Rosmarinic Acid, a Polyphenolic Phytochemical, Inhibits Seasonal Allergic Rhinoconjunctivitis in Humans." *Experimental Biology and Medicine* 229 (2004): 247-254.

Ueda, H., and C. Yamazaki. "Luteolin as an Anti-inflammatory and Antiallergic Constituent of *Perilla frutescens*." *Biological and Pharmaceutical Bulletin* 25 (2002): 1197-1202.

Youn, J., et al. "Beneficial Effects of Rosmarinic Acid on Suppression of Collagen Induced Arthritis." *Journal of Rheumatology* 30 (2003): 1203-1207.

See also: Herbal medicine; Rosemary.

Periodontal disease

CATEGORY: Condition

RELATED TERMS: Gingivitis, gum disease

DEFINITION: Treatment of gum inflammation that can progress to pockets of infection, bone loss, and loosening of the teeth.

PRINCIPAL PROPOSED NATURAL TREATMENTS: None

OTHER PROPOSED NATURAL TREATMENTS: Beta-glucan, bloodroot, calcium, caraway, coenzyme Q_{10}, cranberry juice, essential oil mouthwash, eucalyptus, folate mouthwash, gamma-linolenic acid, green tea chew candy, herbal mouthwash containing chamomile, echinacea, hops, myrrh, mint, sage, and ratania, honey leather, lycopene, magnesium, mangosteen, oligomeric proanthocyanidins, *Macleya cordata* (plume poppy) and *Prunella vulgaris*, propolis, sea cucumber, tea tree oil, vitamin B_{12}, vitamin C, witch hazel, xylitol, zinc

INTRODUCTION

Periodontal disease begins with gum inflammation and progresses to pockets of infection, bone loss, and loosening of the teeth. It is present in 90 percent of people older than age sixty-five years.

Conventional prevention and treatment include regular flossing, using mouthwash that contains extracts of the herb thyme (such as thymol, which is found in Listerine), and using special tooth-brushing appliances. If the condition becomes advanced, special deep-cleaning techniques and even surgery may be necessary.

PROPOSED NATURAL TREATMENTS

According to one small, double-blind, placebo-controlled study, the supplement lycopene, taken at a dose of 8 milligrams (mg) per day, may be helpful for the treatment of periodontal disease, whether taken alone or used to augment the effectiveness of standard treatment. A double-blind study of eighty-nine people tested a European herbal mouthwash (used with a special gum irrigator) containing chamomile, echinacea, myrrh, mint, sage, and ratania. The herbal preparation proved more effective than a conventional mouthwash at reducing gingival inflammation.

Oligomeric proanthocyanidins (OPCs) have antioxidant and anti-inflammatory properties. A fourteen-day, double-blind, placebo-controlled trial of forty people evaluated the potential benefits of a chewing-gum product containing 5 mg of OPCs from pine bark. The use of the OPC gum resulted in significant improvements in gum health and reductions in plaque formation; no similar benefits were seen in the placebo group.

A double-blind study of thirty people found weak evidence that the use of borage oil (a source of gamma-linolenic acid) at a dose of 3,000 mg daily may reduce gingival inflammation. The study also

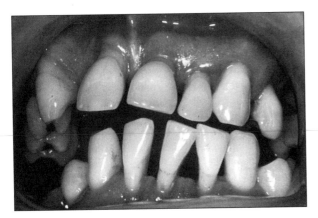

A patient suffering from chronic periodontal disease. (Bio-photo Associates/Getty Images)

examined fish oil at a dose of 3,000 mg daily, or combined fish oil and borage oil at a dose of 1,500 mg each, but failed to find significant benefits with these treatments compared with placebo.

Other natural dental products that have shown promise in small double-blind studies include a toothpaste containing *Macleya cordata* (plume poppy) and *Prunella vulgaris* (also known as heal-all or self-heal), a chew candy containing green tea, an irrigation fluid containing propolis extract, a toothpaste containing sea cucumber, and a gel containing tea tree oil.

Preliminary studies suggest that folate mouthwash may help in periodontal disease. Oral folate supplementation does not appear to be especially effective. However, one small double-blind study found potential benefit with a mixed vitamin-B complex supplement (containing 50 mg of each of thiamin, riboflavin, niacinamide, pantothenate, and pyridoxine; 50 micrograms [mcg] each of biotin and vitamin B_{12}; and 400 mcg of folate).

One test-tube study suggests that cranberry juice might be useful for treating or preventing gum disease. However, there is one problem to work out before cranberry could be practical for this purpose: The sweeteners added to cranberry juice are not good for the teeth, but without them cranberry juice is very bitter.

The supplement coenzyme Q_{10} is sometimes claimed to be an effective treatment for periodontal disease. However, the studies on which this idea is based are too flawed to be taken as meaningful.

Xylitol is a naturally occurring sugar that appears to help suppress the development of cavities when it is used in gum, candy, or toothpaste. Preliminary evidence suggests that it may help prevent gum disease too.

A thorough review of eleven randomized-controlled trials found that the use of mouth rinses containing essential oils is effective against gingivitis and dental plaque formation when used in combination with regular oral hygiene. In one double-blind study, chewing gum containing eucalyptus extract was more beneficial for moderate gingivitis compared with a placebo gum.

One study suggests that chewing honey leather can reduce inflammation of the gums. A special extract of the hops, called hops bract polyphenols, has shown some promise for preventing or treating periodontal disease. A study failed to find that an herbal mouthwash containing the herb mangosteen significantly improved gum health. Other treatments that are sometimes proposed for periodontal disease, but lack meaningful scientific support, include beta-glucan, bioflavonoids, bloodroot, calcium, caraway, magnesium, vitamin C, witch hazel, and zinc.

EBSCO CAM Review Board

FURTHER READING

Chandra, R. V., et al. "Efficacy of Lycopene in the Treatment of Gingivitis." *Oral Health and Preventive Dentistry* 5 (2007): 327-336.

Gebaraa, E. C., et al. "Propolis Extract as an Adjuvant to Periodontal Treatment." *Oral Health and Preventive Dentistry* 1 (2005): 29-35.

Nagata, H., et al. "Effect of Eucalyptus Extract Chewing Gum on Periodontal Health." *Journal of Periodontology* 79 (2008): 1378-1385.

Neiva, R. F., et al. "Effects of Vitamin-B Complex Supplementation on Periodontal Wound Healing." *Journal of Periodontology* 76 (2005): 1084-1091.

Patel, R. M., and Z. Malaki. "The Effect of a Mouthrinse Containing Essential Oils on Dental Plaque and Gingivitis." *Evidence-Based Dentistry* 9 (2008): 18-19.

Rassameemasmaung, S., et al. "Effects of Herbal Mouthwash Containing the Pericarp Extract of *Garcinia mangostana* L. on Halitosis, Plaque, and Papillary Bleeding Index." *Journal of the International Academy of Periodontology* 9 (2007): 19-25.

Shinada, K., et al. "Hop Bract Polyphenols Reduced Three-Day Dental Plaque Regrowth." *Journal of Dental Research* 86 (2007): 848-851.

Soukoulis, S., and R. Hirsch. "The Effects of a Tea Tree Oil-Containing Gel on Plaque and Chronic Gingivitis." *Australian Dental Journal* 49 (2004): 78-83.

See also: Bone and joint health; Canker sores; Cavity prevention.

Peyronie's disease

CATEGORY: Condition
DEFINITION: Treatment of the condition in which a thickened, hardened piece of tissue forms on one side of the penis.
PRINCIPAL PROPOSED NATURAL TREATMENTS: Acetyl-L-carnitine, para-aminobenzoic acid
OTHER PROPOSED NATURAL TREATMENTS: Gotu kola, vitamin E

INTRODUCTION

Peyronie's disease is a condition in which a plaque (a thickened, hardened piece of tissue) forms on one side of the penis. If the plaque becomes large enough, it reduces flexibility of the penis. During erection, the less flexible part of the penis expands to a lesser extent, causing the penis to bend. Pain also may occur. Severe curvature of the penis can make intercourse difficult or even impossible.

The cause of Peyronie's disease is unknown, but it may involve injury to the penis that causes local bleeding, which in turn leads to the formation of fibrous tissue. However, the majority of cases occur without any obvious preceding injury.

Men with Peyronie's disease may have a generalized tendency to form fibrous tissue, as shown by a higher-than-average incidence of Dupuytren's contracture (a condition in which fibrous tissue develops in the hands among men with Peyronie's). The condition also appears to be partially heritable.

Treatment of Peyronie's disease consists first and foremost of watchful waiting. In many cases, the disease never becomes severe enough to cause serious difficulty. Pain on erection generally decreases with time, and in some cases the extent of curvature also decreases.

When the condition is too severe to ignore, a variety of methods may be tried, including injection of various drugs into the fibrous plaque, the use of radiation therapy, and surgery. Of all these, only surgery is widely accepted as effective. However, because surgery can cause complications, such as shortening of the penis, it is usually reserved for serious cases.

PRINCIPAL PROPOSED NATURAL TREATMENTS

Acetyl-L-carnitine. L-carnitine is an amino acid the body uses to turn fat into energy. It is not usually considered a nutrient because the body can manufacture all it needs. Two forms of L-carnitine, acetyl-L-carnitine and propionyl-L-carnitine, have been tried as treatments for Peyronie's disease.

A three-month double-blind study compared the effectiveness of acetyl-L-carnitine to the drug tamoxifen in forty-eight men with Peyronie's disease. Acetyl-L-carnitine (at a dose of 1 gram [g] daily) reduced penile curvature, while tamoxifen did not. In addition, the supplement reduced pain and slowed disease progression to a greater extent than tamoxifen.

Another study evaluated the potential benefits of combination therapy with propionyl-L-carnitine and an injected medication (verapamil). In this trial, sixty men with severe Peyronie's disease were given verapamil injections plus three months of treatment with either propionyl-L-carnitine (2 g per day) or tamoxifen. The use of propionyl-L-carnitine plus verapamil significantly reduced penile curvature, plaque size, and the need for surgery, while tamoxifen plus verapamil had little effect. These studies remain preliminary, but their results are definitely encouraging.

Paraminobenzoic acid. Para-aminobenzoic acid (PABA) has been suggested for a variety of diseases, including Peyronie's disease, in which abnormal fibrous tissue is involved. However, there has been only one reported double-blind study. This trial enrolled 103 men with Peyronie's disease and followed them for one year. The results showed that the use of PABA at a dose of 3 g taken four times daily significantly slowed the progression of Peyronie's disease; it did not, however, reduce preexisting plaque.

OTHER PROPOSED NATURAL TREATMENTS

Vitamin E also has been advocated for the treatment of Peyronie's disease and for the related condition Dupuytren's contracture, but there is no meaningful evidence that it is effective. The herb gotu kola is used to treat various conditions in which fibrous scar tissue causes problems, and for that reason it has been advocated for Peyronie's disease. However, there is no meaningful evidence that it is effective.

HERBS AND SUPPLEMENTS TO USE WITH CAUTION

Various herbs and supplements may interact adversely with drugs used to treat Peyronie's disease, so one should consult a doctor before using any herb or supplement.

EBSCO CAM Review Board

FURTHER READING

Biagiotti, G., and G. Cavallini. "Acetyl-L-Carnitine vs Tamoxifen in the Oral Therapy of Peyronie's Disease." *BJU International* 88 (2001): 63-67.

Cavallini, G., et al. "Oral Propionyl-L-Carnitine and Intraplaque Verapamil in the Therapy of Advanced and Resistant Peyronie's Disease." *BJU International* 89 (2002): 895-900.

Weidner, W., et al. "Potassium Paraaminobenzoate (PO-TABA) in the Treatment of Peyronie's Disease." *European Urology* 47 (2005): 530-536.

See also: Carnitine; Dupuytren's contracture; Men's health; PABA (para-aminobenzoic acid); Prostatitis; Scar tissue; Soft tissue pain; Warts.

Phaseolus vulgaris

CATEGORY: Herbs and supplements
RELATED TERMS: Carbohydrate blocker, starch blocker
DEFINITION: Natural plant product used to treat specific health conditions.
PRINCIPAL PROPOSED USE: Weight loss

OVERVIEW

Supplements made from white kidney beans (*Phaseolus vulgaris*) are sold as starch blockers, supplements said to interfere with the digestion of carbohydrates and thereby promote weight loss.

THERAPEUTIC DOSAGES

The recommended dose of starch blockers, or amylase inhibitors, varies among products. Label instructions regarding dosage should be followed.

THERAPEUTIC USES

Technically, starch blockers are amylase inhibitors. Amylase is one of the main enzymes the body uses to digest starch. In theory, when amylase is blocked, ingested starch can pass through the body undigested, contributing no calories. However, theory is one thing, reality another. Most studies of amylase inhibitors have generally failed to find them effective.

Several possible reasons for this discrepancy have been proposed, such as that the amylase inhibitor may be broken down in the stomach, the product may supply enough of its own amylase to counteract any benefit, and another enzyme, glucoamylase, may be able to take over when amylase cannot do the job. Whatever the cause, the net results in these studies were poor. Use of amylase inhibitors did not in fact block the digestion of starch. However, according to the manufacturer of a current product, more concentrated extracts of *P. vulgaris*, taken in higher doses, do work. Up until recently, the evidence for this claim rested entirely on unpublished studies that could not be independently verified.

Starch and the Digestive System

Proponents of the use of *Phaseolus vulgaris* for weight loss believe that this white kidney bean can block the digestion of starch by inhibiting amylase, an enzyme that digests starch and, hence, calories. Normally, the digestive system acts in the following way:

The digestive glands that act first are in the mouth—the salivary glands. Saliva produced by these glands contains an enzyme—amylase—that begins to digest the starch from food into smaller molecules. An enzyme is a substance that speeds up chemical reactions in the body.

The digestible carbohydrates—starch and sugar—are broken into simpler molecules by enzymes not only in saliva but also in juice produced by the pancreas and in the lining of the small intestine. Starch is digested in two steps. First, an enzyme in the saliva and pancreatic juice breaks the starch into molecules called maltose. Then an enzyme in the lining of the small intestine splits the maltose into glucose molecules that can be absorbed into the blood. Glucose is carried through the bloodstream to the liver, where it is stored or to provide energy for the work of the body.

In 2007, however, a relevant trial was at last published. In this double-blind, placebo-controlled study, sixty slightly overweight people were given either placebo or a phaseolus extract once daily, thirty minutes before a main meal rich in carbohydrates. Over the thirty days of the study, the results indicated that phaseolus treatment led to a significantly greater reduction of body weight and an improvement of lean-to-fat ratio compared with a placebo. While this is promising, independent confirmation in larger trials will be necessary before phaseolus can be considered a proven weight-loss product. One published study failed to find that use of a phaseolus product reduced the rise in blood sugar that usually follows a meal.

SAFETY ISSUES

On the basis of their widespread presence in commonly consumed foods (beans), amylase inhibitors are believed to be quite safe. One side effect, however, is to be expected: flatulence. It is the amylase inhibitors in beans that are responsible for their notorious gassiness. Maximum safe doses in pregnant or nursing women, young children, and individuals with severe hepatic or renal disease have not been established.

EBSCO CAM Review Board

FURTHER READING

Celleno, L., et al. "A Dietary Supplement Containing Standardized *Phaseolus vulgaris* Extract Influences Body Composition of Overweight Men and Women." *International Journal of Medicine and Science* 4 (2007): 45-52.

Cerovic, A., et al. "The Dry Plant Extract of Common Bean Seed (*Phaseoli vulgari pericarpium*) Does Not Have an Affect on Postprandial Glycemia in Healthy Human Subject." *Bosnian Journal of Basic Medical Science* 6 (2006): 28-33.

See also: Herbal medicine; Obesity and excess weight.

Phenobarbital

CATEGORY: Drug interactions
DEFINITION: Medications used to control seizures.
INTERACTIONS: Biotin, dong quai, folate, ginkgo, glutamine, hops, kava, passionflower, St. John's wort, valerian, vitamin D, vitamin K

TRADE NAMES: Bellatal, Solfoton
RELATED DRUGS: Mebaral, mephobarbital, methylphenobarbital

FOLATE
Effect: Supplementation Possibly Helpful

Phenobarbital can reduce folate levels, perhaps by increasing the rate of breakdown of the vitamin. Over time, such a decrease can cause anemia. Taking folate supplements can correct this anemia. Anticonvulsant-induced folate deficiency might also cause birth defects. Women who plan to become pregnant while on phenobarbital should be sure to take a supplement to prevent deficiency.

VITAMIN D
Effect: Supplementation Possibly Helpful

Phenobarbital appears to interfere with the normal absorption or metabolism of vitamin D. In turn, this can impair calcium absorption. Making sure to get enough vitamin D (and calcium) should help prevent any problems from developing.

VITAMIN K
Effect: Supplementation Helpful for Pregnant Women

Children born to women taking phenobarbital while pregnant may be deficient in vitamin K. This might lead to bleeding disorders and facial bone abnormalities. Supplementing with vitamin K during pregnancy should help; however, physician supervision is recommended.

BIOTIN
Effect: Supplementation Possibly Helpful, but Take at a Different Time of Day

Many antiseizure medications, including phenobarbital, are believed to interfere with the absorption of biotin. For this reason, persons taking phenobarbital may benefit from extra biotin. Biotin should be taken two to three hours apart from antiseizure medication. One should not exceed the recommended daily intake, because it is possible that too much biotin might interfere with the effectiveness of the medication.

DONG QUAI, ST. JOHN'S WORT
Effect: Possible Harmful Interaction

Phenobarbital has been reported to cause increased sensitivity to the sun, amplifying the risk of sunburn or skin rash. Because St. John's wort and dong quai may also cause this problem, taking them during treatment with this drug might add to this risk. One should use sunscreen or wear protective clothing during sun exposure if taking one of these herbs while using this anticonvulsant.

GINKGO

Effect: Possible Harmful Interaction

The herb ginkgo (*Ginkgo biloba*) has been used to treat Alzheimer's disease and ordinary age-related memory loss, among many other conditions. The possible harmful interaction involves potential contaminants in ginkgo, not ginkgo itself.

One study found that a natural nerve toxin present in the seeds of *Ginkgo biloba* made its way into standardized ginkgo extracts prepared from the leaves. This toxin has been associated with convulsions and death in laboratory animals.

The detected amounts of this toxic substance are considered harmless. However, given the lack of satisfactory standardization of herbal formulations in the United States, it is possible that some batches of product might contain higher contents of the toxin, depending on the season of harvest. In light of these findings, taking a ginkgo product that happened to contain significant levels of the nerve toxin might theoretically prevent an anticonvulsant from working as well as expected.

HOPS, KAVA, PASSIONFLOWER, VALERIAN

Effect: Possible Harmful Interaction

The herb kava (*Piper methysticum*) has a sedative effect and is used for anxiety and insomnia. Combining kava with anticonvulsants, which possess similar depressant effects, could result in add-on or excessive physical depression, sedation, and impairment. Because of the potentially serious consequences, one should avoid combining these herbs with anticonvulsants or other drugs that also have sedative or depressant effects, such as phenobarbital, unless advised by a physician.

GLUTAMINE

Effect: Theoretical Harmful Interaction

Because phenobarbital works (at least in part) by blocking glutamate pathways in the brain, high dosages of glutamine might possibly overwhelm the drug and increase the risk of seizures.

EBSCO CAM Review Board

FURTHER READING

Arenz, A., et al. "Occurrence of Neurotoxic 4'-O-Methylpyridoxine in *Ginkgo biloba* Leaves, Ginkgo Medications, and Japanese Ginkgo Food." *Planta Medica* 62 (1996): 548-551.

Cornelissen, M., et al. "Supplementation of Vitamin K in Pregnant Women Receiving Anticonvulsant Therapy Prevents Neonatal Vitamin K Deficiency." *American Journal of Obstetrics and Gynecology* 168 (1993): 884-888.

Kishi, T., et al. "Mechanism for Reduction of Serum Folate by Antiepileptic Drugs During Prolonged Therapy." *Journal of the Neurological Sciences* 145 (1997): 109-112.

Lewis, D. P., et al. "Drug and Environmental Factors Associated with Adverse Pregnancy Outcomes: Part I–Antiepileptic Drugs, Contraceptives, Smoking, and Folate." *Annals of Pharmacotherapy* 32 (1998): 802-817.

See also: Biotin; Dong quai; Epilepsy; Folate; Food and Drug Administration; Ginkgo; Glutamine; Supplements: Introduction; Vitamin K.

Phenothiazines

CATEGORY: Drug interactions

DEFINITION: Drugs used to treat schizophrenia and other forms of psychosis.

INTERACTIONS: Coenzyme Q_{10}, milk thistle, fish oil, ginkgo, vitamin E, vitamin B_6, DHEA, glycine, phenylalanine, kava, St. John's wort and other herbs, yohimbe

DRUGS IN THIS FAMILY: Chlorpromazine hydrochloride (Thorazine), fluphenazine (Permitil, Prolixin), mesoridazine besylate (Serentil), perphenazine (Trilafon), prochlorperazine (Compazine), promazine hydrochloride (Sparine), promethazine hydrochloride (injectable Anergan, Phenergan), thioridazine hydrochloride (Mellaril), trifluoperazine hydrochloride (Stelazine), triflupromazine hydrochloride (injectable Vesprin)

COENZYME Q_{10} (CoQ_{10})

Effect: Supplementation Possibly Helpful

Preliminary studies suggest that phenothiazine drugs might deplete the body of CoQ_{10}. While there is no evidence that taking CoQ_{10} supplements provides any specific benefit, supplementing with CoQ_{10} on general principle might be a good idea if one is also taking phenothiazine drugs.

FISH OIL
Effect: Possible Helpful Interaction

Fish oil contains essential fatty acids in the omega-3 family. Fish oil, its constituents, and a slightly modified fish oil constituent called ethyl-EPA have all been tested for treatment of depression. Incomplete and inconsistent evidence hints that these substances might augment the effectiveness of standard medications used for schizophrenia.

MILK THISTLE
Effect: Possible Helpful Interaction

Milk thistle might protect against the liver toxicity sometimes caused by phenothiazine drugs.

GINKGO
Effect: Possible Helpful Interaction

Preliminary evidence suggests that ginkgo might reduce the side effects and increase the efficacy of various antipsychotic medications.

VITAMIN E
Effect: Possible Helpful Interaction

One of the most feared side effects of phenothiazines is the development of a permanent side effect called tardive dyskinesia (TD). This late-developing (tardy, or tardive) complication consists of annoying uncontrollable movements (dyskinesias), particularly in the face.

In early studies, vitamin E had shown some promise for treating tardive dyskinesia, but the largest and best-designed study failed to find benefit.

VITAMIN B$_6$
Effect: Possible Helpful Interaction

A pilot study suggests that vitamin B$_6$ may be helpful for the treatment of tardive dyskinesia (TD). In this four-week, double-blind crossover trial of fifteen persons, treatment with vitamin B$_6$ significantly improved TD symptoms compared with placebo. Benefits were seen after one week of treatment. However, the dosage of vitamin B$_6$ used in this study was quite high (400 mg daily). Toxicity has been reported with daily intake of vitamin B$_6$ at one-half this dose. Vi-

tamin B$_6$ might also reduce symptoms of akathesia, a type of restlessness associated with phenothiazine antipsychotics.

DEHYDROEPIANDROSTERONE (DHEA)
Effect: Possible Helpful Interaction

One small, double-blind study found that use of DHEA reduced the Parkinson-like movement disorders that may occur in people taking phenothiazine drugs.

GLYCINE
Effect: Possible Helpful Interaction

Phenothiazine drugs are most effective for the "positive" symptoms of schizophrenia, such as hallucinations and delusions. (Such symptoms are called "positive" because they indicate the presence of abnormal mental functions, rather than the absence of normal mental functions.) In general, however, these medications are less helpful for the "negative" symptoms of schizophrenia, such as apathy, depression, and social withdrawal. Some evidence hints that the supplement glycine might enhance the effectiveness of phenothiazines in relation to this latter class of symptoms.

PHENYLALANINE
Effect: Possible Increased Risk of Tardive Dyskinesia

There are some indications that using the supplement phenylalanine while taking antipsychotic drugs might increase one's risk of developing tardive dyskinesia.

KAVA
Effect: Possible Increased Risk of Dystonic Reactions

Besides the late-developing complication of tardive dyskinesia, antipsychotic drugs can cause more immediately another movement disorder: dystonic reactions (sudden intense movements of the neck and eyes). There is some evidence that the herb kava can increase the risk or severity of this side effect.

ST. JOHN'S WORT, OTHER HERBS
Effect: Potential Increased Risk of Photosensitivity

Phenothiazines can cause increased sensitivity to the sun. Various herbs, including St. John's wort and dong quai, can also cause this problem. Combined treatment with herb and drug might increase the risk further.

YOHIMBE

Effect: Possible Dangerous Interaction

The herb yohimbe is relatively toxic and can cause problems if used incorrectly. Phenothiazine medications may increase the risk of toxicity.

EBSCO CAM Review Board

FURTHER READING

Berger, G. E., et al. "Ethyl-Eicosapentaenoic Acid in First-Episode Psychosis." *Journal of Clinical Psychiatry* 68 (2007): 1867-1875.

Emsley, R., et al. "Randomized, Placebo-Controlled Study of Ethyl-Eicosapentaenoic Acid as Supplemental Treatment in Schizophrenia." *American Journal of Psychiatry* 159 (2002): 1596-1598.

Fenton, W. S., et al. "A Placebo-Controlled Trial of Omega-3 Fatty Acid (Ethyl Eicosapentaenoic Acid) Supplementation for Residual Symptoms and Cognitive Impairment in Schizophrenia." *American Journal of Psychiatry* 158 (2001): 2071-2074.

Lerner, V., et al. "Vitamin B6 Treatment in Acute Neuroleptic-Induced Akathisia." *Journal of Clinical Psychiatry* 65 (2004): 1550-1554.

Nachshoni, T., et al. "Improvement of Extrapyramidal Symptoms Following Dehydroepiandrosterone (DHEA) Administration in Antipsychotic Treated Schizophrenia Patients." *Schizophrenia Research* 79, nos. 2/3 (2005): 251-256.

Peet, M. "Eicosapentaenoic Acid in the Treatment of Schizophrenia and Depression: Rationale and Preliminary Double-Blind Clinical Trial Results." *Prostaglandins, Leukotrienes, and Essential Fatty Acids* 69 (2003): 477-485.

Zhang, X. Y., et al. "A Double-Blind, Placebo-Controlled Trial of Extract of *Ginkgo biloba* Added to Haloperidol in Treatment-Resistant Patients with Schizophrenia." *Journal of Clinical Psychiatry* 62 (2001): 878-883.

See also: Food and Drug Administration; Supplements: Introduction.

Phenylalanine

CATEGORY: Herbs and supplements

RELATED TERMS: D-phenylalanine, DL-phenylalanine, L-phenylalanine

DEFINITION: Natural substance of the human body used as a supplement to treat specific health conditions.

PRINCIPAL PROPOSED USE: Depression

OTHER PROPOSED USES: Attention deficit disorder, multiple sclerosis, generalized pain, Parkinson's disease, rheumatoid arthritis, vitiligo

OVERVIEW

Phenylalanine occurs in two chemical forms: L-phenylalanine, a natural amino acid found in proteins, and its mirror image, D-phenylalanine, a form synthesized in a laboratory. Some studies have involved the L-form, others the D-form, and still others a combination of the two known as DL-phenylalanine.

In the body, phenylalanine is converted into another amino acid called tyrosine. Tyrosine in turn is converted into L-dopa, norepinephrine, and epinephrine, three key neurotransmitters (chemicals that transmit signals between nerve cells). Because some antidepressants work by raising levels of norepinephrine, various forms of phenylalanine have been tried as a possible treatment for depression.

D-phenylalanine (but not L-phenylalanine) has been proposed to treat chronic pain. It blocks enkephalinase, an enzyme that may act to increase pain levels in the body.

REQUIREMENTS AND SOURCES

L-phenylalanine is an essential amino acid, meaning that humans need it for life and the body cannot manufacture it from other chemicals. It is found in protein-rich foods such as meat, fish, poultry, eggs, dairy products, and beans. If people eat enough protein, they are likely to get enough L-phenylalanine for their nutritional needs. There is no nutritional need for D-phenylalanine.

THERAPEUTIC DOSAGES

D- and DL-phenylalanine are typically taken at a dose of 100 to 200 milligrams (mg) daily for the treatment of depression. For the treatment of chronic pain, studies have used D-phenylalanine in doses as high as 2,500 mg daily. It is best not to take a phenylalanine supplement at the same time as a high-protein meal, as it may not be absorbed well.

THERAPEUTIC USES

Small double-blind, comparative studies suggest (but do not prove) that both the D- and DL- forms of

Food Sources of Phenylalanine
(Grams per 100 Grams of Food)

Soybeans, mature seeds, raw	1.91
Lentils, raw	1.38
Peanuts, all types, raw	1.34
Nuts, almonds	1.15
Chickpeas (garbanzo beans), mature seeds, raw	1.03
Flax seed, raw	0.96
Seeds, sesame butter, tahini, from raw and stone-ground kernels	0.94
Salami, Italian, pork	0.94
Beef, round, top round, separable lean and fat, trimmed to 1/8 inch fat, select, raw	0.88
Beef, top sirloin, separable lean only, trimmed to 1/8 inch fat, choice, raw	0.87
Crustaceans, shrimp, mixed species, raw	0.86
Chicken, broilers or fryers, thigh, meat only, raw	0.78
Fish, salmon pink, raw	0.78
Nuts, walnuts, English	0.71
Chicken, broilers or fryers, wing, meat and skin, raw	0.70
Egg, white, raw, fresh	0.69
Egg, whole, raw, fresh	0.68
Sausage, Italian, pork, raw	0.48
Hummus	0.26
Pork, fresh, separable fat, raw	0.22
Soy milk, fluid	0.15
Milk, whole, 3.25 percent milk fat	0.15
Asparagus	0.08

phenylalanine might be helpful for depression. Weak and contradictory evidence has been used to advocate the use of D-phenylalanine as a general analgesic (pain-relieving treatment). Preliminary uncontrolled and double-blind studies found that L-phenylalanine may enhance the effectiveness of ultraviolet for vitiligo.

Highly preliminary evidence suggests that D-phenylalanine may be helpful for multiple sclerosis when combined with transcutaneous electrical nerve stimu-

lation (TENS). D-phenylalanine has also been proposed as a treatment for Parkinson's disease.

Although D- and DL- phenylalanine are marketed as treatments for attention deficit disorder, they do not appear to be helpful. Some proponents claim that phenylalanine works better when combined with tyrosine, glutamine, and gamma-aminobutyric acid (GABA), but this has not been proven.

SCIENTIFIC EVIDENCE

Depression. A pair of double-blind comparative studies found that D- or DL-phenylalanine may be as effective as the antidepressant drug imipramine and possibly work more quickly. The larger of the two studies compared the effectiveness of D-phenylalanine at 100 mg daily against the same daily dose of imipramine. Sixty people with depression were randomly assigned to take either imipramine or D-phenylalanine for thirty days. The results in both groups were statistically equivalent, meaning that phenylalanine was about as effective as imipramine. D-phenylalanine worked more rapidly, however, producing significant improvement in only fifteen days. Like most antidepressant drugs, imipramine required several weeks to take effect.

The other double-blind study followed more than two dozen people, one-half of whom received DL-phenylalanine (150 to 200 mg daily) and the other half imipramine (100 to 150 mg daily). When they were reevaluated after thirty days, both groups had improved by a statistically equal amount. L-phenylalanine has also been tried as a treatment for depression, but not in studies that could provide a scientifically meaningful result.

No double-blind, placebo-controlled studies of phenylalanine for depression have been done. Without such evidence, it is impossible to be sure that the supplement is actually effective.

Chronic pain. The enzyme enkephalinase breaks down enkephalins, naturally occurring substances that reduce pain. D-phenylalanine (but not L-phenylalanine) is thought to block enkephalinase; this could lead to increased enkephalin levels, which in turn would tend to reduce pain. On this basis, D-phenylalanine has been proposed as a pain-killing drug.

However, there is no meaningful evidence that it really works in this way. A small double-blind, placebo-controlled study reported evidence for the effectiveness of D-phenylalanine in chronic pain, but a careful reexamination of the math involved showed that it actually proved little. Another small double-blind, placebo-controlled study failed to find any benefits. Another study commonly described as showing D-phenylalanine effective suffered from many flaws (including the fact that it lacked a control group) and, therefore, cannot be trusted.

SAFETY ISSUES

The long-term safety of phenylalanine in any of its forms is not known. Both L- and D-phenylalanine must be avoided by those with the rare metabolic disease phenylketonuria (PKU). The maximum safe dosages of phenylalanine have not been established for young children, pregnant or nursing women, or those with severe liver or kidney disease. There are some indications that the combined use of phenylalanine and antipsychotic drugs might increase the risk of developing the long-term side effect known as tardive dyskinesia, or worsen symptoms in those who already have it. Like other amino acids, phenylalanine may interfere with the absorption or action of the drug levodopa, which is used for Parkinson's disease.

IMPORTANT INTERACTIONS

Phenylalanine might interfere with the action of levodopa and other aminio acids; those taking amino acids should take phenylalanine only under a physician's supervision. Persons taking antipsychotic medications should not use phenylalanine.

EBSCO CAM Review Board

FURTHER READING

Camacho, F., and J. Mazuecos. "Treatment of Vitiligo with Oral and Topical Phenylalanine: Six Years of Experience." *Archives of Dermatology* 135 (1999): 216-217.

Werbach, M. R. *Nutritional Influences on Mental Illness: A Sourcebook of Clinical Research.* Tarzana, Calif.: Third Line Press; 1991.

See also: Attention deficit disorder; Depression, mild to moderate; Herbal medicine; Pain management.

Phenytoin

CATEGORY: Drug interactions

DEFINITION: Phenytoin is an anticonvulsant agent used primarily to prevent seizures in conditions such as epilepsy. In some cases, combination therapy with two or more anticonvulsant drugs may be used.

INTERACTIONS: Biotin, calcium, carnitine, folate, ginkgo, glutamine, hops, ipriflavone, kava, passionflower, valerian, vitamin D, vitamin K, white willow

TRADE NAME: Dilantin

DRUGS IN THIS FAMILY: Carbamazepine, phenobarbital, primidone, valproic acid

RELATED DRUGS: Ethotoin (Peganone), mephenytoin (Mesantoin)

GINKGO

Effect: Possible Harmful Interaction

The herb ginkgo (*Ginkgo biloba*) has been used to treat Alzheimer's disease and ordinary age-related memory loss, among many other conditions. Seizures have been reported with the use of ginkgo leaf extract in people with previously well-controlled epilepsy; in one case, the seizures were fatal. One possible explanation is contamination of ginkgo leaf products with ginkgo seeds. It has also been suggested that ginkgo might interfere with the effectiveness of some antiseizure medications, including phenytoin. Finally, it has been noted that the drug tacrine (also used to improve memory) has been associated with seizures, and ginkgo may affect the brain in ways similar to tacrine.

GLUTAMINE

Effect: Possible Harmful Interaction

The amino acid glutamine is converted to glutamate in the body. Glutamate is thought to act as a neurotransmitter (a chemical that enables nerve transmission). Because anticonvulsants work (at least in part) by blocking glutamate pathways in the brain, high dosages of the amino acid glutamine might theoretically diminish an anticonvulsant's effect and increase the risk of seizures.

IPRIFLAVONE

Effect: Possible Harmful Interaction

Ipriflavone, a synthetic isoflavone that slows bone breakdown, is used to treat osteoporosis. Test-tube studies indicate that ipriflavone might increase blood levels of the anticonvulsants phenytoin and carbamazepine when they are taken therapeutically. Ipriflavone was found to inhibit a liver enzyme involved in the body's normal breakdown of these drugs, thus allowing them to build up in the blood. Higher drug levels increase the risk of adverse effects.

Because anticonvulsants are known to contribute to the development of osteoporosis, a concern is that the use of ipriflavone for this drug-induced osteoporosis could result in higher blood levels of the drugs, with potentially serious consequences. People taking either of these drugs should use ipriflavone only under medical supervision.

HOPS, KAVA, PASSIONFLOWER, VALERIAN

Effect: Possible Harmful Interaction

The herb kava (*Piper methysticum*) has a sedative effect and is used for anxiety and insomnia. Combining kava with anticonvulsants, which possess similar depressant effects, could result in add-on or excessive physical depression, sedation, and impairment. In one case report, a fifty-four-year-old man was hospitalized for lethargy and disorientation, side effects attributed to his having taken the combination of kava and the antianxiety agent alprazolam (Xanax) for three days.

Other herbs having a sedative effect that might cause problems when combined with anticonvulsants include ashwagandha, calendula, catnip, hops, lady's slipper, lemon balm, passionflower, sassafras, skullcap, valerian, and yerba mansa.

Because of the potentially serious consequences, one should avoid combining these herbs with anticonvulsants or other drugs that also have sedative or depressant effects, unless advised by a physician.

WHITE WILLOW

Effect: Possible Harmful Interaction

The herb white willow (*Salix alba*), also known as willow bark, is used to treat pain and fever. White willow contains a substance that is converted by the body into a salicylate similar to aspirin. Higher doses

of aspirin may increase phenytoin levels and toxicity during long-term use of both drugs. This raises the concern that white willow might have similar effects on phenytoin, though this has not been proven.

BIOTIN

Effect: Supplementation Possibly Helpful, but Take at a Different Time of Day

Anticonvulsants may deplete biotin, an essential water-soluble B vitamin, possibly by competing with it for absorption in the intestine. It is not clear, however, whether this effect is great enough to be harmful. Blood levels of biotin were found to be substantially lower in 404 people with epilepsy on long-term treatment with anticonvulsants, compared with 112 untreated people with epilepsy. The effect occurred with phenytoin, carbamazepine, phenobarbital, and primidone. Valproic acid appears to affect biotin to a lesser extent than other anticonvulsants.

A test-tube study suggested that anticonvulsants might lower biotin levels by interfering with the way biotin is transported in the intestine.

Biotin supplementation may be beneficial for persons on long-term anticonvulsant therapy. To avoid a potential interaction, one should take the supplement two to three hours apart from the drug. It has been suggested that the action of anticonvulsant drugs may be at least partly related to their effect of reducing biotin levels. For this reason, it may be desirable to take enough biotin to prevent a deficiency but not an excessive amount.

FOLATE

Effect: Possible Benefits and Risks

Folate (also known as folic acid) is a B vitamin that plays an important role in many vital aspects of health, including preventing neural tube birth defects and possibly reducing the risk of heart disease. Because inadequate intake of folate is widespread, if one is taking any medication that depletes or impairs folate even slightly, one may need supplementation.

Most drugs used for preventing seizures can reduce levels of folate in the body. Phenytoin in particular appears to decrease folate levels by interfering with its absorption in the small intestine, as well as by accelerating its normal breakdown by the body. The low blood levels of folate caused by anticonvulsants can raise homocysteine levels, a condition believed to increase the risk of heart disease.

Adequate folate intake is also necessary to prevent neural tube birth defects, such as spina bifida and anencephaly (absence of a brain). Because anticonvulsant drugs deplete folate, babies born to women taking anticonvulsants are at increased risk for such birth defects. Anticonvulsants may also play a more direct role in the development of birth defects.

However, there can be problems with using folate supplements. High folate levels may speed up the normal breakdown of phenytoin. This can lead to breakthrough seizures. For this reason, folate supplementation during phenytoin therapy should be supervised by a physician.

CALCIUM

Effect: Supplementation Probably Helpful, but Take at a Different Time of Day

Anticonvulsant drugs may impair calcium absorption and, in this way, increase the risk of osteoporosis and other bone disorders. Calcium absorption was compared in twelve people on anticonvulsant therapy (all taking phenytoin and some also taking phenobarbital, primidone, and/or carbamazepine) and twelve people receiving no treatment. Calcium absorption was found to be 27 percent lower in the treated participants.

An observational study found low blood calcium levels in 48 percent of 109 people taking anticonvulsants. Other findings in this study suggested that anticonvulsants might also reduce calcium levels by directly interfering with parathyroid hormone, a substance that helps keep calcium levels in proper balance.

A low level of blood calcium can itself trigger seizures, and this might reduce the effectiveness of anticonvulsants. Calcium supplementation may be beneficial for people taking anticonvulsant drugs. However, some studies indicate that antacids containing calcium carbonate may interfere with the absorption of phenytoin and perhaps other anticonvulsants. For this reason, one should take calcium supplements and anticonvulsant drugs several hours apart if possible.

CARNITINE

Effect: Supplementation Possibly Helpful

Carnitine is an amino acid that has been used for heart conditions, Alzheimer's disease, and intermittent claudication. Long-term therapy with anticonvulsant agents, particularly valproic acid, is associated with low levels of carnitine. However, it is not clear whether the anticonvulsants cause the carnitine deficiency or whether it occurs for other reasons. It has been hypothesized that low carnitine levels may contribute to valproic acid's damaging effects on the liver. The risk of this liver damage increases in children younger than twenty-four months, and carnitine supplementation does seem to be protective. However, in one double-blind crossover study, carnitine supplementation produced no real improvement in "well-being" as assessed by parents of children receiving either valproic acid or carbamazepine.

L-carnitine supplementation may be advisable in certain cases, such as in infants and young children (especially those younger than two years) who have neurologic disorders and are receiving valproic acid and multiple anticonvulsants.

VITAMIN D

Effect: Supplementation Possibly Helpful

Anticonvulsant drugs may interfere with the activity of vitamin D. As proper handling of calcium by the body depends on vitamin D, this may be another way that these drugs increase the risk of osteoporosis and related bone disorders. Anticonvulsants appear to speed up the body's normal breakdown of vitamin D, decreasing the amount of the vitamin in the blood. A survey of forty-eight people taking both phenytoin and phenobarbital found significantly lower levels of calcium and vitamin D in many of them, compared with thrity-eight untreated people. Similar but lesser changes were seen in thirteen people taking phenytoin or phenobarbital alone. This effect may be apparent only after several weeks of treatment.

Another study found decreased blood levels of one form of vitamin D but normal levels of another. Because there are two primary forms of vitamin D circulating in the blood, the body might be able to adjust in some cases to keep vitamin D in balance, at least for a time, despite the influence of anticonvulsants. Adequate sunlight exposure may help overcome the effects of anticonvulsants on vitamin D by stimulating the skin to manufacture the vitamin. Of 450 people on anticonvulsants residing in a Florida facility, none was found to have low blood levels of vitamin D or evidence of bone disease. This suggests that environments providing regular sun exposure may be protective. People regularly taking anticonvulsants, especially those taking combination therapy and those with limited exposure to sunlight, may benefit from vitamin D supplementation.

VITAMIN K

Effect: Supplementation Possibly Helpful for Pregnant Women

Phenytoin, carbamazepine, phenobarbital, and primidone speed up the normal breakdown of vitamin K into inactive byproducts, thus depriving the body of active vitamin K. This can lead to bone problems, such as osteoporosis. In addition, use of these anticonvulsants can lead to a vitamin K deficiency in babies born to pregnant women taking the drugs, resulting in bleeding disorders or facial bone abnormalities in the newborns. Women who take these anticonvulsants may need vitamin K supplementation during pregnancy to prevent these conditions in their newborns.

EBSCO CAM Review Board

FURTHER READING

De Vivo, D. C., et al. "L-carnitine Supplementation in Childhood Epilepsy: Current Perspectives." *Epilepsia* 30 (1998): 1216-1225.

Granger, A. S. "*Ginkgo biloba* Precipitating Epileptic Seizures." *Age and Ageing* 30 (2001): 523-525.

Gregory, P. J. "Seizure Associated with *Ginkgo biloba*?" *Annals of Internal Medicine* 134 (2001): 344.

Kupiec, T., and V. Raj. "Fatal Seizures Due to Potential Herb-Drug Interactions with *Ginkgo biloba*." *Journal of Analytical Toxicology* 29 (2006): 755-758.

See also: Biotin; Calcium; Carnitine; Folate; Food and Drug Administration; Ginkgo; Glutamine; Hops; Ipriflavone; Kava; Passionflower; Supplements: Introduction; Valerian; Vitamin D; Vitamin K; White Willow.

Phlebitis and deep vein thrombosis

CATEGORY: Condition

RELATED TERMS: Saphenous thrombophlebitis, superficial phlebitis, thrombophlebitis

DEFINITION: Treatment of serious inflammation of a vein that is often accompanied by blood clots that adhere to the wall of the vein.

PRINCIPAL PROPOSED NATURAL TREATMENTS: None

OTHER PROPOSED NATURAL TREATMENTS: Bromelain, horse chestnut, mesoglycan, reducing homocysteine, vitamin E

INTRODUCTION

The term "phlebitis" refers to an inflammation of a vein, usually in the leg, and frequently accompanied by blood clots that adhere to the wall of the vein. When the affected vein is close to the surface, the condition is called superficial phlebitis. This condition usually resolves on its own without further complications. However, when phlebitis occurs in a deep vein, a condition called deep vein thrombosis (DVT), a clot could dislodge from the vein and lodge in the lungs. This is a life-threatening condition.

Symptoms of superficial phlebitis include pain, swelling, redness, and warmth around the affected vein. The vein feels hard to the touch because of the

Deep Vein Thrombosis and Its Effects

The most serious complication that can arise from deep vein thrombosis (DVT) is a pulmonary embolism (PE), which occurs in more than one-third of persons with DVT. A PE occurs when a portion of the blood clot breaks loose and travels in the bloodstream, first to the heart and then to the lungs, where it can partially or completely block a pulmonary artery or one of its branches.

A PE is a serious, life-threatening complication with signs and symptoms that include shortness of breath, rapid heartbeat, sweating, and sharp chest pain (especially during deep breathing). Some persons may cough up blood, while others may develop dangerously low blood pressure and pass out. Pulmonary embolism frequently causes sudden death, particularly when one or more of the vessels that supply the lungs with blood are completely blocked by the clot.

Those who survive generally do not have any lasting effects because the body's natural mechanisms tend to resorb (or "lyse") blood clots. However, in some instances, the blood clot in the lung fails to completely dissolve, leading to a chronic serious complication that can cause chronic shortness of breath and heart failure. DVT and PE are commonly grouped together and sometimes referred to as venous thromboembolism.

clotted blood. Deep vein thrombosis is more difficult to diagnose. It can occur without any symptoms until the clot reaches the lungs. However, about one-half of the cases include warning symptoms, such as swelling, pain, and warmth in the entire calf, ankle, foot, or thigh (depending on where the involved vein is located). Although these symptoms can also be caused by more benign conditions, DVT is such a life-threatening disorder that physician consultation is necessary.

Risk factors for any type of phlebitis include recent surgery or childbirth, varicose veins, inactivity, or sitting for long periods (such as during an airline flight). Prolonged placement of intravenous catheters can also cause phlebitis, possibly requiring antibiotic treatment.

Conventional treatments for superficial phlebitis include analgesics for pain, warm compresses, and compression bandages or stockings to increase blood flow. In more severe cases, anticoagulants or minor surgery may be required. DVT requires more aggressive treatment, including hospitalization, strong anticoagulants, and a variety of possible surgical procedures.

PROPOSED NATURAL TREATMENTS

There are no well-established natural treatments for phlebitis. There is some evidence, however, that certain natural treatments might help prevent DVTs. Because phlebitis is a potentially life-threatening disorder, one should seek a doctor's advice before attempting any natural treatments. DVT constitutes a medical emergency and requires immediate medical care.

Oligomeric proanthocyanidins. It is thought, though not proven, that the immobility endured during a long airline flight increases the risk of potentially dangerous blood clots in the legs. Travelers at high risk are often advised to take aspirin to "thin" their blood before flying. Oligomeric proanthocyanidins (OPCs), a derivative of pine bark or grape seed, may have a similar effect.

A large, double-blind, placebo-controlled study was performed to evaluate whether OPCs from pine bark could help reduce risk of blood clots on long flights. The study followed 198 people thought to be at high risk for blood clots. Some participants were given 200 milligrams (mg) of OPCs two to three hours before their flight, 200 mg six hours later, and 100 mg the next day; others received placebo on the same

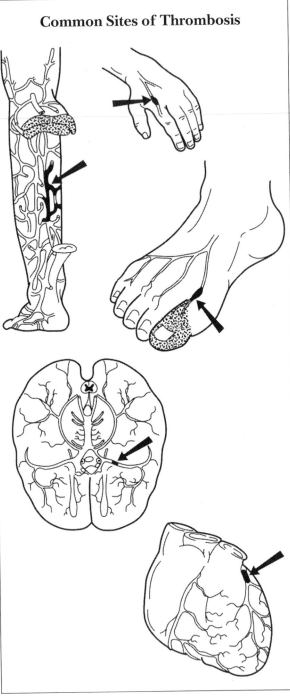

Common Sites of Thrombosis

schedule. The average flight length was about eight hours. The results indicated that the use of OPCs significantly reduced the risk of blood clots. There were five cases of DVTs or superficial thrombosis in the placebo group, compared to none in the OPC group, a difference that was statistically significant.

Another substantial double-blind study (204 participants) suggests preventive benefit in high-risk persons given Flite Tabs, a product that contains pycnogenol (an OPC) combined with nattokinase. Nattokinase, also known as natto, is an extract of fermented soy thought to have some blood-clot-dissolving properties. However, the incidence of DVTs was not reported.

Other treatments. Vitamin E, when taken in high doses, is thought to have a blood-thinning effect. One study found some evidence that regular use of vitamin E at a dose of 600 international units daily may help prevent DVT.

Bromelain is an enzyme found in the stems of pineapple. Because it has anti-inflammatory properties and may be able to prevent blood platelet aggregation, it has been suggested as a treatment for phlebitis. However, there is no good evidence supporting this use.

Mesoglycan is a type of substance found in the tissues of the body, including blood vessels. It is closely related to the anticoagulant drug heparin. Preliminary evidence suggests that mesoglycan might be helpful in treating phlebitis, although not all studies agree. Horse chestnut is often used for chronic venous insufficiency and varicose veins, conditions related to phlebitis. For this reason, horse chestnut is sometimes recommended for phlebitis too, but there is no real evidence that it works.

Homocysteine is a substance that occurs naturally in the body. It has been suggested that when homocysteine levels are too high, the risk of such cardiovascular diseases as heart attack, stroke, and DVT are increased. However, in a very large study, the reduction of homocysteine through the use of folate and vitamins B_{12} and B_6 failed to reduce the risk of DVT.

EBSCO CAM Review Board

FURTHER READING

Belcaro, G., et al. "Prevention of Venous Thrombosis and Thrombophlebitis in Long-Haul Flights with Pycnogenol." *Clinical and Applied Thrombosis/Hemostasis* 10 (2004): 373-377.

Cesarone, M. R., et al. "Prevention of Venous Thrombosis in Long-Haul Flights with Flite Tabs." *Angiology* 54 (2003): 531-539.

Glynn, R. J., et al. "Effects of Random Allocation to Vitamin E Supplementation on the Occurrence of Venous Thromboembolism: Report from the Women's Health Study." *Circulation* 116 (2007): 1497-1503.

Ray, J. G., et al. "Homocysteine-Lowering Therapy and Risk for Venous Thromboembolism." *Annals of Internal Medicine* 146 (2007): 761-767.

Ten Wolde, M., et al. "Travel and the Risk of Symptomatic Venous Thromboembolism." *Thrombosis and Hemostasis* 89 (2003): 499-505.

See also: Bromelain; Horse chestnut; Mesoglycan; Oligomeric proanthocyanidins; Strokes; Vitamin E.

Phosphatidylserine

CATEGORY: Herbs and supplements
RELATED TERMS: Phospholipids, PS
DEFINITION: Natural substance of the human body used as a supplement to treat specific health conditions.
PRINCIPAL PROPOSED USES: Age-related memory loss, Alzheimer's disease
OTHER PROPOSED USES: Depression, enhancing mental function in young people, enhancing sports performance and recovery, stress

OVERVIEW

Phosphatidylserine (PS) is a member of a class of chemical compounds known as phospholipids. PS is an essential component in all human cells; specifically, it is a major component of the cell membrane. The cell membrane is a kind of skin that surrounds living cells. Besides keeping cells intact, this membrane performs vital functions such as moving nutrients into cells and pumping waste products out of them. PS plays an important role in many of these functions.

Good evidence suggests that PS can help declining mental function and depression in the elderly, and it is widely used for this purpose in Italy, Scandinavia, and other parts of Europe. PS has also been marketed as a brain booster for people of all ages, said to sharpen memory and increase thinking ability. However, the evidence to support this use is incomplete and inconsistent.

REQUIREMENTS AND SOURCES

The human body makes all the PS it needs. However, the only way to get a therapeutic dosage of PS is to take a supplement. PS was originally manufactured from the brains of cows, and all the studies described here used this form. However, because animal brain cells can harbor viruses, that form is no longer available. Most PS today is made from soybeans or other plant sources.

There are reasons to expect that plant-source PS should function very similarly to PS made from cows' brains, and some animal studies suggest that it is indeed effective. However, in preliminary trials, soy-based PS and cabbage-based PS failed to prove beneficial.

THERAPEUTIC DOSAGES

For the purpose of improving mental function, PS is usually taken in dosages of 100 milligrams (mg) two to three times daily. After maximum effect is achieved, the dosage can reportedly be reduced to 100 mg daily without losing any benefit. PS can be taken with or without meals. When taking PS for sports purposes, athletes sometimes take as much as 800 mg daily.

THERAPEUTIC USES

Meaningful evidence from numerous double-blind studies suggests that animal-source PS is an effective treatment for Alzheimer's disease and other forms of age-related mental decline. Vegetable-derived PS has little supporting evidence.

PS is widely marketed as a treatment for ordinary age-related memory loss as well. While there is little direct evidence that it works, in studies of severe mental decline, PS appears to have been equally effective whether the cause was Alzheimer's disease or something entirely unrelated, such as multiple small strokes. This certainly suggests that PS may have a positive impact on the brain that is not specific to any one condition. From this observation, it is not a great leap to suspect that it might be useful for much less severe problems with memory and mental function, such as those that seem to occur in nearly all people older than forty. Indeed, double-blind studies have found that phosphatidylserine could improve mental function in people with age-related memory loss. However, two studies failed to find plant-source PS effective for this condition. PS has also been proposed for enhancing mental function in young people, but there is no direct evidence that any form is effec-

tive. Animal-source PS has also shown a slight bit of promise for depression.

Recently, PS has become popular among athletes who hope it can help them build muscle more efficiently. This use is based on weak evidence that PS slows the release of cortisol following heavy exercise. Cortisol is a hormone that causes muscle tissue to break down. For reasons that are unclear, the body produces increased levels of cortisol after heavy exercise. Strength athletes believe that this natural cortisol release works against their efforts to rapidly build muscle mass and hope that PS will help them advance more quickly. However, only two double-blind placebo-controlled studies of PS as a sports supplement have been reported, and neither one found effects on cortisol levels. Of these small trials, one found a possible ergogenic benefit, and the other did not.

Interestingly, PS has also been advocated as an aid to recovery from heavy exercise, according to the theory that use of PS would help reduce muscle soreness. This would seem to contradict the proposed effects on cortisol, as cortisol has anti-inflammatory properties. Nonetheless, researchers performed a double-blind study to evaluate whether 750 mg daily of soy-source PS would reduce muscle soreness following downhill racing; no benefits were seen.

One study found preliminary evidence that a combination of soy-based PS and lecithin may moderate the body's reaction to mental stress. Another study evaluated use of phosphatidylserine for reducing stress in golfers, but the benefits seen failed to reach statistical significance. Participants who were given phosphatidylserine did, however, tee-off successfully at a greater rate than those given a placebo.

SCIENTIFIC EVIDENCE

Alzheimer's disease and other forms of dementia. Overall, the evidence for animal-source PS in dementia is fairly strong. Double-blind studies involving a total of more than one thousand people suggest that phosphatidylserine is an effective treatment for Alzheimer's disease and other forms of dementia.

The largest of these studies followed 494 elderly subjects in northeastern Italy over a course of six months. All suffered from moderate to severe mental decline, as measured by standard tests. Treatment consisted of either 300 mg daily of PS or a placebo. The group that took PS did significantly better in both behavior and mental function than the placebo group. Symptoms of depression also improved.

These results agree with those of numerous other smaller double-blind studies involving a total of more than five hundred people with Alzheimer's and other types of age-related dementia. However, all these studies involved cow-brain PS; studies of plant-source PS for dementia have not been reported.

Ordinary age-related memory loss. There is some evidence that PS can also help people with ordinary age-related memory loss. In one double-blind study that enrolled 149 people with memory loss but not dementia, phosphatidylserine provided significant benefits compared with a placebo. People with the most severe memory loss showed the most improvement. In another study, 131 elderly people with memory problems but no dementia were randomized to receive a combination of PS and omega-3 fatty acids or placebo. Those in the treatment group had improvements in their cognitive abilities compared with those in the placebo group. It is unclear which of the components, if not both of them, produced the beneficial effect.

However, a double-blind trial of 120 older people with memory complaints but not dementia failed to find benefits. This discrepancy may have to do with the type of phosphatidylserine used; this trial used the more modern soy-derived form of the supplement. A cabbage-based source of PS has also failed to prove effective for relatively mild memory loss.

Athletic performance. Weak evidence suggests that PS might decrease the release of the hormone cortisol after intense exercise. Among its many effects, cortisol acts to break down muscle tissue–exactly the opposite of the effect desired by a strength athlete or bodybuilder. This double-blind, placebo-controlled study on eleven intensely trained athletes found that 800 mg of PS taken daily reduced the cortisol rise by 20 percent compared with placebo. Another small study on nine nonathletic males found that daily doses of 400 and 800 mg of PS reduced cortisol levels after exercise by 16 and 30 percent, respectively. Another study found that phosphatidylserine could relieve some overtraining symptoms, including muscle soreness, possibly because of its effects on cortisol.

On the basis of these preliminary trials, PS has been proposed as a sports supplement. However, there is no direct evidence to support the claims that PS actually helps athletes build muscles more quickly and with less training effort. Furthermore, the most recent and best-designed study, using vegetable-source PS, failed to find any effect on cortisol release, muscle soreness, or markers of muscle damage.

SAFETY ISSUES

Phosphatidylserine is generally regarded as safe when used at recommended dosages. Side effects are rare, and when they do occur, they usually consist of nothing much worse than mild gastrointestinal distress. One study found that use of phosphatidylserine did not alter results on standard medical screening tests. However, the maximum safe dosages for young children, pregnant or nursing women, and those with severe liver or kidney disease have not been established.

PS is sometimes taken with ginkgo because they both appear to enhance mental function. However, some caution might be in order: Ginkgo is a blood thinner, and PS might be one as well. PS is known to

The Cell and Its Membrane

The human body is like an electrical company, chemical factory, transportation grid, communications network, detoxification facility, hospital, and battlefield all rolled into one. The workers that drive these activities are the cells.

The body contains trillions of cells, organized into more than two hundred major types. At any given time, each cell is doing thousands of routine jobs, like creating and using energy, manufacturing proteins, and responding to environmental cues. Different cell types also have special duties, like building skin or bone, pumping out hormones, or making antibodies.

Encasing each cell of the human body is a membrane with special gates, channels, and pumps that let in or force out selected molecules. The membrane, which contains a major component—phosphatidylserine—protects the cell's internal environment, a thick brew called the cytosol made of salts, nutrients, and proteins that accounts for about one-half the cell's volume (organelles make up the rest). In addition to the outer membrane, which is made up of proteins and lipids (fats), the cells of humans and other higher organisms have a pair of porous membranes that envelop the nucleus. Each organelle also has an outer membrane.

enhance the effect of heparin, a very strong prescription blood thinner. It is possible that combined use of PS and any drug or supplement that thins the blood could interfere enough with normal blood clotting to cause problems. Some medications and supplements to consider include warfarin (Coumadin), aspirin, pentoxifylline (Trental), clopidogrel (Plavix), ticlopidine (Ticlid), garlic, ginkgo, and vitamin E.

It should be noted that Alzheimer's disease and other types of severe age-related mental impairment are too serious for self-treatment with PS or any other supplement. In some cases, the symptoms of these diseases could be confused with symptoms of other serious conditions. Persons who believe they or a loved one has a severe age-related mental impairment should consult a doctor for diagnosis and treatment.

IMPORTANT INTERACTIONS

Those persons taking prescription blood thinners, such as warfarin (Coumadin), heparin, aspirin, pentoxifylline (Trental), clopidogrel (Plavix), or ticlopidine (Ticlid) should not use phosphatidylserine except on a physician's advice. Taking phosphatidylserine along with ginkgo, garlic, or vitamin E might conceivably thin the blood too much.

EBSCO CAM Review Board

FURTHER READING

Hellhammer, J., et al. "Effects of Soy Lecithin Phosphatidic Acid and Phosphatidylserine Complex (PAS) on the Endocrine and Psychological Responses to Mental Stress." *Stress* 7 (2004): 119-126.

Jager, R., et al. "The Effect of Phosphatidylserine on Golf Performance." *Journal of the International Society of Sports Nutrition* 4, no. 1 (2007): 23.

Jorissen, B. L., et al. "The Influence of Soy-derived Phosphatidylserine on Cognition in Age-Associated Memory Impairment." *Nutritional Neuroscience* 4 (2001): 121-134.

Kingsley, M. I., L. P. Kilduff, et al. "Phosphatidylserine Supplementation and Recovery Following Downhill Running." *Medicine and Science in Sports and Exercise* 38 (2006): 1617-1625.

Kingsley, M. I., D. Wadsworth, et al. "Effects of Phosphatidylserine on Oxidative Stress Following Intermittent Running." *Medicine and Science in Sports and Exercise* 37 (2005): 1300-1306.

Vakhapova, V., et al. "Phosphatidylserine Containing Omega-3 Fatty Acids May Improve Memory Abilities in Non-demented Elderly with Memory Complaints." *Dementia and Geriatric Cognitive Disorders* 29, no. 5 (2010): 467-474.

See also: Aging; Alzheimer's disease and non-Alzheimer's dementia; Ginkgo; Herbal medicine; Memory and mental function impairment; Sports and fitness support: Enhancing performance.

Phosphorus

CATEGORY: Herbs and supplements
RELATED TERM: Phosphate
DEFINITION: Natural substance of the human body used as a supplement to treat specific health conditions.
PRINCIPAL PROPOSED USES: Osteoporosis, sports and fitness support and performance enhancement

OVERVIEW

The mineral phosphorus is an essential part of the diet. In the human body, it is almost always found in an oxidized form known as phosphate. Bone contains the bulk of the body's phosphate. However, innumerable other substances in the body, such as cell membranes, contain phosphate as part of their structure. In addition, phosphate plays a central role in the fundamental energy-producing processes of all life. Indeed, some biochemists believe that phosphate-based reactions in volcanic vents may have occurred before life itself developed, later to be incorporated into the first living cells.

REQUIREMENTS AND SOURCES

In general, most people consume more than enough phosphorus in the diet. It is present in high quantities in milk, other protein sources, and grains. Additionally, it is added to many beverages and packaged foods. Phosphorus deficiency may develop in certain circumstances, however. People with severe alcoholism may become deficient in phosphorus as well as other basic nutrients; deficiency may also occur in people with kidney failure, parathyroid dysfunction, or poorly controlled diabetes.

THERAPEUTIC DOSAGES

In studies of phosphate for enhancing sports performance, a one-time dose of 1 gram (g) of tribasic sodium phosphate has been the most common dose. For ongoing use as treatment for osteoporosis, advocates recommend that phosphate be taken as part of a calcium product that includes phosphate, such as milk products or the supplement tricalcium phosphate.

THERAPEUTIC USES

Because phosphate plays a fundamental role in the body's energy-producing pathways, it has been suggested that taking high doses of phosphate (phosphate loading) before athletic activities might enhance performance. Phosphate-containing chemicals are also part of the process that allows oxygen release from hemoglobin, and this too has intrigued researchers looking for ergogenic aids. However, while some studies have found that phosphate loading improves maximum oxygen utilization, others have not, and flaws in study design cast doubt on the positive results.

Although it has long been stated that high phosphorus intake due to consumption of soft drinks might lead to osteoporosis, there is no solid evidence for this claim; in fact, elevated intake of phosphorus may help prevent osteoporosis. The reason for that is that bone contains both calcium and phosphate.

SAFETY ISSUES

In general, phosphorus is a safe nutritional substance. One-time high intake of some forms of phosphate may cause diarrhea. It is also possible that ongoing intake of phosphorus at high levels may impair absorption of copper, iron, and zinc. Some evidence hints that excessive consumption of phosphorus in the form of soft drinks might increase kidney stone risk, but study results are contradictory, and if there is an effect it appears to be small. Individuals with severe kidney disease should avoid phosphorus supplements, just as they must avoid taking too much of many other minerals.

EBSCO CAM Review Board

FURTHER READING

Heaney, R. P. "Advances in Therapy for Osteoporosis." *Clinical Medicine Research* 1 (2003): 93-99.

Rodgers, A. "Effect of Cola Consumption on Urinary Biochemical and Physicochemical Risk Factors Associated with Calcium Oxalate Urolithiasis." *Urology Research* 27 (1999): 77-81.

See also: Herbal medicine; Osteoarthritis; Sports and fitness support: Enhancing performance.

Photosensitivity

CATEGORY: Condition

RELATED TERMS: Erythropoietic protoporphyria, photoallergy, photodermatitis, phototoxicity, polymorphous light eruptions, porphyria cutanea tarda

DEFINITION: Treatment of the condition in which a person sunburns easily or develops certain skin reactions to sunlight.

PRINCIPAL PROPOSED NATURAL TREATMENT: Beta-carotene

OTHER PROPOSED NATURAL TREATMENTS: Adenosine monophosphate, chocolate, coriander oil, epigallocatechin gallate (from green tea), nicotinamide, vitamin B_6, vitamin C, vitamin E

HERBS AND SUPPLEMENTS TO USE ONLY WITH CAUTION: Artichoke, celery, chrysanthemum, dandelion, dill, endive, essential oils, fennel, fig, lettuce, lime, marigold, parsley, parsnip, St. John's wort, sunflower

INTRODUCTION

All persons will experience sunburn if exposed to enough ultraviolet radiation from the sun or other sources. However, some people burn particularly easily or develop exaggerated skin reactions to sunlight. This condition is called photosensitivity. For some people, consuming certain medications or plant products (or rubbing them on their skin) can cause photosensitivity. Similar reactions are seen in diseases such as lupus and some forms of porphyria (a group of usually hereditary metabolic disorders). In another condition, called polymorphous light eruptions (PLEs), dramatic rashes can develop after fairly limited sun exposure.

The most important step toward treating photosensitivity is to identify whether an external substance is causing the reaction and then to eliminate it if possible. Antibiotics are among the most common photosensitizing drugs. Many other natural substances can also cause this reaction. Another commonsense step is to use sunscreen and wear protective clothing, or simply to stay out of the sun. Some types of photosensitivity may respond to specific treatments such as oral beta-carotene, steroids, or other medications.

PRINCIPAL PROPOSED NATURAL TREATMENTS

Beta-carotene, a plant pigment that gives color to carrots and yams, may be beneficial for a minimum of two kinds of photosensitivity: PLEs and photosensitivity caused by certain types of porphyria. Beta-carotene is the best-studied supplement for photosensitivity, although only four studies on it have been placebo-controlled, and these had conflicting results. According to one theory, beta-carotene prevents skin damage by neutralizing free radicals, harmful chemicals created in the skin by the action of radiation.

One characteristic of beta-carotene is that it gives a deep yellow color to human skin when taken in high doses for several months. Because supplementation must continue for some time to see results, this side effect makes it difficult to conduct a truly double-blind study in which neither researchers nor the participants know who is taking the active compound and who is taking placebo. Once the skin begins to turn yellow, however, those affected are likely to figure out what they are taking, and this may affect the study outcome. Therefore, even the results of placebo-controlled studies of beta-carotene are open to question.

Three controlled trials of beta-carotene for polymorphous light eruptions found mixed results. A ten-week study in fifty people with PLE who were given beta-carotene plus canthaxanthin (another carotene) or placebo found evidence of significant benefit. However, in two other controlled trials of beta-carotene alone, lasting twelve to fifteen weeks (the number of participants was not reported), modest benefits were seen in one study and no benefits in the other. In a preliminary double-blind study, coriander oil applied topically was more beneficial than a placebo cream.

Many uncontrolled studies have reported that beta-carotene extends the time that people with erythropoietic protoporphyria (EPP) can safely spend in the sun. However, studies that lack a control group, as these did, are notorious for producing over-optimistic results; an eleven-month controlled trial found no benefit. A few case reports suggest beta-carotene may also be helpful in another kind of porphyria called porphyria cutanea tarda.

OTHER PROPOSED NATURAL TREATMENTS

Many studies suggest that various antioxidant substances, including chocolate, vitamin C, lycopene, mixed carotenoids, flavonol-enriched green tea extracts, vitamin E, and zeaxanthin taken orally or used topically, may help prevent sunburn in people without photosensitivity.

On this basis, a variety of antioxidants have been tried for photosensitivity. In a double-blind, placebo-controlled trial of twelve people with EPP, 1 gram (g) of oral vitamin C taken daily appeared to help reduce symptoms. However, the study was too small for the results to be statistically significant.

A small, double-blind, placebo-controlled trial of persons with PLE found no benefit with combined vitamin C (3 g per day) and vitamin E (1,500 international units per day). In an uncontrolled study of adenosine monophosphate in twenty-one people with porphyria cutanea tarda, many participants showed decreased photosensitivity, much to the surprise of the investigator.

Two cases of EPP were also reportedly improved by vitamin B_6. In addition, nicotinamide, another B vitamin, was found to help prevent polymorphous light eruptions in an uncontrolled (and, therefore, highly unreliable) study of forty-two people.

HERBS AND SUPPLEMENTS TO USE WITH CAUTION

A number of common herbs and plant products are known to provoke extreme reactions to sunlight in some people. One of the best known of these products is the herb St. John's wort, which has caused fatal photosensitivity reactions in cattle that grazed on it. In one study of highly sun-sensitive people, double doses of the herb produced mild increases in reaction to ultraviolet radiation. There is also one report of a severe skin reaction in a person who used St. John's wort and then received ultraviolet therapy for psoriasis. In addition, topical St. John's wort apparently caused severe sunburn in one person. For this reason, photosensitive people should probably avoid St. John's wort.

Photosensitivity can also result from touching or eating other plants, including celery, dill, fennel, fig, lime, parsley, parsnip, *Arnica*, artichoke, chrysanthemum, dandelion, lettuce, endive, marigold, and sunflower. Most people do not react to these plants. Essential oils of plants may be more problematic than the whole plant itself.

EBSCO CAM Review Board

FURTHER READING

Elmets, C. A., et al. "Cutaneous Photoprotection from Ultraviolet Injury by Green Tea Polyphenols."

Journal of the American Academy of Dermatology 44 (2001): 425-432.

Greul, A. K., et al. "Photoprotection of UV-irradiated Human Skin: An Antioxidative Combination of Vitamins E and C, Carotenoids, Selenium, and Proanthocyanidins." *Skin Pharmacology and Applied Skin Physiology* 15 (2002): 307-315.

Heinrich, U., et al. "Long-Term Ingestion of High Flavanol Cocoa Provides Photoprotection Against UV-Induced Erythema and Improves Skin Condition in Women." *Journal of Nutrition* 136 (2006): 1565-1569.

Palombo, P., et al. "Beneficial Long-Term Effects of Combined Oral/Topical Antioxidant Treatment with the Carotenoids Lutein and Zeaxanthin on Human Skin." *Skin Pharmacology and Applied Skin Physiology* 20 (2007): 199-210.

Reuter, J., et al. "Anti-inflammatory Potential of a Lipolotion Containing Coriander Oil in the Ultraviolet Erythema Test." *Journal of the German Society of Dermatology* 6 (2008): 847-851.

See also: Beta-carotene; Hives; PABA (para-aminobenzoic acid); Skin, aging; Sunburn.

Phyllanthus

CATEGORY: Herbs and supplements
RELATED TERMS: *Phyllanthus amarus, P. niruri, P. urinaria*
DEFINITION: Natural plant product used to treat specific health conditions.
PRINCIPAL PROPOSED USE: Chronic hepatitis B
OTHER PROPOSED USE: Acute hepatitis B

OVERVIEW

Tropical plants in the genus *Phyllanthus* have a long history of use in Ayurvedic medicine (the traditional medicine of India) for the treatment of hepatitis, kidney and bladder problems, intestinal parasites, and diabetes. The most-studied species is *P. amarus.*

THERAPEUTIC DOSAGES

The usual dose of *P. amarus* used in studies is 600 to 900 milligrams (mg) daily.

THERAPEUTIC USES

Hepatitis B is a two-stage illness. It has an acute phase that causes jaundice, severe fatigue, and other symptoms. These symptoms usually resolve in a month or so; however, the infection may then become chronic. Long-term infection with hepatitis B can spread the disease to other people and can also lead to liver injury or liver cancer.

P. amarus has undergone considerable evaluation as a treatment for chronic hepatitis B and a bit of study for acute hepatitis. However, the results have not been promising. The current consensus is that the herb is not helpful for hepatitis. *P. urinaria* also appears to be ineffective.

SCIENTIFIC EVIDENCE

Despite numerous test-tube and animal studies showing efficacy against the hepatitis B virus, *P. amarus* has generally not done well in human trials. Only one study clearly found benefits, and it was seriously flawed. In this thirty-day double-blind, placebo-controlled trial of sixty people with chronic hepatitis B, treatment with phyllanthus (200 mg three times daily) dramatically increased the odds of full recovery. In the treated group, almost 60 percent were hepatitis B-negative at follow-up, compared with only 4 percent in the placebo group. However, the high drop-out rate in the placebo group significantly reduces the reliability of the results. Furthermore, multiple follow-up studies attempting to reproduce these findings have not found any benefits.

Another double-blind, placebo-controlled trial enrolled fifty-seven people with acute hepatitis B to see whether treatment with *P. amarus* (300 mg three times daily for one week) could improve speed of recovery. The results showed no benefit. However, because acute hepatitis B usually lasts a month or more, the duration of treatment in this study was oddly short.

One highly preliminary study suggested that *P. urinaria*, a related species, might be more effective against hepatitis than other species of phyllanthus. However, a subsequent double-blind, placebo-controlled study designed to test this hypothesis failed to find benefit.

SAFETY ISSUES

There are no indications that *P. amarus* is toxic when used at recommended doses, but comprehensive safety studies have not been performed. In double-blind studies, significant side effects have not been reported. Safety in pregnant or nursing women, and individuals with severe liver or kidney disease, has not been established.

EBSCO CAM Review Board

FURTHER READING

Calixto, J. B., et al. "A Review of the Plants of the Genus *Phyllanthus*: Their Chemistry, Pharmacology, and Therapeutic Potential." *Medical Research Review* 18 (1998): 225-258.

Chan, H. L., et al. "Double-Blinded Placebo-Controlled Study of *Phyllanthus urinaris* for the Treatment of Chronic Hepatitis B." *Alimentary Pharmacology and Therapeutics* 18 (2003): 339-345.

Narendranathan, M., et al. "A Trial of *Phyllanthus amarus* in Acute Viral Hepatitis." *Tropical Gastroenterology* 20 (1999): 164-166.

See also: Hepatitis, viral; Herbal medicine.

Picrorhiza

CATEGORY: Herbs and supplements
RELATED TERMS: Kadu, katuka, kuru, kutki, *Picrorhiza kurroa*
DEFINITION: Natural plant product used to treat specific health conditions.
PRINCIPAL PROPOSED USES: None
OTHER PROPOSED USES: Asthma, liver protection, viral hepatitis, vitiligo

OVERVIEW

The rhizome (underground extension of the stalk) of picrorhiza has a long history of use in Indian Ayurvedic medicine for the treatment of digestive problems. Other traditional uses include treatment of scorpion sting, asthma, liver diseases, and febrile infections.

THERAPEUTIC DOSAGES

A typical recommended dose of powdered picrorhiza ranges from 400 to 1,500 milligrams (mg) daily, or an equivalent amount in extract form. Like all plants, picrorhiza contains a variety of chemicals. Some of the more investigated of these constituents are picroside I, kutkoside, androsin, and apocynin. Some picrorhiza extracts are standardized to contain a stated amount of one or more of these substances. However, since no constituent of picrorhiza has any established medicinal benefit, such standardization has no known practical implication.

THERAPEUTIC USES

There are no scientifically established medicinal uses of picrorhiza. Picrorhiza is often advocated as a treatment for asthma, based primarily on two studies conducted in the 1970s. However, neither of these studies was conducted in such a manner as to produce reliable results in the modern sense. Only double-blind, placebo-controlled studies can actually show a treatment effective, and the two such studies of picrorhiza for asthma failed to find the herb more effective than a placebo.

One small, double-blind study found picrorhiza root (375 mg, three times daily) more effective than a placebo for reducing signs of liver damage in people with acute viral hepatitis. However, this study was highly preliminary and suffered from numerous flaws. The other evidence used to support the use of picrorhiza as a liver protectant is even weaker, consisting of test-tube studies, animal studies, and open studies in humans.

Picrorhiza has undergone some study for other proposed uses, but at present there is no meaningful evidence that it is effective for enhancing response to vaccinations, speeding the healing of wounds, or enhancing the effectiveness of conventional treatment for vitiligo.

SAFETY ISSUES

Based on its long history of traditional use, picrorhiza appears to be relatively safe. However, systematic, scientifically modern safety studies of picrorhiza are lacking. For this reason, the use of this herb is not recommended.

Many herbs and other treatments considered safe based on traditional use have later turned out to present severe, previously unrecognized risks. Herbalists would be expected to notice immediate, dramatic reactions to herbal formulas, and one can assume with some confidence that treatments used for thousands of years are at least unlikely to cause such problems in very many people who take them. However, certain types of harm could be expected to easily elude the detection of traditional herbalists. These include safety problems that are delayed, occur relatively rarely, or are difficult to detect without scientific instruments. Because of the lack of comprehensive safety evaluation, it is not recommended that pregnant or nursing women, young children, or people with severe liver or kidney disease use picrorhiza.

EBSCO CAM Review Board

FURTHER READING

Khajuria, A., et al. "RLJ-NE-299A: A New Plant Based Vaccine Adjuvant." *Vaccine* 25 (2007): 2706-2715.

Thomas, M., et al. "AKL1, a Botanical Mixture for the Treatment of Asthma." *BMC Pulmonary Medicine* 7 (2007): 4.

See also: Asthma; Dyspepsia; Herbal medicine.

Placebo effect

CATEGORY: Issues and overviews
RELATED TERM: Placebo response
DEFINITION: An observable or measurable improvement in health or relief of symptoms that is attributable to something other than an administered medicine, medical procedure, or treatment.

OVERVIEW

Since the beginning of medicine, physicians have observed that the very act of prescribing treatments, even worthless or fake treatments, can sometimes make people feel better. Such false treatments were used to palliate patients, albeit temporarily, when little else could be done.

The first known use of the term "placebo" to describe these false treatments can be found in a 1785

medical dictionary. The word "placebo" derives from the Latin "I shall please." Placebos have been commonly used for some time. During the 1950s and 1960s, for example, sugar tablets and saline injections were used by hospitals as fake treatments.

In 1955, an American anesthesiologist, Henry K. Beecher, found the first scientific evidence for the placebo effect. His article "The Powerful Placebo," which was published in the *Journal of the American Medical Society*, reports on how he analyzed fifteen different clinical studies that examined treatments for different diseases. He discovered that 35 percent of 1,082 patients who had received a placebo treatment responded positively. His work strongly suggested the need for clinical studies to be "double-blinded"; that is, studies needed to ensure that neither the experimental subject nor the treating physician knew if the subject received the experimental or placebo treatment. Double-blinding would eliminate the chance that patient improvement would be caused by the expectation of receiving a potentially efficacious treatment.

ETHICS

In 1974, medical ethicist Sissela Bok published the article "The Ethics of Giving Placebos" in *Scientific American*. Bok's immensely influential article argued that the use of placebos in clinical practice is unethical. Consequently, many physicians stopped prescribing placebo treatments, and many hospital pharmacies stopped stocking placebos.

Regardless, to some extent, placebos are still used. A 2003 study published in the journal *Evaluations and the Health Professions* showed that 86 percent of Danish health care providers had used a minimum of one placebo treatment during the previous year. Such placebos included antibiotics for viral infections, sedatives for conditions other than depression, B vitamins for conditions other than multiple sclerosis and hair loss, saline injections, and physical therapy. Despite this finding, little doubt exists that the common use of placebos is no longer regarded favorably in medicine.

FURTHER STUDIES

In 1997, researchers reexamined the same studies analyzed by Beecher in the 1950s and concluded that the improvements observed in patients were caused by typical data fluctuations and not by the placebo effect. This 1997 cast doubt on the existence of the placebo effect.

However, a 2001 study by the research group of Fabrizio Benedetti and colleagues at the University of Torino Medical School in Italy, which was published in the journal *Pain*, provided direct evidence for the existence of the placebo effect. Benedetti and colleagues used three groups of patients who had undergone major surgery and who were all given an intravenous infusion of saline without an anesthetic. The first group was not informed of the infusion, the second group was told that the infusion was either a powerful painkiller or a placebo, and the third group was told that the saline infusion was a potent painkiller. Over three days, those in the group that had been told that they were being given a powerful painkiller required 34 percent less pain relief than the group that had not been told anything about the infusion and required 16 percent less than the group that was told that the infusion could be a placebo or a painkiller. Only the placebo effect could explain these results.

Also in 1997, Benedetti's group conducted pain-tolerance tests on patients while treating them with a nonopioid painkiller called ketorolac or with a drug called naloxone (which blocks the activity of opioid painkillers), or both. Some of these patients were told about their treatments and others were not. The results clearly showed that the presence of naloxone decreased the pain tolerance of those patients who knew they were being treated with ketorolac. Because ketorolac is not an opioid painkiller, the ability of naloxone to decrease pain tolerance shows that the pain reduction caused by the placebo effect is caused by endogenously produced opioid molecules. Brain scans have confirmed this result, because, in general, study subjects who experience an experimentally induced placebo effect show increased brain activity in areas of the brain that are rich in opioid receptors.

COMPLEMENTARY AND ALTERNATIVE MEDICINE

Complementary and alternative medical (CAM) therapies have much in common with placebo effects in that both are given to patients who expect to benefit from them by health care practitioners who expect them to work. To ensure that CAM treatments actually relieve symptoms and improve measurable physiological parameters, it is imperative that all CAM studies properly account for the placebo effect.

Michael A. Buratovich, Ph.D.

FURTHER READING

Bausell, Barker R. *Snake Oil Science: The Truth About Complementary and Alternative Medicine.* New York: Oxford University Press, 2007. A statistician with extensive experience in the design of clinical trials and data analysis describes the placebo effect, how to account for it when designing clinical trials, and why failing to properly account for it invalidates some of the clinical trials that examine the efficacy of complementary and alternative medicine.

Benedetti, Fabrizio. *Placebo Effects: Understanding the Mechanisms in Health and Disease.* New York: Oxford University Press, 2009. A highly respected placebo-effect researcher discusses the neurological basis for the placebo effect and proposes several potential biochemical explanations.

Evans, Dylan. *Placebo: Mind over Matter in Modern Medicine.* New York: Oxford University Press, 2004. A science writer provides an entertaining review of the history of the placebo effect and its use in medicine.

See also: Clinical trials; Double-blind, placebo-controlled studies; Insurance coverage; Pseudoscience; Scientific method; Self-care.

Plantain

CATEGORY: Herbs and supplements
RELATED TERMS: *Plantago lanceolata, P. major*
DEFINITION: Natural plant product used to treat specific health conditions.
PRINCIPAL PROPOSED USES: None
OTHER PROPOSED USES: Anti-inflammatory, chronic bronchitis, skin conditions

OVERVIEW

Plantain (not to be confused with the relative of the banana known by the same name) is a small weed often found in cultivated fields and at the edge of lawns. Traditionally, the crushed leaves were applied to the skin to treat wounds and bites, a leaf tincture was used for coughs, and the dried leaf was taken internally for the treatment of bronchitis, ulcers, epilepsy, and liver problems.

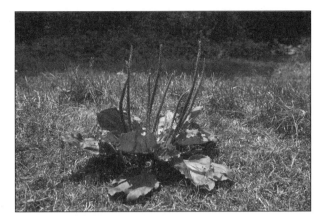

Plantain has been used to treat skin conditions. (Jerome Wexler/Photo Researchers, Inc.)

THERAPEUTIC DOSAGES

A typical dose of plantain for oral use is 1 to 3 grams (g) three times daily. Syrups and tinctures are used for coughs.

Plantain contains active substances in the iridoid glycoside family, especially aucubin, catalpol, and acteoside. The highest levels are found when the plant is collected in mid-fall. Other potentially active ingredients fall in the phenolic category, such as caffeic acid. Some plantain products are standardized to levels of one or more of these ingredients, but it is not clear whether this produces a better product.

THERAPEUTIC USES

Evidence too weak to rely upon has been used to indicate that topical plantain is helpful for skin conditions, including poison ivy and eczema. Similarly weak evidence from two studies performed in Bulgaria hint that oral plantain may be helpful for chronic bronchitis.

Plantain extracts do appear to have anti-inflammatory effects, at least in the test tube. However, unlike most pharmaceutical anti-inflammatory drugs, which work on the cyclooxygenase-1 (COX-1) and cyclooxygenase-2 (COX-2) systems, one study suggests that plantain may work in a different fashion, by decreasing levels of nitric oxide. Whether this indicates any real potential benefit in people remains unknown.

Other possible actions of plantain constituents based on test-tube studies include anticancer effects and antiviral actions. Contrary to some reports, one study found that plantain does not have diuretic (kidney-stimulating) effects.

SAFETY ISSUES

Plantain appears to be relatively safe, but comprehensive safety studies have not been performed. Plantain grown in soil contaminated with heavy metals such as thallium or antimony may develop relatively high concentrations of these potential toxins. Safety in pregnant or nursing women, young children, and individuals with liver or kidney disease has not been established. In 1997, the FDA reported that some plantain available for sale on the herb market was contaminated with similar-appearing foxglove (digitalis), an herb with potent and potentially toxic effects on the heart.

EBSCO CAM Review Board

FURTHER READING

Baroni, F., et al. "Antimony Accumulation in *Achillea ageratum, Plantago lanceolata,* and *Silene vulgaris* Growing in an Old Sb-Mining Area." *Environmental Pollution* 109 (2004): 347-352.

Chiang, L. C., et al. "Antiviral Activity of *Plantago major* Extracts and Related Compounds In Vitro." *Antiviral Research* 55 (2002): 53-62.

Galvez, M., et al. "Cytotoxic Effect of *Plantago* spp. on Cancer Cell Lines." *Journal of Ethnopharmacology* 88 (2003): 125-130.

Gomez-Flores, R., et al. "Immunoenhancing Properties of *Plantago major* Leaf Extract." *Phytotherapy Research* 14 (2001): 617-622.

Herold, A., et al. "Hydroalcoholic Plant Extracts with Anti-inflammatory Activity." *Roumanian Archives of Microbiology and Immunology* 62 (2004): 117-129.

Tamura, Y., and S. Nishibe. "Changes in the Concentrations of Bioactive Compounds in Plantain Leaves." *Journal of Agricultural and Food Chemistry* 50 (2002): 2514-2518.

Vigo, E., et al. "In-Vitro Anti-inflammatory Activity of *Pinus sylvestris* and *Plantago lanceolata* Extracts: Effect on Inducible NOS, COX-1, COX-2 and Their Products in J774A.1 Murine Macrophages." *Journal of Pharmacy and Pharmacology* 57 (2005): 383-391.

See also: Herbal medicine.

Pokeroot

CATEGORY: Herbs and supplements
RELATED TERMS: *Phytolacca americana*, pokeweed
DEFINITION: Natural plant product used to treat specific health conditions.
PRINCIPAL PROPOSED USES: None recommended

OVERVIEW

The herb pokeroot grows wild in many parts of North America. The name comes from a Native American word, *pocan*, a term that indicates any plant used to provide a red-colored dye. Pokeroot is a source of a blood-red pigment. Medicinally, it was used as an "alterative", a substance that supposedly removes toxins from the body and restores overall health. Like other alteratives, pokeroot was used for the treatment of cancer, skin conditions, and many other diseases attributed to toxins. Pokeroot causes vomiting and diarrhea, and these effects were also traditionally considered salutary. However, in modern times, it has become clear that pokeroot causes vomiting and diarrhea because it is toxic; it should not be used.

THERAPEUTIC DOSAGES

The use of pokeroot in any dosage is not recommended.

THERAPEUTIC USES

Pokeroot itself is not sold in the United States. However, substances found in pokeroot have shown promise for drug development. One of these, pokeroot antiviral protein, has shown potential as a treatment for human immunodeficiency virus (HIV) infection and other viral infections. Note, however, that these findings on one ingredient of pokeroot do not indicate that the whole herb is useful for HIV infection.

Another substance in pokeroot, pokeweed mitogen, forces cells to divide, a property that has led to a great deal of scientific investigation. These mitogenic effects are potentially quite dangerous and are more an argument against the use of pokeroot than for it. Other pokeroot constituents have shown potential anti-inflammatory, diuretic, and blood-pressure-lowering effects.

SAFETY ISSUES

Pokeroot is a toxic herb. Ingestion can lead to symptoms such as nausea, vomiting (sometimes with

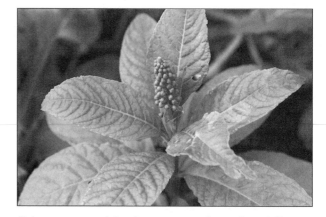

Pokeroot was used for the treatment of a variety of diseases. However, it has been determined to be a toxic plant. (Colin Cuthbert/Dilston Physic Garden/Photo Researchers, Inc.)

blood), diarrhea, rapid heart rate, a dangerous fall in blood pressure, difficult breathing, confusion, and death. Symptoms may develop with one-time use or insidiously over time. Fresh root is more toxic than dried root. The juice of pokeweed berries is even more toxic and can cause severe damage to blood cells even when it is applied only to the skin. Pokeroot should definitely not be used by pregnant or nursing women or young children.

EBSCO CAM Review Board

FURTHER READING

D'Cruz, O. J., et al. "Mucosal Toxicity Studies of a Gel Formulation of Native Pokeweed Antiviral Protein." *Toxicologic Pathology* 32 (2004): 212-221.

Hudak, K. A., et al. "Pokeweed Antiviral Protein Binds to the Cap Structure of Eukaryotic mRNA and Depurinates the mRNA Downstream of the Cap." *RNA* 8 (2002): 1148-1159.

Parikh, B. A., et al. "Evidence for Retro-translocation of Pokeweed Antiviral Protein from Endoplasmic Reticulum into Cytosol and Separation of Its Activity on Ribosomes from Its Activity on Capped RNA." *Biochemistry* 44 (2005): 2478-2490.

Picard, D., et al. "Pokeweed Antiviral Protein Inhibits Brome Mosaic Virus Replication in Plant Cells." *Journal of Biological Chemistry* 280 (2005) 20069-20075.

Turpin, J. A. "Considerations and Development of Topical Microbicides to Inhibit the Sexual Transmission of HIV." *Expert Opinion on Investigational Drugs* 11 (2002): 1077-1097.

Yamaguchi, K., et al. "Mitogenic Properties of Poke-weed Lectin-D Isoforms on Human Peripheral Blood Lymphocytes: Non-mitogen PL-D1 and Mitogen PL-D2." *Bioscience, Biotechnology, and Biochemistry* 68 (2004): 1591-1593.

Wang, S., et al. "The Effects of Pokeweed Mitogen (PWM) and Phytohemagglutinin (PHA) on Bovine Oocyte Maturation and Embryo Development In Vitro." *Animal Reproductive Science* 67 (2001): 215-220.

See also: Herbal medicine.

Policicosanol

CATEGORY: Herbs and supplements
RELATED TERMS: 1-octacosanol, N-octacosanol, octacosanol alcohol, octacosanol, wheat germ oil
DEFINITION: Natural substance promoted as a dietary supplement for specific health benefits.
PRINCIPAL PROPOSED USE: High cholesterol
OTHER PROPOSED USES: Intermittent claudication, Parkinson's disease, sports performance enhancement

OVERVIEW

Policicosanol is a mixture of waxy substances generally manufactured from sugarcane. It contains about 60 percent octacosanol and many related chemicals. In some cases, the terms "octacosanol" and "policicosanol" are used interchangeably.

Numerous studies have reported that sugarcane policicosanol can substantially improve cholesterol profile, with an efficacy approximately equal to that of the most effective drugs used for this purpose. On this basis, policicosanol has been approved as a treatment for high cholesterol in about two dozen countries, most of them in Latin America.

However, essentially all positive studies of policicosanol were performed and reported by a single Cuban research group, a group with a financial relationship to the product. Independent verification of the product's effectiveness was delayed for several years by various legal obstacles. In 2006 and 2007, several independent studies of sugarcane policicosanol were at last reported. In none of these trials has policicosanol proved more effective than placebo.

SOURCES

The tested Cuban policicosanol product is manufactured from sugarcane. Octacosanol and related substances are also found in wheat germ oil, vegetable oils, alfalfa, and various animal products.

Because of political and patent issues, sugarcane policicosanol has not been widely available in the United States. Products sold in the American market as policicosanol are generally derived from beeswax or wheat germ. These products have a significantly different mixture of constituents and could have substantially different effects.

THERAPEUTIC DOSAGES

Typical dosages of policicosanol in Cuban studies have ranged from 5 milligrams (mg) to 10 mg twice daily.

THERAPEUTIC USES

The Cuban research group that holds the patent on sugarcane-derived policicosanol has published approximately eighty double-blind studies on its product. If these reports are to be believed, several thousand people with elevated cholesterol levels have been enrolled in clinical trials ranging in length from six weeks to twelve months. In virtually every one of these trials, policicosanol proved both more effective than placebo and just as effective as statin drugs.

However, in science, it is always necessary to have independent confirmation of results before a treatment can be considered proven to work. The first truly independent trials of policicosanol as a treatment for high cholesterol began to appear in 2006. Of the eighty-nine studies (enrolling more than fifty-seven thousand people) published since then, not one found policicosanol more effective than placebo. These results have raised serious doubts about the effectiveness of sugarcane policicosanol. In addition, questions are being raised about other scientific claims made by the patent-holding Cuban research group.

Wheat-germ policicosanol, sold in the United States as a substitute for sugarcane policicosanol, failed to prove more effective than placebo in the one published clinical trial of this product. There is no published evidence to indicate that beeswax-derived policicosanol affects cholesterol profile. A study published in Croatia reportedly found benefit with rice-source policosanol, but it had significant problems in design and reporting. Considerable doubt exists regarding whether any form of policosanol offers cholesterol-related benefits.

One study, again conducted by the patent-holding Cuban research group, reported that policosanol is helpful for intermittent claudication. Other potential uses of policosanol have been proposed by researchers outside Cuba. A small double-blind trial found marginal evidence that policosanol might enhance sports performance. Marginal benefits were also seen in a small double-blind trial of persons with Parkinson's disease; however, this study also reported that policosanol can increase the side effects of levodopa, the standard drug used for Parkinson's disease. Finally, in a small double-blind trial, policosanol failed to produce any benefits in amyotrophic lateral sclerosis.

SAFETY ISSUES

Virtually all statements regarding the safety of policosanol derive from studies reported by the patent-holding Cuban research group. Because the reliability of these researchers is in question, all of the following statements are similarly open to question.

Given the above caveat, policosanol is said to be safe at the maximum recommended dose. In double-blind trials, only mild short-term side effects, such as nervousness, headache, diarrhea, and insomnia, have been reported. A safety study of 27,879 people followed for two to four years showed that the use of policosanol produced adverse effects, primarily weight loss, excessive urination, and insomnia, in only 0.31 percent of participants. In animal studies, no toxic signs were seen even at 620 times the maximum recommended dose. In addition, policosanol does not adversely affect the liver. Finally, policosanol does not interact with three types of medications used for high blood pressure: calcium-channel antagonists, diuretics, and beta-blockers.

On the other hand, policosanol may be a blood thinner, and it appears to enhance the blood-thinning effects of aspirin, though one study failed to confirm this adverse effect. Still, to be on the safe side, policosanol should not be combined with aspirin or other blood-thinning drugs, such as warfarin (Coumadin), heparin, clopidogrel (Plavix), ticlopidine (Ticlid), or pentoxifylline (Trental). There is also a remote chance that policosanol might cause excessive bleeding if combined with natural supplements that thin the blood, such as garlic, ginkgo, and high-dose vitamin E. Similarly, persons with clotting problems should avoid policosanol, and the supplement should not be used during the period immediately before or after surgery or labor and delivery. One non-Cuban report suggests that policosanol might increase the action of levodopa, a medication used for Parkinson's disease, leading to increased side effects called dyskinesias.

The maximum safe dosages for young children, pregnant or nursing women, and persons with severe liver or kidney disease have not been established.

IMPORTANT INTERACTIONS

Persons taking blood-thinning medications such as aspirin, warfarin, heparin, clopidogrel, ticlopidine, or pentoxifylline should not use policosanol except on medical advice. Also, persons using natural supplements that thin the blood, such as garlic, ginkgo, or high-dose vitamin E, should not use policosanol except under physician supervision. Finally, one should note that policosanol may increase both the effects and the side effects of levodopa.

EBSCO CAM Review Board

FURTHER READING

Francini-Pesenti, F., et al. "Sugar Cane Policosanol Failed to Lower Plasma Cholesterol in Primitive, Diet-Resistant Hypercholesterolaemia." *Complementary Therapies in Medicine* 16 (2008): 61-65.

Kassis, A. N. "Evaluation of Cholesterol-Lowering and Antioxidant Properties of Sugar Cane Policosanols in Hamsters and Humans." *Applied Physiology, Nutrition, and Metabolism* 33 (2008): 540-541.

_____, and P. J. Jones. "Changes in Cholesterol Kinetics Following Sugar Cane Policosanol Supplementation." *Lipids in Health and Disease* 7 (2008): 17.

_____. "Lack of Cholesterol-Lowering Efficacy of Cuban Sugar Cane Policosanols in Hypercholesterolemic Persons." *American Journal of Clinical Nutrition* 84 (2006): 1003-1008.

Reiner, Z., and E. Tedeschi-Reiner. "Rice Policosanol Does Not Have Any Effects on Blood Coagulation Factors in Hypercholesterolemic Patients." *Collegium Antropologicum* 31 (2007): 1061-1064.

See also: Cholesterol, high; Intermittent claudication; Parkinson's disease; Sports and fitness support: Enhancing performance.

Polycystic ovary syndrome

CATEGORY: Condition

DEFINITION: Treatment of a chronic endocrine disorder in women, which is marked by elevated levels of male hormones and infertility and other conditions.

PRINCIPAL PROPOSED NATURAL TREATMENTS: Inositol, N-acetylcysteine

OTHER PROPOSED NATURAL TREATMENTS: B vitamins, chromium, cinnamon, green tea, spearmint tea

INTRODUCTION

Polycystic ovary syndrome (PCOS) is a chronic endocrine disorder in women. It is characterized by elevated levels of male hormones (androgens) and by infertility, obesity, insulin resistance, hair growth on the face and body, and anovulation, a condition in which the ovaries produce few or no eggs.

Ovaries normally produce follicles that develop into eggs. In women with PCOS, the ovaries produce the follicles, but the eggs may not mature or leave the ovary. The immature follicles can develop into fluid-filled sacs called cysts. Most women with PCOS have cysts, but all women with ovarian cysts do not necessarily have PCOS.

The cause of PCOS is unknown, though genetics may play a role. Some evidence suggests the problem is related to insulin resistance with elevated levels of insulin. These high insulin levels may stimulate excess production of androgens from the ovaries. This could

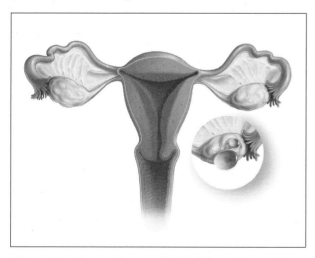

Illustration of an ovarian cyst. (BSIP/Photo Researchers, Inc.)

prevent ovulation and lead to enlarged, polycystic ovaries. Treatments for PCOS include drugs to improve insulin sensitivity, along with hormonal treatments and fertility drugs when pregnancy is desired.

PROPOSED NATURAL TREATMENTS

Inositol. The supplement inositol has shown some promise for PCOS. In a double-blind, placebo-controlled trial, 136 women were given inositol at a dose of 100 milligrams twice daily, while 147 were given placebo. In fourteen weeks, participants given inositol showed improvement in ovulation frequency compared to those given placebo. Benefits were also seen in terms of weight loss and levels of HDL (good) cholesterol. A subsequent study of ninety-four women with PCOS found similar results. However, both of the studies were performed by the same research group. Independent confirmation will be necessary before inositol can be considered an effective treatment for PCOS.

N-acetylcysteine. The supplement N-acetylcysteine (NAC) has shown some promise for the treatment of female infertility caused by PCOS. A double-blind, placebo-controlled study evaluated the effectiveness of NAC in 150 women with PCOS who had previously failed to respond to the fertility drug clomiphene. Participants were given clomiphene plus placebo or clomiphene plus 1.2 grams (g) daily of NAC. The results indicated that combined treatment with NAC plus clomiphene was dramatically more effective than clomiphene taken with placebo. Almost 50 percent of the women in the combined treatment group ovulated, compared to about 1 percent in the clomiphene-alone group. The pregnancy rate in the combined treatment group was 21 percent, compared to 0 percent in the clomiphene-alone group.

However, partially negative results were seen in another study. This trial compared NAC at a dose of 1.8 grams daily with the drug metformin in sixty-one infertile women with PCOS who had, as in the foregoing study, failed to respond to clomiphine. NAC proved far less effective than the drug at inducing ovulation; nonetheless, the data from this study do not rule out the possibility that NAC provided some slight benefit.

Other treatments. The herb cinnamon has shown some promise as a treatment for diabetes. On this basis, it has been tried in PCOS. In a small placebo-controlled study, cinnamon appeared to improve insulin sensitivity.

The supplement chromium has shown promise for improving insulin sensitivity, and on this basis, it has been tried as a treatment for PCOS. However, in a small pilot study, the use of chromium at 200 micrograms daily did not have a positive effect in PCOS.

A mixture of B vitamins has shown some promise for improving pregnancy rates in people with PCOS. Green tea has been tried in PCOS, but the one small published study failed to show benefit of any kind. Daily spearmint tea consumption was reported to improve patient-assessed hirsutism and testosterone and other hormone levels in a small trial of women with PCOS.

EBSCO CAM Review Board

FURTHER READING

Chan, C. C., et al. "Effects of Chinese Green Tea on Weight, and Hormonal and Biochemical Profiles in Obese Patients with Polycystic Ovary Syndrome." *Journal of the Society for Gynecologic Investigation* 13 (2005): 63-68.

Grant, P. "Spearmint Herbal Tea Has Significant Anti-Androgen Effects in Polycystic Ovarian Syndrome." *Phytotherapy Research* 24 (2010): 186-188.

Lucidi, R. S., et al. "Effect of Chromium Supplementation on Insulin Resistance and Ovarian and Menstrual Cyclicity in Women with Polycystic Ovary Syndrome." *Fertility and Sterility* 84 (2005): 1755-1757.

Rizk, A. Y., et al. "N-acetyl-cysteine Is a Novel Adjuvant to Clomiphene Citrate in Clomiphene Citrate-Resistant Patients with Polycystic Ovary Syndrome." *Fertility and Sterility* 83 (2005): 367-370.

Schachter, M., et al. "Prospective Randomized Trial of Metformin and Vitamins for the Reduction of Plasma Homocysteine in Insulin-Resistant Polycystic Ovary Syndrome." *Fertility and Sterility* 88 (2007): 227-230.

Wang, J. G., et al. "The Effect of Cinnamon Extract on Insulin Resistance Parameters in Polycystic Ovary Syndrome." *Fertility and Sterility* 88 (2007): 240-243.

See also: Inositol; N-acetylcysteine.

Popular health movement

CATEGORY: Issues and overviews
RELATED TERMS: Eclectic medicine, Grahamism, Thomsonianism

DEFINITION: An early nineteenth-century health movement in the United States that promoted nontraditional medical treatment, in particular the use of herbal remedies, and opposed traditional medicine.

OVERVIEW

The popular health movement of the early nineteenth century led many Americans to react with scepticism to doctors and to medical practices that were common at the time. People turned instead to forms of treatment that did not involve doctors and often involved herbal remedies. Several factors led to this scepticism.

Beginning in the eighteenth century, doctors claimed knowledge, or expertise, beyond common understanding. This specialized knowledge led to a rise in status and authority for doctors and was symbolized by the increasing use of Latin terms to describe medical conditions, placing the language of doctors beyond the grasp of most people. In spite of claims to expertise, medical practice of the time was often harsh to the point of brutality, and it was still common for a physician to use techniques such as bloodletting by cutting veins or applying leeches. One of the most common prescribed drugs was calomel (mercurous chloride), which was acknowledged to have severe toxic side effects.

A second factor influencing the popular health movement was the mood of the country with the election of Andrew Jackson to the U.S. presidency in 1828. People denounced elitism and elites, including politicians and doctors. Just as politics during this time promoted the idea of democracy as a popular movement and expanded the vote to all white men, the country reacted against the specialized authority of doctors. One effect of this reaction was the abolition by most states of requirements that doctors be licensed.

During this time, too, the country saw philosophical and artistic movements toward nature and the idea of letting nature affect healing; this was a third factor in development of the popular health movement. Nature was embraced, especially with the wide interest in botanical remedies.

THOMSONIANISM

One of the leading figures of the popular health movement was Samuel Thomson, born in New Hampshire to a farming family. Thomson became a leading proponent of herbal cures, which he began learning from a woman who lived nearby. He had seen his mother die of measles; conventional doctors were unable to cure her. Later, after his wife grew ill and doctors had stopped treating her, Thomson called in herbal healers, who were able to help her. He later used his own cures to heal a son and a daughter, strengthening his belief in herbal cures.

Thomson's cures were largely plant-based. His book describing his system was published as *New Guide to Health: Or, Botanic Family Physician* (1822). The use of plants was part of a more complex system of belief, however.

Thomson, who believed that illness came from exposure to cold, argued that keeping the body warm would prevent illness. He applied heat to the body externally and internally with steam baths and cayenne peppers. His system also included the idea of expurgating the body of toxins, which involved the use of laxatives and emetics such as Lobelia plant for therapeutic vomiting. Thomson's relationship with conventional physicians was not good, as he arrogantly rejected treatments not based on his own system.

Eclectic Medicine and Grahamism

Eclectic medicine. Eventually, healers who were interested in Thomson's herbal cures, but also in more conventional medicine, found themselves breaking with Thomson. The physician Wooster Beach, who used Thomson's botanical idea but disagreed with him on other issues, founded a medical school in 1829 as part of the new eclectic medicine movement. This movement argued that physicians should choose freely from any idea or medical system they believed would help their patients. Within the eclectic movement, Thomson's ideas on the use of plants could be used without Thomson's restrictions, which included rejecting the study of physiology and anatomy. The eclectic medicine movement remained influential for a century, lasting until the 1920s.

Grahamism. Probably the most influential health reformer of the early nineteenth century after Thomson was Sylvester Graham, a Presbyterian preacher from Connecticut. Although Graham had no medical training, he had great public influence, particularly on dietary practices. His name is perhaps best known in relation to "Graham crackers," which he invented. Graham also was a strong proponent of vegetarianism and of temperance in general, advocating restrictions

on alcohol consumption and sexual activity. In diet, he urged the use of dark, whole-wheat breads free of the chemical additives that were common even at that time.

Other philosophies of medicine and treatment also became popular. These included hydropathy, with baths as a basic element, and homeopathy, operating from the idea that like treats like. Homeopathy opposed the methods of allopathy, or traditional medicine, which treated disease with substances unrelated to the illness.

David Hutto, Ph.D.

Further Reading

Burbick, Joan. *Healing the Republic: The Language of Health and the Culture of Nationalism in Nineteenth-Century America*. New ed. New York: Cambridge University Press, 2009. First published in 1994, this social and cultural history examines the national dialogue and mood that helped to define the popular health movement.

Cabrera, Chanchal. "The History of Western Herbal Medicine." This brief but detailed history of herbal medicine is available at http://www.chanchalcabrera.com/articles. Of particular note is the discussion of Samuel Thomson and his influence.

"Every Man His Own Physician: Thomsonianism." In *Nature Cures: A History of Alternative Medicine in America*, edited by James C. Whorton. New York: Oxford University Press, 2004. This chapter describes the influence of Samuel Thomson on the popular health movement. Includes a detailed description of what led him to his beliefs about herbal cures.

Whorton, James C. "The History of Complementary and Alternative Medicine." In *Essentials of Complementary and Alternative Medicine*, edited by Wayne B. Jonas and Jeffrey S. Levin. Philadelphia: Lippincott Williams & Wilkins, 1999. Discusses the history of alternative medicine in the United States, with an emphasis on its relationship to conventional medicine. The discussion puts Thomsonianism into a broader context.

See also: Alternative versus traditional medicine; Health freedom movement; Herbal medicine; History of alternative medicine; History of complementary medicine; Homeopathy; Popular practitioners; Samuel Thomson.

Popular practitioners

CATEGORY: Issues and overviews

RELATED TERMS: Alternative health practitioners, clinicians, holistic healers, holistic health practitioners, integrative medical doctors and physicians, natural health practitioners

DEFINITION: Popularly known practitioners of complementary, alternative, and integrative medicine.

OVERVIEW

Numerous health professionals have chosen to include the principles and therapies of complementary and alternative medicine (CAM) in their health care practices. Some do so while maintaining their traditional medical practices. Certain practitioners have become well known in the field of CAM. The following sections highlight the key CAM practitioners Samuel Hahnemann, Edward Bach, John Harvey Kellogg, Andrew Weil, and Deepak Chopra.

KEY PRACTITIONERS

Samuel Hahnemann. Samuel Hahnemann, born April 10, 1755, in East Germany, is best known for his work in homeopathy, a medical system he defined. Homeopathy considers physical symptoms to be guides to the underlying causes of illness and disease.

Hahnemann was a brilliant student who excelled in science and languages, including German, French, Greek, Hebrew, Spanish, English, and Latin. He became a medical student in 1975 and graduated four years later with his doctor of medicine degree from the University of Erlangen in Bavaria. As a practicing physician, Hahnemann became disenchanted with traditional medicine and became a reformer. He advocated the importance of fresh air, regular exercise, a healthy diet, and restful sleep for patients, and of maintaining public hygiene, adequate housing, and proper sewage disposal. He was a writer, intuitively recognizing the role of microorganisms and genetics in disease before other scientists documented these concepts. Hahnemann opposed the abuse of persons with mental illness and employed compassion when working with psychiatric patients.

As the founder of homeopathy, he established a system of holistic treatments that supported the importance of the mind/body connection. His treatments used the law of similars, or "like cures like" (*similia similibus curentur*). He developed a sophisticated laboratory process, a shaking process, to develop medicines that became stronger through dilutions and succession. These homeopathic medicines encouraged the body to respond and heal itself. This approach was unlike traditional Western medicine, which relied on the management and suppression of symptoms rather than on effecting a cure. To prove his ideas, Hahnemann tested his solutions on himself, with repeated success.

Hahnemann served as the chosen physician to the wealthy and famous while providing free care to the poor. Homeopathy demonstrated positive clinical results across Europe, India, and Russia, where it was preferred to other treatments of the day, such as purging and bloodletting.

Edward Bach. Edward Bach was born in 1886 in the United Kingdom. Early in his successful career, Bach practiced as a traditional physician with conventional approaches. He found that an individual's personality and attitude affected his or her health and thought

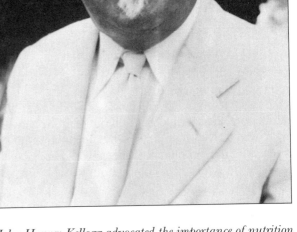

John Harvey Kellogg advocated the importance of nutrition in the management of disease. (AP Photo)

that this should be considered as a part of medical treatment. Like Samuel Hahnemann, he believed that the focus of treating illness should be not on symptom suppression but on addressing the root cause of disease. His dissatisfaction with traditional medicine led him to pursue advanced education in immunology as a bacteriologist.

In 1917, Bach was diagnosed with a severe illness and was told he had three months to live. He focused on his work and lived years past those expected three months. Bach believed that his extended life was helped by following his passion and avocation, and that this was a key to spiritual and physical health.

While working at Royal London Homeopathic Hospital from 1919 to 1922, Bach discovered that Hahnemann had connected the personality to disease more than one hundred years earlier. Bach sought a holistic approach to his medical practice. He used his skills and knowledge from traditional medicine to develop oral vaccines, which he called the Seven Bach Nosodes, from intestinal bacteria, and used them to successfully treat chronic diseases and promote health. The medical profession embraced the concept of vaccines from bacteria, but Bach wanted to develop plant-based therapies. He developed flower essences from *Impatiens* and *Clematis*, among other flowering plants. He eventually produced close to forty essences that addressed negative states of mind, and he formulated what he called Rescue Remedy for stress and other conditions.

Bach provided treatment free of charge to the poor until he died at the age of fifty years, some twenty years after he was told he had three months to live. The Dr. Edward Bach Centre in England offers education and practitioner referrals.

John Harvey Kellogg. John Harvey Kellogg, born in Michigan on February 26, 1852, was one of the first physicians to advocate the importance of nutrition in the management of disease. Kellogg graduated in 1875 with a medical degree from New York University Medical College, Bellevue Hospital.

Kellogg's recognition as a medical physician was connected to his work at Battle Creek Sanitarium, a facility originally operated by the Seventh-day Adventist Church as Western Health Reform Institute. Here the wealthy and famous would stay and seek ways to improve their health. Among those who came for therapy at the sanitarium were U.S. president William Howard Taft, businessmen John D. Rockefeller and Henry Ford, aviator Amelia Earhart, playwright George Bernard Shaw, and inventor Thomas Edison. Activities provided at the sanitarium included education and lectures on healthy lifestyles. Approaches included healthy nutrition through simple vegetarian diets with nuts, prescribed exercise, breathing exercise with fresh air, and abstinence from smoking and drinking alcohol. Residents of Battle Creek Sanitarium could receive enemas, hydrotherapy, phototherapy through sunbaths, and other treatments.

Kellogg taught that a meatless diet was preferred for health. He produced the first meatless "meat" made from nuts and was one of the first to advocate the use of soy-based products. Understanding that the body had natural disease defenses through friendly bacteria in the intestine, he supported the use of acidophilus milk, which included the helpful bacterium *Lactobacillus acidophilus*. Kellogg and his brother were instrumental in developing a healthy breakfast cereal that later became Kellogg's Corn Flakes, still popular today.

Kellogg died on December 14, 1943, at the age of ninety-one, famous for his energy and vision. He authored more than fifty books and was a generous philanthropist.

Andrew Weil. Andrew Weil, one of the most popular CAM practitioners, was born on June 8, 1942, in Philadelphia. He is best known for fusing conventional and alternative medicines into what he called integrative medicine, emphasizing preferred natural ways to health while supporting traditional medical approaches in a health crisis. He recommended boosting the body's natural immune system through activities such as healthy diet, regular exercise, and stress management.

From his early years, Weil had demonstrated diverse abilities and talents. His academic achievements led him to Harvard University, where he majored in biology. His academic mentor, Richard Schultes, an ethnobotanist, influenced his life path. In 1964, Weil graduated from Harvard with a degree in biology and a concentration in botany. Four years later, he graduated from medical school.

As a staff member of the Harvard Botanical Museum, Weil secured independent funding to study medicinal plants and traditional health practices of peoples in the Americas and in Africa. He wrote the first of his many books, *The Natural Mind*, during this time. His research led him to examine the differences

Kellogg's Toasted Corn Flakes

John Harvey Kellogg, in his book The New Dietetics: What To Eat and How—A Guide to Scientific Feeding in Health and Disease *(1921), outlines the preparation of corn flakes in the following passage about the cereal product that made his name famous.*

Toasted corn flakes is a breakfast food prepared from white corn grits by a process of which the following constitute the several successive steps:

1. Cooking at a temperature above the boiling point.
2. Drying.
3. Tempering by the addition of water or steam.
4. Milling by means of mills specially constructed for the purpose by means of which the grits are flattened out into large flakes.
5. Toasting in a traveling oven.
6. Salt and other flavorings are added in the process of cooking.

This product, devised by the author many years ago, in an effort to provide palatable dextrinized cereal foods for the patients of the Battle Creek Sanitarium, was at first designed to be eaten dry as the best means of stimulating the action of the salivary glands and to encourage the practice of thorough mastication. Eaten with milk, corn flakes constitute an excellent breakfast food. It must be acknowledged, however, that when eaten moist with milk or cream it offers no better nutrient than the old-fashioned brose of the Scotch peasantry, or the corn meal mush of our childhood days. It cannot be doubted that all our efforts to improve upon Nature's products by artificial manipulations are more or less futile and often result in a denaturing which lessens their value as food-stuffs.

between conventional medicine and alternative practices, such as the use of organic compounds rather than synthetic drugs.

In 1983, Weil accepted a position as clinical professor at the University of Arizona College of Medicine, while maintaining his private practice. He founded the Program for Integrative Medicine at Arizona, where health professionals can train in the practices of integrative medicine.

Weil bridged the gap between traditional medicine and CAM. He was featured on the October 17, 2005, cover of *Time* magazine. Weil's ideas have influenced the establishment of integrative medicine programs at various colleges and health care agencies across the United States.

Deepak Chopra. Deepak Chopra, born on October 22, 1947, in New Delhi, India, is an advocate of mind/body healing and emotional wellness. His father, a cardiologist, encouraged him to enter medicine by appealing to the young Chopra's love of reading.

Chopra completed medical school at All India Institute of Medical Sciences and did his internship at New Jersey's Muhlenberg Hospital. He served as chief of staff at Boston Regional Medical Center. He is a successful board-certified internal medicine physician and endocrinologist. He has written more than fifty-five books, fourteen of which have been best sellers. Chopra also is a columnist for the *San Francisco Chronicle* and the *Washington Post.*

In 2008, *Time* magazine lauded Chopra's diverse career in CAM, including his work with Ayurveda, Transcendental Meditation, Eastern spirituality, and New Age philosophy. In 1996, with David Simon, he opened the Chopra Center for Well Being in La Jolla, California. This center provides retreats, education, and training programs that merge the best of modern Western medicine with the Eastern principles of healing. The center's signature program, Perfect Health, offers retreats in which guests may participate in Panchakarma detoxification and in cleansing, yoga, and meditation.

Marylane Wade Koch, M.S.N., R.N.

FURTHER READING

Bradford, Thomas Lindsley. *The Life and Letters of Dr. Samuel Hahnemann* (1895). Ninety-two chapters on the life of Samuel Hahnemann, the founder of homeopathy. Available as a public domain work at http://www.homeoint.org/books4/bradford/index.htm.

Kellogg, John Harvey. *The Battle Creek Sanitarium System: History, Organization, Methods, Battle Creek, Michigan* (1908). Describes holistic approaches to wellness and health practiced by Kellogg at the Battle Creek Sanitarium. Available as a public domain work at http://www.archive.org/details/battlecreeksani00kellgoog.

Leary, B. "The Early Work of Dr. Edward Bach." *British Homeopathic Journal* 88, no. 1 (1999): 28-30. Discusses Bach's early scientific work.

Tompkins, Ptolemy. "New Age Super Sage." *Time*, November 14, 2008. Details the life of Deepak Chopra from his early years to his success as a CAM practitioner and a writer.

Weil, Andrew. "On Integrative Medicine and the Nature of Reality." Interview by Bonnie Horrigan. *Alternative Therapies in Health and Medicine* 7, no. 4 (2001): 96-104. An interview with Weil, in which he discusses integrative medicine and other topics.

See also: Alternative versus traditional medicine; Functional foods: Overview; Health freedom movement; History of alternative medicine; History of complementary medicine; Integrative medicine; Mind/body medicine; Optimal health; Popular Health movement; Traditional healing; Wellness, general; Wellness therapies; Whole medicine.

Potassium

CATEGORY: Herbs and supplements
RELATED TERMS: Chelated potassium (potassium aspartate, potassium citrate), potassium bicarbonate, potassium chloride
DEFINITION: Natural substance essential for health and promoted as a dietary supplement for specific health benefits.
PRINCIPAL PROPOSED USE: Hypertension

OVERVIEW

Potassium is a mineral found in many foods and supplements. Pure potassium is not seen in health food stores or pharmacies because it is a highly reactive metal that bursts into flames when exposed to water. The potassium that is eaten or taken as a supplement is composed of potassium atoms bound to other, nonmetallic substances.

Potassium is one of the major electrolytes in the body, along with sodium and chloride. Potassium and sodium work together like a molecular seesaw: When the level of one goes up, that of the other goes down. Together, the three dissolved minerals play an intimate chemical role in every function of the body.

REQUIREMENTS AND SOURCES

Potassium is an essential mineral obtained from many common foods. True potassium deficiencies are rare except in cases of prolonged vomiting or diarrhea or with the use of diuretic drugs. However, in one sense, potassium deficiency is common when compared to the amount of sodium in the diet. It is

probably healthy to consume a minimum of five times as much potassium as sodium (and perhaps fifty to one hundred times as much), but the standard American diet contains twice as much sodium as potassium. Therefore, taking extra potassium may be a good idea to balance the sodium consumed to such excess.

Bananas, orange juice, potatoes, avocados, lima beans, cantaloupes, peaches, tomatoes, flounder, salmon, and cod all contain more than 300 milligrams (mg) of potassium per serving. Other good sources include chicken, meat, and various other fruits, vegetables, and fish.

Over-the-counter potassium supplements typically contain 99 mg of potassium per tablet. There is some evidence that, of the different forms of potassium supplements, potassium citrate may be most helpful for those with high blood pressure.

Research indicates that it is important also to get enough magnesium when one is taking potassium. It might be wise to also take extra vitamin B_{12}.

THERAPEUTIC DOSAGES

When used by physicians, potassium is usually measured in milliequivalents (meqs) rather than in the more common milligrams. A typical therapeutic dosage of potassium is between 10 and 20 meq, taken three to four times daily.

THERAPEUTIC USES

The most common use of potassium supplements is to make up for potassium depletion caused by diuretic drugs. These medications are often used to help regulate blood pressure, but by depleting the body of potassium, they may inadvertently make blood pressure harder to control.

SCIENTIFIC EVIDENCE

High blood pressure. According to a review of thirty-three double-blind studies, potassium supplements can produce a slight but definite drop in blood pressure. However, two large studies found no benefit. The explanation is probably that potassium is only slightly helpful. When a treatment has only a small effect, it is not unusual for some studies to show no effect while others find a modest benefit. It is possible that potassium may help only those people who are a bit deficient in this mineral. Evidence suggests that potassium supplements may be most effective for people who eat too much salt.

SAFETY ISSUES

As an essential nutrient, potassium is safe when taken at appropriate dosages. If too much is taken, the body will simply excrete it in the urine. However, people who have severe kidney disease cannot excrete potassium normally and should consult a physician before taking a potassium supplement. Similarly, persons taking potassium-sparing diuretics (such as spironolactone), ACE inhibitors (such as captopril), or trimethoprim-sulfamethoxazole should not also take potassium supplements except under doctor supervision. Potassium pills can cause injury to the esophagus if they get stuck on the way down, so one should make sure to take them with plenty of water.

IMPORTANT INTERACTIONS

Persons taking loop diuretics or thiazide diuretics may need more potassium. Persons taking ACE inhibitors (such as captopril, lisinopril, and enalapril), potassium-sparing diuretics (such as triamterene or spironolactone), or trimethoprim-sulfamethoxazole should not take potassium except on the advice of a physician.

EBSCO CAM Review Board

FURTHER READING

Gu, D., et al. "Effect of Potassium Supplementation on Blood Pressure in Chinese." *Journal of Hypertension* 19 (2001): 1325-1331.

He, F. J., et al. "Effects of Potassium Chloride and Potassium Bicarbonate on Endothelial Function, Cardiovascular Risk Factors, and Bone Turnover in Mild Hypertensives." *Hypertension* 55 (2010): 681-688.

Savica, V., G. Bellinghieri, and J. D. Kopple. "The Effect of Nutrition on Blood Pressure." *Annual Review of Nutrition* 30 (2010): 365-401.

See also: Heart attack; Hypertension.

Potassium-sparing diuretics

CATEGORY: Drug interactions
DEFINITION: An alternative diuretic used to avoid the potassium loss common with loop and thiazide diuretics.
INTERACTIONS: Arginine, magnesium, potassium, white willow, zinc

POTASSIUM

Effect: Likely Harmful Interaction

Potassium-sparing diuretics cause the kidneys to hold potassium in the body. Persons taking these medications generally should not take potassium supplements because potassium levels might rise too high.

Treatments that combine thiazide diuretics (which cause potassium loss) and potassium-sparing diuretics can affect potassium levels unpredictably. Persons taking such a combination medication should not take potassium except on the advice of a physician.

MAGNESIUM

Effect: Possible Harmful Interaction

Preliminary evidence from animal studies suggests that the potassium-sparing diuretic amiloride might cause the body to retain magnesium also, along with potassium. Therefore, taking magnesium supplements might conceivably present the risk of excessive magnesium levels.

ARGININE

Effect: Possible Harmful Interaction

Based on experience with intravenous arginine, it is possible that the use of high-dose oral arginine might alter potassium levels in the body, especially in people with severe liver disease. This is a potential concern for persons who take potassium-sparing diuretics.

WHITE WILLOW

Effect: Possible Negative Interaction

The herb white willow contains substances that are similar to aspirin. On this basis, it might not be advisable to combine white willow with potassium-sparing diuretics.

ZINC

Effect: Possible Harmful Interaction

The potassium-sparing diuretic amiloride was found to significantly reduce zinc excretion from the body. This means that if one takes zinc supplements at the same time as amiloride, zinc accumulation could occur. This could lead to toxic side effects. However, the potassium-sparing diuretic triamterene does not seem to cause this problem.

EBSCO CAM Review Board

FURTHER READING

Reyes, A. J., et al. "Urinary Zinc Excretion, Diuretics, Zinc Deficiency, and Some Side-Effects of Diuretics." *South African Journal of Medical Sciences* 64 (1983): 936-941.

Wester, P. O. "Urinary Zinc Excretion During Treatment with Different Diuretics." *Acta Medica Scandinavica* 208 (1980): 209-212.

See also: Arginine; Food and Drug Administration; Magnesium; Potassium; Supplements: Introduction; Thiazide diuretics; White willow; Zinc.

Preeclampsia and pregnancy-induced hypertension

CATEGORY: Condition

RELATED TERMS: Eclampsia, gestational hypertension, hypertension of pregnancy, pregnancy-induced hypertension, toxemia of pregnancy

DEFINITION: Treatment of increased blood pressure, protein in the urine, and other symptoms during pregnancy.

PRINCIPAL PROPOSED NATURAL TREATMENT: Calcium

OTHER PROPOSED NATURAL TREATMENTS: Arginine, coenzyme Q_{10}, evening primrose oil, folate, lycopene, magnesium, N-acetylcysteine, omega-3 fatty acids, vitamin C and vitamin E in combination, zinc

INTRODUCTION

Pregnant women occasionally experience an increase in blood pressure known as gestational hypertension or pregnancy-induced hypertension (PIH). In a more severe condition called preeclampsia, a rise in blood pressure is accompanied by protein in the urine and sometimes by sudden weight gain, swelling in the face or hands, and other symptoms. When left untreated, preeclampsia can lead to seizures (called eclampsia) or to liver, kidney, or bleeding problems in the pregnant woman and distress or growth retardation in the fetus. Unless preeclampsia is mild, doctors usually seek to deliver the baby early.

PRINCIPAL PROPOSED NATURAL TREATMENTS

Although there are no fully established natural treatments for the prevention of preeclampsia or PIH, calcium has shown significant promise.

Calcium. A meta-analysis (statistical review) of eleven studies of calcium supplementation in pregnancy, involving more than six thousand women, found that calcium slightly reduced the risk of preeclampsia and hypertension, particularly in two groups of women: those at high risk for hypertension and those with low calcium intakes.

However, by far the largest single study in the meta-analysis found no benefits. In this double-blind study, researchers gave either 2 grams (g) of calcium or placebo daily to 4,589 women from weeks thirteen to twenty-one of their pregnancy onward. In the end, researchers found no significant decreases in rates of hypertension or preeclampsia, not even when they looked specifically at women whose daily calcium consumption mirrored that of women in developing countries. The meta-analysis included this negative study in its calculations but still found that calcium seemed to be helpful.

In a subsequent double-blind, placebo-controlled study published in 2006 and conducted by the World Health Organization, calcium supplements (1.5 g per day) were tried in 8,325 pregnant women whose calcium intake was inadequate. Calcium failed to reduce the incidence of preeclampsia, but it did appear to reduce the severity of preeclampsia episodes. Calcium might be of some benefit for those pregnant women who are at high risk for hypertension or deficient in calcium. However, for well-nourished, low-risk women, effects are likely to be minimal or nonexistent.

One double-blind, placebo-controlled study suggests that calcium supplements are not effective for treating preeclampsia that has already developed. Calcium does, however, appear to offer the additional benefit of reducing blood levels of lead during pregnancy. Weak evidence hints that the use of calcium by pregnant women might reduce the risk of hypertension in their children.

OTHER PROPOSED NATURAL TREATMENTS

Antioxidants are substances that fight free radicals, dangerous and naturally occurring molecules that may play a role in preeclampsia. For various theoretical reasons, it has been proposed that the use of antioxidants by pregnant women may help stop preeclampsia from developing. One double-blind, placebo-controlled study found evidence that a combination of the antioxidant vitamin E (400 international units [IU] daily) and vitamin C (1,000

Calcium Supplements

Calcium supplements are available without a prescription in a wide range of preparations and strengths, which can make selecting one a confusing experience. The best supplement to take is the one that meets an individual's specific needs. Other important things to consider include the following:

Purity. Choose calcium supplements with familiar brand names. Look for labels that state "purified" or have the USP (United States Pharmacopeia) symbol. Avoid supplements made from unrefined oyster shell, bone meal, or dolomite that do not have the USP symbol, because they may contain high levels of lead or other toxic metals.

Absorbability. The body easily absorbs most brand-name calcium products. One can find out how well a particular calcium product dissolves by placing the product in a small amount of warm water for thirty minutes and stirring it occasionally. If it has not dissolved within this time, it probably will not dissolve in your stomach. Chewable and liquid calcium supplements dissolve well because they are broken down before they enter the stomach.

The body best absorbs calcium, whether from food or supplements, when it is taken several times a day in amounts of not more than 500 milligrams (mg), but taking it all at once is better than not taking it at all. Calcium carbonate is absorbed best when taken with food. Calcium citrate can be taken anytime.

Tolerance. Some calcium supplements may cause side effects, such as gas or constipation, for some people. If simple measures (such as increasing one's intake of fluids and high-fiber foods) do not solve the problem, one should try another form of calcium. Also, it is important to increase the dose of the supplement gradually: Take just 500 mg a day for a week, and then slowly add more calcium. Do not take more than the recommended amount of calcium without a doctor's approval.

Calcium interactions. Calcium supplements may interact with over-the-counter and prescription medications. For example, calcium supplements may reduce the absorption of the antibiotic tetracycline. Calcium also interferes with iron absorption. One should not take a calcium supplement at the same time as an iron supplement, unless the calcium supplement is calcium citrate or the iron supplement is taken with vitamin C. Any medications that need to be taken on an empty stomach should not be taken with calcium supplements.

---

milligrams [mg] daily) reduced the incidence of preeclampsia. Benefits were also seen in another study of this combination and in a study using a mixture of numerous antioxidants with other nutrients. Additionally, a double-blind trial found potential preventive effects with the antioxidant substance lycopene (taken at 2 mg twice daily). However, researchers caution that further study is necessary: Many other treatments have shown initial promise for preventing preeclampsia, but these treatments lost luster when subsequent studies were performed.

The most prominent of these once-promising substances include folate, magnesium, omega-3 fatty acids (fish oil), and zinc. Furthermore, a large follow-up study of vitamin E combined with vitamin C failed to find any benefit, and in a review of ten studies involving 6,533 persons, antioxidant supplementation (of mostly vitamins E and C) during pregnancy did not reduce the risk of preeclampsia or any of its complications. In addition, a high-quality randomized trial of 1,365 high-risk pregnant women found that daily supplementation with combination vitamin E (400 IU) and vitamin C (1,000 mg) through delivery was not associated with reduced risk of preeclampsia or other serious outcomes.

One study involving 235 pregnant women in Ecuador (average age 17.5 years) suggests that daily supplementation with 200 mg of coenzyme Q_{10} during the second half of pregnancy may reduce the risk of developing preeclampsia. Though promising, the reliability of these results is in question because of low compliance with the supplements.

Other studies have looked at possible treatments of preeclampsia once it has already occurred. Results are somewhat positive, though mixed, on the potential benefits of arginine for this purpose. Evening primrose oil has failed to prove helpful, as has a combination of vitamin C, vitamin E, and the drug allopurinol. However, magnesium, taken by injection (but not orally) appears to provide meaningful benefits. One study failed to find N-acetylcysteine helpful for severe preeclampsia.

EBSCO CAM Review Board

FURTHER READING

Bergel, E., and A. J. Barros. "Effect of Maternal Calcium Intake During Pregnancy on Children's Blood Pressure." *BMC Pediatrics* 7 (2007): 15.

Roes, E. M., et al. "Oral N-acetylcysteine Administration Does Not Stabilise the Process of Established Severe Preeclampsia." *European Journal of Obstetrics, Gynecology, and Reproductive Biology* 127 (2006): 61-67.

Rumbold A. R., and C. A. Crowther et al. "Vitamins C and E and the Risks of Pre-eclampsia and Perinatal Complications." *New England Journal of Medicine* 354 (2006): 1796-1806.

Rumbold, A. R., and L. Duley et al. "Antioxidants for Preventing Pre-eclampsia." *Cochrane Database of Systematic Reviews* (2008): CD004227. Available through *EBSCO DynaMed Systematic Literature Surveillance* at http://www.ebscohost.com/dynamed.

Rumiris, D., et al. "Lower Rate of Pre-eclampsia After Antioxidant Supplementation in Pregnant Women with Low Antioxidant Status." *Hypertension and Pregnancy* 25 (2006): 241-253.

Sibai, B. M. "Magnesium Sulfate Prophylaxis in Preeclampsia." *American Journal of Obstetrics and Gynecology* 190 (2004): 1520-1526.

Staff, A. C., et al. "Dietary Supplementation with L-Arginine or Placebo in Women with Pre-eclampsia." *Acta Obstetricia et Gynecologica Scandinavica* 83 (2004): 103-107.

Teran, E., et al. "Coenzyme Q10 Supplementation During Pregnancy Reduces the Risk of Pre-eclampsia." *International Journal of Gynaecology and Obstetrics* 105 (2009): 43-45.

Villar, J., H. Abdel-Aleem, et al. "World Health Organization Randomized Trial of Calcium Supplementation Among Low Calcium Intake Pregnant Women." *American Journal of Obstetrics and Gynecology* 194 (2006): 639-649.

Villar, J., M. Purwar, et al. "World Health Organisation Multicentre Randomised Trial of Supplementation with Vitamins C and E Among Pregnant Women at High Risk for Pre-eclampsia in Populations of Low Nutritional Status from Developing Countries." *BJOG: An International Journal of Obstetrics and Gynaecology* 116 (2009): 780-788.

See also: Calcium; Pregnancy support; Women's health.

Pregnancy support

CATEGORY: Condition

RELATED TERMS: Anemia in pregnancy, birth defects, birth disorders, childbirth support, constipation in pregnancy, gestational diabetes, gingivitis in pregnancy, hemorrhoids in pregnancy, jaundice of pregnancy, leg cramps in pregnancy, low birth weight, miscarriage, neural tube defects, prematurity, varicose veins in pregnancy

DEFINITION: Treatment of medical conditions related to fetal development, pregnancy, and childbirth.

PRINCIPAL PROPOSED NATURAL TREATMENTS

- *Anemia:* Iron (if deficient)
- *Hemorrhoids:* Citrus bioflavonoids, oxerutins
- *Prevention of neural tube defects and other birth disorders:* Folate, multivitamin-multimineral supplements
- *Varicose veins:* Citrus bioflavonoids, gotu kola, horse chestnut, oxerutins

OTHER PROPOSED NATURAL TREATMENTS

- *Assisting or initiating childbirth:* Acupuncture, aromatherapy, castor oil, hypnotherapy, massage, proteolytic enzymes, red raspberry
- *Bladder infections:* Vitamin C
- *Constipation:* Dandelion, fiber supplements, flaxseed, glucomannan, lactulose
- *Diabetes in pregnancy:* Chromium, vitamin B_6
- *Gingivitis:* Folate
- *Jaundice of pregnancy:* S-adenosylmethionine
- *Leg cramps:* Calcium, magnesium, vitamin B_1 plus vitamin B_6
- *Prevention of low birth weight:* B vitamins, calcium, fish oil, folate, iron, magnesium, vitamin D, zinc
- *Prevention of miscarriage:* Vitamin B_{12}
- *Prevention of prematurity:* Calcium, fish oil, iron, magnesium, zinc
- *Support of healthy mental function in infant:* Fish oil

INTRODUCTION

Pregnancy is a time of dramatic transitions. Body systems that once sustained a single human now support two. Organs, blood vessels, body chemistry, and even the solid supporting structures of a woman's body all go through changes; in the meantime, the fetus's body grows from a tiny bundle of cells to a full-sized baby.

Since ancient times, women have tried herbs and other natural treatments to ease discomfort or assist with pregnancy, childbirth, and breast-feeding. However, pregnancy is also a circumstance when the potential risk of any treatment rises dramatically. Seemingly benign medications, even natural ones, have been found to cause birth defects or disorders or to increase the risk of complications. Some traditional remedies, such as blue cohosh for labor stimulation, must be discontinued for safety reasons.

Thorough study is needed before any treatment can be considered absolutely safe in pregnancy, and in many cases this research may never be done because of insurmountable ethical considerations regarding the safety of the fetus. It is important to talk with a doctor before deciding to use any treatment, whether it is natural or conventional.

PRINCIPAL PROPOSED NATURAL TREATMENTS

Many natural treatments have shown promise for conditions related to pregnancy. This section will discuss those treatments (except those for nausea and vomiting and preeclampsia) with the most scientific support. The safety of the following treatments has not been confirmed, except for nutrients such as vitamins and minerals, for which appropriate dosages for pregnancy have been established.

Venous insufficiency. Increased pressure from the expanding abdomen and other factors can lead to the pooling of fluid in the legs, a condition called venous insufficiency (closely related to varicose veins).

Venous insufficiency occurs outside pregnancy too, and a variety of natural treatments, including buckwheat, butcher's broom, citrus bioflavonoids, gotu kola, horse chestnut, oligomeric proanthocyanidins, and red vine leaf, have shown promise in their treatment. Only one natural treatment, oxerutins, has been studied in a double-blind trial enrolling pregnant women with venous insufficiency. In this study of sixty-nine women, researchers found oxerutins more effective than placebo.

Hemorrhoids. Hemorrhoids are actually varicose veins in or around the anus. Oxerutins and citrus bioflavonoids have been studied for hemorrhoids during pregnancy. A double-blind study enrolling ninety-seven pregnant women found oxerutins (1,000 milligrams [mg] daily) significantly better than placebo at reducing the pain, bleeding, and inflammation of hemorrhoids. Evidence for citrus bioflavonoids is lim-

ited to one open trial. Other natural treatments for varicose veins are often recommended for hemorrhoids too, although research on their use for this condition in pregnancy is lacking.

Anemia. Anemia is common during pregnancy and is usually caused by a deficiency in iron. However, iron supplements can be hard on the stomach, thereby aggravating morning sickness. One study found evidence that a fairly low supplemental dose of iron (20 mg daily) is nearly as effective for treating anemia of pregnancy as 40 mg or even 80 mg daily and is less likely to cause gastrointestinal side effects. (A daily dosage of 20 mg is lower than the amount contained in standard prenatal vitamins.)

Pregnant women who are not anemic should not take more than the recommended daily allowance of iron in pregnancy, as excess iron intake may be harmful for both pregnant women and their fetuses. One study suggests that iron plus folate is more effective for the treatment of iron-deficiency anemia in pregnancy than iron alone, even in women who do not appear to be folate-deficient.

Prevention of neural tube defects and other birth defects. Folate supplements can help prevent a serious and common type of birth defect known as neural tube defects (NTDs). Folate, or folate plus multivitamin-multimineral supplements, may help prevent other birth defects too, including cleft palate and anomalies of the heart and urinary tract. One preliminary study of 859 babies suggests that zinc may help prevent NTDs, but evidence of this is weak.

OTHER PROPOSED NATURAL TREATMENTS

Other natural remedies have been recommended for treating discomforts and complications of pregnancy or decreasing risks to the fetus and baby.

Assisting childbirth. Castor oil. Castor bean oil was noted by the ancient Egyptians to stimulate labor, and it is still used by some conventional physicians and midwives to induce contractions (for example, it is used when labor does not occur spontaneously after the woman's water has broken). A recent controlled trial of one hundred pregnant women compared oral castor oil to no treatment and found that 57.7 percent of those given castor oil began labor within twenty-four hours, compared to only 4.2 percent of those without treatment. Other preliminary studies also suggest that castor oil may help. Castor oil is a strong laxative, and diarrhea is a nearly universal effect.

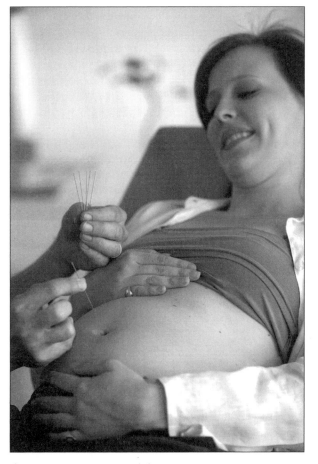

A pregnant woman receiving an acupuncture treatment.
(Philippe Garo/Photo Researchers, Inc.)

In addition, considering how common this treatment is, research on its safety and effectiveness is surprisingly scant. One case of a potentially fatal complication linked to the use of castor oil has been reported, though some have questioned whether the castor oil was responsible. In addition, an observational study of South African women found that those self-treating with castor oil or other traditional herbs (or both) had a higher incidence of meconium (fetal feces) in the amniotic fluid, a sign of fetal distress.

Acupuncture. Acupuncture has shown some promise for reducing pain in labor, but the quality of most of the supporting evidence is relatively poor. In one study, sterile water injections were found to be more effective than acupuncture for lower back pain and relaxation during labor. It is unclear whether or not the persons in the study knew what treatment they were receiving at the time.

In one placebo-controlled trial, real acupuncture was no better than sham acupuncture in relieving pelvic pain before labor. A carefully conducted review of ten randomized, controlled trials involving 2,038 women could not uncover consistent evidence of acupuncture's effectiveness for labor pain either alone or with other treatments. In one study involving sixty women, postoperative acupuncture or electro-acupuncture reduced pain within the first two hours (but no longer) and demand for pain medication within the first twenty-four hours after cesarean section.

A study of forty-five pregnant women found that women who received acupuncture on the mathematically calculated birth "due date" gave birth sooner than those who did not received acupuncture. However, this trial used a no-treatment control group instead of sham acupuncture, making its results unreliable. Another study suggested that the use of acupuncture may help stimulate normal term labor. A third study of 106 women with premature rupture of membranes (water breaking too early) found that acupuncture did not effectively speed up delivery. It should be noted that none of these three studies used sham acupuncture as a control, making their results unreliable. However, in a subsequent trial that attempted to address this problem, real acupuncture administered for two days before a planned induction of labor (artificial stimulation of labor) was no better than sham acupuncture at preventing the need for induction or shortening the time of labor.

Two studies suggest that acupuncture and associated therapies can help "turn" a breech presentation of the fetus. In 2008, researchers published a review of six randomized, controlled trials that investigated acupuncture-like therapies (moxibustion, acupuncture, or electro-acupuncture) applied to a specific acupuncture point (BL 67). They concluded that these therapies were effective at decreasing the incidence of breech presentations at the time of delivery. Again, however, not all of these studies employed a sham-acupuncture group for comparison.

Other natural treatments. One double-blind, placebo-controlled trial evaluated the effects of red raspberry in 192 pregnant women. Treatment (placebo or 2.4 grams [g] of raspberry leaf daily) began at thirty-two weeks of pregnancy and was continued until the onset of labor. The results failed to show any statistically meaningful differences between the groups. Red raspberry did not significantly shorten labor, reduce pain, or prevent complications.

Blue cohosh is a toxic herb and should not be used. One published case report documents profound heart failure in a baby born to a mother who used blue cohosh to induce labor. Severe medical consequences were also seen in a child whose mother took both black and blue cohosh.

Proteolytic enzymes may reduce inflammation and discomfort following episiotomy. Hypnotherapy and massage therapy have shown some promise for assisting labor. In a large controlled trial (more than six hundred participants), lavender oil aromatherapy failed to improve pain after childbirth.

Constipation. Constipation frequently occurs during pregnancy, for reasons that are not entirely clear. Fiber supplements, such as psyllium seed, are commonly recommended for the treatment of constipation in pregnancy because of their apparent safety. Flaxseed is another high-fiber seed, and alternative practitioners often recommend it. However, flaxseed contains estrogen-like substances that might pose hazards to the fetus; one study found an effect on reproductive organs and function in baby rats whose mothers ate large amounts of flaxseed during pregnancy.

Other natural remedies for constipation during pregnancy include dandelion root and a combination of glucomannan and lactulose. However, there is no meaningful evidence to indicate that they are effective.

One should avoid the use of powerful laxatives, including natural remedies such as buckthorn, cascara, rhubarb, castor bean oil, and *Senna,* because they can induce uterine contractions. The traditional remedy yellow dock, though milder, might warrant similar caution.

Leg cramps. Pregnant women sometimes experience painful leg cramps. A double-blind study of seventy-three women with this symptom found that magnesium was significantly more effective than placebo in decreasing their distress. Calcium has also been studied for this problem, but research gives little indication that it helps. A combination of vitamins B_1 and B_6 has also been suggested for leg cramps, but evidence that it helps remains minimal.

Prevention of prematurity. Not entirely consistent evidence suggests that the use of fish oil or its constituents by pregnant women might help prevent prema-

ture births. Double-blind studies have evaluated the minerals calcium, zinc, and magnesium for this purpose too, but the results have been mixed. A number of trials suggest that anemia is linked to prematurity; however, evidence as to whether iron supplements can help remains inconclusive. Several studies have evaluated folate but did not find it effective for preventing premature birth.

One study failed to find vitamin C helpful for preventing premature birth. However, another study found that vitamin C (100 mg per day after twenty weeks of pregnancy) helped prevent early rupture of the chorioamniotic membrane (water breaking). Another study found that the use of vitamin E (400 international units daily) and vitamin C (500 mg per day) after premature water breaking helped hold off delivery by several days.

Prevention of low birth weight. Babies born below a specific weight (5.5 pounds), called low birth weight, are at greater risk for complications. A meta-analysis of seven controlled studies looked at the effects of calcium supplementation on birth weight. These studies predominantly focused on preventing hypertension or preeclampsia (or both) in the pregnant woman, both of which can result in low-birth-weight babies. Overall, calcium appeared to decrease the percentage of babies weighing less than 5 pounds 8 ounces. However, other analysts looking at a somewhat different group of studies came to the opposite conclusion.

Quite a few double-blind studies have examined zinc and magnesium for preventing low birth weight, with mixed results. Results have been similarly mixed in other controlled trials of folate and fish oil or one of its fatty acids. Vitamin D and B vitamins have also been proposed, but evidence of their usefulness is weak.

It was earlier believed that iron was helpful in preventing low birth weight. However, a large-scale unblinded study of well-nourished women found that routine iron supplements in pregnancy had no effect on birth weight. Iron supplementation in pregnant women who are not anemic may not be good for either the woman or the fetus. In another study, a double-blind, placebo-controlled study of 1,877 women, the use of combined vitamin E and vitamin C failed to prove helpful in preventing low birth weight.

Other uses of natural treatments. A common problem in pregnancy is an increased tendency toward swollen or bleeding gums, a condition known as gingivitis.

Two small double-blind studies suggest that folate mouthwash may help. However, folate supplements do not appear to be especially effective against gingivitis.

A condition called intrahepatic cholestasis may occur during pregnancy, causing jaundice and other complications. Preliminary evidence suggests that the supplement S-adenosylmethionine might be helpful for preventing this.

A single-blind trial found suggestive evidence that vitamin C, taken at a dose of 100 mg daily, might help prevent bladder infections in pregnancy. A placebo-controlled study of thirty women suggested that the mineral chromium may be useful for gestational diabetes, the term for diabetes that occurs during pregnancy. Vitamin B_6 has also been proposed for this condition, but evidence in support of its effectiveness is minimal.

The use of fish oil or its constituents docosahexaenoic acid (DHA) and eicosapentaenoic acid by pregnant women might help support healthy cognitive and visual function in their children. Also, low levels of vitamin B_{12} may increase the risk of miscarriage, and B_{12} supplements may help.

A small preliminary study found that fish oil was significantly more effective than placebo at alleviating postpartum depression. However, two other studies failed to find either fish oil or one of its chief components, DHA, helpful for preventing perinatal (including postpartum) depression.

HERBS AND SUPPLEMENTS TO AVOID DURING PREGNANCY AND BREAST-FEEDING

Virtually no medicinal herb has been established as safe in pregnancy or breast-feeding, and even herbs that might seem safe because of their wide use in cooking could cause problems when they are taken in the form of highly concentrated extracts. For example, based on food use, it is unlikely that cooked garlic presents much risk; however, garlic supplements contain certain rather potent and potentially toxic ingredients present only in raw garlic. Few people eat large quantities of raw garlic on a regular basis, so there is no history of its long-term use to show its effects.

Other herbs that are traditionally regarded with caution during pregnancy include andrographis, boldo, catnip, chasteberry, essential oils, feverfew, juniper, licorice, nettle, red clover, rosemary, shepherd's purse, and yarrow. For example, chasteberry has shown a theoretical potential for inhibiting milk supply. In addition, herbs with estrogen-like properties could possibly affect the fetus; these herbs include soy, isoflavones, red clover, flaxseed, lignans, and hops.

These products have been found on occasion to contain toxic heavy metals, poisonous herbs, or unlabeled prescription drugs. In one case report, a brain-damaged child born to a woman using an Ayurvedic formula was found to have the highest bloods levels of lead ever recorded in a living newborn. Analysis of the formula revealed a very high lead content and toxic levels of mercury. In general, it is probably accurate to say that no herb can be regarded as definitely benign.

However, other supplements that are not essential nutrients are in much the same position as herbs, and they could conceivably cause harm. For example, the supplement conjugated linoleic acid appears to reduce the fat content of breast milk, with potentially harmful effects on the nursing infant. Chitosan may cause impaired nutrient absorption and at times may contain arsenic. (Contamination with toxic substances is also a real possibility with certain calcium supplements, which have been found to contain high levels of lead.) Nonetheless, many herbs and supplements have a high enough safety factor that researchers have felt comfortable recommending their use by pregnant women.

EBSCO CAM Review Board

FURTHER READING

Borna, S., et al. "Vitamins C and E in the Latency Period in Women with Preterm Premature Rupture of Membranes." *International Journal of Gynaecology and Obstetrics* 90 (2005): 16-20.

Casanueva, E., et al. "Vitamin C Supplementation to Prevent Premature Rupture of the Chorioamniotic Membranes." *American Journal of Clinical Nutrition* 81 (2005): 859-863.

Chang, M. Y., S. Y. Wang, and C. H. Chen. "Effects of Massage on Pain and Anxiety During Labour." *Journal of Advanced Nursing* 38 (2002): 68-73.

Cho, S. H., H. Lee, and E. Ernst. "Acupuncture for Pain Relief in Labour." *BJOG: An International Journal of Obstetrics and Gynaecology* 117 (2010): 907-920.

Decsi, T., and B. Koletzko. "N-3 Fatty Acids and Pregnancy Outcomes." *Current Opinion in Clinical Nutrition and Metabolic Care* 8 (2005): 161-166.

Elden, H., et al. "Acupuncture as an Adjunct to Standard Treatment for Pelvic Girdle Pain in Pregnant Women." *BJOG: An International Journal of Obstetrics and Gynaecology* 115 (2008): 1655-1668.

Ernst, E. "Herbal Medicinal Products During Pregnancy: Are They Safe?" *BJOG: An International Journal of Obstetrics and Gynaecology* 109 (2002): 227-235.

Goh, Y. I., et al. "Prenatal Multivitamin Supplementation and Rates of Congenital Anomalies." *Journal of Obstetrics and Gynaecology Canada* 28 (2006): 680-689.

Knudsen, V. K., et al. "Fish Oil in Various Doses or Flax Oil in Pregnancy and Timing of Spontaneous Delivery." *BJOG: An International Journal of Obstetrics and Gynaecology* 113 (2006): 536-543.

Llorente, A. M., et al. "Effect of Maternal Docosahexaenoic Acid Supplementation on Postpartum Depression and Information Processing." *American Journal of Obstetrics and Gynecology* 188 (2003): 1348-1353.

Martensson, L., E. Stener-Victorin, and G. Wallin. "Acupuncture Versus Subcutaneous Injections of Sterile Water as Treatment for Labour Pain." *Acta Obstetricia et Gynecologica Scandinavica* 87 (2008): 171-177.

Ochoa-Brust, G. J., et al. "Daily Intake of 100 Mg Ascorbic Acid as Urinary Tract Infection Prophylactic Agent During Pregnancy." *Acta Obstetricia et Gynecologica Scandinavica* 86 (2007): 783-787.

Olsen, S. F., et al. "Duration of Pregnancy in Relation to Fish Oil Supplementation and Habitual Fish Intake." *European Journal of Clinical Nutrition* 8 (2007): 976-985.

Rees, A. M., M. P. Austin, and G. B. Parker. "Omega-3 Fatty Acids as a Treatment for Perinatal Depression." *Australian and New Zealand Journal of Psychiatry* 42 (2008): 199-205.

Rumbold, A. R., et al. "Vitamins C and E and the Risks of Preeclampsia and Perinatal Complications." *New England Journal of Medicine* 354 (2006): 1796-1806.

Smith, C. A., et al. "Acupuncture to Induce Labor." *Obstetrics and Gynecology* 112 (2008): 1067-1074.

Su, K. P., et al. "Omega-3 Fatty Acids for Major Depressive Disorder During Pregnancy." *Journal of Clinical Psychiatry* 69 (2008): 644-651.

Van den Berg, I., et al. "Effectiveness of Acupuncture-Type Interventions Versus Expectant Management to Correct Breech Presentation." *Complementary Therapies in Medicine* 16 (2008): 92-100.

Zhou, S. J., et al. "Should We Lower the Dose of Iron When Treating Anaemia in Pregnancy?" *European Journal of Clinical Nutrition* 63 (2009): 183-190.

See also: Breast-feeding support; Childbirth support: Homeopathic remedies; Childbirth techniques; Citrus bioflavonoids; Folate; Gotu kola; Hemorrhoids; Horse chestnut; Iron; Oxerutins; Pain management; Preeclampsia and pregnancy-induced hypertension; Women's health.

Pregnenolone

CATEGORY: Herbs and supplements
RELATED TERMS: Hormones, steroids
DEFINITION: Natural substance of the human body used as a supplement to treat specific health conditions.
PRINCIPAL PROPOSED USES: None
OTHER PROPOSED USES: Aging in general, Alzheimer's disease, depression, enhancing memory and mental function, fatigue, menopausal symptoms, osteoporosis, Parkinson's disease, rheumatoid arthritis, stress, weight loss

OVERVIEW

Pregnenolone has been called the grandmother of all steroid hormones. The body manufactures it from cholesterol and then uses it to make testosterone, cortisone, progesterone, estrogen, DHEA (5-dehydroepiandrosterone), androstenedione, aldosterone, and all other hormones in the steroid family.

One reason given for using pregnenolone is that the level of many of these hormones declines with age. By taking pregnenolone supplements, proponents say, people can keep all their hormones at youthful levels. However, pregnenolone levels themselves do not decline with age, and there is no indication that taking extra pregnenolone will increase the levels of any other hormones. Furthermore, even if it did, that does not mean using pregnenolone is a great idea.

Steroid hormones are powerful substances, and they can cause harm as well as benefit. Long-term use of cortisone causes severe osteoporosis. Estrogen can increase the risk of cancer, and anabolic steroids (used by athletes) may cause liver problems and stress the heart. Experts have very little idea what long-term consequences the use of pregnenolone might entail.

Actually, it is ironic that pregnenolone is legally classified as a dietary supplement. Pregnenolone is not a nutrient. It is a drug, just as estrogen, cortisone, and aldosterone are drugs. It use is not recommended until scientists know more about what it really does.

At present, there is only one effect of pregnenolone that has been documented via double-blind, placebo-controlled studies: For reasons that are not clear, regular use of pregnenolone may greatly decrease the sedative effect of drugs in the Valium family (benzodiazepines).

REQUIREMENTS AND SOURCES

Pregnenolone is not normally obtained from foods. The human body manufactures it from cholesterol. Supplemental pregnenolone is made synthetically in a lab from substances found in soybeans.

THERAPEUTIC DOSAGES

A typical recommended dosage of pregnenolone is 30 milligrams (mg) daily, but some studies have used as much as 700 mg.

THERAPEUTIC USES

On the Internet and in health magazines, pregnenolone is described as a treatment for an enormous list of health problems, including Alzheimer's disease, menopausal symptoms, Parkinson's disease, osteoporosis, fatigue, stress, depression, and rheumatoid arthritis. It is also supposed to help people lose weight, improve brain power, and make people feel young again. However, like so many overhyped new supplements, there is little to no scientific evidence for any of these uses. Studies involving rats suggest that pregnenolone may enhance memory, but there have been no human studies.

SAFETY ISSUES

Pregnenolone is a powerful hormone, not a nutrient that people naturally get in their food. This supplement should be approached with caution, as if it were a drug, because for all intents and purposes, it is a drug. Persons thinking about taking it should consult a doctor first. Pregnenolone is definitely not recommended for children, pregnant or nursing women, or those with liver or kidney disease.

IMPORTANT INTERACTIONS

As noted earlier, pregnenolone may decrease the effectiveness of sedatives in the Valium family (benzodiaz-

epines). People using benzodiazepine drugs for sleep or for anxiety find that these drugs do not work as well if they take pregnenolone.

EBSCO CAM Review Board

FURTHER READING

Flood, J. F., J. E. Morley, and E. Roberts. "Pregnenolone Sulfate Enhances Post-training Memory Processes When Injected in Very Low Doses into Limbic System Structures: The Amygdala Is by Far the Most Sensitive." *Proceedings of the National Academy of Science USA* 92 (1995): 10806-10810.

Meieran, S. E., et al. "Chronic Pregnenolone Effects in Normal Humans: Attenuation of Benzodiazepine-Induced Sedation." *Psychoneuroendocrinology* 29 (2004): 486-500.

See also: Benzodiazepines; Herbal medicine.

Premenstrual syndrome (PMS)

CATEGORY: Condition

RELATED TERM: Premenstrual dysphoric disorder

DEFINITION: Treatment of symptoms related to the onset of menstruation.

PRINCIPAL PROPOSED NATURAL TREATMENTS: Calcium, chasteberry

OTHER PROPOSED NATURAL TREATMENTS: Acupuncture, chiropractic, ginkgo, gamma-linolenic acid, grass pollen (plus grass pistils and royal jelly), inositol, krill oil, magnesium, massage, multivitamin-multimineral supplements, oligomeric proanthocyanidins, progesterone cream, soy isoflavones (plus dong quai and black cohosh), vitamin E

PROBABLY INEFFECTIVE TREATMENT: Vitamin B_6

INTRODUCTION

Many women experience a variety of unpleasant symptoms, commonly called premenstrual syndrome (PMS), in the week or two before menstruating. These symptoms include irritability, anger, headaches, anxiety, depression, fatigue, fluid retention, breast tenderness, and cramps. When emotional symptoms related to depression predominate in PMS, the condition is sometimes called premenstrual dysphoric disorder (PMDD). These symptoms undoubtedly result from hormonal changes of the menstrual cycle, but medical researchers do not know the exact cause of PMS or how to treat it.

Conventional treatments for PMS and PMDD include antidepressants, beta-blockers, diuretics, oral contraceptives, and other hormonally active formulations. Of these, antidepressants such as selective serotonin reuptake inhibitors (Prozac, for example) are perhaps the most effective.

PRINCIPAL PROPOSED NATURAL TREATMENTS

There is fairly good evidence that calcium supplements can significantly reduce all the major symptoms of PMS. There is also some evidence for the herbs chasteberry and ginkgo. Vitamin B_6 is widely recommended too, but its scientific record is mixed at best.

Calcium. A large double-blind, placebo-controlled study found positive results using calcium for the treatment of PMS symptoms. Participants took 300 milligrams (mg) of calcium (as calcium carbonate) four times daily. Compared to placebo, calcium significantly reduced mood swings, pain, bloating, depression, back pain, and food cravings. Similar findings were also seen in earlier preliminary studies of calcium for PMS.

Chasteberry. The herb chasteberry is widely used in Europe as a treatment for PMS symptoms. More than most herbs, chasteberry is frequently called by its Latin name, *Vitex* or *Vitex agnus-castus.*

A double-blind, placebo-controlled study of 178 women found that treatment with chasteberry during three menstrual cycles significantly reduced PMS symptoms. The dose used was one tablet three times daily of a chasteberry dry extract. Women in the treatment group experienced significant improvements in symptoms, including irritability, depression, headache, and breast tenderness.

There is little corroborating evidence for this one well-designed study. An earlier double-blind trial compared chasteberry to vitamin B_6 (pyridoxine) instead of placebo. The two treatments proved equally effective. However, because vitamin B_6 itself has not been shown effective for PMS, these results mean little. Even better evidence indicates that chasteberry can help the cyclic breast tenderness that is often, but not necessarily, connected with PMS.

Vitamin B_6. Vitamin B_6 has been used for PMS for many decades, by both European and American physicians. However, the results of scientific studies are

---

What Are the Symptoms of PMS?

Premenstrual syndrome (PMS) often includes both physical and emotional symptoms. These symptoms, such as the following, vary from woman to woman:

- Acne
- Swollen or tender breasts
- Feeling tired
- Trouble sleeping
- Upset stomach, bloating, constipation, or diarrhea
- Headache or backache
- Appetite changes or food cravings
- Joint or muscle pain
- Trouble with concentration or memory
- Tension, irritability, mood swings, or crying spells
- Anxiety or depression

---

mixed at best. The latest and best-designed double-blind study, enrolling 120 women, found no benefit. In this trial, three prescription drugs were compared with vitamin B_6 (pyridoxine, at 300 mg daily) and placebo. All study participants received three months of treatment and three months of placebo. vitamin B_6 proved to be no better than placebo.

Approximately one dozen other double-blind studies have investigated the effectiveness of vitamin B_6 for PMS, but none were well designed, and the results were mixed. Some books on natural medicine report that the negative results in some of these studies were caused by insufficient vitamin B_6 dosage, but in reality there was no clear link between dosage and effectiveness. It has been suggested too that the combination of vitamin B_6 and magnesium might be more effective than either treatment alone, but this remains to be proven.

OTHER PROPOSED NATURAL TREATMENTS

Ginkgo. One double-blind, placebo-controlled study evaluated the benefits of *Ginkgo biloba* extract for women with PMS symptoms. This trial enrolled 143 women, eighteen to forty-five years of age, and monitored them for two menstrual cycles. Each woman received either the ginkgo extract (80 mg twice daily) or placebo on day sixteen of the first cycle. Treatment was continued until day five of the next cycle and resumed again on day sixteen of that cycle. Compared to placebo, ginkgo significantly relieved major symptoms of PMS, especially breast pain and emotional disturbance. In another, similarly designed trial involving eighty-five university students, Ginkgo biloba L. significantly reduced PMS symptom severity compared with placebo.

Magnesium. Preliminary studies suggest that magnesium may also be helpful for PMS. A double-blind, placebo-controlled study of thirty-two women found that magnesium taken from day fifteen of the menstrual cycle to the onset of menstrual flow could significantly improve premenstrual mood changes.

Another small, double-blind, preliminary study found that the regular use of magnesium could reduce symptoms of PMS-related fluid retention. In this study, thirty-eight women were given magnesium or placebo for two months. The results showed no effect after one cycle, but by the end of two cycles, magnesium significantly reduced weight gain, swelling of extremities, breast tenderness, and abdominal bloating.

In addition, one small double-blind study (twenty participants) found that magnesium supplementation might help prevent menstrual migraines. Preliminary evidence suggests that combining vitamin B_6 with magnesium might improve the results.

Additional treatments. Several double-blind, placebo-controlled studies, enrolling about 400 women, found evidence that multivitamin-multimineral supplements may be helpful for PMS. It is not clear what ingredients in these supplements played a role. Preliminary double-blind trials also suggest that vitamin E may be helpful for PMS.

A product containing grass pollen, royal jelly (made by bees), and the pistils (seed-bearing parts) of grass has been proposed for use in PMS. In a double-blind, placebo-controlled, crossover trial of thirty-two women, the use of the product for two menstrual cycles appeared to significantly improve PMS symptoms compared to the use of placebo.

A double-blind, placebo-controlled study of thirty women with premenstrual fluid retention found that the use of oligomeric proanthocyanidins at a dose of 320 mg daily significantly reduced the sensation of fluid retention in the leg; however, actual leg swelling as measured was not significantly improved. One poorly designed human trial hints that krill oil may be helpful for some PMS symptoms.

In a twenty-four-week double-blind study, forty-nine women with menstrual migraines received either placebo or a combination supplement containing soy isoflavones, dong quai, and black cohosh extracts. The treatment proved at least somewhat more effective than placebo. Soy isoflavones alone have also shown some potential benefit.

Evening primrose oil, a source of the omega-6 fatty acids, was once thought to be helpful for cyclic breast pain. However, it probably does not work for this purpose. It has also been proposed as a treatment for general PMS symptoms, but there is only minimal supporting evidence. Preliminary evidence suggests that St. John's wort might be helpful for mood changes in PMS.

One study often cited as evidence that massage therapy is helpful for PMS was fatally flawed by the absence of a control group. However, a better-designed trial compared reflexology (a special form of massage involving primarily the foot) with fake reflexology in thirty-eight women with PMS symptoms and found evidence that real reflexology was more effective. A small crossover trial of chiropractic manipulation for PMS symptoms found equivocal results at best. In a 2010 review of nine clinical trials, researchers could not conclusively determine the effectiveness of acupuncture for premenstrual syndrome because of the poor quality of the studies.

Progesterone cream is sometimes recommended for PMS, but there is no meaningful evidence that it is effective. One study failed to find the supplement inositol helpful for PMS.

EBSCO CAM Review Board

FURTHER READING

Bryant, M., et al. "Effect of Consumption of Soy Isoflavones on Behavioural, Somatic, and Affective Symptoms in Women with Premenstrual Syndrome." *British Journal of Nutrition* 93 (2005): 731-739.

Burke, B. E., R. D. Olson, and B. J. Cusack. "Randomized, Controlled Trial of Phytoestrogen in the Prophylactic Treatment of Menstrual Migraine." *Biomedicine and Pharmacotherapy* 56 (2002): 283-288.

Cho, S. H., and J. Kim. "Efficacy of Acupuncture in Management of Premenstrual Syndrome." *Complementary Therapies in Medicine* 18 (2010): 104-111.

Christie, S., et al. "Flavonoid Supplement Improves Leg Health and Reduces Fluid Retention in Premenopausal Women in a Double-Blind, Placebo-Controlled Study." *Phytomedicine* 11 (2004): 11-17.

Hernandez-Reif, M., et al. "Premenstrual Symptoms Are Relieved by Massage Therapy." *Journal of Psychosomatic Obstetrics and Gynaecology* 21 (2000): 9-15.

Ozgoli, G., et al. "A Randomized, Placebo-Controlled Trial of *Ginkgo biloba* L. in Treatment of Premenstrual Syndrome." *Journal of Alternative and Complementary Medicine* 15 (2009): 845-851.

Sampalis, F., et al. "Evaluation of the Effects of Neptune Krill Oil on the Management of Premenstrual Syndrome and Dysmenorrhea." *Alternative Medicine Review* 8 (2003): 171-179.

See also: Calcium; Chasteberry; Ginkgo; Magnesium; Menopause; Pain management; Vitamin B$_6$; Women's health.

Premenstrual syndrome (PMS): Homeopathic remedies

CATEGORY: Homeopathy
DEFINITION: The use of highly diluted remedies to treat symptoms related to the onset of menstruation.
STUDIED HOMEOPATHIC REMEDIES: *Calcarea carbonica, Chamomilla*, classical homeopathic remedy, *Pulsatilla*

SCIENTIFIC EVALUATIONS OF HOMEOPATHIC REMEDIES

According to one small trial, classical homeopathic therapy may be helpful for PMS. A three-month, double-blind, placebo-controlled trial tested the effects of a homeopathic remedy given in a single dose at the beginning of the trial. Each of the twenty women with PMS symptoms who participated in the trial received a classical homeopathic interview and was prescribed a personalized homeopathic remedy. Then, one-half the women received the remedy prescribed to them, and the other one-half received placebo. The results showed significantly fewer symptoms in the treated group.

Another double-blind, placebo-controlled trial evaluated the effectiveness of daily treatment with an individualized homeopathic remedy. However, the dropout rate was too high for the results to be interpreted in a meaningful way.

TRADITIONAL HOMEOPATHIC TREATMENTS

Classical homeopathy offers possible homeopathic treatments for PMS. These therapies are chosen based on various specific details of the person seeking treatment.

The homeopathic remedy *Calcarea carbonica* is often used for PMS when the symptom picture includes fluid retention, headaches, breast tenderness, and a feeling of being overwhelmed. Other symptoms associated with this remedy include feeling extremely fatigued and depleted, a feeling of cold limbs, and difficulty climbing stairs or even walking. Furthermore, these symptoms should worsen with exposure to coldness or dampness in the morning and should worsen with exertion.

Homeopathic *Chamomilla* is often used in forms of PMS where anger and irritability are predominant features. Menstrual flow is typically heavy, with dark, clotted blood. Heat worsens symptoms, while aerobic exercise reduces them.

Pulsatilla may be helpful for PMS in young women. The symptom picture for *Pulsatilla* is moodiness and a tendency to tears, along with nausea and mild dizziness.

EBSCO CAM Review Board

FURTHER READING

Chapman, E. H., et al. "Results of a Study of the Homoeopathic Treatment of PMS." *Journal of the American Institute of Homeopathy* 87 (1994): 14-21.

Jones, A. "Homeopathic Treatment for Premenstrual Symptoms." *Journal of Family Planning and Reproductive Health Care* 29 (2003): 25-28.

Klein-Laansma, C. T., et al. "Semi-standardised Homeopathic Treatment of Premenstrual Syndrome with a Limited Number of Medicines." *Homeopathy* 99 (2010): 192-204.

Yakir, M., et al. "Effects of Homeopathic Treatment in Women with Premenstrual Syndrome." *British Homeopathic Journal* 90 (2001): 148-153.

See also: Chamomile; Homeopathy; Premenstrual syndrome (PMS); Women's health.

Prickly ash

CATEGORY: Herbs and supplements
RELATED TERMS: *Zanthoxylum americanum, Z. clavaherculis*
DEFINITION: Natural plant product used to treat specific health conditions.

PRINCIPAL PROPOSED USES: None

OTHER PROPOSED USES: Dry mouth, intermittent claudication, osteoarthritis, Raynaud's syndrome, toothache

OVERVIEW

The prickly ash tree has a long history of use in Native American medicine. The bark was used to treat intestinal cramps, dry mouth, muscle and joint pain, toothache, nervous disorders, arthritis, and leg ulcers. The berries were used for circulatory problems such as intermittent claudication and Raynaud's syndrome.

THERAPEUTIC DOSAGES

Prickly ash is often taken in the form of tea, made by boiling 5 to 10 grams (g) of the bark in a cup of water for ten to fifteen minutes. For toothache, the pieces of the bark may be chewed. Tinctures are also available.

THERAPEUTIC USES

There are no documented medical uses of prickly ash bark. In test-tube studies, substances called furano-coumarins in prickly ash have shown antifungal properties. Another prickly ash constituent, chelerythrine, has shown activity against antibiotic-resistant staph bacteria. However, it is a long way from studies like these to actual evidence of efficacy. Only double-blind, placebo-controlled studies can show that a treatment actually works, and none have been performed on prickly ash.

SAFETY ISSUES

Prickly ash has not undergone any modern scientific safety evaluation. It contains potentially toxic alkaloids; whether these lead to any harmful effects remains unknown. Safety in young children, pregnant or nursing women, or people with severe liver or kidney disease has not been established.

EBSCO CAM Review Board

FURTHER READING

Bafi-Yeboa, N. F., et al. "Antifungal Constituents of Northern Prickly Ash, *Zanthoxylumamericanum mill.*" *Phytomedicine* 12 (2005): 370-377.

Gibbons, S., et al. "Activity of *Zanthoxylum clava-herculis* Extracts Against Multi-drug Resistant Methicillin-Resistant *Staphylococcus aureus* (mdr-MRSA)." *Phytotherapy Research* 17 (2003): 274-275.

See also: Folk medicine; Herbal medicine.

Primidone

CATEGORY: Drug interactions

DEFINITION: Like phenobarbital, to which it is closely related, primidone is used to control epileptic seizures.

INTERACTIONS: Biotin, dong quai, folate, ginkgo, glutamine, hops, kava, passionflower, St. John's wort, valerian, vitamin B_3, vitamin D, vitamin K

TRADE NAME: Mysoline

FOLATE

Effect: Supplementation Possibly Helpful

Primidone can reduce folate levels, perhaps by increasing the rate of breakdown of the vitamin. Over time, such a decrease can cause anemia. Taking folate supplements will correct this anemia. Anticonvulsant-induced folate deficiency might also cause birth defects. Women who plan to become pregnant while on primidone should be sure to take a supplement to prevent deficiency.

VITAMIN D

Effect: Supplementation Possibly Helpful

Primidone appears to interfere with the normal absorption or metabolism of vitamin D. This in turn impairs calcium absorption, with many potential complications. To help avoid this problem, one should consume adequate amounts of vitamin D.

VITAMIN K

Effect: Supplementation Possibly Helpful for Pregnant Women

Children born to women taking primidone while pregnant may be deficient in vitamin K. This might lead to bleeding disorders and facial bone abnormalities. Supplementing with vitamin K during pregnancy should help; however, physician supervision is also recommended.

BIOTIN

Effect: Supplementation Possibly Helpful, but Take at a Different Time of Day

Many antiseizure medications, including primidone, are believed to interfere with the absorption of biotin. For this reason, persons taking primidone may benefit from extra biotin. Biotin should be taken two to three hours apart from antiseizure medication. One should not exceed the recommended daily intake, because it is possible that too much biotin might interfere with the effectiveness of the medication.

GLUTAMINE
Effect: Theoretical Harmful Interaction

Because many antiepilepsy drugs, including primidone, work by blocking glutamate stimulation in the brain, high dosages of glutamine might counteract the drugs' effects and pose a risk of increased seizures.

VITAMIN B₃
Effect: Potentially Dangerous Interaction

Niacinamide (a form of vitamin B_3) might increase blood levels of primidone, possibly requiring reduction in drug dosage.

DONG QUAI, ST. JOHN'S WORT
Effect: Possible Harmful Interaction

Primidone has been reported to cause increased sensitivity to the sun, amplifying the risk of sunburn or skin rash. Because St. John's wort and dong quai may also cause this problem, taking them during treatment with this drug might add to this risk. One should wear sunscreen or protective clothing during sun exposure if also taking one of these herbs while using this anticonvulsant.

GINKGO
Effect: Possible Harmful Interaction

The herb ginkgo (*Ginkgo biloba*) has been used to treat Alzheimer's disease and ordinary age-related memory loss, among many other conditions. The interaction with primidone involves potential contaminants in ginkgo, not ginkgo itself.

A recent study found that a natural nerve toxin present in the seeds of *Ginkgo biloba* made its way into standardized ginkgo extracts prepared from the leaves. This toxin has been associated with convulsions and death in laboratory animals.

The detected amounts of this toxic substance are considered harmless. However, given the lack of satisfactory standardization of herbal formulations in the United States, it is possible that some batches of product might contain higher contents of the toxin, depending on the season of harvest. In light of these findings, taking a ginkgo product that happened to contain significant levels of the nerve toxin might theoretically prevent an anticonvulsant from working as well as expected.

HOPS, KAVA, PASSIONFLOWER, VALERIAN
Effect: Possible Harmful Interaction

The herb kava (*Piper methysticum*) has a sedative effect and is used for anxiety and insomnia. Combining kava with anticonvulsants, which possess similar depressant effects, could result in add-on or excessive physical depression, sedation, and impairment. Because of the potentially serious consequences, one should avoid combining these herbs with anticonvulsants or other drugs that also have sedative or depressant effects, such as primidone, unless advised by a physician.

EBSCO CAM Review Board

FURTHER READING

Kishi, T., et al. "Mechanism for Reduction of Serum Folate by Antiepileptic Drugs During Prolonged Therapy." *Journal of the Neurological Sciences* 145 (1997): 109-112.

Kupiec, T., and V. Raj. "Fatal Seizures Due to Potential Herb-Drug Interactions with *Ginkgo biloba*." *Journal of Analytical Toxicology* 29 (2006): 755-758.

Lewis, D. P., et al. "Drug and Environmental Factors Associated with Adverse Pregnancy Outcomes: Part 1–Antiepileptic Drugs, Contraceptives, Smoking, and Folate." *Annals of Pharmacotherapy* 32 (1998): 802-817.

Tyagi, A., and N. Delanty. "Herbal Remedies, Dietary Supplements, and Seizures." *Epilepsia* 44 (2003): 228-235.

See also: Biotin; Dong quai; Epilepsy; Folate, Food and Drug Administration; Ginkgo; Glutamine; Hops; Kava; Passionflower; Phenobarbital; Pregnancy support; St. John's wort; Supplements: Introduction; Valerian; Vitamin B₃; Vitamin D; Vitamin K.

Probiotics

CATEGORY: Herbs and supplements

RELATED TERMS: *Bifidobacterium bifidum, Lactobacillus acidophilus, L. bulgaricus, L. casei, L. gasseri, L. plantarum, L. reuteri, L. sakei, Lactobacillus* GG, *Lactobacillus* LB, *Saccharomyces boulardii, Streptococcus salivarius, S. thermophilus*

DEFINITION: Helpful, "friendly" bacteria that offer specific health benefits.

PRINCIPAL PROPOSED USES: Various forms of diarrhea, including travelers' diarrhea, diarrhea caused by antibiotics, and viral diarrhea (in children); gastrointestinal side effects of cancer therapy; irritable bowel syndrome; ulcers (as an adjunct to standard therapy)

OTHER PROPOSED USES: Allergic rhinitis, Behçet's syndrome, canker sores, colds (prevention), colon cancer prevention, chronic constipation, diverticular disease, dyspepsia, eczema, high cholesterol, immune support, inflammatory bowel disease (ulcerative colitis and Crohn's disease), insomnia, milk allergies, probiotics, rheumatoid arthritis, ulcers, vaginal infection, yeast hypersensitivity syndrome

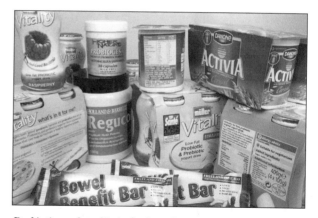

Probiotic and prebiotic food products. (Cordelia Molloy/ Photo Researchers, Inc.)

OVERVIEW

Lactobacillus acidophilus is a friendly strain of bacteria used to make yogurt and cheese. Although humans are born without it, acidophilus soon establishes itself in the intestines and helps prevent intestinal infections. Acidophilus also flourishes in the vagina, where it protects girls and women from yeast infections.

Acidophilus is one of several microbes known collectively as probiotics (meaning "pro life"), indicating that they are bacteria and yeasts that help rather than harm. Other helpful microbes include the yeast *Saccharomyces boulardii* and the bacteria *L. bulgaricus*, *L. reuteri*, *L. plantarum*, *L. casei*, *B. bifidum*, *Streptococcus salivarius*, and *S. thermophilus*.

The digestive tract contains billions of bacteria and yeasts. Some of these internal inhabitants are more helpful to the body than others. Acidophilus and related probiotics not only help the digestive tract function but also reduce the presence of less healthful organisms by competing with them for the limited space available. For this reason, the use of probiotics can help prevent infectious diarrhea.

Antibiotics can disturb the balance of the digestive tract by killing friendly bacteria. When this happens, harmful bacteria and yeasts can move in and flourish. This can lead to vaginal yeast infections (*Candida albicans*). Conversely, it appears that the regular use of probiotics can help prevent vaginal infections and generally improve the health of the gastrointestinal system. Persons taking antibiotics should probably take probiotics too and should continue probiotics for some time after treatment with antibiotics.

SOURCES

Although probiotic bacteria are helpful and perhaps even necessary for human health, no daily requirement exists. Probiotics are living creatures, not chemicals, so they can sustain themselves in the body unless something comes along to damage them, such as antibiotics.

Cultured dairy products such as yogurt and kefir are good sources of acidophilus and other probiotic bacteria. Supplements are widely available in powder, liquid, capsule, or tablet form. Grocery stores and natural food stores sell milk that contains live acidophilus. In addition to probiotics, related substances known as prebiotics may enhance the colonization of healthy bacteria in the intestinal tract.

THERAPEUTIC DOSAGES

Dosages of acidophilus are expressed not in grams or milligrams (mg) but in billions of organisms. A typical daily dose should supply about three to five billion live organisms. Other probiotic bacteria are used similarly. The typical dose of *S. boulardii* yeast is 500 mg twice daily (standardized to provide 3×10^{10} colony-forming units per gram), to be taken while traveling or at the start of using antibiotics and to be continued for a few days after antibiotics are stopped.

Because probiotics are not drugs but rather living organisms that a person is trying to transplant to the digestive tract, it is necessary to take the treatment regularly. Each time this is done, beneficial bacterial colonies in the body are reinforced, so that they can gradually push out harmful bacteria and yeasts.

Probiotics, as living organisms, may die on the store shelf. A study reported in 1990 found that most acidophilus capsules on the market contained no living acidophilus. The situation has improved in subsequent evaluations, but some products remain substandard. The container label should guarantee living organisms at the time of purchase, not just at the time of manufacture. Another approach is to eat acidophilus-rich foods such as yogurt, in which the bacteria are most likely still alive.

To treat or prevent vaginal infections, one can mix two tablespoons of yogurt or the contents of a couple of capsules of acidophilus with warm water. This mixture can then be used as a douche.

Finally, in addition to increasing one's intake of probiotics, a person can take fructo-oligosaccharides, supplements that can promote thriving colonies of helpful bacteria in the digestive tract. Fructo-oligosaccharides are carbohydrates found in fruit. *Fructo* means "fruit" and an "oligosaccharide" is a type of carbohydrate. Taking this supplement is like putting manure in a garden; it is thought to foster a healthy environment for the bacteria. The typical daily dose of fructo-oligosaccharides is between 2 and 8 grams.

THERAPEUTIC USES

Evidence from many double-blind, placebo-controlled trials suggests that probiotics may be helpful for many types of diarrhea and for irritable bowel syndrome. Additionally, probiotics have shown some promise for preventing or treating eczema.

Probiotics may be helpful for controlling symptoms and maintaining remission in ulcerative colitis. However, probiotics may be less useful for inducing remission. For example, when probiotics were added to standard medications used for induction of remission, no additional benefits were seen in a study of people with mild-to-moderate ulcerative colitis.

Probiotics might help prevent colds, possibly by improving immunity. On a related note, one small double-blind study found evidence that the use of the probiotic bacterium *L. fermentum* improved the effectiveness of the influenza vaccine. The probiotic supplement was taken in two doses. One was taken two weeks before the vaccine, and the other was taken two weeks after.

Although probiotics are widely used to prevent or treat vaginal yeast infections, evidence regarding potential benefit remains incomplete and inconsistent.

A small trial of fifty-five women with vulvovaginal candidiasis did demonstrate that daily *L. rhamnosus* and *L. reuteri* supplementation for four weeks, combined with single-dose fluconazole (an antifungal medication), decreased symptoms compared with fluconazole alone. Another large and well-designed trial, however, failed to find a *Lactobacillus* preparation helpful for preventing yeast infections caused by antibiotics. One study did find that probiotics might reduce levels of *C. albicans* in the mouth.

The bacterium *Gardnerella vaginalis* can cause a different type of vaginal infection. As with vaginal yeast infections, probiotics have shown some promise for this condition, but evidence remains inconclusive. A trial of sixty-four women taking a single dose of tinidazole for bacterial vaginosis suggests that women who also took daily probiotics capsules had better cure rates at four weeks. A larger trial involving 120 women with a history of bacterial vaginosis found that taking one capsule daily of the probiotics *L. rhamnosus*, acidophilus, and *S. thermophilus* reduced recurrence.

The bacterium *Helicobacter pylori* is the main cause of ulcers in the stomach and duodenum. Antibiotics can kill *H. pylori*, but more than one type of antibiotic must be used at the same time. Even in this case, the bacteria are not necessarily eradicated. Probiotics may be helpful for this. Evidence suggests that various probiotics can inhibit the growth of *H. pylori*. While this effect does not appear to be strong enough for probiotic treatment to eradicate *H. pylori* on its own, preliminary evidence, including several small double-blind trials, suggests that various probiotics may help standard antibiotic therapy work better, reducing side effects and possibly increasing the rate of eradication.

Some preliminary double-blind trials suggest that probiotics might improve cholesterol profile. Various probiotics might be helpful for allergic rhinitis (hay fever).

Milk fermented by probiotics may slightly improve blood pressure levels. While there is some evidence that probiotics can help reduce symptoms of milk allergies, one study found that adding probiotics to cow's milk formula for infants was not helpful. One study found that the use of probiotics during pregnancy and breast-feeding may decrease the likelihood that a highly allergic nursing mother will pass her allergic tendencies to her breast-fed infant.

One double-blind, placebo-controlled study of seventy people with chronic constipation found some evidence of benefit with *L. casei* Shirota. Another study found that *L. rhamnosus* was helpful for chronic constipation in children. A small trial also found benefits in children, this time with a mixture of bifidobacteria and lactobacilli. In another study, a combination of *B. lactis* and *B. longus* showed promise for improving bowel regularity in residents of nursing homes. Finally, in a six-week, double-blind, placebo-controlled trial of 274 people with constipation-predominant irritable bowel syndrome, the use of a probiotic formula containing *B. animalis* significantly improved stool frequency.

A preliminary double-blind, placebo-controlled study found evidence that *Lactobacillus* GG might potentially be helpful for treating antibiotic-resistant bacteria. This small study followed twenty-three people with severe kidney disease who tested positive for vancomycin-resistant bacteria in the stool. (Vancomycin is one of the main final-option antibiotics for the treatment of resistant bacteria.) The use of a yogurt product containing *L. rhamnosus* appeared to be more effective at ridding the gastrointestinal tract of these bacteria than did placebo. However, the study had a number of flaws, especially its small size. Note also that participants in this study did not have active infection with antibiotic-resistant bacteria; they were carriers for it. One should not attempt to use probiotics as the sole treatment for active infection with resistant bacteria. The preventive use of probiotics does not appear to help prevent the development of resistant bacterial strains that may arise during antibiotic treatment.

Probiotic treatment has also been proposed as a treatment for canker sores and as a preventive measure against colon cancer, but there is no solid evidence that it is effective. One study found that giving probiotics to certain critically ill people could help prevent multiple organ failure.

Probiotics have shown some promise for helping to prevent cavities by antagonizing cavity-causing bacteria. An open study found hints that probiotics might be helpful for mouth sores caused by Behçet's syndrome. One small, placebo-controlled study found that the use of *L. helveticus* might improve sleep quality in the elderly, for reasons that are not clear.

Probiotics have shown some promise in the treatment of infections with the yeast *C. albicans*. Probiotics are also proposed for the treatment of a theoretically related, but markedly controversial, condition known as yeast hypersensitivity syndrome (also known as chronic candidiasis, chronic candida, systemic candidiasis, and candida). As described by some alternative medicine practitioners, yeast hypersensitivity syndrome is a common problem that consists of a population explosion of the normally benign candida yeast that live in the vagina and elsewhere in the body, coupled with a type of allergic sensitivity to it. Probiotic supplements are widely recommended for this condition because they establish large, healthy populations of friendly bacteria that compete with the candida. However, there is no evidence that yeast hypersensitivity is a common problem and virtually no evidence that it exists at all.

In one small, twelve-week study, *Lactobacillus* GG failed to prove more effective than placebo for the treatment of rheumatoid arthritis. Another study failed to find *Lactobacillus* GG helpful for dyspepsia (generic stomach pain of unknown origin) in children.

A one-year-long open trial of 150 women failed to find *Lactobacillus* probiotics effective for preventing urinary tract infections, compared with cranberry juice or no treatment. Other studies, however, including a large (453-participant), three-month, double-blind, placebo-controlled study of a special healthful *Escherichia coli* probiotic did find benefits.

A substantial study failed to find a mixture of *L. casei, L. bulgaricus,* and *S. thermophilus* in yogurt and milk helpful for asthma in children. However, another study found that the combination of a probiotic (*B. breve*) and a prebiotic (galacto- and fructo-oligosaccharide) may help reduce wheezing in infants with eczema.

SCIENTIFIC EVIDENCE

Travelers' diarrhea. According to several studies, it appears that the regular use of acidophilus and other probiotics can help prevent travelers' diarrhea, an illness caused by eating contaminated food, usually in developing countries. One double-blind, placebo-controlled study followed 820 people traveling to southern Turkey and found that the use of *Lactobacillus* GG significantly protected against intestinal infection.

Other studies using *S. boulardii,* including a double-blind, placebo-controlled trial enrolling three thousand Austrian travelers, found similar benefits. The greatest benefits were seen in travelers who visited

North Africa and Turkey. The researchers noted that the benefit depended on consistent use of the product, and that a dosage of 1,000 mg daily was more effective than 250 mg daily.

Infectious diarrhea. Probiotics may also help prevent or treat acute infectious diarrhea in children and adults. A review of the literature published in 2001 found thirteen double-blind, placebo-controlled trials on the use of probiotics for acute infectious diarrhea in infants and children; ten of these trials involved treatment, and three involved prevention. Overall, the evidence suggests that probiotics can significantly reduce the duration of diarrhea and perhaps help prevent it. The evidence is strongest for the probiotic *Lactobacillus* GG and for infection with a particular virus, rotavirus, which causes severe diarrhea in children.

One double-blind, placebo-controlled trial of 269 children (aged one month to three years) with acute diarrhea found that those treated with *Lactobacillus* GG recovered more quickly than those given placebo. The best results were seen among children with rotavirus infection. Similar results with *Lactobacillus* GG were seen in a double-blind study of seventy-one children. However, 224 young Chinese children with severe, acute diarrhea found no benefit from lactose-free formula supplemented with bifidobacteria and *S. thermophilus*, suggesting that probiotics may not be as useful for cases of severe, dehydrating diarrhea. Also, *L. rhamnosus* GG is not always associated with improvement. When given for ten days to 229 infants from rural India who were hospitalized with acute diarrhea, the probiotic did not reduce the severity of the diarrhea during that time period.

In addition, a double-blind study evaluated the possible benefits of the probiotic *L. reuteri* in sixty-six children with rotavirus diarrhea. The study found that treatment shortened the duration of symptoms and that the higher the dose, the better the effect. Similar benefits were seen in a placebo-controlled trial of 151 infants and children given the probiotic *E. coli Nissle* 1917 (a safe strain of *E. coli*) for twenty-one days for nonspecific (presumably viral) cases of mild to moderate diarrhea.

A double-blind, placebo-controlled study of eighty-one hospitalized children found that treatment with *Lactobacillus* GG reduced the risk of developing diarrhea, particularly rotavirus infection. A double-blind, placebo-controlled study found that *Lactobacillus* GG helped prevent diarrhea in 204 undernourished children.

Other studies generally (though not consistently) indicate that the probiotics *B. bifidum*, *S. thermophilus*, *L. casei*, *Lactobacillus* LB, and *S. boulardii* (individually and combined with *L. reuteri* and *L. rhamnosus*) may also help prevent or treat diarrhea in infants and children. One study found that bacteria in the *B. bifidum* family can kill numerous bacteria that cause diarrhea.

A large (211-participant), double-blind, placebo-controlled study found that adults with diarrhea also can benefit from probiotic treatment. Another study found that the regular use of probiotics could help prevent gastrointestinal infections in adults.

Antibiotic-related diarrhea. The results of many double-blind and open trials suggest that probiotics, especially *S. boulardii* and *Lactobacillus* GG, may help prevent or treat antibiotic-related diarrhea. For example, one study evaluated 180 people, who received either placebo or 1,000 mg of *Saccharomyces* daily with their antibiotic treatment, and found that the treated group developed diarrhea significantly less often. A similar study of 193 people also found benefit.

A minimum of three more studies involving adults found that various species of *Lactobacillus*, taken either alone or in combination, were beneficial, even in cases of *Clostridium difficile* infection, the most serious type of antibiotic-induced diarrhea. However, a study of 302 people found no benefit with *Lactobacillus* GG. A review of four probiotic studies found insufficient evidence for their effectiveness in the treatment of *C. difficile*. Finally, although taking probiotic organisms in the proper concentration may be beneficial for antibiotic-induced diarrhea, one study found that consuming fresh yogurt during antibiotic treatments had no significant effect on the incidence of diarrhea.

Other forms of diarrhea. Two double-blind, placebo-controlled studies enrolling almost seven hundred people undergoing radiation therapy for cancer found that the use of probiotics significantly improved radiation-induced diarrhea. Similar evidence supports the use of *L. rhamnosus* and a special, nonpathogenic form of *E. coli*. However, of eighty-five women receiving pelvic radiation for cervical or uterine cancer, those who consumed a liquid yogurt preparation enriched with *L. casei* had no less diarrhea than those who took a placebo drink. Small double-blind studies suggest that *S. boulardii* might be helpful for treating chronic diarrhea in people with human immunodeficiency virus infection, in persons hospitalized and being fed through a tube, and in people with Crohn's disease.

Premature infants weighing less than 2,500 grams (5.5 pounds) are at risk for a life-threatening intestinal condition called necrotizing enterocolitis (NEC). In a study that pooled the results of nine randomized, placebo-controlled trials involving 1,425 infants, probiotic supplementation significantly reduced the occurrence of NEC and death associated with it. A subsequent study found similar benefits in very low-birth-weight infants weighing less than 1,500 grams (3.3 pounds).

Inflammatory bowel disease. The conditions Crohn's disease and ulcerative colitis are in the family of conditions known as inflammatory bowel disease. Chronic diarrhea is a common feature of these conditions.

A double-blind trial of 116 people with ulcerative colitis compared probiotic treatment with a relatively low dose of the standard drug mesalazine. The results suggest that probiotic treatment might be just as effective as low-dose mesalazine for controlling symptoms and maintaining remission. Evidence of benefit was seen in other trials too.

One preliminary study found *S. boulardii* helpful for mild diarrhea in stable Crohn's disease. However, two studies failed to find benefit with *Lactobacillus* probiotics, and in an analysis of eight randomized, placebo-controlled studies, probiotics were ineffective at maintaining remission in persons with Crohn's disease.

Probiotics might be useful for people with ulcerative colitis who have had part or all of their colon removed. Such people frequently develop a complication called pouchitis, the inflammation of part of the remaining intestine. A nine-month, double-blind trial of forty people found that a combination of three probiotic bacteria could significantly reduce the risk of a pouchitis flare-up in people with chronic pouchitis. Participants were given either placebo or a mixture of probiotics, including four strains of lactobacilli, three strains of bifidobacteria, and one strain of *S. salivarius*. The results showed that treated people were far less likely to have relapses of pouchitis.

Another study found that probiotics used right after surgery can help prevent pouchitis from developing. One study, however, failed to find benefit with *L. johnsonii* in people with Crohn's disease who had undergone a similar operation. Finally, some evidence hints that probiotics might reduce the joint pain that commonly occurs in people with either kind of inflammatory bowel disease.

Irritable bowel syndrome. People with irritable bowel syndrome (IBS) experience crampy digestive pain and alternating diarrhea and constipation and other symptoms. Although the cause of IBS is not known, one possibility is a disturbance in healthy intestinal bacteria. Based on this theory, probiotics have been tried as a treatment for IBS, with some success.

In a six-week, double-blind, placebo-controlled trial of 274 people with constipation-predominant IBS, the use of a probiotic formula containing *B. animalis* significantly reduced discomfort and increased stool frequency. Also, 266 women with constipation who consumed yogurt containing *B. animalis* and the prebiotic fructo-oligosaccharides twice daily for two weeks experienced significant improvement compared with women consuming regular yogurt as a placebo. Finally, in another trial of 298 persons with IBS, eight weeks of treatment with beneficial *E. coli* reduced typical symptoms compared with placebo.

Benefits were seen in eight other small, double-blind trials too, using *L. plantarum*, *L. acidophilus*, *L. rhamnosus*, *L. salivarius*, and *Bifidobacterium*, and using proprietary probiotic combinations of various strains. Benefits have also been seen with combination prebiotic and probiotic formulas and prebiotics alone. Other studies have failed to find probiotics more effective than placebo.

Two studies that pooled previous randomized trials on the use of probiotics for IBS came to similar conclusions: Probiotics appear to offer some benefit, most notably for global symptoms and abdominal discomfort. However, these two studies were unable to determine what probiotic species were most effective.

Eczema. The use of probiotics during pregnancy and after childbirth may reduce the risk of childhood eczema. In a large, long-term, double-blind study, 1,223 pregnant women were given either placebo or a probiotic mixture (containing lactobacilli and bifidobacteria) beginning two to four weeks before delivery. Their newborn children then received either probiotics or placebo for six months. The results showed that the probiotics mixture markedly reduced the incidence of eczema (though not of other allergic diseases). However, in a follow-up to this study, researchers found that the probiotic supplementation was not associated with reduced eczema in children followed through the age of five years. The probiotics also had no effect on allergic rhinitis or asthma.

Another study also yielded marginal results, and a third study involving only *Lactobacillus* found no benefit for the prevention of eczema. This latter study actually demonstrated a modestly increased risk of wheezing bronchitis in infants who took the probiotic. However, some probiotics combined with prebiotics may help to reduce wheezing in infants with eczema. For example, *B. breve* and a galacto- and fructo-oligosaccharide mixture showed benefit in one randomized study involving ninety infants.

B. longum and *L. rhamnosus* supplementation did not reduce the incidence of eczema atopic dermatitis or allergic sensitization at twelve months among Asian infants at risk of allergic diseases. Researchers in another study concluded that not all probiotics are created equal. In this placebo-controlled study, *L. rhamnosus* reduced the incidence of eczema in the children, but a strain of *B. animalis* did not.

According to some studies, infants who already have eczema may benefit from probiotics. However, a careful review of twelve studies involving 781 children found no convincing evidence that probiotics can effectively treat eczema in this age group.

If probiotics are beneficial for childhood eczema, they are probably more effective at preventing the condition than at treating it. A carefully conducted review of numerous studies cautiously concluded that probiotics may help reduce the risk of eczema in infants and children, particularly those at high risk. Also, two subsequent reviews found that probiotics were more effective at preventing childhood eczema, particularly when given before birth to the pregnant woman and the fetus.

Immunity. A number of studies suggest that various probiotics can enhance immune function. One twelve-week, double-blind, placebo-controlled trial evaluated twenty-five healthy elderly people, half of whom were given milk containing a particular strain of *B. lactis* and the other half of whom were given milk alone. The results showed various changes in immune parameters, which the researchers took as possibly indicating improved immune function. Another double-blind, placebo-controlled study of fifty people using *B. lactis* had similar results.

A seven-month, double-blind, placebo-controlled study of 571 children in day care centers in Finland found that the use of milk fortified with *Lactobacillus* GG reduced the number and severity of respiratory infections. In another controlled trial, probiotics (*L. rhamnosus* GG and *B. lactis* Bb-12) given daily to infants in their formula significantly reduced the risk of acute otitis media and of recurrent respiratory infections during the first year of life, compared with placebo.

Benefits were seen in three other large studies, in which probiotics combined with multivitamins and multiminerals helped prevent colds (or helped reduce their duration and severity) in adults. However, a smaller and shorter study failed to find any effect on respiratory infections. Similarly, *L. fermentum* given to twenty healthy, elite distance runners for four months during winter training was significantly more effective at reducing the number and severity of respiratory symptoms compared with placebo. One study found that *Lactobacillus* GG or *L. acidophilus* may improve the immune response to vaccinations.

Cholesterol. An eight-week, double-blind, placebo-controlled trial of seventy overweight people found that a probiotic treatment containing *S. thermophilus* and *Enterococcus faecium* could reduce LDL (bad) cholesterol by about 8 percent. Similarly positive results were seen in other short-term trials of various probiotics. However, a six-month, double-blind, placebo-controlled trial found no long-term benefit. Researchers speculate that participants stopped using the product regularly in the later parts of the study.

SAFETY ISSUES

Probiotics may occasionally cause a temporary increase in digestive gas. However, beyond that, they do not present any known risks for most people. In one trial of 140 healthy infants, formula supplemented with long-chain polyunsaturated fatty acids and probiotics appeared as safe as standard formula and did not have any effect on infant growth by the end of the seven-month trial.

However, persons who are immunosuppressed could conceivably be at risk for developing a dangerous infection with the probiotic organism itself; at least one person taking immunosuppressive medications has died in this manner.

In a detailed review of four studies, researchers concluded that the use of probiotics did not benefit persons with severe acute pancreatitis. Furthermore, according to one study, the use of probiotics led to an increased risk of mortality in persons with severe acute pancreatitis and should, therefore, be avoided under these circumstances.

Drug interactions. It may be beneficial for persons taking antibiotics to take probiotic supplements at the same time and to continue the probiotics for a couple of weeks after finishing the course of drug treatment. Doing so will help restore the balance of natural bacteria in the digestive tract.

EBSCO CAM Review Board

FURTHER READING

Do, V. T., B. G. Baird, and D. R. Kockler. "Probiotics for Maintaining Remission of Ulcerative Colitis in Adults." *Annals of Pharmacotherapy* 44 (2010): 565-571.

Gao, X. W., et al. "Dose-Response Efficacy of a Proprietary Probiotic Formula of *Lactobacillus acidophilus* CL1285 and *Lactobacillus casei* LBC80R for Antibiotic-Associated Diarrhea and *Clostridium difficile*-Associated Diarrhea Prophylaxis in Adult Patients." *American Journal of Gastroenterology* 105 (2010): 1636-1641.

Gibson, R. A., et al. "Safety of Supplementing Infant Formula with Long-Chain Polyunsaturated Fatty Acids and *Bifidobacterium lactis* in Term Infants." *British Journal of Nutrition* 101 (2009): 1706-1713.

Kim, J. Y., et al. "Effect of Probiotic Mix (*Bifidobacterium bifidum, Bifidobacterium lactis, Lactobacillus acidophilus*) in the Primary Prevention of Eczema." *Pediatric Allergy and Immunology* 21 (2010): 386-393.

McFarland, L. V., and S. Dublin. "Meta-analysis of Probiotics for the Treatment of Irritable Bowel Syndrome." *World Journal of Gastroenterology* 14 (2008): 2650-2661.

Misra, S., T. K. Sabui, and N. K. Pal. "A Randomized Controlled Trial to Evaluate the Efficacy of *Lactobacillus* GG in Infantile Diarrhea." *Journal of Pediatrics* 155 (2009): 129-132.

Park, S. K., et al. "The Effect of Probiotics on *Helicobacter pylori* Eradication." *Hepatogastroenterology* 54 (2007): 2032-2036.

Pillai, A., et al. "Probiotics for Treatment of *Clostridium difficile*-Associated Colitis in Adults." *Cochrane Database of Systematic Reviews* (2008): CD004611. Available through *EBSCO DynaMed Systematic Literature Surveillance* at http://www.ebscohost.com/dynamed.

Rautava, S., S. Salminen, and E. Isolauri. "Specific Probiotics in Reducing the Risk of Acute Infections in Infancy." *British Journal of Nutrition* 101 (2009): 1722-1726.

Tubelius, P., et al. "Increasing Work-Place Healthiness with the Probiotic *Lactobacillus reuteri*." *Environmental Health* 4 (2005): 25.

Underwood, M. A., et al. "A Randomized Placebo-Controlled Comparison of Two Prebiotic/Probiotic Combinations in Preterm Infants: Impact on Weight Gain, Intestinal Microbiota, and Fecal Short-Chain Fatty Acids." *Journal of Pediatric Gastroenterology and Nutrition* 48 (2009): 216-225.

Woo, S. I., et al. "Effect of *Lactobacillus sakei* Supplementation in Children with Atopic Eczema-Dermatitis Syndrome." *Annals of Allergy, Asthma, and Immunology* 104 (2010): 343-348.

Ya, W., C. Reifer, and L. E. Miller. "Efficacy of Vaginal Probiotic Capsules for Recurrent Bacterial Vaginosis." *American Journal of Obstetrics and Gynecology* 203 (2010): 120.

See also: Crohn's disease; Diarrhea; Dyspepsia; Gas, intestinal; Gastrointestinal health; Irritable bowel syndrome (IBS); Lactose intolerance; Ulcerative colitis; Ulcers.

Progesterone

CATEGORY: Herbs and supplements
RELATED TERMS: Micronized progesterone, progesterone cream
DEFINITION: Natural substance of the human body used as a supplement to treat specific health conditions.
PRINCIPAL PROPOSED USES: Replacement for standard progestins
OTHER PROPOSED USES: Menopausal symptoms, opposing estrogen, preventing or treating osteoporosis

OVERVIEW

Progesterone is one of the two primary female hormones. As the name implies, progesterone prepares (pro) the womb for pregnancy (gestation). Progesterone works in tandem with estrogen; indeed, if estrogen is taken as a medication without being balanced by progesterone (so-called unopposed estrogen), there is an increased risk of uterine cancer.

However, progesterone is not well absorbed orally. For this reason, pharmaceutical manufacturers developed progestins, substances similar to progesterone that are more easily absorbed. Most of the time, a woman prescribed progesterone is really being given a progestin. Two of the most commonly used progestins are medroxyprogesterone and norethindrone. However, it has been suggested that actual progesterone may offer benefits over progestins, such as fewer side effects.

Progesterone can be absorbed through the skin to some extent, and some alternative practitioners have, for years, promoted the use of progesterone creams. Such progesterone creams are typically, but misleadingly, said to contain natural progesterone. This is an oddly chosen term, as the progesterone in these creams is actually produced in a laboratory, just like other synthetic hormones. To avoid confusion in this article, herein progesterone will be called true progesterone, or just progesterone. Besides creams, a special form of true progesterone that can be absorbed orally, micronized progesterone, has recently become available as a prescription drug.

Inconsistent evidence suggests that progesterone cream might help reduce menopausal symptoms. However, it does not appear to be strong enough to balance the effects of estrogen, thus reducing the risk of uterine cancer. (Oral micronized progesterone is strong enough for this purpose.) Contrary to numerous books and magazine articles, there is no more than weak, inconsistent evidence that progesterone cream offers any benefits for osteoporosis.

REQUIREMENTS AND SOURCES

Progesterone is synthesized in the body and is not found in appreciable quantities in food. For use as a drug or dietary supplement, progesterone is synthesized from chemicals found in soy or Mexican yam.

Another aspect of the widespread misinformation involving progesterone cream is the concept that Mexican yam itself contains progesterone or substances that the body can convert into progesterone. This is incorrect. Industrial chemists can convert a constituent of Mexican yam (diosgenin) into progesterone, but only by using chemical pathways not found in the body.

THERAPEUTIC DOSAGES

The usual dose of progesterone in cream form is 20 milligrams (mg) daily. Although this dose might decrease menopausal hot flashes, most studies found that even doses as high as 64 mg daily do not provide

enough progesterone to protect the uterus from the effects of estrogen. However, one study found that use of micronized progesterone cream at 80 mg daily produced about the same progesterone levels in the body as an oral dose of 200 mg daily; oral micronized progesterone taken at a dose of 200 to 400 mg daily is approximately as effective as the standard dosage of the more commonly used progestins.

THERAPEUTIC USES

Progesterone cream was widely promoted in the 1990s as a treatment for osteoporosis, on the basis of meaningless studies whose designs were too poor to establish anything. When properly designed studies were performed, the results were at best inconsistent.

Studies conflict on whether progesterone cream can help hot flashes. One double-blind, placebo-controlled study failed to find any improvements in mood or general well-being in menopausal women using progesterone cream. Like progestins, oral progesterone protects the uterus from the stimulating effects of unopposed estrogen. However, standard doses of progesterone cream probably provide too little progesterone to serve this purpose.

SCIENTIFIC EVIDENCE

Osteoporosis. Despite widespread reporting that true progesterone is effective for treating or preventing osteoporosis, the evidence for such an effect is at best inconsistent. This notion originated with test-tube and other preliminary studies suggesting that progesterone or progestins can stimulate the activity of cells that build bone. Subsequently, a poorly designed and uncontrolled study (really, a series of case histories from one physician's practice) purportedly demonstrated that progesterone cream can slow or even reverse osteoporosis.

However, a one-year double-blind trial of 102 women given either progesterone cream (providing 20 mg progesterone daily) or placebo cream, along with calcium and multivitamins, found no evidence of any improvements in bone density attributable to progesterone. A smaller, short-term trial found that progesterone cream has no effect on bone metabolism.

In contrast to these negative results, benefits were seen in a small two-year double-blind, placebo-controlled study in which twenty-two women were given progesterone cream. (Interestingly, in this study, use of progesterone cream plus soy isoflavones produced benefits inferior to those of progesterone cream alone.) It is, therefore, at least possible that progesterone cream is helpful for osteoporosis if taken for a long enough period; however, more research is needed.

Menopausal symptoms. In the one-year double-blind trial of 102 women described above, use of progesterone cream was found to significantly reduce hot flashes and related symptoms. However, a slightly smaller twelve-week double-blind trial failed to find progesterone cream helpful for reducing menopausal symptoms. The authors of this second study point out that the first study was statistically flawed.

Opposing estrogen. Unless a woman has had a hysterectomy, if she takes estrogen she needs to take progesterone too, or run the risk of uterine cancer. Two twelve-week double-blind studies enrolling a total of about one hundred women found that progesterone cream (at doses up to 64 mg) did not have the required protective effect on the cells of the uterus. One study, however, did find benefit at dosages of either 15 or 40 mg daily. The explanation for these disparate results may lie in the results of two other studies, which suggest that progesterone cream is erratically absorbed.

SAFETY ISSUES

Even though progesterone is sold as a dietary supplement, it is a hormone, not a food. Its use is not recommended except under a physician's supervision. Like progestins, true progesterone causes side effects. In one study, oral micronized progesterone at a dose of 400 mg per day was associated with dizziness, abdominal cramping, headache, breast pain, muscle pain, irritability, nausea, fatigue, diarrhea, and viral infections.

EBSCO CAM Review Board

FURTHER READING

Hermann, A. C., et al. "Over-the-counter Progesterone Cream Produces Significant Drug Exposure Compared to a Food and Drug Administration-Approved Oral Progesterone Product." *Journal of Clinical Pharmacology* 45, no. 6 (2005): 614-619.

Leonetti, H. B., K. J. Wilson, and J. N. Anasti. "Topical Progesterone Cream Has an Antiproliferative Effect on Estrogen-Stimulated Endometrium." *Fertility and Sterility* 79 (2003): 221-222.

Lydeking-Olsen, E., et al. "Soymilk or Progesterone for Prevention of Bone Loss." *European Journal of Nutrition* 4, no. 4 (2004): 246-257.

Wren, B. G., et al. "Transdermal Progesterone and Its Effect on Vasomotor Symptoms, Blood Lipid Levels, Bone Metabolic Markers, Moods, and Quality of Life for Postmenopausal Women." *Menopause* 10 (2003): 13-18.

See also: Estrogen; Herbal medicine; Menopause; Osteoporosis.

Progressive muscle relaxation

CATEGORY: Therapies and techniques

RELATED TERMS: Autonomic nervous system, behavioral medicine, vasodilation

DEFINITION: A technique that promotes physiologic relaxation and reduced stress by systematically tensing and relaxing major muscle groups of the body.

PRINCIPAL PROPOSED USES: Anxiety, chronic pain, fears and phobias, headaches, hypertension, respiratory disorders, sleep disorders, stress reduction, temperomandibular disorders

OTHER PROPOSED USES: General health and wellness, stress management

OVERVIEW

The positive effects of relaxation and the contributory influences of prolonged stress and tension on illness have long been recognized. Progressive muscle relaxation (PMR) is a technique aimed at reducing the somatic (bodily) consequences of stress, such as muscle tension, by lowering physiologic arousal and, thereby, inducing relaxation.

Commonly used models of progressive relaxation are based on the principles identified by American psychiatrist Edmund Jacobson in the 1930s. The basic technique developed by Jacobson involves alternately tensing and relaxing major muscle groups of the body, while concurrently focusing on sensations associated with the tensing and relaxing.

Regardless of the reasons for its application, current PMR methods begin with a rationale for its use. The fundamental premise is that muscle tension, even when it is not overtly perceived, causes anxiety (and often pain, discomfort, and agitation) and that significant a reduction in associated symptoms will result if tense muscles are relaxed.

Participants learning PMR are requested to loosen tight clothing and to sit in a comfortable chair in a quiet setting relatively free from distraction. A trained therapist then instructs and demonstrates how to isolate, tense, and relax muscles, and then systematically guides the person through the different muscle groups in a fixed order.

During the "tensing" phase of the procedure, the person is directed to constrict the identified muscle as tightly as possible while keeping other muscle groups loose and relaxed. Attention is directed to the sensations associated with tensing, such as tightness and discomfort. The tensing phase lasts approximately ten seconds and is followed by the "relaxing" or "releasing" phase, wherein muscles tension is "let go" and muscles are allowed to become limp. The participant then focuses on the feeling of tension and discomfort draining from the muscle and takes notice of the contrast between the warmth and comfort of relaxed muscles and the discomfort of tensed muscles.

After about ten to fifteen seconds of relaxing, the sequence is repeated with another muscle group. A typical sequence of muscle groups addressed in the technique is the following: hands, biceps and triceps, shoulders, chest, neck, mouth and lips, eyes, forehead and scalp, back, stomach, thighs, calves, feet, and toes. After completing the sequence of tensing and releasing phases, participants take an "inventory" of their muscle groups and relax those with remaining tension. The procedure takes about twenty to thirty minutes to complete.

During the procedure, participants are encouraged to avoid blocking thoughts that might intrude upon their consciousness, and either to allow these thoughts to flow through their mind or to shift their focus toward their breathing if they find themselves distracted. For a period of time following the exercise, participants may engage in slow, steady, and even breathing as a means of enhancing the relaxation response. They may also repeat a calming word or phrase such as "relax," "release," or "let go" each time they exhale so that the word or phrase becomes a cue for promoting relaxation, a practice known as cue-controlled relaxation.

Typically, two or three guided relaxation sessions are conducted to develop basic proficiency with the exercise. Nonguided practice sessions are encouraged to further enhance skills, with the goal of the person being able to achieve a highly relaxed state

Relaxation Techniques

Relaxation techniques include a number of practices, such as progressive muscle relaxation, guided imagery, biofeedback, self-hypnosis, and deep breathing exercises. The goal is similar in all: to consciously produce the body's natural relaxation response, characterized by slower breathing, lower blood pressure, and a feeling of calm and well-being.

Relaxation is more than a state of mind; it physically changes the way the body functions. Being able to produce the relaxation response using relaxation techniques may counteract the effects of long-term stress, which may contribute to or worsen a range of health problems including depression, digestive disorders, headaches, high blood pressure, and insomnia.

When a person is under stress, the body releases hormones that produce the fight-or-flight response: Heart rate and breathing rate go up, and blood vessels narrow (restricting the flow of blood). This response allows energy to flow to parts of the body, such as the muscles and the heart, that need to take action. However useful this response may be in the short term, evidence shows that when the body remains in a stress state for a long time, emotional or physical damage can occur. Long-term or chronic stress (lasting months or years) may reduce the body's ability to fight illness and can lead to or worsen certain health conditions. Chronic stress may lead to high blood pressure, headaches, stomachache, and other symptoms. Stress may worsen certain conditions, such as asthma. Stress also has been linked to depression, anxiety, and other mental illnesses.

In contrast to the stress response, the relaxation response slows the heart rate, lowers blood pressure, and decreases oxygen consumption and levels of stress hormones. Because relaxation is the opposite of stress, the theory is that voluntarily creating the relaxation response through regular use of relaxation techniques could counteract the negative effects of stress.

without guidance. Common variations to the procedure include abbreviated protocols such as "release only" methods, whereby the tensing phase is eliminated or emphasis is directed at specific muscle groups that are identified as particularly key in inducing overall relaxation. Audiotapes of the relaxation procedure may also be used to develop relaxation skills.

MECHANISM OF ACTION

PMR has been found to affect the autonomic nervous system, which, among other functions, regulates how the body reacts to changes in the environment. These effects include decreases in heart rate, blood pressure, and muscle tension, and general arousal. Vasodilation of blood vessels also occurs, causing increased blood flow throughout the body, most noticeably in the extremities. These responses are the opposite of those produced by anxiety and lead to subjective feelings of warmth, comfort, and calmness.

USES AND APPLICATIONS

PMR has a long history of use in psychiatry, psychology, and behavioral medicine. The procedure has been employed as a stand-alone therapy and as a component of multifaceted protocols treating psychiatric and medical illnesses. In nonmedical settings, the procedure is commonly used to promote overall wellness and healthy adaptation to life stressors.

SCIENTIFIC EVIDENCE

A large body of research has demonstrated that PMR is effective in reducing symptoms stemming from a variety of medical and psychiatric conditions. A double-blind, placebo-controlled study in 2005 examined the technique as applied in a medical setting. The study showed that asthmatic female adolescents' lung function, heart rate, and blood pressure improved after learning and employing PMR. Another double-blind, placebo-controlled study, in 2009, examined the technique's psychiatric application. The study found that PMR improved anxiety symptoms in hospitalized adults with schizophrenia.

CHOOSING A PRACTITIONER

Trained and licensed mental health or medical professionals should be consulted for persons seeking PMR treatment for psychiatric, psychological, or medical conditions. For nonmedical applications, trained nonprofessionals and audiotapes are usually appropriate.

SAFETY ISSUES

Before participating in PMR, interested persons should consult a physician or other health care provider.

Paul F. Bell, Ph.D.

FURTHER READING

Chen, W. C., et al. "Efficacy of Progressive Muscle Relaxation Training in Reducing Anxiety in Patients with Acute Schizophrenia." *Journal of Clinical Nursing* 18, no. 15 (2009): 2187-2196.

Neumann, Donald A. *Kinesiology of the Musculoskeletal System: Foundations for Rehabilitation.* 2d ed. St. Louis, Mo.: Mosby/Elsevier, 2010.

Nickel, C., et al. "Effect of Progressive Muscle Relaxation in Adolescent Female Bronchial Asthma Patients." *Journal of Psychosomatic Research* 59 (2005): 393-398.

See also: Alexander technique; Aston-Patterning; Dance movement therapy; Exercise; Exercise-based therapies; Feldenkrais method; Fibromyalgia: Homeopathic remedies; Manipulative and body-based practices; Massage therapy; Mind/body medicine; Pain management; Reflexology; Relaxation response; Rolfing; Shiatsu; Soft tissue pain.

Prolotherapy

CATEGORY: Therapies and techniques
RELATED TERM: Sclerotherapy
DEFINITION: Treatment involving injections of chemical irritant solutions into the area around a loose ligament.
PRINCIPAL PROPOSED USES: Back pain, osteoarthritis
OTHER PROPOSED USES: Fibromyalgia, plantar fasciitis, sciatica, sports injuries, temporomandibular joint disorder, tendonitis, tension headaches

OVERVIEW

Invented in the 1950s by George Hackett, prolotherapy is based on the theory that chronic pain is often caused by laxness of the ligaments that are responsible for keeping a joint stable. When ligaments and associated tendons are loose, the body is said to compensate by using muscles to stabilize the joint. The net result, according to prolotherapy theory, is muscle spasms and pain.

Prolotherapy treatment involves injections of chemical irritant solutions into the area around such ligaments. These solutions are believed to cause tissue to proliferate (grow), increasing the strength and thickness of ligaments. In turn, this presumably serves to tighten up the joint and relieve the burden on associated muscles, stopping muscle spasms. In the case of arthritic joints, increased ligament strength would allow the joint to function more efficiently, thus reducing pain.

Prolotherapy has not been widely accepted in conventional medicine. The technique is used by prolotherapy practitioners to treat many conditions, including back pain, osteoarthritis, fibromyalgia, plantar fasciitis, sciatica, sports injuries, temporomandibular joint disorder, tendonitis, and tension headaches. Most studies have focused on its use in back pain and osteoarthritis, but the evidence does not clearly support its effectiveness.

How is prolotherapy performed? Prolotherapy is generally administered at intervals of four to six weeks, although studies have used a more frequent schedule. The treatment involves injection of a mixture containing an irritant and a local anesthetic. A total of four to six treatments is typical. When treating back pain, prolotherapy practitioners frequently use a form of manipulation somewhat similar to chiropractic. However, the manipulation is applied after local anesthetic has been injected, and it is somewhat intense.

There are several irritant solutions used in prolotherapy. Concentrated dextrose or glucose has become increasingly popular because it is completely nontoxic. Phenol (a potentially toxic substance) and glycerin are also sometimes used. Other, nonirritant substances may be added to the solution, such as vitamin B_{12}, corn extracts, cod liver oil extracts, zinc, and manganese; however, there is no evidence that these substances add any benefit.

SCIENTIFIC EVIDENCE

Some animal and human studies have found that prolotherapy injections increase the strength and thickness of ligaments. Six double-blind human trials of prolotherapy have been reported: four involving back pain (with mixed results) and the other two involving osteoarthritis (with positive results).

Back pain. Although two studies have suggested prolotherapy may be effective for low back pain, two more recent studies found prolotherapy to be ineffective. In a review of five studies, three found prolotherapy to be no more effective than control treatments for low back pain. The other two studies suggested that prolotherapy was more effective than

control treatments when used with therapies such as spinal manipulation and exercise. Another review suggested that prolotherapy may be effective when used with other therapies, but not when used alone.

When used alone, prolotherapy is probably no more effective than a placebo injection for the treatment of low back pain. However, there is some evidence that the technique may be beneficial when combined with other therapies.

Osteoarthritis. A double-blind, placebo-controlled study evaluated the effects of three prolotherapy injections (using a 10 percent dextrose solution) at two-month intervals in sixty-eight people with osteoarthritis of the knee. At the six-month follow-up, participants who had received prolotherapy showed significant improvements in pain at rest and while walking. These participants also showed reduced swelling and fewer episodes of "buckling" than those who had received placebo treatment.

The same research group performed a similar double-blind trial of twenty-seven people with osteoarthritis in the hands. The results at the six-month follow-up showed that range of motion and pain with movement improved significantly in the treated group compared with the placebo group.

SAFETY ISSUES

In studies, prolotherapy has not caused any serious, irreversible injury. After each injection there is usually discomfort that lasts for a few minutes to several days, but this discomfort is seldom severe. Of more concern is that severe headaches have been reported in treatment of low back pain in a minority of patients. Also, because phenol is a potentially toxic substance, treatment with a dextrose solution alone is preferable.

CHOOSING A PRACTITIONER

Prolotherapy is practiced by a medical doctor or a doctor of osteopathy. Generally, physicians specializing in orthopedics or physical medicine and rehabilitation are most likely to practice prolotherapy.

EBSCO CAM Review Board

FURTHER READING

Coombes, B. K., L. Bisset, and B. Vicenzino. "Efficacy and Safety of Corticosteroid Injections and Other Injections for Management of Tendinopathy." *The Lancet* 376 (2010): 1751-1767.

Dagenais, S., J. Mayer, et al. "Evidence-Informed Management of Chronic Low Back Pain with Prolotherapy." *Spine Journal* 8 (2008): 203-212.

Dagenais, S., M. Yelland, et al. "Prolotherapy Injections for Chronic Low-Back Pain." *Cochrane Database of Systematic Reviews* (2007): CD004059. Available through *EBSCO DynaMed Systematic Literature Surveillance* at http://www.ebscohost.com/dynamed.

Hauser, R. A. "Punishing the Pain: Treating Chronic Pain with Prolotherapy." *Rehab Management* 12 (1999): 26-30.

Yelland, M. J., et al. "Prolotherapy Injections, Saline Injections, and Exercises for Chronic Low-Back Pain." *Spine* 29 (2004): 9-16.

See also: Back pain; Bone and joint health; Corticosteroids; Enzyme potentiated desensitization; Exercise; Osteoarthritis; Pain management.

Prostatitis

CATEGORY: Condition

RELATED TERMS: Acute bacterial prostatitis, chronic pelvic pain syndrome, chronic prostatitis, prostatalgia, prostatodynia

DEFINITION: Treatment of inflammation of the prostate.

PRINCIPAL PROPOSED NATURAL TREATMENTS: None

OTHER PROPOSED NATURAL TREATMENTS: Acupuncture, biofeedback, bromelain, buchu, couch grass, cranberry, echinacea, *Eleutherococcus*, garlic, goldenseal, grass pollen extract, lapacho, marshmallow, multivitamin-multimineral supplements, pipsissewa, proteolytic enzymes, pygeum, quercetin, saw palmetto, vitamin C, watermelon seed, zinc

INTRODUCTION

Prostatitis is inflammation of the prostate. The prostate is a walnut-sized gland in males that surrounds the urethra. It produces a fluid that is part of semen. There are three main types of prostatitis: acute bacterial, chronic bacterial, and chronic nonbacterial.

Acute bacterial prostatitis is the easiest form to treat, but it is also the least common. Symptoms include chills, fever, pain in the lower back and genital area, urinary frequency and urgency (often at night), burning or painful urination, and body aches. Examination of the urine shows white blood cells. Antibiotic treatment is highly successful for this form of prostatitis.

Chronic bacterial prostatitis resembles acute prostatitis, but it is milder and may continue for a long time (months or years). It is believed that chronic bacterial prostatitis is caused by a problem in the prostate that makes the gland a focus for infection. Antibiotic treatment usually relieves symptoms, but the symptoms often come back after treatment is stopped.

Chronic nonbacterial prostatitis, also known as chronic pelvic pain syndrome or prostatodynia, is the most common form of prostatitis. It is also the least understood and the most difficult to treat. Symptoms include urinary urgency, urinary frequency (especially at night), pain or burning while urinating, difficulty urinating, lower abdominal pain or pressure, rectal or perineal discomfort, lower back pain, painful ejaculation, and impotence. These symptoms may wax and wane for no obvious reason. Conventional medicine lacks a specific treatment for chronic nonbacterial prostatitis. Supportive treatments may be used, including stool softeners, pain medications, and warm sitz baths.

PROPOSED NATURAL TREATMENTS

Quercetin belongs to a class of water-soluble plant coloring agents called bioflavonoids, which have anti-inflammatory and antioxidant properties. Bioflavonoids have been investigated for a wide variety of medical uses. A study published in 1999 suggests that quercetin may be helpful for chronic nonbacterial prostatitis. In this double-blind trial, thirty men with fairly severe chronic nonbacterial prostatitis were given either quercetin (500 milligrams [mg] twice daily) or placebo for one month. The results showed that participants given quercetin improved to a significantly greater extent than those in the placebo group. The greatest gains were seen in the reduction of pain.

A special grass pollen extract has also shown promise. In a six-month double-blind study of sixty men with nonbacterial prostatitis, the use of the grass pollen extract was more effective than placebo. Grass pollen is better known as a treatment for benign prostatic hypertrophy (BPH). All the other commonly used natural treatments for this condition have also been suggested for prostatitis. However, while there is reasonably good supporting evidence that some of these help BPH, the evidence regarding their use in prostatitis remains weak. For example, uncontrolled trials and other highly preliminary forms of evidence hint that the herb pygeum might be helpful for prostatitis. Also, an open controlled trial (using a no-treatment group) found indications that saw palmetto might be helpful for prostatitis; however, an open comparative study found the drug finasteride more effective than the herb for this purpose.

A combination of herbal extracts, including *Serenoa repens* (saw palmetto), *Urtica dioica* (neetle), curcumin, and quercitin, may turn out to be modestly beneficial as additional treatment. In a trial of 143 men with chronic bacterial prostatitis, the preparation enhanced the effectiveness of a two-week course of antibiotic (prulifloxacin).

Other herbs and supplements sometimes recommended for prostatitis, but almost entirely lacking any supporting evidence, include bromelain, buchu, couch grass, cranberry, echinacea, *Eleutherococcus*, garlic, goldenseal, lapacho, marshmallow, multivitamin-multimineral supplements, pipsissewa, proteolytic enzymes, vitamin C, watermelon seed, and zinc.

Acupuncture and biofeedback have been tried too. In a study involving eighty-nine men with chronic nonbacterial prostatitis, a ten-week trial of acupuncture was modestly more effective than sham (fake) acupuncture at relieving symptoms, both during treatment and for six months following treatment.

HERBS AND SUPPLEMENTS TO USE WITH CAUTION

Various herbs and supplements may interact adversely with drugs used to treat prostatitis, so persons should be cautious when considering the use of herbs and supplements.

EBSCO CAM Review Board

FURTHER READING

Cai, T., et al. "*Serenoa repens* Associated with *Urtica dioica* (ProstaMEV) and Curcumin and Quercitin (FlogMEV) Extracts Are Able to Improve the Efficacy of Prulifloxacin in Bacterial Prostatitis Patients." *International Journal of Antimicrobial Agents* 33 (2009): 549-553.

Elist, J. "Effects of Pollen Extract Preparation Prostat/Poltit on Lower Urinary Tract Symptoms in Patients with Chronic Nonbacterial Prostatitis/Chronic Pelvic Pain Syndrome." *Urology* 67 (2006): 60-63.

Kaplan, S. A., M. A. Volpe, and A. E. Te. "A Prospective, One-Year Trial Using Saw Palmetto Versus Finasteride in the Treatment of Category III Prostatitis/Chronic Pelvic Pain Syndrome." *Journal of Urology* 171 (2004): 284-288.

Lee, S. W., et al. "Acupuncture Versus Sham Acupuncture for Chronic Prostatitis/Chronic Pelvic Pain." *American Journal of Medicine* 121 (2008): 79.

See also: Bladder infection; Infertility, male; Men's health; Pain management.

Protease inhibitors

CATEGORY: Drug interactions
DEFINITION: Drugs used to treat or prevent infection by viruses, including the human immunodeficiency virus (HIV) and the hepatitis C virus.
INTERACTIONS: Garlic, glutamine, grapefruit juice, milk thistle, St. John's wort, vitamin C
DRUGS IN THIS FAMILY: Amprenavir (Agenerase), indinavir (Crixivan), nelfinavir (Viracept), ritonavir (Norvir), saquinavir (Fortovase and Invirase)

GLUTAMINE
Effect: Possible Helpful Interaction

The amino acid glutamine is thought to have protective effects on the digestive tract. One small double-blind study found that the use of glycine at 30 grams daily reduced diarrhea caused by nelfinavir.

ST. JOHN'S WORT
Effect: Dangerous Interaction

St. John's wort has been found to decrease blood levels of the HIV drug indinavir by an average of 57 percent. The reduction is substantial, and it could lead to failure of the drug to keep HIV in check. Similar effects are expected to occur with other protease inhibitors. Furthermore, St. John's wort also appears to interact with another category of drugs used for HIV, reverse transcriptase inhibitors.

Persons who are HIV-positive should not take St. John's wort. Furthermore, a person who has been stabilized on HIV medications (while also taking St. John's wort) should note that if he or she stops taking the herb, blood levels of the drugs could rise, potentially leading to increased side effects.

GRAPEFRUIT JUICE
Effect: Possible Harmful Interaction

Grapefruit juice impairs the body's normal breakdown of several drugs, allowing them to build up to

---

Warning: St. John's Wort

The U.S. Food and Drug Administration issued a public health advisory in 2000 concerning the risk of drug interactions between the herb St. John's wort and the protease inhibitor indinavir and other drugs. That advisory is excerpted here.

The Food and Drug Administration would like to inform you [the public] about results from a study conducted by the National Institutes of Health (NIH) that showed a significant drug interaction between St. John's wort (*Hypericum perforatum*), an herbal product sold as a dietary supplement, and indinavir, a protease inhibitor used to treat HIV [human immunodeficiency virus] infection. In this study, concomitant administration of St. John's wort and indinavir substantially decreased indinavir plasma concentrations, potentially due to induction of the cytochrome P450 metabolic pathway. . . .

At this time, pharmacokinetic data are available only for concomitant administration of indinavir with St. John's wort. However, based on these results, it is expected that St. John's wort may significantly decrease blood concentrations of all of the currently marketed HIV protease inhibitors (PIs) and possibly other drugs (to varying degrees) that are similarly metabolized, including the non-nucleoside reverse transcriptase inhibitors (NNRTIs). Consequently, concomitant use of St. John's wort with PIs or NNRTIs is not recommended because this may result in suboptimal antiretroviral drug concentrations, leading to loss of virologic response and development of resistance or class cross-resistance.

Because herbal products are widely used in the United States and are available in various forms, such as combination products and teas, it is important that health care professionals ask patients about concomitant use of products that could contain St. John's wort (*Hypericum perforatum*).

In addition, FDA is working closely with drug manufacturers to ensure that product labeling of antiretrovirals is revised to highlight the potential for drug interactions with St. John's wort.

---

potentially excessive levels in the blood. Saquinavir mesylate and other protease inhibitors may be affected. One study indicates this effect can last for three days or more after one drinks the juice. If one is taking protease inhibitors, the safest approach to avoid side effects is to avoid grapefruit juice altogether.

VITAMIN C
Effect: Possible Harmful Interaction

One study found that the use of vitamin C at a dose of 1 gram daily significantly reduced levels of indinavir. This was the first report of such an interaction with vitamin C, but the study was well designed and deserves to be taken seriously. People taking any protease inhibitor should avoid taking vitamin C or should have their protease inhibitor levels checked whenever they start (or stop) taking vitamin C.

GARLIC
Effect: Possible Harmful Interaction

The herb garlic is widely used in the belief that it can help prevent heart disease. However, it may not be safe to combine garlic supplements with protease inhibitors.

Two people with HIV reportedly experienced severe gastrointestinal toxicity from the drug ritonavir after taking garlic supplements. Garlic might also reduce the effectiveness of some drugs used for HIV.

MILK THISTLE
Effect: Possible Helpful Interaction

The herb milk thistle is thought to have liver-protective properties, and some people with HIV may take milk thistle in hopes of minimizing liver-related side effects of HIV medications. While there is no evidence that milk thistle provides any benefit in this regard, one study did find that it does not interfere with levels of indinavir.

EBSCO CAM Review Board

FURTHER READING
Huffman, F. G., and M. E. Walgren. "L-glutamine Supplementation Improves Nelfinavir-Associated Diarrhea in HIV-Infected Individuals." *HIV Clinical Trials* 4 (2003): 324-329.

Piscitelli, S. C. "Use of Complementary Medicines by Patients with HIV: Full Sail into Uncharted Waters." *Medscape HIV/AIDS* 6, no. 3 (2000).

Piscitelli, S. C., A. H. Burstein, D. Chaitt, et al. "Indinavir Concentrations and St. John's Wort." *The Lancet* 355 (2000): 547-548.

Piscitelli, S. C., A. H. Burstein, N. Welden, et al. "The Effect of Garlic Supplements on the Pharmacokinetics of Saquinavir." *Clinical Infectious Diseases* 34 (2002): 234-238.

Takanaga, H., et al. "Relationship Between Time After Intake of Grapefruit Juice and the Effect on Pharmacokinetics and Pharmacodynamics of Nisoldipine in Healthy Subjects." *Clinical Pharmacology and Therapeutics* 67 (2000): 201-214.

See also: Angiotensin-converting enzyme (ACE) inhibitors; Food and Drug Administration; Garlic; Glutamine; HIV/AIDS support; Milk thistle; St. John's wort; Reverse transcriptase inhibitors; Vitamin C.

Proteolytic enzymes

CATEGORY: Herbs and supplements

RELATED TERMS: Bromelain, chymotrypsin, digestive enzymes, pancreatin, papain, serrapeptase, trypsin

DEFINITION: Natural substance of the human body and of plants used as a supplement to treat specific health conditions.

PRINCIPAL PROPOSED USES: Dyspepsia, neck pain and other forms of chronic musculoskeletal pain, osteoarthritis, pancreatic insufficiency, shingles (herpes zoster), sports injuries, surgery support

OTHER PROPOSED USES: Breast engorgement, food allergies, reducing side effects of radiation therapy for cancer, rheumatoid arthritis, sports and fitness support and recovery

OVERVIEW

Proteolytic enzymes (proteases) help the body digest the proteins in food. Although the body produces these enzymes in the pancreas, certain foods also contain proteolytic enzymes. Papaya and pineapple are two of the richest plant sources, as attested by their traditional use as natural tenderizers for meat. Papain and bromelain are the names for the proteolytic enzymes found in these fruits. The enzymes made in the human body are called trypsin and chymotrypsin.

The primary use of proteolytic enzymes is as a digestive aid for people who have trouble digesting proteins. However, proteolytic enzymes may also be absorbed internally to some extent and may reduce pain and inflammation.

REQUIREMENTS AND SOURCES

People do not need to get proteolytic enzymes from food, because the body manufactures them (primarily trypsin and chymotrypsin). However, deficiencies in proteolytic enzymes do occur, usually resulting from diseases of the pancreas (pancreatic insufficiency). Symptoms include abdominal discomfort, gas, indigestion, poor absorption of nutrients, and passing undigested food in the stool.

For use as a supplement, trypsin and chymotrypsin are extracted from the pancreas of various animals. Bromelain extracted from pineapple stems and papain made from papayas can also be purchased.

THERAPEUTIC DOSAGES

The amount of an enzyme is expressed not only in grams or milligrams but also in activity units or international units. These terms refer to the enzyme's potency (specifically, its digestive power). Recommended dosages of proteolytic enzymes vary with the form used. Because of the wide variation, label instructions regarding dosage should be followed.

Proteolytic enzymes can be broken down by stomach acid. To prevent this from happening, supplemental enzymes are often coated with a substance that does not dissolve until it reaches the intestine. Such a preparation is called enteric-coated.

THERAPEUTIC USES

The most obvious use of proteolytic enzymes is to assist digestion. However, a small double-blind, placebo-controlled trial found no benefit from proteolytic enzymes as a treatment for dyspepsia (indigestion).

Proteolytic enzymes can also be absorbed into the body whole and may help reduce inflammation and pain; however, the evidence is inconsistent. Several studies found that proteolytic enzymes might be helpful for neck pain, osteoarthritis, and post-herpetic neuralgia (an aftereffect of shingles). However, all of these studies suffer from significant limitations (such as the absence of a placebo group), and none provide substantially reliable information.

Studies performed decades ago suggest that proteolytic enzymes may help reduce the pain and discomfort that follow injuries (especially sports injuries). However, a more recent, better-designed, and far larger study failed to find any benefit. Proteolytic enzymes have also been evaluated as an aid to recovery from the pain and inflammation caused by surgery, but most studies are decades old, and in any case, the results were mixed.

A double-blind, placebo-controlled trial published in the 1960s found that use of proteolytic enzymes helped reduce the discomfort of breast engorgement in lactating women. A study tested bromelain for enhancing recovery from heavy exercise by decreasing delayed-onset muscle soreness, but it found no benefits. Another study, this one using a mixed proteolytic enzyme supplement, also failed to find any benefits. Two studies failed to find proteolytic enzymes helpful for reducing side effects of radiation therapy for cancer.

Some alternative medicine practitioners believe that proteolytic enzymes may help reduce symptoms of food allergies, presumably by digesting the food so well that there is less to be allergic to; however, there is no scientific evidence for this proposed use.

Another theory popular in certain alternative medicine circles suggests that proteolytic enzymes can aid rheumatoid arthritis, multiple sclerosis, lupus, and other autoimmune diseases. Supposedly, these diseases are made worse when whole proteins from foods leak into the blood and cause immune reactions. Digestive enzymes are said to help foil this so-called leaky gut problem. Again, however, there is no meaningful evidence to substantiate this theory. Furthermore, one fairly large (301-participant) study failed to find proteolytic enzymes helpful for multiple sclerosis.

SCIENTIFIC EVIDENCE

Most of the studies described in this section used combination products containing various proteolytic enzymes plus other substances, such as the bioflavonoid rutin.

Papain

The papaya (also called papaw, pawpaw, mamao, or tree melon) is the source of one of nature's own digestive aids: papain. The papaya is believed to have originated in southern Mexico, Central America, or the West Indies but is now grown in tropical and subtropical areas around the world. It is a pear-shaped fruit with skin that turns from green to a bright orange-yellow as it ripens.

What Is Papain? Papain is a milky latex that is collected by making incisions in unripe papayas. It is one of a group of proteolytic enzymes found in papayas, pineapples, and certain other plants. Proteolytic enzymes help you digest the proteins in food. Papaya and pineapple stems are two of the richest plant sources of proteolytic enzymes.

Where Does Papain Come From? Papain comes from the papaya, a tropical fruit that is about six inches long and can range from 1 to 20 pounds in weight, depending on the variety. Inside, the papaya has silky smooth, orange-yellow flesh and a large center cavity full of shiny grayish-black seeds. The flesh is juicy and has a subtle, sweet-tart or musky taste, somewhat like a cantaloupe.

Papaya is now widely cultivated in tropical and subtropical countries. There are about forty-five species of papaya. The most common variety in the United States is the Solo papaya, which is grown in Hawaii and Florida. Mexican papayas are much larger than the Hawaiian types and may be more than 15 inches long.

To extract papain latex from a papaya, the skin of an unripe papaya is cut. After the latex is collected, it is dried either by the sun or in ovens and sold in powdered form.

What Is Papain Used For? The primary use of papain is as a meat tenderizer. It also has been used as a digestive aid for people who have trouble digesting proteins. However, a small double-blind, placebo-controlled trial found no benefit from proteolytic enzymes as a treatment for dyspepsia (indigestion).

There is weak evidence to suggest that papain, taken with other enzymes, might improve the rate of recovery from various types of injuries and might reduce the chronic pain and discomfort of such conditions as neck pain and osteoarthritis. Proteolytic enzymes have also had mixed results as an aid to recovery from surgery and as a treatment for shingles.

Many practitioners of alternative medicine believe that papain may be helpful for food allergies and autoimmune diseases. However, there is little to no meaningful evidence supporting the claim that papain actually works for these conditions.

Some Precautions to Consider. In clinical studies, papain and other proteolytic enzymes have been found to be quite safe, though they may occasionally cause digestive upset and allergic reactions. Also, persons taking warfarin, aspirin, or other drugs that thin the blood should not take proteolytic enzymes without first consulting a doctor.

Elizabeth A. Peterson, M.F.A.

Chronic musculoskeletal pain. Several studies provide preliminary evidence that proteolytic enzymes might be helpful for various forms of chronic pain, including neck pain and osteoarthritis. A double-blind, placebo-controlled trial of thirty people with chronic neck pain found that use of a proteolytic enzyme mixture modestly reduced pain symptoms compared with a placebo.

Osteoarthritis. Studies enrolling a total of more than four hundred people compared proteolytic enzymes to the standard anti-inflammatory drug diclofenac for the treatment of osteoarthritis-related conditions of the shoulder, back, or knee. The results generally showed that the supplement had benefits equivalent to those of the medication. However, all of these studies suffered from various flaws that limit their reliability; the most important flaw was the absence of a placebo group.

Shingles (herpes zoster). Shingles is an acute, painful infection caused by the varicella-zoster virus, the organism that causes chickenpox. Proteolytic enzymes have been suggested as treatment. However, there is little evidence to support their use. A double-blind study of 190 people with shingles compared proteolytic enzymes to the standard antiviral drug acyclovir. Participants were treated for fourteen days and their pain was assessed at intervals. Although both groups had similar pain relief, the enzyme-treated group experienced fewer side effects. However, since acyclovir offers minimal benefit at most, these results do not mean very much. Similar results were seen in another double-blind study in which 90 people were given an injection of either acyclovir or enzymes, followed by a course of oral medication for seven days.

Sports injuries. Several small studies have found proteolytic enzyme combinations helpful for the treatment of sports injuries. However, the best and largest trial by far failed to find benefit. A double-blind, placebo-controlled study of 44 people with sports-related ankle injuries found that treatment with proteolytic enzymes resulted in faster healing and reduced the time away from training by about 50 percent. Based on these results, a very large (721-participant), double-blind, placebo-controlled trial of people with sprained ankles was undertaken. This study failed to find benefit with rutin, bromelain, or trypsin, separately or in combination.

Three other small double-blind studies, involving a total of about eighty athletes, found that treatment with proteolytic enzymes significantly speeded healing of bruises and other mild athletic injuries, compared with placebo. In another double-blind trial, one hundred people were given an injection of their own blood under the skin to simulate bruising following an injury. Researchers found that treatment with a proteolytic enzyme combination significantly speeded up recovery. In addition, a double-blind, placebo-controlled trial of seventy-one people with finger fractures found that treatment with proteolytic enzymes significantly improved recovery. However, these studies were performed decades ago and are not quite up to modern standards.

Surgery. Numerous studies have evaluated various proteolytic enzymes as an aid to recovery from surgery, but the results have been mixed. Again, most of these studies are not up to modern standards. A double-blind, placebo-controlled trial of eighty people undergoing knee surgery found that treatment with mixed proteolytic enzymes after surgery significantly improved rate of recovery, as measured by mobility and swelling.

Another double-blind, placebo-controlled trial evaluated the effects of a similar mixed proteolytic enzyme product in eighty individuals undergoing oral surgery. The results showed reduced pain, inflammation, and swelling in the treated group compared with the placebo group. Benefits were also seen in another trial of mixed proteolytic enzymes for dental surgery, as well as in one study involving only bromelain.

A double-blind, placebo-controlled study of 204 women receiving episiotomies during childbirth found evidence that a mixed proteolytic enzyme product can reduce inflammation. Bromelain was also found helpful for reducing inflammation following episiotomy in one double-blind, placebo-controlled trial of 160 women, but a very similar study found no benefit.

Other double-blind, placebo-controlled studies have found that bromelain reduces inflammation and pain following nasal surgery, cataract removal, and foot surgery. However, a study of 154 individuals undergoing facial plastic surgery found no benefit.

A small double-blind, placebo-controlled trial of twenty-four people having surgical extraction of third molars found that serrapeptase given during the procedure reduced postoperative pain and swelling (significant differences on days two, three, and seven).

SAFETY ISSUES

In studies, proteolytic enzymes are believed to have proven to be quite safe, although they can occasionally cause digestive upset and allergic reactions. One proteolytic enzyme, pancreatin, may interfere with folate absorption. In addition, the proteolytic enzyme papain might increase the blood-thinning effects of warfarin and possibly other anticoagulants. The proteolytic enzyme bromelain might also cause problems if combined with drugs that thin the blood. In addition, there are concerns that bromelain should not be mixed with sedative drugs. Finally, bromelain may increase blood concentrations of certain antibiotics.

IMPORTANT INTERACTIONS

People taking the proteolytic enzyme pancreatin may need extra folate. People taking warfarin (Coumadin), aspirin, or other drugs that thin the blood should not take the proteolytic enzymes papain or bromelain except under a doctor's supervision. Those taking sedative drugs should not take bromelain, except under a physician's supervision.

EBSCO CAM Review Board

FURTHER READING

Akhtar, N. M., et al. "Oral Enzyme Combination Versus Diclofenac in the Treatment of Osteoarthritis of the Knee." *Clinical Rheumatology* 23 (2004): 410-415.

Al-Khateeb, T. H., and Y. Nusair. "Effect of the Proteolytic Enzyme Serrapeptase on Swelling, Pain, and Trismus after Surgical Extraction of Mandibular Third Molars." *International Journal of Oral Maxillofacial Surgery* 37 (2008): 264-268.

Baumhackl, U., et al. "A Randomized, Double-Blind, Placebo-Controlled Study of Oral Hydrolytic Enzymes in Relapsing Multiple Sclerosis." *Multiple Sclerosis* 11 (2005): 166-168.

Beck, T. W., et al. "Effects of a Protease Supplement on Eccentric Exercise-Induced Markers of Delayed-Onset Muscle Soreness and Muscle Damage." *Journal of Strength and Conditioning Research* 21 (2007): 661-667.

Kerkhoffs, G. M., et al. "A Double-Blind, Randomised, Parallel Group Study on the Efficacy and Safety of Treating Acute Lateral Ankle Sprain with Oral Hydrolytic Enzymes." *British Journal of Sports Medicine* 38 (2004): 431-435.

Klein, G., et al. "Efficacy and Tolerance of an Oral Enzyme Combination in Painful Osteoarthritis of the Hip: A Double-Blind, Randomised Study Comparing Oral Enzymes with Non-steroidal Anti-inflammatory Drugs." *Clinical and Experimental Rheumatology* 24 (2006): 25-30.

See also: Bromelain; Herbal medicine; Osteoarthritis; Shingles.

Proton pump inhibitors

CATEGORY: Drug interactions
DEFINITION: Drugs used to reduce levels of stomach acid.
INTERACTIONS: Folate, minerals, St. John's wort, vitamin B_{12}
DRUGS IN THIS FAMILY: Lansoprazole (Prevacid), omeprazole (Prilosec)

ST. JOHN'S WORT

Effect: Possible Harmful Interactions

The herb St. John's wort is known to interact with numerous drugs. There are two potential harmful interactions between St. John's wort and proton pump inhibitors.

One study found that the use of St. John's wort greatly decreases levels of omeprazole (such as Prilosec) in the body. This would be expected to lead to markedly reduced efficacy.

The other potential risk is more theoretical. When taken to excess, the herb St. John's wort can cause an increased risk of sunburn. Some evidence hints that proton pump inhibitors might increase this risk.

VITAMIN B_{12}

Effect: Supplementation Likely Helpful

Vitamin B_{12} deficiency is a concern with the use of all drugs that reduce stomach acidity. In food, vitamin B_{12} is always accompanied by proteins, and it must be separated from them before it can begin to be absorbed. Following separation, B_{12} is then attached to a substance called intrinsic factor, which allows B_{12} to be absorbed in the intestines.

Stomach acid plays a role in this separation. If one does not have enough stomach acid, the process of freeing vitamin B_{12} from protein so that it can be bound to intrinsic factor may be impaired.

Studies suggest that treatment with proton pump inhibitors might significantly reduce the absorption of vitamin B_{12}. There is some evidence that cranberry juice might increase B_{12} absorption in persons taking proton pump inhibitors, possibly because the juice is somewhat acidic.

FOLATE
Effect: Supplementation Possibly Helpful

Research on related medications suggests that proton pump inhibitors may slightly reduce the body's absorption of folate. The decrease in folate absorption should be quite small, but because folate deficiency is quite common and potentially harmful, taking extra folate might make sense as insurance.

MINERALS
Effect: Supplementation Possibly Helpful

By reducing stomach acid levels, proton pump inhibitors might interfere with the absorption of iron, zinc, and perhaps other minerals. Taking mineral supplements to meet the U.S. Dietary Reference Intake (formerly known as the Recommended Dietary Allowance) levels for these nutrients should help.

EBSCO CAM Review Board

FURTHER READING
Aymard, J. P., et al. "Haematological Adverse Effects of Histamine H2-Receptor Antagonists." *Medical Toxicology and Adverse Drug Experience* 3 (1988): 430-448.

Mirossay, A., et al. "Potentiation of Hypericin and Hypocrellin-Induced Phototoxicity by Omeprazole." *Phytomedicine* 6 (1999): 311-317.

Wang, L. S., et al. "St. John's Wort Induces Both Cytochrome P450 3a4-Catalyzed Sulfoxidation and 2c19-Dependent Hydroxylation of Omeprazole." *Clinical Pharmacology and Therapeutics* 75 (2004): 191-197.

See also: Betaine hydrochloride; Cranberry; Folate; Food and Drug Administration; Gastrointestinal health; Iron; St. John's wort; Supplements: Introduction; Ulcers; Vitamin B_{12}; Vitamins and minerals; Zinc.

Pseudoscience

CATEGORY: Issues and overviews
RELATED TERMS: Ad hoc hypotheses, anecdotal evidence, burden of proof, confirmation, mantra of holism, refutation
DEFINITION: Discussion of key warning signs of pseudoscience in CAM

OVERVIEW
Pseudoscience exhibits the superficial appearance of science but lacks its substance. In the case of complementary and alternative medicine (CAM), pseudoscientific procedures appear to play by the rules of science but in fact do not. Pseudoscientific procedures rarely possess the crucial safeguards against confirmation bias that characterize the mature sciences. Instead they exhibit the tendency to seek evidence consistent with hypotheses and to deny, dismiss, and distort evidence that is not. As a consequence, pseudoscience leaves itself vulnerable to errors.

The distinction between science and pseudoscience is not absolute or clear-cut; some sciences engage in pseudoscientific practices, and vice versa. Nevertheless, as philosopher of science Mario Bunge and others have observed, numerous indicators, or warning signs, of pseudoscience can be pinpointed. It should be noted that these indicators do not prove the presence of a pseudoscience, but the more such indicators accompany a discipline, the more skeptical one should be of that discipline. In particular, there are ten warning signs of pseudoscience, all of which are relevant to certain CAM practices.

KEY WARNING SIGNS
Overuse of ad hoc hypotheses. An ad hoc hypothesis is an escape hatch or loophole that allows proponents of claims to discount negative results. Although developed sciences sometimes make use of ad hoc hypotheses, pseudosciences routinely invoke them as ploys to immunize their claims from refutation. For example, a proponent of a new form of meditation found to be ineffective in ten independent studies might maintain that all of these investigations were flawed because they were not conducted by the technique's developer, who is the only person qualified to perform them.

Absence of self-correction. Sciences tend to change over time in response to new data; pseudosciences rarely do. For example, despite extensive scientific data showing that an herbal remedy is ineffective for severe depression, a practitioner might continue to insist that the treatment should be prescribed for this condition.

Focus on confirmation rather than refutation. As philosopher of science Karl Popper observed, science progresses most efficiently when investigators strive to disprove their claims rather than to prove them. In contrast, pseudosciences tend to focus on confirming rather than disconfirming instances. For example, when confronted with evidence that an initial positive finding could not be replicated in five other investigations, a proponent of using acupuncture to treat diabetes might focus exclusively on the positive result, and ignore the replication failures.

Reversed burden of proof. In science, the onus of proof lies with the proponent of a claim, not with skeptics. In contrast, pseudosciences tend to place the burden of proof on skeptics rather than on proponents. For example, an advocate of using shark cartilage to treat cancer might insist that critics have not proven conclusively that shark cartilage is ineffective. In science, it is up to the advocate to show that shark cartilage works, not up to the critic to show that it does not.

Evasion of peer review. Sciences rely on a procedure called peer review, in which journal manuscripts reporting original findings are sent to several independent scholars to evaluate the merits of the studies. Many, or most, manuscripts submitted to premier journals are rejected for publication; others are accepted only after multiple rounds of substantial revision. Although peer review is not a perfect process, it weeds out many errors in researchers' methodology or conclusions. Some pseudoscientific CAM procedures circumvent the peer review process, thereby bypassing one of the key safeguards of science. For example, many advocates of energy therapies for anxiety disorders have advanced claims that have not been subjected to independent scrutiny by other scholars.

Mantra of holism. Many pseudosciences invoke the mantra of holism; that is, they argue that a claim cannot be tested in isolation and must be tested only in the context of all other claims. Holism is invoked to insulate assertions against refutation. For example, a believer in naturopathy might insist that a study showing that naturopathy is ineffective be dismissed because persons who use naturopathy almost always do so along with other treatments.

Over-reliance on anecdotal evidence. A familiar saying in science is that "the plural of anecdote is not fact." Anecdotes, which usually take the form of "I know a person who" stories, can be helpful in science, especially when they suggest fruitful hypotheses that can later be tested in rigorous investigations. However, anecdotes rarely, if ever, justify a definitive claim that a CAM technique works. For example, a practitioner who asserts that homeopathy must be effective because he or she has witnessed several persons "get better after receiving homeopathic remedies" is operating in a pseudoscientific fashion.

Absence of boundary conditions. Pace University psychologist Terence Hines noted that almost all scientific procedures possess boundary conditions: limitations on when the technique works and when it does not work. In contrast, pseudoscientific treatments frequently lack boundary conditions. Their proponents often maintain that they are effective for virtually every condition and every person. For example, an advocate of chiropractic might contend that this method is effective not only for back problems but also for cancer, multiple sclerosis, diabetes, and schizophrenia.

Use of scientific-sounding language. Many pseudosciences utilize scientific-sounding terms to create an aura of legitimacy. In doing so, however, they often use these terms incorrectly. For example, in explaining how their methods seem to work, they may refer to "quantum fields," "neural networks," or "complexity theory" yet also may strip these terms of much of their accurate meaning.

Absence of connectivity. In science, new ideas tend to build on, or connect with, earlier ideas. In contrast, many pseudosciences purport to construct entirely new paradigms from whole cloth. For example, the developer of a new magnet therapy might insist that his treatment relies on entirely undiscovered electromagnetic principles.

CONCLUSION

These ten warning signs of pseudoscience are not exhaustive. Social work researchers Bruce Thyer and Monica Pignotti have identified other features of pseudoscience, including a tendency to make extraordinary claims that go far beyond scientific evidence (such as claims of miracle cures), insistence that a technique is being unfairly suppressed by establishment scientists, and requirements that practitioners of the technique agree to vows of secrecy. In all cases, pseudosciences purport to be something they are not. Therefore, consumers should be wary of CAM procedures that display any of the warning signs presented here.

Scott O. Lilienfeld, Ph.D.

FURTHER READING

Bausell, R. Barker. *Snake Oil Science: The Truth About Complementary and Alternative Medicine.* New York: Oxford University Press, 2007. A critical examination of CAM practices, with particular emphasis on factors that can lead physicians, consumers, and others to be fooled by techniques that claim effectiveness.

Bunge, Mario. "What Is Pseudoscience?" *Skeptical Inquirer* 9 (1984): 36-46. A scholarly examination of the core characteristics of pseudoscience and how it differs from common definitions of science.

Lilienfeld, Scott O., Steven J. Lynn, and Jeffrey M. Lohr, eds. *Science and Pseudoscience in Clinical Psychology.* New York: Guilford Press, 2003. A comprehensive examination of the problem of pseudoscience in mental health treatment, along with discussions of the criteria for pseudoscience.

See also: Clinical trials; Double-blind, placebo-controlled studies; Placebo effect; Popular practitioners of CAM; Regulation of CAM; Scientific method.

Psoriasis

CATEGORY: Condition

DEFINITION: Treatment of a skin condition that leads to an intensely itchy rash with clearly defined borders and scales.

PRINCIPAL PROPOSED NATURAL TREATMENT: Oregon grape

OTHER PROPOSED NATURAL TREATMENTS: Acupuncture, aloe vera cream, balneotherapy (spa therapy), capsaicin cream, cetylated fatty acids, fish oil, folate (to reduce side effects of methotrexate), fumaric acid, hypnotherapy, seal oil, vitamin A, vitamin D

INTRODUCTION

Up to 2 percent of Americans have psoriasis, a skin condition that leads to an intensely itchy rash with clearly defined borders and scales that resemble silvery mica. The fingernails are also frequently involved, showing pitting or thickening.

Medical treatment for psoriasis includes applications of topical steroids and peeling agents that expose the underlying skin for the steroid to contact. Ultraviolet light can also be used, sometimes combined with coal tar applications or medications called psoralens. Synthetic relatives of vitamins A and D are also used.

PRINCIPAL PROPOSED NATURAL TREATMENTS

Oregon grape. Evidence from two double-blind, placebo-controlled trials and one comparative trial suggests that cream made from the herb Oregon grape (*Mahonia*) may help reduce symptoms of psoriasis, although it does not seem to be as effective as standard medications. In a double-blind study published in 2006, two hundred people were given either a cream containing 10 percent Oregon grape extract or placebo twice a day for three months. The results indicate that those using Oregon grape experienced greater benefits than those in the placebo group, and the difference was statistically significant. The treatment was well tolerated, although it caused a rash or a burning sensation in a few people.

Benefits were also seen in a double-blind, placebo-controlled study of eighty-two people with psoriasis. However, the study design had a significant flaw: The treatment salve was darker in color than the placebo, possibly allowing participants to guess which was which.

Another study found that dithranol, a conventional drug used to treat psoriasis symptoms, was more effective than Oregon grape. The authors failed to state whether this study was double-blind. Forty-nine participants applied one treatment to their left side and the other to their right for four weeks. Skin biopsies were then analyzed and compared with samples taken at the beginning of the study. The physicians evaluating changes in skin tissue were unaware what treatments had been used on the samples. Greater improvements were seen in the dithranol group.

A large open study in which 443 participants with psoriasis used Oregon grape topically for twelve weeks

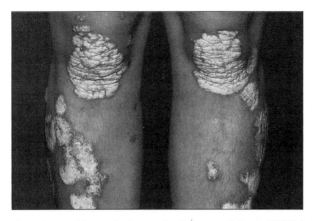

A patient with psoriasis on the knees and legs. (BSIP/ Photo Researchers, Inc.)

found the herb to be helpful for 73.7 percent of the group. Without a placebo group, it is not possible to know whether Oregon grape was truly responsible for the improvement seen, but the trial does help to establish the herb's safety and tolerability. Laboratory research suggests Oregon grape has some effects at the cellular level that might be helpful in psoriasis, such as slowing the rate of abnormal cell growth and reducing inflammation.

OTHER PROPOSED NATURAL TREATMENTS

Aloe vera. Aloe vera cream may be helpful for psoriasis, according to a double-blind study performed in Pakistan that enrolled sixty men and women with mild to moderate symptoms of psoriasis. Participants were treated with either topical aloe vera extract (0.5 percent) or a placebo cream, applied three times daily for four weeks. Aloe treatment produced significantly better results than placebo, and these results were said to endure for almost one year after treatment was stopped. The study authors also reported a high level of complete "cure," but what exactly they meant by this was not reported clearly. A follow-up study of forty people that attempted to replicate these results failed to find aloe more effective than placebo.

Capsaicin. Capsaicin is the "hot" in cayenne pepper. Creams made from capsaicin are used to treat a number of pain-related conditions. Some evidence indicates that capsaicin cream may also be helpful for psoriasis. A double-blind, placebo-controlled trial of almost two hundred people found that the use of topical capsaicin can improve itching and the overall se-

verity of psoriasis. Benefits were also seen in a smaller double-blind trial.

Fish oil. The evidence regarding fish oil's effectiveness for psoriasis remains incomplete and contradictory. An eight-week double-blind study followed twenty-eight people with chronic psoriasis. One-half received ten capsules of fish oil daily, and one-half received a placebo. By the end of the study, researchers saw significant improvement in itching, redness, and scaling, but not in the size of the psoriasis patches. However, another double-blind study followed 145 people with moderate to severe psoriasis for four months and found no benefit compared with placebo.

Other natural treatments. Based on preliminary evidence, shark cartilage and cetylated fatty acids have also been proposed for treatment of psoriasis. Beta-carotene, barberry, burdock, chromium, cleavers, *Coleus forskohlii*, goldenseal, topical licorice cream, milk thistle, red clover, selenium, taurine, vitamin E, yellow dock, and zinc are also sometimes mentioned as possible treatments for psoriasis. However, there is no meaningful evidence that they work.

A somewhat toxic natural substance called fumaric acid is sometimes recommended for psoriasis. Vitamin A or special forms of vitamin D taken at high levels may improve symptoms, but these are dangerous treatments that should be used only under the supervision of a physician.

People using the drug methotrexate for psoriasis frequently develop nausea, mouth sores, and other side effects. Evidence indicates that taking folate supplements may help.

Seal oil has shown some promise for the treatment of psoriatic arthritis (a type of joint pain and inflammation that can occur in association with psoriasis). Another study found that hypnosis may improve psoriasis symptoms. Balneotherapy (spa therapy) might also have value.

Although case reports suggest that acupuncture might be useful for psoriasis, a controlled trial failed to find acupuncture more effective than fake acupuncture. Another small study suggested that the Chinese herbal decoction Qinzhu Liangxue may be helpful in selected persons with psoriasis, though this finding is highly preliminary.

HERBS AND SUPPLEMENTS TO USE WITH CAUTION

Various herbs and supplements may interact adversely with drugs used to treat psoriasis, so persons considering the use of herbs and supplements should first consult a physician.

EBSCO CAM Review Board

FURTHER READING

Bernstein, S., et al. "Treatment of Mild to Moderate Psoriasis with Relieva, a *Mahonia aquifolium* Extract." *American Journal of Therapeutics* 13 (2006): 121-126.

Dawe, R. S., et al. "A Randomized Controlled Comparison of the Efficacy of Dead Sea Salt Balneophototherapy vs. Narrowband Ultraviolet B Monotherapy for Chronic Plaque Psoriasis." *British Journal of Dermatology* 153 (2005): 613-619.

Gambichler, T., N. S. Tomi, and A. Kreuter. "Controlled Clinical Trials on Balneophototherapy in Psoriasis." *British Journal of Dermatology* 154 (2006): 802-803.

Madland, T. M., et al. "Subjective Improvement in Patients with Psoriatic Arthritis After Short-Term Oral Treatment with Seal Oil: A Pilot Study with Double Blind Comparison to Soy Oil." *Journal of Rheumatology* 33 (2006): 307-310.

Paulsen, E., et al. "A Double-Blind, Placebo-Controlled Study of a Commercial Aloe Vera Gel in the Treatment of Slight to Moderate Psoriasis Vulgaris." *Journal of the European Academy of Dermatology and Venereology* 19 (2005): 326-331.

See also: Aloe; Cayenne; Fish oil; Oregon grape.

Pulse diagnosis

CATEGORY: Therapies and techniques

RELATED TERM: *Mai*

DEFINITION: A technique used in Asian acupuncture and herbal medicine to assess a person's state of health.

PRINCIPAL PROPOSED USES: Disease etiology, nature, and prognosis

OTHER PROPOSED USE: Ensuring proper insertion of acupuncture needles

OVERVIEW

The pulse represents the arterial palpation of the heartbeat by trained fingertips. A pulse is taken at a site on the body that allows an artery to be compressed against a bone, such as at the neck (carotid artery), at the wrist (radial artery), and at the inside of the elbow (brachial artery).

In modern medicine, a human pulse is a convenient tactile method to determine systolic blood pressure. Stethoscope and blood-pressure-cuff measurements reveal a person's pulse rate and possible irregularities in the heart. In contrast to pulse diagnosis in complementary and alternative medicine (CAM), pulse diagnosis in Western medicine is used to determine conditions of the heart and major vessels only; it is not used to determine a person's overall state of health.

MECHANISM OF ACTION

In Chinese medicine, the pulse determines if a syndrome is hot or cold in nature or is caused by an excess or deficiency, and it determines which of the humors (qi, moisture, blood) and which organ systems are affected. The strengths and weaknesses and the different qualities and speed of the pulse are used to assess a person diagnostically. Chinese medical diagnosis generally uses the wrist pulse, looking at six different pulses in each wrist, each corresponding to specific organs of the body.

The Chinese method of taking the pulse is based on touching the wrist with three levels of pressure: superficial palpation (almost no pressure; detects bounding of the pulse up to the skin surface), intermediate palpation (light pressure; reveals basic pulse forms), and deep palpation (firm pressure; indicates how the pulse can emerge from the physical constraint).

USES AND APPLICATIONS

Although practitioners trained in pulse diagnosis can discover much about a person by using this method alone, pulse diagnosis is generally used in conjunction with other diagnostic methods.

SCIENTIFIC EVIDENCE

Investigations of pulse diagnosis indicate that certain features, such as pulse speed, are objective and repeatable. However, other features range in level of reliability. Rigorous, double-blind studies of pulse diagnosis are difficult to conduct because diagnostic variables and disease subcategories are often subjective. There are ongoing attempts to more clearly define pulse forms and make pulse diagnosis objective (for example, by developing medical equipment that can detect and record pulse forms and by developing statistical analyses of pulse types by disease).

CHOOSING A PRACTITIONER

A medical doctor's taking of a person's pulse is not equivalent to pulse diagnosis in CAM. Pulse diagnosis in CAM is performed by practitioners in traditional Asian medicine. One should choose a practitioner who is certified by the National Certification Commission for Acupuncture and Oriental Medicine and who is licensed by the state in which he or she practices.

SAFETY ISSUES

Pulse diagnosis is noninvasive and has no known side effects.

Anita P. Kuan, Ph.D.

FURTHER READING

Dharmananda, Subhuti. "The Significance of Traditional Pulse Diagnosis in the Modern Practice of Chinese Medicine" (2000). Available at http://www.itmonline.org/arts/pulse.htm.

National Center for Complementary and Alternative Medicine. http://www.nccam.nih.gov/health/whatiscam/chinesemed.htm.

Walsh, Sean, and Emma King. *Pulse Diagnosis: A Clinical Guide.* New York: Churchill Livingstone/Elsevier, 2007.

Wiseman, Nigel, and Andy Ellis. *Fundamentals of Chinese Medicine: Zhong Yi Xue Ji Chu.* Rev. ed. Brookline, Mass.: Paradigm, 1997.

See also: Acupuncture; Ayurveda; Hara diagnosis; Herbal medicine; Traditional Chinese herbal medicine; Traditional healing; Tongue diagnosis.

Pumpkin seed

CATEGORY: Functional foods
RELATED TERMS: *Cucurbita maxima, C. pepo*
DEFINITION: Natural food product promoted as a dietary supplement for specific health benefits.
PRINCIPAL PROPOSED USE: Benign prostatic hyperplasia
OTHER PROPOSED USES: Kidney stones, parasites

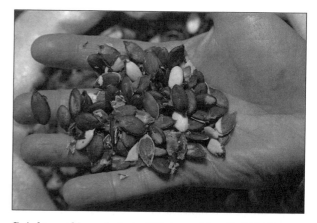

Dried pumpkin seeds that will be pressed for oil. (AP Photo)

OVERVIEW

The familiar Halloween pumpkin is a member of the squash family, native to North and Central America. The seeds of the pumpkin were used medicinally in Native American medicine, primarily for the treatment of kidney, bladder, and digestive problems. From 1863 to 1936, the United States Pharmacopoeia listed pumpkin seeds as a treatment for intestinal parasites.

USES AND APPLICATIONS

Pumpkin seed oil has become popular today as a treatment for prostate enlargement (benign prostatic hyperplasia, or BPH), and it was approved for this use in 1985 by Germany's Commission E. However, there is no meaningful evidence that pumpkin seed is helpful for this condition. Only double-blind, placebo-controlled studies can prove a treatment effective, and none have been reported for pumpkin seed oil alone. However, two such studies evaluated a combination product containing pumpkin seed oil and the herb saw palmetto.

These studies did suggest benefit with the combination product, but because saw palmetto is thought to be effective for BPH, it is not clear whether pumpkin seed oil made any additional contribution. The only reported study on pumpkin seed oil alone lacked a placebo group, and for this reason its results prove little. (BPH is a condition that responds greatly to the power of suggestion, so it could have been assumed, even before conducting this trial, that people given pumpkin seed oil would show improvement.)

In highly preliminary research, pumpkin seed or its constituent cucurbitin has shown some activity against intestinal parasites. These studies, however, can only be regarded as preliminary investigations of a traditional use; they were not designed in such a way that they could prove effectiveness.

Two studies performed in Thailand hint that pumpkin seed snacks might help prevent kidney stones among children at high risk for developing them. However, this research looked only at chemical changes in the urine suggestive of a possible preventive effect, not at actual reduction of stones. Furthermore, the design of the studies did not reach modern standards.

DOSAGE

In studies, the dose of pumpkin seed oil used for the treatment of BPH was 160 milligrams three times daily. For the prevention of kidney stones, the dose of pumpkin seed snack tried was 5 to 10 grams per day.

SAFETY ISSUES

As a widely eaten food, pumpkin seeds are presumed to be safe (though there have been cases in which incompletely chewed seeds have lodged in the esophagus). There are no known or suspected safety risks with pumpkin seed oil.

EBSCO CAM Review Board

FURTHER READING

Caili, F., S. Huan, and L. Quanhong. "A Review on Pharmacological Activities and Utilization Technologies of Pumpkin." *Plant Foods for Human Nutrition* 61 (2006): 73-80.

Naghii, M. R., and M. Mofid. "Impact of Daily Consumption of Iron Fortified Ready-to-eat Cereal and Pumpkin Seed Kernels (*Cucurbita pepo*) on Serum Iron in Adult Women." *Biofactors* 30 (2007): 19-26.

Suphiphat, V., et al. "The Effect of Pumpkin Seeds Snack on Inhibitors and Promoters of Urolithiasis in Thai Adolescents." *Journal of the Medical Association of Thailand* 76 (1993): 487-493.

See also: Benign prostatic hyperplasia; Functional foods: Introduction; Kidney stones; Prostatitis.

Pygeum

CATEGORY: Herbs and supplements
RELATED TERM: *Pygeum africanus*
DEFINITION: Natural plant product used to treat specific health conditions.
PRINCIPAL PROPOSED USE: Benign prostatic hyperplasia
OTHER PROPOSED USES: Impotence, male infertility, prostatitis

OVERVIEW

The pygeum tree is a tall evergreen native to central and southern Africa. Its bark has been used since ancient times to treat problems with urination.

THERAPEUTIC DOSAGES

The usual dosage of pygeum is 50 milligrams (mg) twice per day (occasionally 100 mg twice daily) of an extract standardized to contain 14 percent triterpenes and 0.5 percent n-docosanol. A dose of 100 mg once daily appears to be as effective as the most common dosage of 50 mg twice daily. There is some reason to believe that pygeum's effectiveness might be enhanced when it is combined with nettle root, another natural treatment for BPH.

THERAPEUTIC USES

Pygeum is primarily used as a treatment for benign prostatic hyperplasia (BPH), or prostate enlargement. This use is supported by scientific evidence about as strong as that for the more famous natural BPH remedy, saw palmetto. However, saw palmetto is probably the better treatment to use. The pygeum tree has been so devastated by collection for use in medicine that some regard it as a threatened species. Saw palmetto is cultivated rather than collected in the wild. Besides BPH, pygeum is also sometimes proposed for prostatitis, as well as impotence and male infertility; however, there is little real evidence that it works for these conditions.

SCIENTIFIC EVIDENCE

At least seventeen double blind trials of pygeum for BPH have been performed, involving a total of almost one thousand individuals and ranging in length from forty-five to ninety days. Many of these studies were poorly reported or designed. Nonetheless, overall the results make a meaningful case that pygeum can reduce symptoms such as nighttime urination, urinary frequency, and residual urine volume.

The best of these studies was conducted at eight sites in Europe and included 263 men between fifty and eighty-five years of age. Participants received 50 mg of a pygeum extract or a placebo twice daily. The results showed significant improvements in residual urine volume, voided volume, urinary flow rate, nighttime urination, and daytime frequency.

It is not known how pygeum works. Unlike the standard drug finasteride, it does not appear to work by affecting the conversion of testosterone to dihydrotestosterone. Rather it is thought to reduce inflammation in the prostate and also to inhibit prostate growth factors, substances implicated in inappropriate prostate enlargement.

Safety Issues

Pygeum appears to be essentially nontoxic, both in the short and long term. The most common side effect is mild gastrointestinal distress. However, safety in young children, pregnant or nursing women, and those with severe liver or kidney disease has not been established.

EBSCO CAM Review Board

Further Reading

Bombardelli, E., and P. Morazzoni. "*Prunus africana* (Hook. f.) Kalkm." *Fitoterapia* 68 (1997): 205-218.

Chatelain, C., W. Autet, and F. Brackman. "Comparison of Once and Twice Daily Dosage Forms of *Pygeum africanum* Extract in Patients with Benign Prostatic Hyperplasia: A Randomized, Double-Blind Study, with Long-term Open Label Extension." *Urology* 54 (1999): 473-478.

Wilt, T., et al. "*Pygeum africanum* for Benign Prostatic Hyperplasia." *Cochrane Database of Systemic Reviews* 1 (2002): CD001044.

See also: Benign prostatic hyperplasia; Herbal medicine; Nettle; Saw palmetto.

Pyruvate

Category: Herbs and supplements
Related terms: Calcium pyruvate, dihydroxyace-

tone pyruvate, magnesium pyruvate, potassium pyruvate, sodium pyruvate

Definition: Natural substance of the human body used as a supplement to treat specific health conditions.
Principal proposed use: Weight loss
Other proposed use: Sports performance enhancement

Overview

Pyruvate supplies the body with pyruvic acid, a natural compound that plays important roles in the manufacture and use of energy. Pyruvate supplements have become popular with bodybuilders and other athletes, based on claims that pyruvate can reduce body fat and enhance the body's ability to use energy efficiently. However, at the present time, there is only preliminary evidence that it really works.

Requirements and Sources

Pyruvate is not an essential nutrient, since the body makes all it needs. It can be found in food, however, with an average diet supplying anywhere from 100 milligrams (mg) to 2 grams (g) daily. Apples are the best source: A single apple contains about 450 mg of pyruvate. Beer and red wine contain about 75 mg per serving.

Therapeutic dosages are usually much higher than what can be obtained from food: A person would have to eat almost seventy apples a day to get the proper amount. To use pyruvate for therapeutic purposes, one must take a supplement.

Although most pyruvate products on the market contain pyruvate only (or are almost all pyruvate), some also contain a related compound, dihydroxyacetone, which the body converts into pyruvate. The combination of the two products is known as DHAP.

Therapeutic Dosages

A typical therapeutic dosage of pyruvate is 30 g daily, although dosages of 6 to 44 g daily have been used in studies. Dihydroxyacetone dosages in studies of DHAP (pyruvate plus dihydroxyacetone) have ranged from 12 to 75 g daily.

Therapeutic Uses

Evidence from several small placebo-controlled studies suggests that pyruvate may enhance weight loss. Pyruvate is also marketed as a sports performance supplement, but the supporting evidence for this use is weak and contradictory at best.

SCIENTIFIC EVIDENCE

Several small studies enrolling a total of about 150 persons have found evidence that pyruvate or DHAP can aid weight loss and improve body composition (the proportion of fat to muscle tissue). For example, in a six-week, double-blind, placebo-controlled trial, fifty-one persons were given either pyruvate (6 g daily), placebo, or no treatment. All participated in an exercise program. In the treated group, significant decreases in fat mass (2.1 kilograms [kg]) and percentage body fat (2.6 percent) were seen, along with a significant increase in muscle mass (1.5 kg). No significant changes were seen in the placebo and no-treatment groups.

Another placebo-controlled study (blinding not stated) used a much higher dose of pyruvate: 22 to 44 g daily, depending on total calorie intake. In this trial, thirty-four slightly overweight persons were put on a mildly weight-reducing diet for four weeks. Subsequently, one-half were given a liquid dietary supplement containing pyruvate. Over the course of six weeks, individuals in the pyruvate group lost a small amount of weight (about 1.5 pounds each), while those in the placebo group did not lose weight. Most of the weight loss came from fat.

A third placebo-controlled study evaluated the effects of combined dihydroxyacetone and pyruvate (DHAP) when individuals who had previously lost weight increased their calorie intake. Seventeen severely overweight women were put on a restricted diet as inpatients for three weeks, during which time they lost an average of approximately 17 pounds. They were then given a high-calorie diet. Approximately one-half of the women also received 15 g of pyruvate and 75 g of dihydroxyacetone daily. The results showed that after three weeks of this weight-gaining diet, individuals receiving the supplements gained only about 4 pounds, compared with about 6 pounds in the placebo group. Close evaluation showed that pyruvate specifically blocked regain of fat weight.

While all these studies are intriguing, large studies (one hundred participants or more) are needed to establish the potential benefits of pyruvate for weight loss.

SAFETY ISSUES

Both pyruvate and dihydroxyacetone appear to be quite safe, apart from mild side effects, such as occasional stomach upset and diarrhea. Very weak evidence (too weak to be of much concern) hints that pyruvate supplements might adversely affect cholesterol profile by negating the positive effects of exercise on HDL (good cholesterol). Maximum safe dosages for children, women who are pregnant or nursing, and persons with liver or kidney disease have not been established.

It should be noted that any contaminants present in a pyruvate product, even in very small percentages, could lead to harmful results because of the enormous dosages used. For this reason, individuals should always be certain to use only high-quality pyruvate products.

EBSCO CAM Review Board

FURTHER READING

Kalman, D., et al. "The Effects of Pyruvate Supplementation on Body Composition in Overweight Individuals." *Nutrition* 15 (1999): 337-340.

Koh-Banerjee, P. K., et al. "Effects of Calcium Pyruvate Supplementation During Training on Body Composition, Exercise Capacity, and Metabolic Responses to Exercise." *Nutrition* 21 (2005): 312-319.

Morrison, M. A., L. L. Spriet, and D. J. Dyck. "Pyruvate Ingestion for Seven Days Does Not Improve Aerobic Performance in Well-Trained Individuals." *Journal of Applied Physiology* 89 (2000): 549-556.

See also: Herbal medicine; Low-carbohydrate diet; Obesity and excess weight; Sports and fitness support: Enhancing performance.

Q

Qigong

CATEGORY: Therapies and techniques

RELATED TERMS: Chi Kung, external qigong, internal qigong, qi therapy

DEFINITION: A group of techniques that use various breathing exercises and physical postures.

PRINCIPAL PROPOSED USE: General wellness

OTHER PROPOSED USES: Asthma, cancer treatment support, depression, fibromyalgia, hypertension, neck pain, Parkinson's disease

OVERVIEW

The term *qigong* refers to various systems of breathing exercises and physical postures that are thought to improve general health by following the principles of traditional Chinese medicine. More precisely, this practice is known as internal qigong, or qigong practiced by a person for his or her own benefit. Expert qigong practitioners may also use their training to treat other people, a practice called external qigong, or qi therapy.

Internal qigong is said to increase one's overall vitality and health by facilitating the free flow of qi in the body. The term *qi* refers to the underlying "energy" in the body, as conceptualized in the ancient medical systems of East Asia. (There is no scientific evidence for the existence of qi.) Those who practice external qigong claim to have developed so much mastery of qi that they can project it into others.

Methods related to modern qigong are mentioned in Chinese texts dating back more than three millennia. Qigong bears a close relationship to the martial arts traditions of East Asia, but like Tai Chi, it has been adapted primarily for health rather than for fighting. Qigong also has strong historical connections with metaphysical and religious traditions, but it has become popular more recently as a purely secular exercise. This evolution is similar to that of yoga.

Cults may form around practitioners of external qigong. Reportedly, the present-day qigong master Li

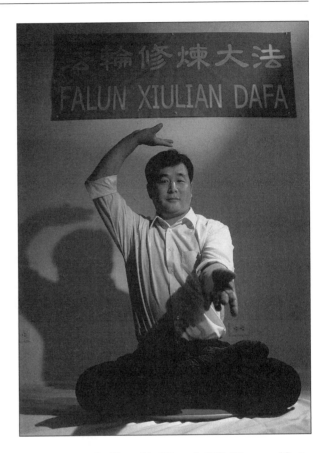

Qigong master Li Hongzhi. (Time & Life Pictures/Getty Images)

Hongzhi can turn invisible, levitate, teleport himself through space, and control people's thoughts. His tens of millions of followers, known collectively as the Falun Gong, have achieved sufficient political power in China to have been banned.

SCIENTIFIC EVIDENCE

Mainstream scientists do not accept the concept of qi, but internal qigong can be considered a form of exercise and studied as such. External qigong, however, does not strike most scientists as plausible; it has nonetheless undergone some study.

All of the research published on either type of qigong suffers from significant flaws. This is to some extent the fault of researchers who may possess a type of personal devotion to qigong that impairs scientific objectivity. However, even with the best of intentions and the most implacable dedication to objectivity, a researcher will find it difficult to properly study qigong. This results from a problem intrinsic to the treatment: It is difficult, if not impossible, to conduct a true double-blind, placebo-controlled study of qigong.

For the results of a study to be truly reliable, some participants must receive real treatment (the active group), while others receive placebo treatment (the control group). In addition, both participants and researchers must not know which group is which. Without this "blinding," the placebo effect and other confounding factors will inevitably and significantly skew the results.

When conducting studies of herbs, supplements, or drugs, it is relatively easy to achieve blinding: Some participants receive the real treatment in a capsule, while others receive a fake treatment in an identical capsule, and neither researchers nor participants know which is which. The capsules are coded, and the code is not broken until after the study has been completed. With qigong exercises, however, as with many other alternative therapies, there is no simple equivalent.

Consider internal qigong. While some participants can be assigned fake qigong exercises, it is difficult to make sure they do not know that the exercises they are practicing are fake. One would need to first train a group of people to teach the fake exercises, and to do so without letting this group know that the exercises are fake; in turn, they would teach the participants in the placebo group. However, the duped participants and duped teachers would have to be prevented from learning about real qigong, because such knowledge would destroy the necessary deception. Such a complex feat would be challenging to achieve. Perhaps it would be more practical to compare qigong exercises with an equally impressive but ineffective intervention, such as fake ultraviolet laser acupuncture or fake ultrasound treatment. However, a review of the literature failed to find any such study of qigong.

External qigong presents a somewhat different but related challenge. Because qi is said to be invisible, a practitioner of external qigong could simply convey qi to certain participants and only pretend to

Study Shows Health Benefits Combining Qigong and Tai Chi

A review of scientific literature suggests that there is strong evidence of beneficial health effects of qigong and tai chi, including for bone health, cardiopulmonary fitness, balance, and quality of life. Both qigong and tai chi have origins in China and involve physical movement, mental focus, and deep breathing. Because of the apparent similarities between tai chi and qigong, the researchers reviewed the literature on both practices together. The review was published in the *American Journal of Health Promotion* in 2010.

Researchers from Arizona State University, the University of North Carolina, and the Institute of Integral Qigong and Tai Chi in Santa Barbara, California, analyzed seventy-seven articles reporting the results of sixty-six randomized controlled trials of tai chi and qigong. The studies involved a total of 6,410 participants. A majority of the studies compared tai chi or qigong with a nonexercise control group, but some included a comparison group that practiced other forms of exercise, while others included both exercise and nonexercise groups to evaluate the effects of tai chi and qigong.

Of the many outcomes identified by the reviewers, current research suggests that the strongest and most consistent evidence of health benefits for tai chi or qigong is for bone health, cardiopulmonary fitness, balance, and factors associated with preventing falls and improving quality of life and self-efficacy (the confidence in and perceived ability to perform a behavior). Evidence is mixed, according to the review, about tai chi or qigong's effects on psychological factors and patient-reported outcomes (reports from patients of symptoms related to disease).

The reviewers concluded that the evidence is sufficient to suggest that tai chi and qigong together represent a viable alternative to conventional forms of exercise. Reviewers also noted that because of the similarities in philosophy and critical elements between tai chi and qigong, the outcomes can be analyzed across both types of studies.

convey it to others. However, practitioners would know what they themselves were doing, and the history of medical research indicates that by subtle, even unconscious, cues these practitioners would convey emotional confidence when providing real therapy and lack of confidence when providing fake therapy. In turn, this "confidence differential" would create placebo effects and other confounding factors. One proposed method to overcome this problem involves using actors to confidently provide a fake therapy; however, again, no such study could be found in the published literature. Given these caveats, a summary of the evidence is provided here.

Internal qigong. In controlled studies, the use of internal qigong has shown some potential benefit for asthma, cancer treatment support, depression, fibromyalgia, hypertension, Parkinson's disease, and enhancing general wellness. However, consistent and convincing evidence of effectiveness is lacking for all of these conditions.

In one study, qigong was no more effective than conventional physical therapy exercise techniques in the treatment of chronic, nonspecific neck pain. A review of nine clinical trials and observational studies found insufficient evidence to support qigong for the treatment of type 2 diabetes.

External qigong. One study reported that, compared with placebo treatment, external qigong affects heart rate in a positive way. Another study reported that, compared with placebo treatment, external qigong reduces symptoms of premenstrual syndrome. Both of these studies had problems in statistical analysis. A third randomized trial compared the effects of two qigong practitioners and a sham practitioner (administering fake or placebo qigong) on 106 persons with osteoarthritis of the knee. Compared with the sham group, only those persons treated by one of the true qigong practitioners showed significant improvement. This suggests that something other than the qigong itself imparted benefit. Intuitively, it would seem that internal qigong would be a better choice for osteoarthritis, though there is no scientific support for this belief.

SAFETY ISSUES

Qigong, when practiced in moderation, is most likely generally safe. However, people with severe heart or lung conditions may put themselves through excessive stress by attempting vigorous breathing exercises.

There are numerous anecdotes in which practitioners of qigong have developed serious mental problems ("qigong psychosis") as a result of practicing the method to an extreme or with insufficient or inept guidance. However, it has been suggested that some people with latent mental illnesses have been drawn to extreme forms of qigong, rather than that the qigong practice itself caused the mental illness.

EBSCO CAM Review Board

FURTHER READING

Chen, K. W., et al. "Effects of External Qigong Therapy on Osteoarthritis of the Knee." *Clinical Rheumatology* 27 (2008): 1497-1505.

Guo, X., et al. "Clinical Effect of Qigong Practice on Essential Hypertension." *Journal of Alternative and Complementary Medicine* 14 (2008): 27-37.

Hui, P. N., et al. "An Evaluation of Two Behavioral Rehabilitation Programs, Qigong Versus Progressive Relaxation, in Improving the Quality of Life in Cardiac Patients." *Journal of Alternative and Complementary Medicine* 12 (2006): 373-378.

Lansinger, B., et al. "Qigong and Exercise Therapy in Patients with Long-Term Neck Pain." *Spine* 32 (2007): 2415-2422.

Lee, M. S., M. K. Kim, and H. Ryu. "Qi-Training (Qigong) Enhanced Immune Functions: What Is the Underlying Mechanism?" *International Journal of Neuroscience* 115 (2005): 1099-1104.

Lee, M. S., et al. "Qigong for Type 2 Diabetes Care." *Complementary Therapies in Medicine* 17 (2009): 236-242.

Lee, T. I., H. H. Chen, and M. L. Yeh. "Effects of Chan-Chuang Qigong on Improving Symptom and Psychological Distress in Chemotherapy Patients." *American Journal of Chinese Medicine* 34 (2006): 37-46.

Mannerkorpi, K., and M. Arndorw. "Efficacy and Feasibility of a Combination of Body Awareness Therapy and Qigong in Patients with Fibromyalgia." *Journal of Rehabilitative Medicine* 36 (2004): 279-281.

Oh, B., et al. "Impact of Medical Qigong on Quality of Life, Fatigue, Mood, and Inflammation in Cancer Patients." *Annals of Oncology* 21 (2010): 608.

Witt, C., et al. "Qigong for Schoolchildren." *Journal of Alternative and Complementary Medicine* 11 (2005): 41-47.

See also: Chinese medicine; Exercise; Pain management; Reiki; Wellness, general.

Quercetin

CATEGORY: Herbs and supplements

RELATED TERM: Quercetin chalcone

DEFINITION: Natural plant product used to treat specific health conditions.

PRINCIPAL PROPOSED USES: None

OTHER PROPOSED USES: Allergies (hay fever), antiviral, asthma, cancer prevention, eczema, heart disease prevention, high blood pressure, hives, interstitial cystitis, prostatitis (chronic pelvic pain syndrome), stroke prevention

OVERVIEW

Quercetin belongs to a class of water-soluble plant coloring substances called bioflavonoids. Bioflavonoids have strong antioxidant effects when they are studied in the test tube, and this is the basis for some of the health claims attached to them. However, growing evidence suggests that bioflavonoids do not in fact act as antioxidants in human beings. Nonetheless, as widely available plant substances, they are considered possible seminutrients, substances that are not essential for life but might help promote optimal health.

REQUIREMENTS AND SOURCES

Quercetin is not an essential nutrient. It is found in red wine, grapefruit, onions, apples, and black tea and, in lesser amounts, in leafy green vegetables and beans. However, to get a therapeutic dosage, one needs to take a supplement. Quercetin supplements are available in pill and tablet form.

THERAPEUTIC DOSAGES

A typical dosage is 200 to 400 milligrams (mg) three times daily. A special type of quercetin, quercetin chalcone, is claimed to be absorbed better, but there is little reliable evidence to prove this.

THERAPEUTIC USES

Quercetin is widely marketed as a treatment for allergic conditions such as asthma, hay fever, eczema, and hives. These proposed uses are based on test-tube research showing that quercetin prevents certain immune cells from releasing histamine, the chemical that triggers an allergic reaction. Quercetin may also block other substances involved with allergies. However, this evidence is far too preliminary to rely upon.

Scientists have found no direct evidence that the ingestion of quercetin supplements will reduce allergy symptoms.

A different proposed use of quercetin does have some meaningful supporting evidence: the treatment of prostatitis. This condition is an inflammation or infection of the prostate gland. Prostatitis, sometimes called chronic pelvic pain syndrome, causes chronic pain and difficulty with urination. Conventional treatment for this condition is often unsatisfactory. One small double-blind, placebo-controlled study has found preliminary evidence that quercetin might be useful for treating prostatitis. Another small, double-blind, placebo-controlled trial found that a supplement containing quercetin reduced symptoms of interstitial cystitis.

As noted, it has been suggested that quercetin's antioxidant properties might make it helpful for preventing heart disease and strokes. However, the evidence that it works is highly incomplete. It should be noted that other powerful antioxidants, such as vitamin E and beta-carotene, have been ineffective for preventing these conditions. There is limited evidence, however, from a single small, double-blind trial, that quercetin might have the separate effect of lowering blood pressure when it is high. Test-tube studies and animal research have additionally suggested that quercetin might have cancer-preventive properties.

An animal study found that quercetin might protect rodents with diabetes from forming cataracts. Another intriguing finding from test-tube research is that quercetin seems to prevent a wide range of viruses from infecting cells and reproducing once they are inside cells. One study found that quercetin produced this effect against herpes simplex, polio virus, and various respiratory viruses, including influenza. However, such studies have been too indirect to determine whether humans taking quercetin supplements can hope for benefits against diseases caused by those viruses.

SCIENTIFIC EVIDENCE

Prostatitis. A one-month double-blind, placebo-controlled trial of thirty men with chronic pelvic pain (prostatitis) tested the potential effectiveness of quercetin. Participants received either placebo or 500 mg of the supplement twice daily. The results showed that those who received quercetin experienced a statistically significant improvement in symptoms (such as pain); those given placebo did not improve.

While these are promising results, the study was small and cannot be regarded as definitive. Furthermore, the researchers failed to provide the usual statistical evaluation required for such studies (a statistical analysis that directly compares the results in the treatment group against those in the placebo group). Thus further study will be necessary to discover whether quercetin is actually effective for prostatitis.

Interstitial cystitis. People with interstitial cystitis experience pain and discomfort in the bladder that is reminiscent of a bladder infection, but without the actual presence of such an infection. In a six-week double-blind, placebo-controlled study, twenty people received either placebo or a supplement containing quercetin and other bioflavonoids. The results appeared to indicate better results in the quercetin group. However, this study has been presented only as an abstract, and it is not clear from the write-up whether the results were statistically meaningful.

SAFETY ISSUES

Quercetin appears to be quite safe. However, concerns have been raised that, under some circumstances, it might raise cancer risk. Quercetin "fails" a standard laboratory test called the Ames test, which is designed to identify chemicals that might be carcinogenic. Nonetheless, a bad showing on the Ames test does not definitely mean a chemical causes cancer. Most other evidence suggests that quercetin does not cause cancer and may, in fact, help prevent cancer. Still, one highly preliminary study suggests that quercetin combined with other bioflavonoids in the diet of pregnant women might increase the risk of infant leukemia. On this basis, pregnant women should probably avoid quercetin supplements. Maximum safe dosages for young children, nursing women, and people with serious liver or kidney disease have not been established.

Evidence suggests that the use of quercetin supplements can elevate urine and blood levels of the substance homovanillic acid. While this itself should be harmless, lab tests for homovanillic acid are used to diagnose a rare and dangerous condition called neuroblastoma; for this reason, use of quercetin supplements could potentially cause a false positive diagnosis of this condition.

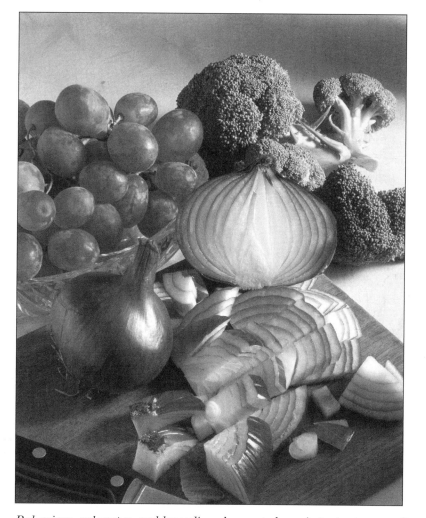

Red onions, red grapes, and broccoli are known to be an important source of quercetin. Quercetin is widely promoted as a treatment for allergic conditions such as asthma, hay fever, eczema, and hives. However, in order to get the therapeutic dosage, one must take a supplement. (Sheila Terry/Photo Researchers, Inc.)

EBSCO CAM Review Board

FURTHER READING

Edwards, R. L., et al. "Quercetin Reduces Blood Pressure in Hypertensive Subjects." *Journal of Nutrition* 137 (2007): 2405-2411.

Lotito, S. B., and B. Frei. "Consumption of Flavonoid-Rich Foods and Increased Plasma Antioxidant Capacity in Humans: Cause, Consequence, or Epiphenomenon?" *Free Radical Biology and Medicine* 41 (2006): 1727-1746.

Strick, R., et al. "Dietary Bioflavonoids Induce Cleavage in the MLL Gene and May Contribute to Infant Leukemia." *Proceedings of the National Academy of Sciences* 97 (2000): 4790-4795.

Weldin, J., et al. "Quercetin, an Over-the-Counter Supplement, Causes Neuroblastoma-like Elevation of Plasma Homovanillic Acid." *Pediatric and Developmental Pathology* 5 (2004): 547-551.

See also: Citrus bioflavonoids; Prostatitis.

R

Radiation therapy support: Homeopathic remedies

CATEGORY: Homeopathy
DEFINITION: The use of highly diluted remedies to treat the side effects of radiation therapy.
STUDIED HOMEOPATHIC REMEDIES: Belladonna, combination homeopathic remedy containing belladonna and irradiated water plus alcohol, *Ledum palustre*, sulphur

INTRODUCTION

Radiation therapy is one of the most important methods to treat cancer. However, while it generally causes fewer side effects than chemotherapy, it can still cause problems, including skin damage, diarrhea, and fatigue. Homeopathic remedies have been proposed for minimizing these side effects.

SCIENTIFIC EVALUATIONS OF HOMEOPATHIC REMEDIES

Radiation therapy can cause significant skin damage, similar to that of a severe sunburn. A ten-week, double-blind, placebo-controlled trial of sixty-one women with breast cancer evaluated the possible benefits of homeopathic treatment for reducing the severity of this side effect. Researchers used a combination of belladonna 7c (centesimals) and a novel homeopathic remedy made from water and alcohol that had been subjected to radiation. However, no benefits were seen in the treated group as compared with the placebo group.

TRADITIONAL HOMEOPATHIC TREATMENTS

According to the principles of classical homeopathy, there are many possible homeopathic treatments for radiation therapy support. These therapies are chosen based on various specific details of the person seeking treatment.

Homeopathic belladonna is traditionally used to treat skin conditions that are red and hot and possibly accompanied by fever. The homeopathic remedy sulphur might be used for radiation skin damage that involves red and irritated skin with scaly patches that may be dry or moist. The symptom picture includes the worsening of the irritated area of the skin by application of heat or water and by contact with clothing. Homeopathic *Ledum palustre* is traditionally used for conditions involving puffy, swollen skin that feels cold to the touch and feels better when cold compresses are applied.

EBSCO CAM Review Board

FURTHER READING

Balzarini, A., et al. "Efficacy of Homeopathic Treatment of Skin Reactions During Radiotherapy for Breast Cancer." *British Homeopathic Journal* 89 (2000): 8-12.

Guethlin, C., et al. "Characteristics of Cancer Patients Using Homeopathy Compared with Those in Conventional Care." *Annals of Oncology* 21 (2010): 1094-1099.

Kassab, S., et al. "Homeopathic Medicines for Adverse Effects of Cancer Treatments." *Cochrane Database of Systematic Reviews* (2009): CD004845. Available through *EBSCO DynaMed Systematic Literature Surveillance* at http://www.ebscohost.com/dynamed.

Rajendran, E. S. "Homeopathy as a Supportive Therapy in Cancer." *Homeopathy* 93 (2004): 99-102.

See also: Cancer treatment support; Homeopathy.

Radionics

CATEGORY: Therapies and techniques
RELATED TERMS: Applied kinesiology, energy medicine, homeopathy, parapsychology, psionics, radiesthesia, vibrational medicine
DEFINITION: The detection of vital energy patterns from physical matter that is unique to a person to diagnose disease and to promote healing.

PRINCIPAL PROPOSED USES: Disease diagnosis and therapy

OTHER PROPOSED USES: Allergies, bleeding, bruises, fractures, sexual dysfunction, sinus infection

OVERVIEW

Developed by San Francisco physician Albert Abrams in the early twentieth century, radionics focuses on the electronic detection of vital energy (radiation) patterns as a means of diagnosing and treating disease. The method claims that healing can be produced from a distance. The term "radionics" comes from combining the words "radiation" and "electronics."

MECHANISM OF ACTION

Abrams claimed that he could detect particular energies or vibrations emitted from healthy and diseased tissue in all living things. A specimen of blood, hair, or other physical substances, and even a person's signature, is placed in an electronic black box. Rates associated with energy flows in the body are measured as indicators of health or disease.

USES AND APPLICATIONS

Radionic instruments diagnose the health state of the body; they also reportedly heal the disease by transmitting healthy vibrations to the sick tissue or organs. Sending "good" energy to the diseased area of the body counteracts "bad" energy, thus providing energy that heals bruises, fractures, and allergies and also cures diseases such as pneumonia and cancer.

SCIENTIFIC EVIDENCE

Radionic practitioners claim that when the right frequencies of radiation are applied to the body, treatment goes beyond the cellular tissues to the electronic structures of the atoms; this affects the electrons in a characteristic, healing manner. Although radionic devices produce measurable readings, there is no scientific basis for claiming that the readings (rates) have anything to do with healthy or diseased vibrations of electrons or body energy. In 1950, a radionic device developed by Ruth Drown, a noted advocate of radionics, was tested at the University of Chicago and did not work as promised. Rigorous double-blind studies conducted to test radionics have failed to prove its validity.

The Body Electric

The developer of radionics, San Francisco physician Albert Abrams, wrote in his book New Concepts in Diagnosis and Treatment: Physico-Clinical Medicine—The Practical Application of the Electronic Theory in the Interpretation and Treatment of Disease *(1922) that "physiologists have established the following" with regard to the human body's "electric" composition:*

1. Electrical currents appear in the body when a muscle or nerve is active, and such currents are intimately associated with the functional condition of the tissue.
2. These action currents correspond to the general law that every active portion of nerve or muscle maintains a negative relation toward the resting part, *i.e.*, the active muscle and nerve show a negative electrical reaction toward the resting structures.
3. The action currents are sufficiently strong to have a stimulating action of their own.

Of the many radionic instruments that have been developed during the past several decades, none have been found to be effective in diagnosing or treating disease. The U.S. Food and Drug Administration does not recognize radionic devices for any legitimate medical use. Most physicians classify radionics as pseudoscience and quackery. It is a controversial form of complementary and alternative medicine because neither the external energy fields nor their therapeutic effects have been demonstrated to have any biophysical merit.

SAFETY ISSUES

Although radionics is generally safe, the advertised strengths of radionics, namely noninvasive diagnosis and avoidance of surgery and drugs, are safety concerns. There is the risk that serious illness will remain undetected and untreated. It could delay the time it takes for a patient to see a qualified health-care provider about a potentially life-threatening condition. If used, radionics should be used only as a complement to proven medical care.

Alvin K. Benson, Ph.D.

FURTHER READING

Mason, Keith. *The Radionics Handbook: How to Improve Your Health with a Powerful Form of Energy Therapy.* London: Piatkus Books, 2001.

Radionic Association. http://radionic.co.uk.

"Radionics." In *The Skeptic's Dictionary.* Available at http://www.skepdic.com/radionics.html.

Russell, Edward W. *Report on Radionics: The Science Which Can Cure Where Orthodox Medicine Fails.* New York: Random House, 2004.

See also: Applied kinesiology; Bioenergetics; Energy medicine; Homeopathy; Pulse diagnosis.

Raw foods diet

CATEGORY: Therapies and techniques
RELATED TERMS: Living foods diet, raw foodism
DEFINITION: Vegan diet consisting of uncooked vegetables and fruits, nuts, seeds, and sprouted grains and beans.
PRINCIPAL PROPOSED USES: Cancer, fatigue, fibromyalgia, general health, illness prevention, rheumatoid arthritis
OTHER PROPOSED USES: Digestion, weight loss

OVERVIEW

The raw foods diet began in the mid-nineteenth century, when health reformer Sylvester Graham claimed that illness could be avoided by consuming only uncooked foods. In the 1940s, German physician Max Gerson claimed that his particular raw foods regimen could cure advanced forms of cancer. The popularity of the diet has grown in recent years, perhaps because of its use among celebrities.

Raw food consumption can vary, according to the specific diet, from 50 to 100 percent of a person's food consumption. Experts recommend that the diet's foods be unprocessed. Many elements of the diet can be prepared in unique ways, such as presoaking nuts and grains. Food may be "cooked" using a food dehydrator, but the temperature of the food should not exceed 118° Fahrenheit. Because beverages including coffee, tea, alcohol, soda, and bottled juice are processed, raw food dieters generally drink only water and freshly made juices.

MECHANISM OF ACTION

Proponents of the raw foods diet note that a key benefit of the diet is the preservation of health-promoting enzymes in uncooked foods; these enzymes are deactivated by cooking. However, sources in the medical community note that enzymes in food are destroyed by stomach acids. Raw food diet proponents counter that the enzymes are later reactivated in the small intestine.

USES AND APPLICATIONS

Proponents of the raw foods diet view it as a lifestyle rather than as a time-limited diet or one chiefly intended for weight loss. The diet is often credited by proponents with promoting general health and improved energy and with helping to alleviate chronic illnesses, including cancer and fibromyalgia.

SCIENTIFIC EVIDENCE

A limited body of published scientific research exists on the rationale for the raw foods diet or associated outcomes. Research findings suggest that a raw foods, vegan diet may help to reduce symptoms of fibromyalgia and rheumatoid arthritis and to promote weight loss. In one study of Americans who had been on the raw foods diet a long time, respondents reported improved health and quality of life. The study found that the average nutrient intake while on the diet was higher for some components (such as vitamins A and C) and lower for others (such as protein and vitamin B_{12}).

SAFETY ISSUES

Extremely restrictive diets such as the raw foods diet can impair growth and are not recommended for infants and children. Fresh produce can be a source of food-borne illness, and a raw foods diet can increase the risk of infection in persons whose immune systems are compromised, such as persons undergoing bone marrow or stem cell transplantation.

Katherine Hauswirth, M.S.N., R.N.

FURTHER READING

Cunningham, C. "What Is a Raw Foods Diet and Are There Any Risks or Benefits Associated with it?" *Journal of the American Dietetic Association* 104 (2004): 1623.

Havala Hobbs, S. "Raw Foods Diets: A Review of the Literature." *Vegetarian Times,* issue 4 (2002): 30-31.

"Living and Raw Foods: Frequently Asked Questions." http://www.living-foods.com/faq.html.

See also: Anti-inflammatory diet; Diet-based therapies; Food allergies and sensitivities; Functional foods:

Introduction; Functional foods: Overview; Low-carbohydrate diet; Low-glycemic-index diet; Macrobiotic diet; Vegan diet; Vegetarian diet.

Raynaud's phenomenon

CATEGORY: Condition
RELATED TERMS: Primary Raynaud's, Raynaud's disease, secondary Raynaud's
DEFINITION: Treatment of a condition in which the fingers and toes are extra-sensitive to cold.
PRINCIPAL PROPOSED NATURAL TREATMENTS: None
OTHER PROPOSED NATURAL TREATMENTS: Acupuncture, arginine, biofeedback, fish oil, gamma-linolenic acid, ginkgo, inositol hexaniacinate, vitamin C

INTRODUCTION

Raynaud's phenomenon is a little-understood condition in which the fingers and toes show an exaggerated sensitivity to cold. Classic cases show a characteristic white, blue, and red color sequence as the digits lose blood supply and then warm up again. Some people develop only one or two of these signs.

The cause of Raynaud's phenomenon is unknown. It can occur by itself, as primary Raynaud's (also called Raynaud's disease), or as a consequence of other illnesses, such as scleroderma. In the latter case, it is called secondary Raynaud's.

Conventional treatment consists mainly of reassurance and the recommendation to avoid exposure to cold and the use of tobacco (which can worsen Raynaud's). In severe cases, a variety of drugs can be tried.

PROPOSED NATURAL TREATMENTS

Preliminary evidence supports the use of several natural supplements in the treatment of Raynaud's phenomenon. Most of the positive evidence regards primary Raynaud's.

In a seventeen-week, double-blind, placebo-controlled trial of thirty-five people with Raynaud's, fish oil (taken at a dose that provided a total of 3.96 grams [g] of eicosapentaenoic acid and 2.64 g of docosahexaenoic acid daily) reduced reaction to cold among those with primary Raynaud's disease, but it did not seem to help those with Raynaud's caused by other illnesses. In an eighty-four-day, double-blind, placebo-controlled study of twenty-three people with primary Raynaud's, the use of inositol hexaniacinate significantly reduced the frequency of attacks.

The herb *Ginkgo biloba* has been found to increase circulation in the fingertips and thus has been proposed as a treatment for Raynaud's. A ten-week, double-blind, placebo-controlled trial of twenty-two people with primary Raynaud's found that the use of ginkgo at the very high dose of 120 milligrams three times daily reduced the number of Raynaud's attacks.

One small double-blind study found suggestions that evening primrose oil might help primary or secondary Raynaud's. A double-blind, placebo-controlled, crossover trial of ten people failed to find arginine at 8 g daily helpful for primary Raynaud's.

A small double-blind trial tested the effects of a single dose of 2 g of vitamin C on Raynaud's caused by scleroderma and found no benefit. Finally, evidence suggests that biofeedback is at most no more than marginally effective for Raynaud's; the same is true of acupuncture.

EBSCO CAM Review Board

FURTHER READING

Hahn, M., et al. "Is There a Vasospasmolytic Effect of Acupuncture in Patients with Secondary Raynaud Phenomenon?" *Journal of the German Society of Dermatology* 2 (2005): 758-762.

Mavrikakis, M. E., et al. "Ascorbic Acid Does Not Improve Endothelium-Dependent Flow-Mediated Dilatation of the Brachial Artery in Patients with Raynaud's Phenomenon Secondary to Systemic Sclerosis." *International Journal of Vitamin and Nutrition Research* 73 (2003): 3-7.

Muir, A. H., et al. "The Use of *Ginkgo biloba* in Raynaud's Disease." *Vascular Medicine* 7 (2002): 265-267.

See also: Acupuncture; Arginine; Biofeedback; Fish oil; Gamma-linolenic acid; Ginkgo; Inositol; Restless legs syndrome; Vitamin C.

Red clover

CATEGORY: Herbs and supplements
RELATED TERM: *Trifolium pratense*
DEFINITION: Natural plant product used to treat specific health conditions.
PRINCIPAL PROPOSED USE: Menopausal symptoms

OTHER PROPOSED USES: Acne, cyclic mastalgia, eczema, enhancement of mental function, high blood
pressure, high cholesterol, osteoporosis, psoriasis

OVERVIEW

Red clover has been cultivated since ancient times,
primarily to provide a favorite grazing food for animals. Like many other herbs, however, red clover was
also a valued medicine. Although it has been used for
many purposes worldwide, the one condition most
consistently associated with red clover is cancer. Chinese physicians and Russian folk healers have also
used it to treat respiratory problems.

In the nineteenth century, red clover became popular among herbalists as an "alternative," or "blood
purifier." This medical term, long since defunct, refers
to an ancient belief that toxins in the blood are the
root cause of many illnesses. Cancer, eczema, and the
eruptions of venereal disease were all seen as manifes-
tations of toxic buildup. Red clover was considered
one of the best herbs to "purify" the blood. For this
reason, it is included in many of the famous treatments
for cancer, including Jason Winters's cancer-cure tea.

Recently, special red clover extracts high in substances called isoflavones have arrived on the market.
These isoflavones produce effects in the body somewhat similar to those of estrogen, and for this reason
they are called phytoestrogens ("phyto" indicates a
plant source). The major isoflavones in red clover include genistein and daidzen, also found in soy, as well
as formononetin and biochanin.

THERAPEUTIC DOSAGES

A typical dosage of red clover extract provides 40 to
160 milligrams (mg) of isoflavones daily. In the positive study described below, 80 mg daily was a sufficient
dosage to reduce menopausal hot flashes.

THERAPEUTIC USES

Evidence is inconsistent regarding whether red
clover isoflavones are helpful for menopausal hot
flashes, with the largest trial failing to find benefits. A
small and poorly reported double-blind, placebo-controlled study provides weak evidence that red clover
isoflavones might be helpful for cyclic mastalgia.

Although soy and, possibly, soy isoflavones have
been found to reduce cholesterol levels, two trials enrolling a total of more than one hundred women
failed to find red clover isoflavones helpful for this

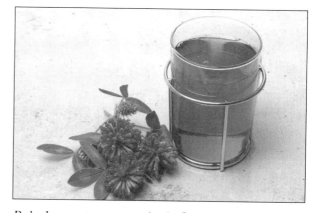

*Red clover extracts contain isoflavones, which produce
effects similar to estrogen.* (Bildagentur-online/TH Foto-
Werbung/ Photo Researchers, Inc.)

purpose. However, in a double-blind, placebo-controlled comparative study of eighty people (both men
and women), a red clover extract modified to be rich
in biochanin did reduce LDL (bad) cholesterol, while
one enriched in formononetin did not.

One very small double-blind study found hints that
red clover isoflavones might slightly improve blood
pressure in postmenopausal women with diabetes.
Preliminary evidence suggests that red clover isoflavones may help prevent or treat osteoporosis. In a six-
month, double-blind study, use of red clover isoflavones failed to enhance or harm mental function.

There is no evidence that red clover can help treat
cancer. However, its usage in many parts of the world
as a traditional cancer remedy has prompted scientists to take a close look at the herb. It turns out that
the isoflavones in red clover may possess antitumor
activity in the test tube. However, such preliminary research does not prove that red clover can treat cancer.

Red clover is sometimes recommended for the treatment of acne, eczema, psoriasis, and other skin diseases.

SCIENTIFIC EVIDENCE

Menopausal hot flashes. In a twelve-week double-
blind, placebo-controlled trial of thirty postmenopausal women, use of red clover isoflavones at a dose of
80 mg daily significantly reduced hot flash symptoms
compared with placebo. Benefits were also seen in a
ninety-day study of sixty postmenopausal women given
placebo or 80 mg of red clover isoflavones. However,
a much larger study (252 participants) failed to find
benefit with 82 or 57 mg of red clover isoflavones daily.

Two other studies also failed to find benefit. One, a twenty-eight-week double-blind, placebo-controlled crossover study of fifty-one postmenopausal women, found no reduction in hot flashes among those given 40 mg of red clover isoflavones daily. No benefits were seen in another double-blind, placebo-controlled trial that involved thirty-seven women given isoflavones from red clover at a dose of either 40 or 160 mg daily.

SAFETY ISSUES

Red clover is on the U.S. Food and Drug Administration's Generally Recognized As Safe (GRAS) list and is included in many beverage teas. However, detailed safety studies have not been performed.

Because of its blood-thinning and estrogen-like constituents, red clover should not be used by pregnant or nursing women or by women who have had breast or uterine cancer. A study investigating the safety of red clover in women with a family history of breast cancer found no changes in breast density or thickness of the uterine lining over a three-year period, which is somewhat reassuring. However, the study was much too short to determine red clover's long-term effect on cancer risk. Safety in young children and in those with severe liver or kidney disease has also not been established.

Based on their constituents, red clover extracts may conceivably interfere with hormone treatments and anticoagulant drugs. One double-blind study of postmenopausal women found that the use of red clover isoflavones at a dose of 80 mg daily for ninety days resulted in increased levels of testosterone. The potential significance of this is unclear. The same study found that red clover isoflavones reduced the thickness of the uterine lining, a finding that suggests low possibility for increasing the risk of endometrial cancer.

IMPORTANT INTERACTIONS

Persons who are taking hormones or blood-thinning drugs–such as warfarin (Coumadin), heparin, clopidogrel (Plavix), ticlopidine (Ticlid), pentoxifylline (Trental), or even aspirin–should not use red clover unless they are under a physician's supervision.

EBSCO CAM Review Board

FURTHER READING

Atkinson, C., et al. "The Effects of Phytoestrogen

Isoflavones on Bone Density in Women." *American Journal of Clinical Nutrition* 79 (2004): 326-333.

Blakesmith, S. J., et al. "Effects of Supplementation with Purified Red Clover (*Trifolium pratense*) Isoflavones on Plasma Lipids and Insulin Resistance in Healthy Premenopausal Women." *British Journal of Nutrition* 89 (2003): 467-475.

Hidalgo, L. A., et al. "The Effect of Red Clover Isoflavones on Menopausal Symptoms, Lipids and Vaginal Cytology in Menopausal Women." *Gynecological Endocrinology* 21 (2005): 257-264.

Howes, J. B., K. Bray, et al. "The Effects of Dietary Supplementation with Isoflavones from Red Clover on Cognitive Function in Postmenopausal Women." *Climacteric* 7 (2004): 70-77.

Howes, J. B., D. Tran, et al. "Effects of Dietary Supplementation with Isoflavones from Red Clover on Ambulatory Blood Pressure and Endothelial Function in Postmenopausal Type 2 Diabetes." *Diabetes, Obesity, and Metabolism* 5 (2003): 325-332.

Nestel, P., et al. "A Biochanin-Enriched Isoflavone from Red Clover Lowers LDL Cholesterol in Men." *European Journal of Clinical Nutrition* 58 (2004): 403-408.

Tice, J. A., et al. "Phytoestrogen Supplements for the Treatment of Hot Flashes: The Isoflavone Clover Extract (ICE) Study." *Journal of the American Medical Association* 290 (2003): 207-214.

See also: Isoflavones; Menopause; Women's health.

Red raspberry

CATEGORY: Herbs and supplements
RELATED TERM: *Rubus idaeus*
DEFINITION: Natural plant product used to treat specific health conditions.
PRINCIPAL PROPOSED USES: None
OTHER PROPOSED USE: Prevention of complications of pregnancy

OVERVIEW

Herbalists have long believed that raspberry leaf tea, taken regularly during pregnancy, can prevent complications and make delivery easier. Raspberry has also been used to reduce excessive menstruation and relieve symptoms of diarrhea. However, there is no evidence that it is safe or effective for these uses.

THERAPEUTIC DOSAGES

A typical dosage of raspberry leaf tea is made with 1 cup of boiling water poured over 1 or 2 teaspoons of dried leaf; the tea is steeped for ten minutes and then sweetened to taste. Unlike many medicinal herbs, raspberry leaf actually has a pleasant taste. Pregnant women may be advised to drink 2 to 3 cups of the tea daily.

THERAPEUTIC USES

Red raspberry tea is still commonly recommended for pregnant women. However, while there is weak preliminary evidence from animal studies that raspberry might have an effect on the uterus, the only real clinical study trial reported to date found no benefit. This double-blind, placebo-controlled study evaluated the effects of red raspberry in 192 pregnant women. Treatment (placebo or 2.4 grams of raspberry leaf daily) began at the thirty-second week of pregnancy and was continued until the onset of labor. The results failed to show any statistically meaningful differences between the groups. Red raspberry did not significantly shorten labor, reduce pain, or prevent complications. Thus, at present, it appears that red raspberry does not work in the manner ascribed to it by tradition.

SAFETY ISSUES

Raspberry is believed to be safe. The double-blind, placebo-controlled trial above found no evidence of harm in the ninety-six pregnant women given red raspberry. However, this does not exclude the possibility of rare side effects or toxicity with excessive dosages. Safety in young children and in those with severe liver or kidney disease has also not been established.

EBSCO CAM Review Board

FURTHER READING

Simpson, M., et al. "Raspberry Leaf in Pregnancy: Its Safety and Efficacy in Labor." *Journal of Midwifery and Women's Health* 46 (2001): 51-59.

See also: Childbirth support: Homeopathic remedies; Pregnancy support; Women's health.

Red tea

CATEGORY: Herbs and supplements
RELATED TERMS: *Aspalathus linearis*, Rooibos
DEFINITION: Natural plant product consumed for specific health benefits.
PRINCIPAL PROPOSED USE: Beverage tea
OTHER PROPOSED USES: Allergies, antioxidant, cancer prevention, dyspepsia, eczema, infantile colic, insomnia, minor injuries, preventing liver damage, warts

OVERVIEW

Rooibos, or red tea, is a plant native to the Cape Town region of South Africa. Long used as a beverage tea, it was popularized as a medicinal herb in the late 1960s by Annique Theron, who claimed that it could help relieve colic and other infant-related problems. Since then, it has been advocated for a variety of additional conditions, including stomach distress (dyspepsia), allergies, warts, eczema, anxiety, insomnia, and minor injuries.

The tea is harvested during the summer. It is green when it is picked, but then it becomes red during a fermentation process similar to that used for making black tea.

USES AND APPLICATIONS

Rooibos tea is marketed as a treatment for a wide variety of conditions. However, no proposed uses of this herb have any meaningful supporting scientific evidence. Like other forms of tea, red tea contains antioxidant substances in the phenol family. This alone is the basis for many of the health claims attached to it. However, innumerable substances contain antioxidants; furthermore, the theory that antioxidants provide widespread health benefits has largely collapsed.

Nonetheless, test-tube studies hint that red tea might be helpful for preventing heart disease, preventing liver injury, and reducing cancer risk. Other test-tube studies hint that constituents of red tea might have activity against the human immunodeficiency virus.

However, all of this evidence remains far too weak to be relied upon. In general, only double-blind, placebo-controlled studies can prove that a treatment is effective. Test-tube studies are at the opposite end of

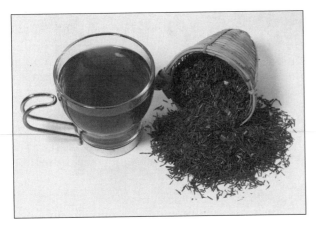

Tea made from rooibos leaves, some of which are seen at right. (TH Foto-Werbung/Photo Researchers, Inc.)

the spectrum; they are useful as basic research, but the overwhelming majority of potential benefits seen in the test tube are not seen in human trials. Therefore, while rooibos may be a pleasant beverage tea, any medicinal claims attached to it are without scientific foundation.

DOSAGE

Rooibos tea is made by steeping one teaspoon, or one tea bag, of the herb in a cup of water.

SAFETY ISSUES

As a widely used beverage tea, rooibos is presumed to be safe. It does not contain caffeine. Maximum safe doses in pregnant or nursing women, young children, and those with severe liver or kidney disease has not been determined.

EBSCO CAM Review Board

FURTHER READING

Bramati, L., F. Aquilano, and P. Pietta. "Unfermented Rooibos Tea: Quantitative Characterization of Flavonoids by HPLC-UV and Determination of the Total Antioxidant Activity." *Journal of Agricultural and Food Chemistry* 51 (2003): 7472-7474.

González-Gallego, J., et al. "Fruit Polyphenols, Immunity, and Inflammation." *British Journal of Nutrition* 104, suppl. 3 (2010): S15-S27.

Joubert, E., et al. "Antioxidant and Pro-oxidant Activities of Aqueous Extracts and Crude Polyphenolic Fractions of Rooibos (*Aspalathus linearis*)." *Journal of Agricultural and Food Chemistry* 53 (2005): 10260-10267.

Nakano, M., et al. "Polysaccharide from *Aspalathus linearis* with Strong Anti-HIV Activity." *Bioscience, Biotechnology, and Biochemistry* 61 (1997): 267-271.

Persson, I. A., et al. "Tea Flavanols Inhibit Angiotensin-Converting Enzyme Activity and Increase Nitric Oxide Production in Human Endothelial Cells." *Journal of Pharmacy and Pharmacology* 58 (2006): 1139-1144.

See also: Black tea; Folk medicine; Functional beverages; Green tea; Herbal medicine; Hypertension; Kombucha tea.

Red yeast rice

CATEGORY: Herbs and supplements
RELATED TERMS: *Monascus purpureus*, angkak, benikoju, hong qu, monacolin K, xuezhikang, zhitai
DEFINITION: Natural plant product used to treat specific health conditions.
PRINCIPAL PROPOSED USE: High cholesterol
OTHER PROPOSED USE: Heart attack prevention

OVERVIEW

Red yeast rice is a traditional Chinese substance made through the fermentation of a type of yeast called *Monascus purpureus* over rice. Various formulations of this product have been used in China since at least 800 C.E. as a food and also as a medicinal substance within the context of traditional Chinese herbal medicine. This ancient preparation contains naturally occurring substances similar (in some cases, identical) to cholesterol-lowering prescription drugs in the statin family.

THERAPEUTIC DOSAGES

The dosage of red yeast rice used in most studies is 1.2 to 2.4 grams (g) of red yeast rice powder daily. However, owing to patent-infringement suits by the manufacturer of a statin drug that is naturally present in red yeast rice, the most-studied red yeast rice product has been taken off the market, and it is not clear whether the remaining products have greater or lesser potency. The herb St. John's wort is known to reduce the effectiveness of drugs in the statin family. There is every reason to believe it would have the same effect on the action of red yeast rice.

THERAPEUTIC USES

Red yeast rice is thought to be effective for lowering cholesterol, presumably because of its statin constituents. There is evidence to support this use.

SCIENTIFIC EVIDENCE

An eight-week double-blind, placebo-controlled trial of eighty-three people with high cholesterol evaluated red yeast rice. At the end of the treatment period, levels of total cholesterol had decreased significantly in the red yeast rice group compared with the placebo group. Benefits were also seen in LDL (bad cholesterol) and triglycerides as well. No significant differences were noted in HDL (good cholesterol) levels from baseline or between groups. In an eight-week study of seventy-nine people, use of red yeast rice was noted to improve the LDL/HDL ratio, along with several other measures of cardiac risk.

In a carefully conducted review of ninety-three randomized trials involving almost ten thousand persons, researchers concluded that red yeast rice can significantly lower levels of total cholesterol, LDL, and triglycerides, and raise levels of HDL, compared with placebo.

A double-blind study performed in China compared an alcohol extract of red yeast rice (Xuezhikang) against placebo in almost five thousand people with heart disease. In a four-year study period, the use of the supplement reportedly reduced the heart attack rate by about 45 percent compared with placebo, and total mortality by about 35 percent. However, these levels of reported benefit are so high as to raise questions about the study's reliability. At least three other studies, all from this same original population of participants, have found similar results in diabetics with heart disease and in patients with previous heart attack, with surprisingly large reductions in the rates of coronary events (for example, heart attack) and mortality. These levels of reported benefit, however, are so high and so similar as to raise questions about their reliability.

SAFETY ISSUES

In clinical trials, use of red yeast rice has not been associated with any significant side effects. However, red yeast rice contains naturally occurring statin drugs, and use of statin drugs can cause side effects ranging from minor to life-threatening. Some of the most common include muscle pain, joint pain, liver

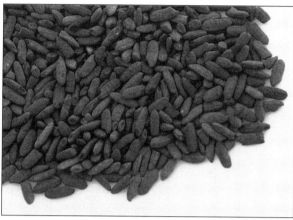

Red yeast rice has been used in China since at least 800 C.E. as a food and also as part of traditional Chinese herbal medicine. (Scimat/Photo Researchers, Inc.)

inflammation, and peripheral nerve damage; severe breakdown of muscle tissue (rhabdomyolysis) leading to kidney failure has also occurred. It is almost certain that red yeast rice can cause the same problems if it is used by enough people, and there are at least two case reports in the literature of muscle injury caused by red yeast rice; in one case, rhabdomyolosis developed. Due to the relative lack of regulation of supplement manufacture, the statin content of red yeast rice products is unpredictable, and this could increase potential risk. In addition, red yeast rice may at times contain the toxic substance citrinin.

Based on the known effects of statins, pregnant or nursing women, women likely to become pregnant, young children, and people with liver or kidney disease should not use red yeast rice. Furthermore, red yeast rice should not be combined with fibrate drugs, cyclosporine, erythromycin-family drugs, antifungal drugs, or high-dose niacin. Finally, it does not make sense to combine red yeast rice with standard statin drugs.

Statin drugs are known to interfere with the body's ability to produce the natural substance CoQ_{10}, and one animal study found the same effect with red yeast rice. For this reason, people taking red yeast rice could conceivably benefit from CoQ_{10} supplementation; however, this has not been proven.

Because red yeast rice is essentially a drug supplied by a natural product, and this drug has many potential side effects, it is recommended that red yeast rice be used only under physician supervision.

IMPORTANT INTERACTIONS

Persons who are taking fibrate drugs, cyclosporine, erythromycin-family drugs, antifungal drugs, or high-dose niacin should not use red yeast rice. In persons who are using red yeast rice to keep their cholesterol levels down, taking the herb St. John's wort may impair the effectiveness of red yeast rice and cause cholesterol levels to rise.

EBSCO CAM Review Board

FURTHER READING

Andrén, L., A. Andreasson, and R. Eggertsen. "Interaction Between a Commercially Available St. John's Wort Product (Movina) and Atorvastatin in Patients with Hypercholesterolemia." *European Journal of Clinical Pharmacology* 63 (2007): 913-916.

Du, B. M., et al. "The Beneficial Effects of Lipid-Lowering Therapy with Xuezhikang on Cardiac Events and Total Mortality in Coronary Heart Disease Patients With or Without Hypertension." *Zhonghua Xin Xue Guan Bing Za Zhi* 34 (2006): 890-894.

Huang, C. F., et al. "Efficacy of *Monascus purpureus* Went Rice on Lowering Lipid Ratios in Hypercholesterolemic Patients." *European Journal of Cardiovascular Prevention and Rehabilitation* 14 (2007): 438-440.

Liu, J., et al. "Chinese Red Yeast Rice (*Monascus purpureus*) for Primary Hyperlipidemia." *Chinese Medicine* 1 (2006): 4.

Lu, Z., et al. "Effect of Xuezhikang, an Extract from Red Yeast Chinese Rice, on Coronary Events in a Chinese Population with Previous Myocardial Infarction." *American Journal of Cardiology* 101 (2008): 1689-1693.

Ye, P., et al. "Effect of Xuezhikang on Cardiovascular Events and Mortality in Elderly Patients with a History of Myocardial Infarction: A Subgroup Analysis of Elderly Subjects from the China Coronary Secondary Prevention Study." *Journal of the American Geriatrics Society* 55 (2007): 1015-1022.

Zhao, S. P., et al. "Xuezhikang, an Extract of Cholestin, Reduces Cardiovascular Events in Type 2 Diabetes Patients with Coronary Heart Disease: Subgroup Analysis of Patients with Type 2 Diabetes from China Coronary Secondary Prevention Study (CCSPS)." *Journal of Cardiovascular Pharmacology* 49 (2007): 81-84.

See also: Cholesterol, high; Heart attack.

Reflexology

CATEGORY: Therapies and techniques
RELATED TERMS: Reflex therapy, zone reflex, zone therapy
DEFINITION: A therapeutic method of relieving pain and tension by stimulating predefined pressure points on the feet and hands by the use of finger pressure.
PRINCIPAL PROPOSED USES: Allergy symptoms, asthma, back pain, boosting circulation, chronic fatigue syndrome, diabetes, fibromyalgia, gastrointestinal disorders, headaches, premenstrual syndrome, respiratory infections, restoring bodily functions, skin disorders, stimulation of internal organs
OTHER PROPOSED USES: Complementary to treatments for conditions such as anxiety, asthma, cardiovascular issues, diabetes, headaches, kidney function, premenstrual syndrome, sinusitis

OVERVIEW

Reflexology is based on the belief that reflex points on the feet and hands are connected to and correspond to every part of the body. Charts with organs superimposed on the foot and hand are said to map these points. Reflexology promotes healing by stimulating the nerves in the body and by encouraging the flow of blood, a process that not only quells the sensation of pain but also relieves the source of the pain.

Reflexology traces its roots to ancient Egypt and China. In the early twentieth century, American physician William Fitzgerald concluded that the foot was the best place to map parts of the body for diagnosis and treatment. He divided the body into ten zones and determined which section of the foot controlled each particular zone. Fitzgerald believed gentle pressure on a particular area of the foot would generate relief in the targeted zone. This process was originally named "zone therapy." A few years later, another doctor, Joe Shelby Riley, published drawings of zones of both the feet and the hands to promote what he named "zone reflex." In the 1930s, Eunice Ingham, a physiotherapist, further developed Fitzgerald's maps to include reflex points, which were much more specific than the zones used in Fitzgerald's maps. It was Ingham who changed the name of zone therapy to "reflexology."

Reflexology is based on the theory that reflex points, located in the feet or hands, are linked to or correspond to various organs and parts of the body. According to this theory, stimulation of these points is thought to affect the connected organ or body part. By stimulating the reflex points, reflexologists believe they can relieve a variety of health problems and promote well-being and relaxation.

To represent how the body's systems correspond to one another, reflexologists use reflexology maps. A good example of a reflexology map exists for the feet. Each foot represents a vertical half of the body. The left foot corresponds to the left side of the body and all organs found there, while the right foot corresponds to the right side of the body and all organs found there. For example, the liver is on the right side of the body, so the corresponding reflex area is on the right foot.

Reflexology is similar to acupuncture and acupressure in that it works with the body's vital energy through the stimulation of points on the body. However, acupuncture and acupressure points do not always coincide with the reflex points used in reflexology. Reflexology and acupressure are both "reflex" therapies in that they work with points on one part of the body to affect other parts of the body. While reflexology uses reflexes that are in an orderly arrangement and resemble a shape of the human body on the feet and hands, acupressure uses more than eight hundred reflex points that are found along long, thin energy lines called meridians that run the length of the entire body.

Reflexology is sometimes confused with massage. While both massage and reflexology use touch, the approaches are very different. Massage is the systematic manipulation of the soft tissues of the body, using specific techniques (for example, tapping, kneading, stroking, and friction) to relax the muscles. Reflexology focuses on reflex maps of points and areas of the body represented on the feet and hands, using unique "micromovement" techniques to create a response throughout the body. Massage therapists work from the outside in; that is, they manipulate specific muscle groups or fascia to release tension. Reflexology practitioners see themselves as working from the inside out, stimulating the nervous system to release tension.

MECHANISM OF ACTION

Several theories purport to explain the mechanisms of action involved in reflexology, but none of

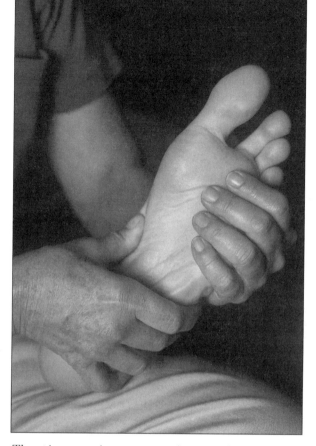

Therapist massaging pressure points on a foot. (Will and Deni McIntyre/Photo Researchers, Inc.)

these have been scientifically proven. Reflexologists propose that when invisible forces or energy fields in the body are blocked, illness can result. Reflexology promotes healing by stimulating the foot, which increases the flow of vital energy to various parts of the body. Reflexology may also promote healing by releasing endorphins, which are natural pain killers in the body. Reflexology could also stimulate nerve circuits and promote lymphatic flow.

According to the beliefs of reflexologists, energy travels from the foot to the spine, where it is released to the rest of the body. They believe that reflexology releases endorphins and detoxifies the body by dissolving uric acid crystals in the feet. Some reflexologists maintain that a tender or gritty area of the foot or hand reflects a current or past disease in the organ linked to that area.

SCIENTIFIC EVIDENCE

Available scientific evidence does not support claims that reflexology cures any disease. However, it has been shown to help promote relaxation and reduce pain in some people. The vast majority of what is written about reflexology is anecdotal or from small uncontrolled studies. Of the more than three thousand citations found on PubMed (a medical literature database) with reference to reflexology, only one was a randomized clinical trial. That study compared two groups of persons with multiple sclerosis: one receiving reflexology and the other a sham (fake) treatment. The study concluded that reflexology treatment provided statistically significant improvements in motor, sensory, and urinary symptoms.

A 2003 study looked at persons with cancer pain and found that reflexology seemed to help symptoms for a short time. However, the effects were gone three hours after the treatment was completed. A recheck at twenty-four hours showed no difference between the groups. A 2007 study of eighty-six people with metastatic cancer compared reflexology administered by patients' partners with reading to patients by their partners. The reflexology group reported less anxiety and less pain. Early evidence suggests foot reflexology may help manage some pain and fatigue in persons with cancer.

Reflexology may also reduce anxiety and improve general quality of life in persons with cancer. However, some studies have shown that reflexology is no better than foot massage in palliative cancer care. Reflexology may help relieve nausea, vomiting, and fatigue in persons with breast cancer receiving chemotherapy. However, further research is needed before a recommendation can be made.

A 2002 study looked at symptoms of menopause in women. All the women in the study received either a reflexology treatment or a placebo foot massage. Participants reported improved menopausal symptoms; no difference was seen between the foot massage and reflexology groups. Reflexology may relieve premenstrual symptoms or menstrual problems; however, more research is necessary to reach a firm conclusion. Research suggests that reflexology also may have beneficial effects in women with urinary incontinence.

In a Danish study in the early 1990s, 220 people with migraine headaches or tension headaches were evaluated. Eighty-one percent of the participants said they were helped by reflexology. Nineteen percent of those who had been taking medication were able to stop after six months of reflexology treatments. However, because there was no control group, scientists who conducted the study cautioned that the patients' improved well-being could have been caused by other factors. Reflexology may relieve migraines or tension headaches and may reduce the need for pain medications, but, researchers concluded, further study is needed to determine the benefits, if any, of reflexology.

Reflexology may be useful for relaxation, reducing stress, or relieving anxiety related to other medical problems or surgeries. However, it is not clear if reflexology is better than (or equal to) massage or other types of physical manipulation. Research has been inconclusive.

It is not clear if reflexology can help treat bowel problems. One small, controlled clinical trial showed reflexology to be an effective method of treating encopresis (fecal incontinence) and constipation over a six-week period, but further research is needed to confirm these results.

Positive results have been noted when a number of conditions were treated with reflexology. Preliminary research reports that reflexology is a preferred therapy in women with ankle and foot edema in late pregnancy. Early studies suggest that reflexology may help with overall well-being in pregnant women. However, reflexology does not appear to relieve symptoms such as bloating. Further research is needed before reflexology can be recommended for problems related to pregnancy.

Reflexology may possibly help manage type 2 diabetes in some persons, but more clinical trials are necessary to determine whether it is an effective treatment for diabetes. Early research suggests that reflexology may speed recovery after surgery. However, persons who received reflexology also tended to have poorer-quality sleep. It is unclear whether reflexology can benefit persons with lung diseases. Some research suggests that it may reduce fatigue and insomnia in coal miners with lung disease. Preliminary evidence suggests that reflexology is not helpful for chronic lower back pain. Better research is needed to make a firm conclusion.

CHOOSING A PRACTITIONER

One should so some research before choosing a reflexologist. The goal is to find a practitioner who has been properly trained and who has adequate

Headache Pain

William H. Fitzgerald and coauthor Edwin F. Bowers, in their book Zone Therapy: or, Relieving Pain at Home *(1917), discuss how to treat one's own headaches with reflexology, which was then called zone therapy. An excerpt from their discussion is provided here.*

The next time you have a headache, instead of attempting to paralyze the nerves of sensation with an opiate, or a coal tar "pain-deadener," push the headache out through the top of the head. It's surprisingly easy.

It merely requires that you press your thumb—or, better still, some smooth, broad metal surface, as the end of a knife-handle—firmly against the roof of the mouth, as nearly as possible under the battleground—and hold it there for from three to five minutes—by the watch. It may be necessary, if the ache is extensive, to shift the position of the thumb or metal "applicator" so as to "cover" completely the area that aches.

Headaches and neuralgias, of purely nervous origin, not due to poison from toxic absorption from the bowels, or to constipation, or alcoholism, tumors, eye-strain, or some specific organic cause, usually subside under this pressure within a few minutes. . . .

Many patients cure their own or their friend's and relative's headaches or neuralgic attacks in this manner. In their own headaches they use their right or left thumb—depending upon whether they are right- or left-handed. In treating others, they use the first and second fingers, pressing firmly under the seat of pain.

experience. Asking friends, family, and other health care providers for referrals is a good way to find a reflexologist. One can also visit the Web sites of professional associations, which provide information on reflexology. One should be sure to ask practitioners about their training and certification and should seek a nationally certified reflexologist, one who not only has trained at an accredited institution but also has passed a national board examination.

SAFETY ISSUES

As with massage and other forms of bodywork, reflexology can generally be adapted to meet the needs of persons with cancer, for example. Deep pressure and vigorous manipulation of the foot should be avoided during times of active treatment for cancer or if the person has edema in the foot or lower leg. It is recommended that persons with cancer not have pressure applied directly to known tumor sites or to lumps that may be cancerous. People with cancer that has spread to the bone or who have fragile bones should avoid physical manipulation or deep pressure because of the risk of fracture. Bodywork should be provided by a trained professional with expertise in working safely with people who have or had cancer.

People with recent or healing fractures, unhealed wounds, or active gout affecting the foot should avoid reflexology. A person who has osteoarthritis affecting the ankle or foot or who has severe circulation problems in the legs or feet should seek medical consultation before starting reflexology. People with chronic conditions such as arthritis and heart disease should talk to their doctors before having any type of therapy that involves moving joints and muscles. Relying on this type of treatment alone and avoiding or delaying conventional medical care may have serious health consequences.

Gerald W. Keister, M.S.

FURTHER READING

Carter, M., and T. Weber. *Hand Reflexology: Key to Perfect Health.* Paramus, N.J.: Prentice Hall, 2000. This book guides the reader step by step through finger-pressure techniques to send relief to the sources of pain and discomfort. Presented in easy-to-understand language. Contains more than one hundred illustrations.

Dougans, I. *The New Reflexology: A Unique Blend of Traditional Chinese Medicine and Western Reflexology Practice for Better Health and Healing.* New York: Marlowe, 2006. Clearly explains why meridians are essential for reflexology and how to use meridian therapy and the five elements for assessment and treatment.

Seager, A. *Reflexology and Associated Aspects of Health: A Practitioner's Guide.* Berkeley, Calif.: North Atlantic Books, 2005. Written in a user-friendly style, this book is of interest not only to reflexologists but also to a wide range of complementary medicine therapists and to general readers interested in these therapies.

Tiran, D., and P. A. Mackereth. *Clinical Reflexology: A Guide for Integrated Practice.* New York: Churchill Livingstone/Elsevier, 2011. Contains detailed presentations of clinical reflexology and applications for clinical practice.

Wright, J. *Reflexology and Acupressure: Pressure Points for Healing.* Summertown, Tenn.: Hamlyn and Healthy Living, 2003. This book presents basic techniques and easy-to-follow therapies involving both reflexology and acupressure.

See also: Acupressure; Acupuncture; Craniosacral therapy; Energy medicine; Manipulative and body-based practices; Massage therapy; Mind-body medicine; Pain management; Rolfing; Shiatsu; Therapeutic touch.

Regulation of CAM

CATEGORY: Organizations and legislation

DEFINITION: Oversight of complementary and alternative medicine products and therapies to ensure safety and efficacy for health care consumers.

OVERVIEW

Systems of rules and guidelines comprise the legal framework enforced by institutions to regulate economics, politics, and many other aspects of modern society. While all legal systems deal with comparable basic issues, each respective country recognizes, classifies, and interprets its legal components and topics differently. Typically, the purpose of a law is to restrict and control harm to others by serving as a social mediator among the parties involved. Thus, focusing on public protection, which includes patient and health consumer safety, governments regulate affairs in the public health arena and in the care provided by health professionals.

Consumers appropriately want to have confidence in their health professionals, whether those professionals are practicing conventional Western medicine or complementary alternative medicine (CAM). When people need care, they entrust themselves to doctors, nurses, and a whole range of other trained health care professionals, including CAM practitioners. People want to know that their trust is appropriately placed and that they will not be mistreated or harmed. The preservation of trust is the foundation for the care provided. Through regulation and oversight, a framework of guidelines, rules, and controls are built into the system to maintain patient safety and efficacy of treatments, products, therapies, and practices.

CAM is a $34 billion annual industry, according the 2007 National Health Survey conducted by the Centers for Disease Control and Prevention's National Center for Health Statistics. Most of this spending for therapies, products, office visits, classes, and relaxation techniques is not covered by health insurance in the United States. The safety and efficacy of these products and therapies are not the only pressing issues that require regulatory attention.

Despite CAM's popularity, strong debates surround its practice because of the unclear nature of some of its therapies and because of the broad array of claims different practitioners make. Some of the ingredients and claims of natural products and practices contribute to greater controversy because of the lack of formal quality standards and clinical trials, which are normally expected by the scientific community.

Although CAM use has been rising around the world through the years, the evolution of CAM regulation has been ineffective, failing to keep up with the expansion of its use, demands, and needs. Generally, existing CAM regulatory models have either been absent or been inadequate. CAM advocates defend consumer freedom and their right to have access to healing alternatives compatible with their own values, beliefs, and philosophies toward health and life. However, government regulators are still trying to find a regulatory balance to protect consumers from negative outcomes, adulteration, or misbranding of products or therapies. At the same time, regulators are trying to avoid limiting access to holistic, nonbiomedical therapies.

FEDERAL LEGAL AUTHORITY

The U.S. Food and Drug Administration (FDA) issued the "Guidance for Industry: Complementary and Alternative Medicine Products and Their Regulation by the Food and Drug Administration" (2006) in response to the increased use of CAM practices and products in the United States. This document also addresses rising public confusion about whether certain therapies or products used are subject to regulation.

"The Guidance" has two main regulatory points. First, a CAM product might be subject to regulation as a drug, a biological or cosmetic device, or a food (including food additives and dietary supplements) under the Federal Food, Drug and Cosmetic (FFDC) Act or the Public Health Service (PHS) Act. These statutory classifications cover several CAM products.

Second, neither FFDC nor PHS relieves CAM products from regulation. As the FDA receives its laws from the U.S. Congress, it has legal authority based on the legal tools Congress has given the agency. In deciding law-science issues, FDA efforts are based on sound scientific rationale related to ensuring safe therapies and products for consumers, while balancing access to the highest reasonable standard of health.

The FFDC is a federal law enacted by Congress that establishes the legal framework for how the FDA works. The FFDC is found in the United States Code (starting at 21 U.S.C. 301). The FDA develops regulations based on the laws under which it operates. The agency, guided by the Administrative Procedure Act (a federal law), follows procedures to issue its regulations. FDA regulations are also federal laws, although they are not part of the FFDC. FDA regulations are found in Title 21 of the Code of Federal Regulations. The agency adheres to procedures in its "Good Guidance Practice." Guidelines, however, are not legally binding.

Some CAM advocates oppose any legal intervention in their affairs, considering guidances and regulations to be governmental restrictions. Regulation critics state that the FDA's criteria for experimental evaluation methods are orthodox and that it obstructs CAM practioners attempting to bring valuable and effective treatments to the public. CAM advocates argue that their contributions and breakthroughs are often unjustly dismissed, unnoted, or stifled. CAM providers acknowledge that health fraud does occur, and they agree that it should be appropriately addressed and curtailed. However, they also argue that restrictive regulations should not spread to valid CAM health practices and products.

STANDARDS AND SCIENCE-BASED REGULATION

Conventional biomedical drugs obtain FDA market approval only after clinical trials establish their efficacy. Safety testing is another legal requirement. Biopharmaceutical manufacturing standards are strictly regulated to guarantee a given medicine has uniform and standard quantity, identity, purity, and strength of an active ingredient in its formulation, and that it is not contaminated or adulterated. Because alternative health products are not governed by the same quality-control standards as non-CAM products, one might see inconsistencies among doses. As result, CAM products are susceptible to contamination, adulteration, misbranding, and fraud.

Because there are no global, harmonized CAM regulatory guidelines, world commerce amplifies the problem, as each country may or may not have its own quality standards, levels of regulation, and legal authority to enforce compliance. The FDA believes that all of this puts consumers in an unfair and difficult position: how to properly evaluate the risks and qualities of natural treatments.

CAM proponents assure consumers that their healing therapies are natural, harmless, and effective. From the CAM perspective, regulations personify a dividing model within the healing arts flanked by traditional medicine and unconventional health care. Proponents argue that the law endorses and favors biomedicine. Some CAM promoters state that guidance language is confusing to the consumer and is unconstitutional. They are concerned that regulations are restricting access to natural therapies. Proponents want the FDA to better articulate the equilibrium between consumer protection and consumer freedom.

REGULATION OF CAM THERAPIES

The National Center for Complementary and Alternative Medicine (NCCAM) is part of the National Institutes of Health (NIH). The FDA's CAM guidance expanded on the CAM categories of NCCAM for its development and issuance. The five major regulated categories are whole medical systems, mind-body medicine, biologically based practices, manipulative and body-based practices, and energy medicine. The intended use of a product plays a vital role in the way it is regulated. Therefore, when a product satisfies the statutory definition of a drug, device, food, or biological product, it will face regulation under FFDC or PHS, or both.

Manufacturers of natural goods as well as holistic practitioners cannot promote their products or services as cures or treatments. They are allowed only to claim that the products or practices may promote a specific outcome. They also must include on the product's label or on a practitioner's advertisement an FDA disclaimer. Likewise, there is no assurance that natural goods are consistently formulated to guarantee strength, amount, and purity of the active ingredient in each dose. When using health therapies, choosing a suitable manufacturer is vital to confirm safety, intended use, and end result.

FUTURE CHALLENGES AND GOALS

CAM regulation affects a number of constituents, including health care providers trying to reduce the legal risks of integrating CAM into their biomedical practices; FDA officials and judges, attorneys, and legislators; credentialing and licensing agencies and organizations that standardize CAM-practice qualifications; consumers and patients hoping to access available wellness options; and insurers, clinics, and hospitals striving to integrate CAM therapies in health plans. As the FDA's guidance is relatively young, these constituent groups are reshaping the developing legal authority for the coexistence of the safe and effective exercise of integrated health care. The FDA pursues a scientific regulatory model.

For CAM proponents, an ideal future includes forward-thinking regulation that sustains a broad, non-biomedical, holistic, and neutral move that embraces wellness alternatives. The type of regulation needed will help integrate biomedicine and CAM so that consumers will be protected from fraudulent and dangerous therapies.

Ana Maria Rodriguez-Rojas, M.S.

FURTHER READING

Astin, J. A. "Why Patients Use Alternative Medicine." *Journal of the American Medical Association* 279 (1998): 1548-1553. Provides survey results of a study assessing what prompts consumers to use alternative medicine.

Briggs, J. P., and R. L. Nahin. "Cost of Complementary and Alternative Medicine and Frequency of Visits to CAM Practitioners." Atlanta: Centers for Disease Control and Prevention, 2007. Results from the National Health Survey of 2007 regarding CAM-related spending in the United States.

Cohen, M. H., and K. J. Kemper. "Complementary Therapies in Pediatrics: A Legal Perspective." *Pediatrics* 115, no. 3 (2005): 774-780. Examines the legal considerations of CAM therapies for pediatric patients.

Eisenberg, D. M., et al. "Credentialing Complementary and Alternative Medical Providers." *Annals of Internal Medicine* 137, no. 12 (2002): 965-973. A review discussing the status and mechanisms of licensing and the establishment of standards of practice to protect patients.

Fontanarosa, P. B., and G. D. Lundberg. "Alternative Medicine Meets Science." *Journal of the American Medical Association* 280 (1998): 1618-1619. An editorial that promotes scientific evidence-based methods for determining quality medicines and therapies.

Hutt, Peter B., Richard A. Merrill, and Lewis A. Grossman. *Food and Drug Law: Cases and Materials.* 3d ed. New York: Foundation Press, 2007. A brief account of the FDA's administrative law. Deals with governmental attempts to protect public health and individual welfare in the development and marketing of essential products.

National Center for Complementary and Alternative Medicine. "Statistics on CAM Costs: 2007 National Health Interview Survey." Available at http://nccam.nih.gov/news/camstats/costs. Provides statistics on CAM costs in the United States from the 2007 National Health Survey.

U.S. Food and Drug Administration. "Guidance for Industry on Complementary and Alternative Medicine Products and Their Regulation by the Food and Drug Administration." Rockville, Md.: Author, December, 2006. The first FDA guidance on CAM in the United States.

See also: CAM on PubMed; Codex Alimentarius Commission; Dietary Supplement Health and Education Act of 1994; Education and training of CAM practitioners; Food and Drug Administration; Health freedom movement; Insurance coverage; Internet and CAM; Licensing and certification for CAM practitioners; National Center for Complementary and Alternative Medicine; Office of Dietary Supplements; Popular practitioners; Pseudoscience; Scientific method.

Reiki

CATEGORY: Therapies and techniques
DEFINITION: Spiritual healing that involves holding hands in certain positions over parts of the body to improve energy flow.
PRINCIPAL PROPOSED USES: None
OTHER PROPOSED USES: Increasing wellness, treating diseases of all types

OVERVIEW

The Japanese word *reiki* can be translated as "life-force energy." The term refers to a form of spiritual healing that involves holding one's hands above another's body. Many people have taken training in Reiki, and the service is provided in a variety of settings. However, there is no scientific foundation in support of Reiki's effectiveness for any purpose.

History of Reiki. There are two principal stories regarding the origin of Reiki. In both versions, the method was invented in Japan by Mikao Usui. Many Reiki practitioners in the United States believe that Usui was a Christian monk who invented the technique in the mid-nineteenth century. However, according to the more traditional Japanese schools of Reiki, Usui was a member of a Japanese spiritual organization called Rei Jyutsu Ka, and he developed the technique around 1915. (The story that he was a Christian may have been invented to facilitate the acceptance of Reiki in the West.) Both versions of Reiki's history agree that Usui based his technique on methods and philosophies drawn from numerous traditional Asian healing methods.

After Usui's death, various forms of Reiki continued to be taught by his students. One of these students, Chujiro Hayashi, systematized Reiki into three levels and added many hand movements to the technique. In turn, one of Hayashi's students, Hawayo Takata, brought Reiki to the United States.

In the early 1980s, Takata's granddaughter, Phyllis Furumoto, took on the mantle of Hayashi and Takata's line of Reiki and popularized it widely in the West. However, many other forms of Reiki continue to exist, descending through different lineages of teachers. There are considerable differences between the various approaches, and certain groups strongly challenge the validity of others.

What is Reiki? Most types of Asian medicine make use of the concept of qi, a form of vital energy that flows through the body. Free-flowing, abundant qi is said to create health, while stagnant or deficient qi is thought to lead to illness. Reiki practitioners believe that they can improve this energy by holding their hands in certain positions over parts of a person's body; advanced practitioners believe they can produce this effect from a distance. The net result, according to the theory, is accelerated healing and increased wellness.

In many ways, Reiki resembles therapeutic touch, except that the instructions given to its practitioners are more specific. A certified practitioner of Reiki has spent time learning specified hand movements and positions and has also undergone an "attunement" to an already-certified Reiki practitioner. This chain of attunements goes back to Usui, the method's founder.

In its most popular Western form, Reiki is learned in three stages. The first stage involves an attunement

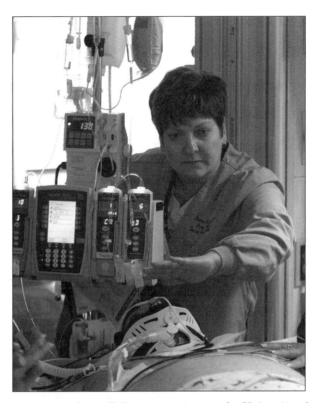

A nurse performs Reiki on a patient at the University of Maryland Medical Center in Baltimore. (AP Photo)

that permits physical healing. The second stage grants the ability to carry out healing over a distance. The third degree of training allows the practitioner to perform healing on a spiritual level and to give attunements to students. Generally, each level is obtained by paying a fee and completing a weekend course.

USES AND APPLICATIONS

Reiki is promoted as a treatment that can accelerate physical, emotional, or spiritual healing in every conceivable situation. It is used as a support for conventional medical care, rather than as a replacement for it.

SCIENTIFIC EVIDENCE

The only truly meaningful way to determine whether a medical therapy works is to perform a double-blind, placebo-controlled trial. For hands-on therapies such as Reiki, however, a truly double-blind study is not possible; the Reiki practitioner will inevitably know whether he or she is administering real

Reiki Training, Licensing, and Certification

No special background or credentials are needed to receive training in the practice of Reiki. However, Reiki must be learned from an experienced teacher or a Reiki master; it cannot be self-taught. The specific techniques taught can vary greatly.

Training in traditional Reiki has three degrees (levels), each focusing on a different aspect of practice. Each degree includes one or more initiations (also called attunements or empowerments). Receiving an initiation is believed to activate the ability to access Reiki energy. Training for first- and second-degree practice is typically given in eight to twelve class hours in about two days. In first-degree training, students learn to perform Reiki on themselves and on others. In second-degree training, students learn to perform Reiki on others from a distance. Some students seek master-level (third-degree) training. A Reiki master can teach and initiate students. Becoming a master can take years of practice.

Reiki practitioners' training and expertise vary. Increasingly, many people who seek training are licensed health care professionals. However, no licensing or professional standards exist for the practice of Reiki.

Reiki rather than fake Reiki. The best that can be hoped for is a single-blind study in which participants do not know whether they received real or fake Reiki and in which the medical outcome is evaluated by an observer who also does not know who is or is not receiving real Reiki and is, therefore, "blinded."

In a 2008 review of nine randomized-controlled trials on the effectiveness of Reiki for various purposes, researchers stated that no firm conclusions could be drawn from any of these studies. In a subsequent controlled trial, one hundred persons with fibromyalgia received Reiki or direct-touch therapy from either a true Reiki master or an actor posing as a Reiki master. There was no difference in symptom improvement between the two groups. In one review of three Reiki studies, researchers found that more experienced practitioners appeared to have a greater effect on pain reduction. This observation could not be explained.

A simpler study design compares Reiki to no treatment. However, studies of this type cannot provide reliable evidence about the efficacy of a treatment: If

a benefit is seen, there is no way to determine whether it was caused by Reiki specifically or just by attention generally. (Attention alone will almost always produce some reported benefit.)

Finally, there are many case reports in which people are given Reiki and then seem to improve. Such reports do not mean anything scientifically; numerous people receiving placebo in placebo-controlled studies also seem to improve. Thus, such reports cannot say anything about whether Reiki itself offers any benefit.

In one study, female nursing students received either real Reiki or a placebo form of the treatment called mimic Reiki. Before-and-after tests failed to find any improvement in general well-being attributable to Reiki treatment.

In another study, researchers evaluated the effectiveness of Reiki (with a related technique called LeShan) in twenty-one people undergoing oral surgery for impacted wisdom teeth. Each participant received two surgeries, one with Reiki and the other without (in random order). People reported less pain when they received Reiki than when they received no treatment; however, because of the lack of a fake treatment group, the results mean little.

Choosing a Practitioner

There are several competing organizations that issue certifications to Reiki practitioners. These include the Reiki Alliance, the Reiki Foundation, and the Awareness Institute.

Safety Issues

There are no known or proposed safety risks with Reiki unless a person chooses to use Reiki instead of, rather than as a support to, standard medical care.

EBSCO CAM Review Board

Further Reading

Assefi, N., et al. "Reiki for the Treatment of Fibromyalgia." *Journal of Alternative and Complementary Medicine* 14 (2008): 1115-1122.

Lee, M. S., M. H. Pittler, and E. Ernst. "Effects of Reiki in Clinical Practice." *International Journal of Clinical Practice* 62 (2008): 947-954.

Richeson, N. E., et al. "Effects of Reiki on Anxiety, Depression, Pain, and Physiological Factors in Community-Dwelling Older Adults." *Research in Gerontological Nursing* 3 (2010): 187-199.

So, P. S., Y. Jiang, and Y. Qin. "Touch Therapies for Pain Relief in Adults." *Cochrane Database of Systematic Reviews* (2008): CD006535. Available through *EBSCO DynaMed Systematic Literature Surveillance* at http://www.ebscohost.com/dynamed.

Thornton, L. C. "A Study of Reiki, an Energy Field Treatment, Using Rogers' Science." *Rogerian Nursing Science News* 8 (1996): 14-15.

See also: Manipulative and body-based therapies; Massage therapy; Metamorphic technique; Pain management; Qigong; Therapeutic touch.

Reishi

CATEGORY: Herbs and supplements
RELATED TERM: *Ganoderma lucidum*
DEFINITION: Natural plant product used to treat specific health conditions.
PRINCIPAL PROPOSED USE: Adaptogen (improve resistance to stress)
OTHER PROPOSED USES: Altitude sickness, autoimmune diseases, cancer prevention, cancer treatment, diabetes, enhancing mental function, high blood pressure, immune support, insomnia, multiple sclerosis, ulcers, viral infections

OVERVIEW

The tree fungus known as reishi has a long history of use in China and Japan as a semimagical healing

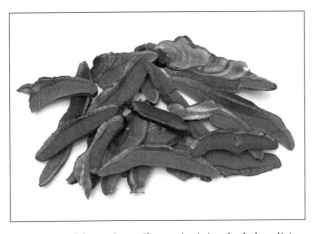

Reishi is used for various ailments in Asian herbal medicine. (Scimat/Photo Researchers, Inc.)

herb. It is more revered than ginseng and, up until recently, was more rare. Many stories tell of people with severe illnesses journeying immense distances to find it. Today, reishi is artificially cultivated and widely available in stores that sell herbal products.

THERAPEUTIC DOSAGES

The usual dosage of reishi is 2 to 6 grams (g) per day of raw fungus, or an equivalent dosage of concentrated extract, taken with meals. In traditional Chinese medicine, reishi is often combined with related fungi, such as shiitake, hoelen, or polyporus. It is often taken continually for its presumed overall health benefits.

THERAPEUTIC USES

Reishi (like its fungi cousins maitake, *Coriolus versicolor*, and shiitake) is marketed as a kind of cure-all said to strengthen immunity, help prevent cancer, and also possibly treat cancer as well. It is also said to be useful for autoimmune diseases (such as myasthenia gravis and multiple sclerosis), viral infections, high blood pressure, diabetes, altitude sickness, ulcers, and insomnia; enhancement of mental function is another claim made.

SCIENTIFIC EVIDENCE

While there has been a great deal of basic scientific research into the chemical constituents of reishi, reliable double-blind, placebo-controlled studies are all but nonexistent. Test-tube studies indicate that reishi has immunomodulatory effects. This means that reishi may affect the immune system, but not necessarily that it strengthens it. (Alternative medicine proponents often blur the difference between these two ideas.) However, one small double-blind, placebo-controlled human trial failed to find any significant immunomodulatory effects. Other weak evidence hints that reishi may have chemopreventive properties, suggesting that it may help prevent cancer. However, a great many substances fight cancer in the test tube, while few actually help people with the disease.

Other highly preliminary forms of evidence suggest that reishi may have antiviral effects and possibly antibacterial effects too. However, it is a long way from studies of this type to meaningful clinical uses.

Contemporary herbalists regard reishi as an adaptogen, a substance believed to be capable of helping the body resist stress of all kinds. However, there is no meaningful evidence to support this claim.

One questionable double-blind study performed in China reportedly found reishi helpful for neurasthenia. The term "neurasthenia" is seldom used in modern medicine; it generally indicates fatigue due to psychological causes.

SAFETY ISSUES

Because it is used as a food in Asia, reishi is generally regarded as safe. One small study evaluating the safety of reishi when taken at a dose of 2 g daily for ten days failed to find any evidence of ill effects. However, another study found indications that reishi impairs blood clotting. For this reason, prudence suggests that individuals with bleeding problems should avoid reishi; the herb should also be avoided in the periods just before and after surgery or labor and delivery. Furthermore, individuals taking medications that impair blood clotting, such as aspirin, warfarin (Coumadin), heparin, clopidogrel (Plavix), pentoxifylline (Trental), or ticlopidine (Ticlid), should use reishi only under a doctor's supervision. Finally, the safety of reishi in young children, pregnant or nursing women, and those with severe liver or kidney disease has not been established.

IMPORTANT INTERACTIONS

Persons who are taking blood-thinning medications, such as aspirin, warfarin (Coumadin), heparin, clopidogrel (Plavix), pentoxifylline (Trental), or ticlopidine (Ticlid), should use reishi only under a doctor's supervision.

EBSCO CAM Review Board

FURTHER READING

Bao, X. F., X. S. Wang, et al. "Structural Features of Immunologically Active Polysaccharides from *Ganoderma lucidum*." *Phytochemistry* 59 (2002): 175-181.

Bao, X. F., Y. Zhen, L. Ruan, and J. N. Fang. "Purification, Characterization, and Modification of T Lymphocyte-Stimulating Polysaccharide from Spores of *Ganoderma lucidum*." *Chemical and Pharmaceutical Bulletin* (Tokyo) 50 (2002): 623-629.

Eo, S. K., et al. "Antiviral Activities of Various Water- and Methanol-Soluble Substances Isolated from *Ganoderma lucidum*." *Journal of Ethnopharmacology* 68 (1999): 129-136.

Min, B. S., et al. "Triterpenes from the Spores of *Ganoderma lucidum* and Their Cytotoxicity Against Meth-A and LLC Tumor Cells." *Chemical and Pharmaceutical Bulletin* (Tokyo) 48 (2000): 1026-1033.

Wang, Y. Y., et al. "Studies on the Immuno-modulating and Antitumor Activities of *Ganoderma lucidum* (Reishi) Polysaccharides: Functional and Proteomic Analyses of a Fucose-Containing Glycoprotein Fraction Responsible for the Activities." *Bioorganic and Medicinal Chemistry* 10 (2002): 1057-1062.

Wu, T. S., L. S. Shi, and S. C. Kuo. "Cytotoxicity of *Ganoderma lucidum* Triterpenes." *Journal of Natural Products* 64 (2001): 1121-1122.

Zhang, J., et al. "Activation of B Lymphocytes by GLIS, a Bioactive Proteoglycan from *Ganoderma lucidum*." *Life Sciences* 71 (2002): 623-638.

See also: Altitude sickness; Cancer risk reduction; Cancer treatment support; Diabetes; Ginseng; Hypertension; Insomnia; Multiple sclerosis; Stress; Ulcers.

Relaxation response

CATEGORY: Therapies and techniques
RELATED TERMS: Integrative medicine, meditation, mind/body medicine, stress reduction
DEFINITION: A self-induced, peaceful, relaxed mental state attained through various techniques.
PRINCIPAL PROPOSED USES: Anxiety, coping, pain, mental and physical stress

OVERVIEW

Herbert Benson, a graduate of Harvard Medical School and director emeritus at Benson-Henry Institute for Mind Body Medicine at Massachusetts General Hospital, published the book *The Relaxation Response* in 1975. The book includes data produced from research Benson conducted at Harvard's Thorndike Memorial Laboratory and at Beth Israel Hospital in Boston. Walter B. Cannon, another researcher who was at Harvard Medical School in the 1920s, had identified what he called the fight-or-flight physical response to stress on body and mind. Cannon found that perceived and actual life-threatening situations produced a flood of stress hormones to prepare a person to fight (confront the situation) or to flee. In such situations the heart pounds, breathing accelerates, and blood flow to the muscles is increased. This response is basically a survival mechanism, a natural physical response elicited when a person's life is endangered.

Frequent situations in daily life, such as traffic jams, waiting in lines, financial difficulties, and family problems, also produce stress-related hormones that over time can take a toll on the body. The relaxation response was developed as a mechanism to counteract this hormonal response to stress.

Benson's therapy was not new, and it was based on the age-old practices and philosophies of Transcendental Meditation (TM). For relaxation response, these practices are simplified and can be performed by anyone. To elicit the response, Benson offers the following instructions: Find a quiet, peaceful environment for practice; muscles should be consciously relaxed; a word such as "one" or "peace," or a phrase, possibly a prayer, should be repeated silently in the mind; any intrusive thoughts should be observed only and then passively dismissed; and breathing should be slow and deep. Benson advises practicing this technique from ten to twenty minutes each day. The process is quite individualized, however, and no single method works for everyone. Other techniques may be equally effective, such as running, yoga, knitting, dance, or playing a musical instrument.

By studying the effects of stress on the human body and the various techniques to counteract them, Benson demonstrated the connection of mind and body and how this connection affects health and well-being. His continuing research includes the possible clinical uses of the response in medicine and psychiatry.

MECHANISM OF ACTION

The release of fight-or-flight hormones when a person is no longer threatened is counteracted through natural activation of the parasympathetic nervous system. Findings from research conducted at Harvard Medical School in the late 1960s showed that Transcendental Meditation could produce profound physiologic changes that were opposite to those produced by stress. Metabolism, blood pressure, heart rate, and rate of breathing could all be decreased. TM and the relaxation response work in essentially the same way and, when practiced, allow the practitioner to counteract stress voluntarily.

USES AND APPLICATIONS

The relaxation response may be practiced at will to counteract stress inherent in daily life, to reduce general stress levels and discomfort, to reduce levels of pain or distress in illness, and to alleviate physical symptoms of stress on the body. Continuing research has broadened possible applications to uses such as reducing stress and improving cognition in healthy aging adults, improving productivity in workers, reducing pain in people with chronic diseases such as human immunodeficiency virus or acquired immune deficiency syndrome (HIV/AIDS) and arthritis, and improving academic performance.

SCIENTIFIC EVIDENCE

A body of scientific evidence exists from continuing research by Benson, his associates, and others. Much of this research has been conducted at Harvard Medical School, Harvard's Thorndike Memorial Laboratory, and the Benson-Henry Institute for Mind Body Medicine.

The practice of meditation has been shown by magnetic resonance imaging to activate neural structures involved in attention and control of the autonomic nervous system. Measurably lower oxygen consumption, heart rate, respiration, and blood lactate indicate a decrease in activity of the sympathetic nervous system, resulting in a restful, or hypometabolic, state. This is the opposite of the increased activity, or hypermetabolic state, produced by stress.

Double-blind studies have been conducted with varying results. One study tried to determine if combining acupuncture treatments with the relaxation response could improve quality of life for persons with human immunodeficiency virus infection or acquired immune deficiency syndrome. Conclusions from the pilot trial confirmed the benefits of combined therapies for some measures of improved quality of life. Although skeptics remain, research is continuing on possible uses of the relaxation response in medicine and psychiatry using improved research tools and methods.

CHOOSING A PRACTITIONER

The relaxation response can be self-taught and does not require a practitioner. Classes, meditation groups, and many instruction books are available for the person who wishes to learn the technique.

SAFETY ISSUES

There are no identified safety issues with the practice of the relaxation response. Benson has warned, however, that if it is used as a medical treatment, it should be practiced only with the knowledge and approval of, and under the supervision of, a qualified physician.

Martha O. Loustaunau, Ph.D.

FURTHER READING

Benson, H. "The Relaxation Response: Its Subjective and Objective Historical Precedents and Physiology." *Trends in Neurosciences* 6 (1983): 281-284. Discusses research at Harvard's Thorndike Memorial Laboratory in defining the physiology and in describing the subjective and objective historical precedents and clinical usefulness of the relaxation response.

_____, and M. Klipper. *The Relaxation Response.* New York: William Morrow, 1975. Benson's explanation and synthesis of research on the relaxation response, based on historical, religious, and literary writings, with related scientific data from research conducted by Benson and associates. This work was expanded and updated in 2000, citing additional information on updated research.

Lazar, S., et al. "Functional Brain Mapping of the Relaxation Response and Meditation." *NeuroReport* 11 (2000): 1581-1585. Discusses how magnetic resonance imaging shows that the practice of meditation activates neural structures affecting attention and control of the autonomic nervous system.

See also: Autogenic training; Hypnotherapy; Meditation; Mind/body medicine; Progressive muscle relaxation; Relaxation therapies; Stress; Transcendental Meditation.

Relaxation therapies

CATEGORY: Therapies and techniques

RELATED TERMS: Autogenic training, guided imagery, guided visualizations, Jacobsen's relaxation technique, meditation, mindfulness meditation, progressive muscular relaxation, relaxation response, Transcendental Meditation

DEFINITION: Techniques to reduce everyday stress.

PRINCIPAL PROPOSED USES: Cancer chemotherapy support, chronic pain, hypertension, insomnia, stress, surgery support

OTHER PROPOSED USES: Angina, asthma, anxiety, back pain, bulimia nervosa, colds (prevention), congestive heart failure, depression, fibromyalgia, herpes prevention, human immunodeficiency virus infection support, immune support, interstitial cystitis, irritable bowel syndrome, menopause, migraine headaches, osteoarthritis, premenstrual syndrome, pregnancy support, psoriasis, rheumatoid arthritis, stroke rehabilitation, tension headaches, ulcerative colitis

OVERVIEW

Constant stress is one of the defining features of modern life and the source of many common health problems. Stress plays an obvious role in nervousness, anxiety, and insomnia, but it is also thought to contribute to a vast number of other illnesses.

In the past, most people engaged in many hours of physical exercise daily, an activity that reduces the effects of psychological stress. Life was also slower then and was more in harmony with the natural cycles of day and season. Today, however, a person is relatively sedentary, while the mind is forced to respond to the rapid pace of a society that never stops. The result is high levels of stress and a reduced ability to cope with that stress.

There are several ways to mitigate the damage caused by stress. Increased physical exercise can help, as can simple, commonsense steps such as taking relaxation breaks and vacations. If these approaches do not have adequate results, more formal methods may be helpful.

This article discusses a group of stress-reduction techniques often called relaxation therapies. In addition to these methods, other methods that can help include yoga, Tai Chi, hypnosis, massage, and biofeedback.

WHAT ARE RELAXATION THERAPIES?

There are many types of relaxation therapies, and they use a variety of techniques. However, most of them share certain related features.

In many relaxation techniques, one begins by either lying down or assuming a relaxed, seated posture in a quiet place and then closing the eyes. The next step differs depending on the method. In autogenic training, relaxation response, and certain forms of meditation, a person focuses his or her mind on internal sensations, such as the breath. Guided-imagery techniques employ deliberate visualization of scenes or actions, such as walking on a quiet beach. Progressive relaxation techniques involve gradual relaxation of the muscles. Finally, some schools of meditation incorporate the repetition of a phrase or sound silently or aloud.

All of these techniques are best learned with the aid of a trained practitioner. The usual format is a group class supplemented by regular home practice. If a person is diligent enough, experience suggests that he or she can develop the ability to call on a relaxed state at will, even in the middle of a very stressful situation.

USES AND APPLICATIONS

Relaxation therapies are most commonly tried in medical circumstances in which stress is believed to play a particularly large role. These circumstances include insomnia, surgery, chronic pain, and cancer chemotherapy. A specific form of guided visualization has also been used in an attempt to actually treat cancer.

SCIENTIFIC EVIDENCE

Although many studies have been performed on relaxation therapies, most of these studies are inadequately designed. To be fair, there are considerable difficulties in the path of any researcher who wishes to scientifically assess the effectiveness of a relaxation therapy such as hypnosis. There are several factors involved, but the most important is fairly fundamental: It is difficult to design a proper double-blind, placebo-controlled study of relaxation therapy. Researchers studying the herb St. John's wort, for example, can use placebo pills that are indistinguishable from the real thing. However, it is difficult to design a form of placebo relaxation therapy that cannot be detected as such by both practitioners and participants.

One clever method used by some researchers involves the use of intentionally neutral visualizations. Instead of imagining lying in bed and sleeping peacefully, participants in the placebo group might be told to visualize something like a green box. The problem here is that researchers teaching the visualization method to participants may inadvertently convey a sense of disbelief in the placebo treatment. This can be solved by using relatively untrained people who are

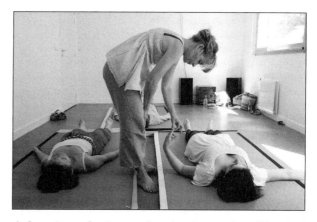

A therapist conductiong a relaxation therapy class. (Phanie/ Photo Researchers, Inc.)

themselves deceived by experimenters to teach the method, but the practical obstacles are significant.

For this reason, many studies of relaxation therapy have made major compromises to the double-blind, placebo-controlled model. Some randomly assigned participants receive either relaxation therapy or no treatment. In the best of these studies, results were rated by examiners who did not know which participants were in which group (in other words, the examiners were "blinded observers"). However, it is not clear whether benefits reported in such studies come from the relaxation therapy or from less specific factors, such as mere attention.

Other studies have compared relaxation therapies to different techniques, such as hypnosis or cognitive psychotherapy. However, the same difficulties arise when trying to study these latter therapies, and the results of a study that compares an unproven treatment to one that is also imperfectly documented are not very meaningful.

Even less meaningful studies of relaxation therapies simply involved giving people the therapy and monitoring them to see whether they improved. Such open-label trials prove nothing. Given these caveats, the following is a summary of what science knows about the medical benefits of relaxation therapy.

POSSIBLE BENEFITS

Insomnia. Numerous controlled studies have evaluated relaxation therapies for the treatment of insomnia. These studies are difficult to summarize because many involved therapy combined with other methods, such as biofeedback, sleep restriction, and paradoxical intent (trying not to sleep). The type of relaxation therapy used in the majority of these trials was progressive muscle relaxation. Many of these trials used the clever form of placebo treatment described in the foregoing section; others simply compared relaxation therapy to no treatment.

Overall, the evidence indicates that relaxation therapies may be somewhat helpful for insomnia, although not dramatically so. For example, in a controlled study of seventy people with insomnia, participants using progressive relaxation showed no meaningful improvement in the time to fall asleep or the duration of sleep, but they reported feeling more rested in the morning. In another study, twenty minutes of relaxation practice was required to increase sleeping time by thirty minutes.

Asthma. A review article published in 2002 found fifteen published controlled trials that evaluated relaxation therapies for the treatment of asthma. Most of the studies were rated as very poor or poor quality. Overall, the results failed to demonstrate improvement, although a muscular relaxation technique called Jacobsen's relaxation did show some benefit.

Anxiety. A fair amount of evidence supports relaxation therapies for treating the symptoms of anxiety, at least in the short term. In a 2008 review of twenty-seven studies, researchers concluded that relaxation therapies (including Jacobson's progressive relaxation, autogenic training, applied relaxation, and meditation) were effective against anxiety. However, not all of the studies were randomized, controlled trials.

Hypertension. It seems intuitive that relaxation should lower blood pressure. Indeed, many studies have evaluated the benefits of relaxation therapies for hypertension and related cardiovascular risks. The results, however, have been mixed at best.

In a review of twenty-five studies of various relaxation therapies for high blood pressure (with 1,198 participants), researchers found that those studies employing a control group had no significant effect on lowering blood pressure compared with sham (placebo) therapies. However, a separate review of nine randomized trials concluded that the regular use of Transcendental Meditation may significantly reduce both systolic and diastolic blood pressure compared with a control. Similarly, an analysis of seventeen randomized-controlled trials of various relaxation therapies found that only Transcendental Meditation resulted in significant reductions in blood pressure; biofeedback, progressive muscle relaxation, and stress management training produced no such benefit. In addition, a trial of eighty-six persons with hypertension suggested that daily, music-guided slow breathing reduced systolic blood pressure measured in a twenty-four-hour period.

Other conditions. Other conditions that have at least minimal supporting evidence for response to relaxation therapies include the following: angina, back pain, bulimia nervosa, cancer treatment support, including cancer pain, chronic pain, congestive heart failure, depression, fibromyalgia, interstitial cystitis, irritable bowel syndrome, menopause, obsessive-compulsive disorder, osteoarthritis, premenstrual syndrome, pregnancy support (reducing perceived stress), psoriasis, rheumatoid arthritis, stress, stroke rehabilitation, surgery support (primarily reducing pain and stress before or after surgery), tension headaches, and ulcerative colitis. In many cases the results are marginal at best, and contradictory outcomes between trials are common.

One study suggests that the use of visualizations before surgery not only reduces the need for pain medications but also reduces the chance of developing hematomas (collections of blood under the skin). However, more study is needed to verify this somewhat difficult-to-believe result. A more easily accepted study found that either relaxation therapy or aerobic exercise can improve symptoms of fatigue after cancer surgery, and that each approach is about as effective as the other.

Another study found that persons with cancer who were exposed to empathetic care along with self-hypnotic relaxation experienced significantly less pain and anxiety during an uncomfortable, invasive procedure than similar persons receiving only empathetic or usual care. These results suggest that pain under these circumstances is more effectively relieved when the patient relies on his or her own self-coping abilities rather than on another person's kindness.

Researchers in Taiwan have also studied the role of relaxing music in reducing cancer pain. Randomly selected were 126 hospitalized persons. In one group, participants listened to music for thirty minutes and were given pain medication; participants in the other group were given the medication only. The group that listened to music experienced significantly more pain relief than the group that did not.

Numerous studies have also investigated the benefits of relaxation therapies for persons with human immunodeficiency virus (HIV) infection. A careful review of thirty-five randomized trials found that relaxation therapies may be generally helpful in improving the quality of life of HIV-positive persons and in reducing their anxiety, depression, stress, and fatigue. These interventions, though, had no significant effect on the growth of the virus, nor did they influence immunologic or hormonal activity. Subsequently, however, a small study involving forty-eight HIV-positive persons found that mindfulness meditation, a popular method for inducing the relaxation response, slowed the loss of the specific immune cells destroyed by the virus, though more research needs to be done to confirm this result.

Some studies have evaluated highly specific guided visualizations, rather than general relaxation. For example, it has been suggested that a systematic program of imagining microscopic soldiers shooting down one's cancer cells can improve the chances of surviving cancer. Despite much enthusiasm, there is still no meaningful evidence to support this appealing idea. Nonetheless, there is some evidence from a set of small trials that specific immune-oriented visualizations can provide enhanced protection against herpes flare-ups and winter colds.

Contrary to common claims, published evidence does not demonstrate that Transcendental Meditation (TM) improves mental functioning. There is some evidence, however, that TM might be helpful for improving exercise capacity and general quality of life in people with congestive heart failure.

A careful review of twenty trials found psychological interventions such as cognitive behavioral therapy, biofeedback, relaxation, and coping were associated with reduced chronic headache or migraine pain in 589 children compared with sham (placebo), standard therapies, waiting list control, or other active treatments.

CHOOSING A PRACTITIONER

There is no widely accepted license for practicing relaxation therapy. However, it is often practiced by licensed therapists and psychologists.

SAFETY ISSUES

There are no known or proposed safety risks with relaxation therapies.

EBSCO CAM Review Board

FURTHER READING

Anderson, J. W., C. Liu, and R. J. Kryscio. "Blood Pressure Response to Transcendental Meditation." *American Journal of Hypertension* 21 (2008): 310-316.

Eccleston, C., et al. "Psychological Therapies for the Management of Chronic and Recurrent Pain in Children and Adolescents." *Cochrane Database of Systematic Reviews* (2009): CD003968. Available through *EBSCO DynaMed Systematic Literature Surveillance* at http://www.ebscohost.com/dynamed.

Hanstede, M., Y. Gidron, and I. Nyklicek. "The Effects of a Mindfulness Intervention on Obsessive-Compulsive Symptoms in a Non-clinical Student Population." *Journal of Nervous and Mental Disease* 196 (2008): 776-779.

Heather, O. D., et al. "Relaxation Therapies for the Management of Primary Hypertension in Adults." *Cochrane Database of Systematic Reviews* (2008): CD004935. *EBSCO DynaMed Systematic Literature Surveillance* at http://www.ebscohost.com/dynamed.

Huang, S. T., M. Good, and J. A. Zauszniewski. "The Effectiveness of Music in Relieving Pain in Cancer Patients." *International Journal of Nursing Studies* 47 (2010): 1354-1362.

Jayadevappa, R., et al. "Effectiveness of Transcendental Meditation on Functional Capacity and Quality of Life of African Americans with Congestive Heart Failure." *Ethnicity and Disease* 17 (2007): 72-77.

Jorm, A. F., A. J. Morgan, and S. E. Hetrick. "Relaxation for Depression." *Cochrane Database of Systematic Reviews* (2008): CD007142. Available through *EBSCO DynaMed Systematic Literature Surveillance* at http://www.ebscohost.com/dynamed.

Lahmann, C., F. Röhricht, and N. Sauer. "Functional Relaxation as Complementary Therapy in Irritable Bowel Syndrome." *Journal of Alternative and Complementary Medicine* 16 (2010): 47-52.

Lahmann, C., et al. "Brief Relaxation Versus Music Distraction in the Treatment of Dental Anxiety." *Journal of the American Dental Association* 139 (2008): 317-324.

Modesti, P. A., et al. "Psychological Predictors of the Antihypertensive Effects of Music-Guided Slow Breathing." *Journal of Hypertension* 28 (2010): 1097-1103.

Scott-Sheldon, L. A., et al. "Stress Management Interventions for HIV+ Adults." *Health Psychology* 27 (2008): 129-139.

See also: Autogenic training; Relaxation response; Stress; Walking, mind/body.

Restless legs syndrome

RELATED TERM: Periodic leg movements in sleep
CATEGORY: Condition
DEFINITION: Treatment of the intense urge to move one's legs, especially when sitting still or when trying to fall asleep.
PRINCIPAL PROPOSED NATURAL TREATMENTS: None
OTHER PROPOSED NATURAL TREATMENTS: Folate, iron, magnesium, vitamin B_{12}, vitamin C, vitamin E

INTRODUCTION

People with restless legs syndrome (RLS) often feel an intense urge to move their legs, particularly when sitting still or trying to fall asleep. Unlike persons with nighttime leg cramps (a different condition), people with RLS do not experience pain. Instead, they may describe an uncomfortable "creepy-crawly sensation" inside their legs. Walking relieves the symptoms, but as soon as the affected person settles down again, the urge to move recurs. The feeling is sometimes described as "wanting to ride a bicycle under the covers."

RLS tends to run in families, often emerging or worsening with age. People with RLS frequently have another condition called periodic leg movements in sleep (PLMS). Persons with PLMS kick their legs frequently during the night, disrupting their own sleep and that of their bed partner.

Because RLS is occasionally linked to other serious diseases, one should consult a doctor if symptoms of RLS emerge. Conventional medical treatment for RLS usually involves taking a levodopa-carbidopa combination, which is a treatment for Parkinson's disease. The drug quinine has been used in the past, but one double-blind study found no benefit. Because of a risk of dangerous side effects, quinine is no longer used for this purpose.

PROPOSED NATURAL TREATMENTS

Preliminary evidence suggests that symptoms of RLS may be relieved by supplementation with one of several minerals or vitamins, including magnesium, folate, iron, and vitamin E. However, there are no double-blind studies to support these treatments; therefore, their use remains speculative.

Magnesium. Preliminary studies suggest that supplemental magnesium may be helpful for RLS, even when magnesium levels are normal. An open study of ten people with insomnia related to RLS or PLMS found that their sleep improved significantly when they took magnesium nightly for four to six weeks. However, open studies are extremely unreliable because they do not factor out the placebo effect. Also, no double-blind studies on magnesium for RLS have been reported.

Folate. Based on numerous case reports of improvement, folate is also sometimes recommended for RLS. Symptoms decreased in one study of forty-five persons given 5 to 30 milligrams of folate daily. However, again this was not a double-blind experiment; therefore, the meaningfulness of the results are questionable. Such high doses of folate should be administered only under medical supervision. Folate taken in nutritional doses may be of benefit to pregnant women with RLS who are deficient in this vitamin.

Iron. A number of studies have linked RLS to low levels of iron in the blood. In one analysis of the medical records of twenty-seven people with RLS, those with the most severe symptoms had lower-than-average levels of serum ferritin, one measure of iron deficiency. In another study in which eighteen elderly people with RLS were compared with eighteen elderly people without the condition, those with RLS also had reduced levels of serum ferritin. When fifteen of the participants were given iron, all but one experienced a reduction in symptoms. Those with the lowest initial ferritin levels improved the most. However, once more, these were not double-blind studies, so the results cannot be trusted.

In contrast to these results, a double-blind study of twenty-eight people found that iron did not relieve RLS any better than did placebo. However, in this particular study, participants had normal levels of iron on average. The study did not effectively measure whether iron might help RLS among people with iron deficiency.

One theory holds that mild iron deficiency may cause RLS by decreasing the amount of a neurotransmitter called dopamine. This theory is supported by findings that conventional drugs that increase dopamine activity (such as the Parkinson's disease drug combination of levodopa-carbidopa) can also alleviate RLS.

Iron supplements might be useful for people with RLS who are also deficient in iron, but this has not been proven. Still, if one is deficient in iron, the deficiency is worth correcting. Note that tests for anemia

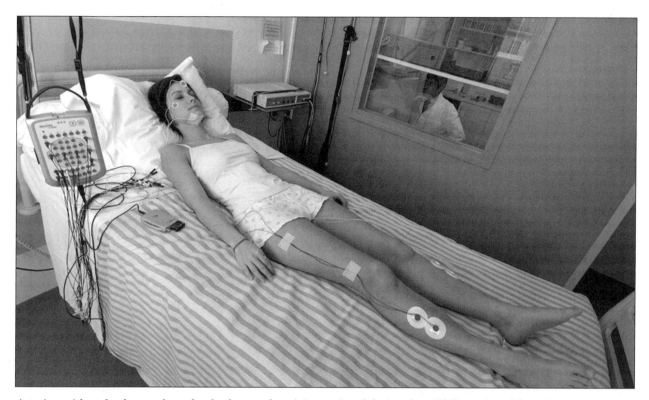

A patient with restless legs syndrome has her leg muscle activity monitored during sleep. (Philippe Garo/Photo Researchers, Inc.)

will not necessarily pick up the low-grade iron deficiency that is linked to RLS. For that purpose, one will need tests that specifically evaluate iron levels, such as ferritin, serum iron, and total iron-binding capacity.

Vitamin E. Vitamin E has also been proposed for RLS. In one report, seven of nine people with RLS given 400 to 800 international units daily of vitamin E experienced virtually complete control of symptoms, while the other two people had partial relief. Other anecdotal reports suggest that vitamin C may be useful and that vitamin B_{12} may benefit people with RLS who are deficient in this nutrient. However, while these reports may sound good, they mean little because they were not double-blind studies.

EBSCO CAM Review Board

FURTHER READING

Davis, B. J., et al. "A Randomized, Double-Blind, Placebo-Controlled Trial of Iron in Restless Legs Syndrome." *European Neurology* 43 (2000): 70-75.

Hornyak, M., et al. "Magnesium Therapy for Periodic Leg Movements-Related Insomnia and Restless Legs Syndrome." *Sleep* 21 (1998): 501-505.

Silber, M. H. "Restless Legs Syndrome." *Mayo Clinic Proceedings* 72 (1997): 261-264.

Sun, E. R., et al. "Iron and the Restless Legs Syndrome." *Sleep* 21 (1998): 371-377.

See also: Fibromyalgia: Homeopathic remedies; Folate; Insomnia; Iron; Magnesium; Vitamin B_{12}; Vitamin C; Vitamin E.

Resveratrol

CATEGORY: Functional foods
RELATED TERM: Grape skin
DEFINITION: Natural substance promoted as a dietary supplement for specific health benefits.
PRINCIPAL PROPOSED USES: None
OTHER PROPOSED USES: Cancer prevention, heart disease

Overview

The French diet is high in saturated fat and cholesterol, yet France has one of the world's lowest rates of heart disease. One theory for this apparent discrepancy is that another major player in the French diet, red wine, protects the arteries of the heart. Another possibility, perhaps even more likely, is that cutting down on saturated fat is less helpful than previously thought.

Resveratrol is a natural antioxidant found in red wine. Antioxidants protect cells in the body from damage by free radicals, naturally occurring but harmful substances that are thought to play a role in cardiovascular disease. Resveratrol is also a phytoestrogen, a substance that mimics some of the effects of estrogen, while blocking others. Soy, another phytoestrogen, is thought to help prevent heart disease and cancer, and resveratrol might have similar effects. However, none of these potential benefits of resveratrol have been documented in any meaningful way, and there is some evidence that resveratrol taken by mouth is broken down by the liver before it enters the bloodstream.

Sources

Resveratrol is not an essential nutrient. It is found in red wine, red grape skins and seeds, and purple grape juice. Peanuts also contain a small amount of resveratrol. Resveratrol supplements are available too.

Therapeutic Dosages

Because no clinical studies have been undertaken to look at the effects of resveratrol, the optimal therapeutic dosage has not been established. Based on animal studies, a reasonable therapeutic dosage might be about 500 milligrams daily.

Therapeutic Uses

Preliminary evidence, such as the results of test-tube studies, suggests that resveratrol may help prevent heart disease and cancer. However, not all studies have been favorable. Furthermore, there is some evidence that resveratrol is immediately broken down by the human liver and therefore does not enter the bloodstream at any significant level. In any case, only double-blind studies can prove a treatment effective, and none have been reported with resveratrol.

Safety Issues

Resveratrol, which has a chemical structure similar to that of the synthetic estrogenic hormone diethylstilbestrol, has estrogenic effects. According to one study, resveratrol might stimulate the growth of breast cancer cells. For this reason, resveratrol should be avoided by women who have had breast cancer or are at high risk of developing it. Maximum safe dosages for children, pregnant or nursing women, or those with severe liver or kidney disease have not been determined.

EBSCO CAM Review Board

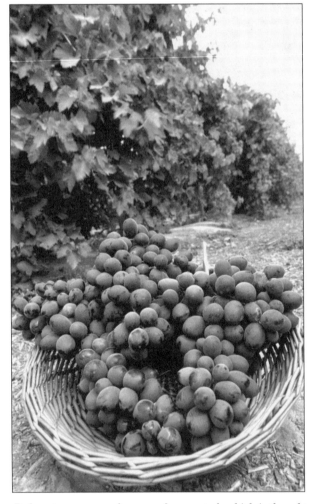

Red grapes are a good source of resveratrol, which is thought to have cancer-preventing properties. (U.S. Department of Agriculture)

Further Reading

El Attar, T. M., and A. S. Virji. "Modulating Effect of Resveratrol and Quercetin on Oral Cancer Cell Growth and Proliferation." *Anticancer Drugs* 10 (1999): 187-193.

Fulda, S. "Resveratrol and Derivatives for the Prevention and Treatment of Cancer." *Drug Discovery Today* 15 (2010): 757-765.

Gullett, N. P., et al. "Cancer Prevention with Natural Compounds." *Seminars in Oncology* 37 (2010): 25-281.

Mgbonyebi, O. P., J. Russo, and I. H. Russo. "Antiproliferative Effect of Synthetic Resveratrol on Human Breast Epithelial Cells." *International Journal of Oncology* 12 (1998): 865-869.

Walle, T., et al. "High Absorption but Very Low Bioavailability of Oral Resveratrol in Humans." *Drug Metabolism and Disposition* 32 (2004): 1377-1382.

See also: Antioxidants; Cholesterol, high.

Retinitis pigmentosa

CATEGORY: Condition

DEFINITION: Treatment of a progressive eye disease that leads to impaired night vision and decreased peripheral vision or decreased central and color vision.

PRINCIPAL PROPOSED NATURAL TREATMENTS: None

OTHER PROPOSED NATURAL TREATMENTS: Docosahexaenoic acid (a component of fish oil), lutein, vitamin A

HERBS AND SUPPLEMENTS TO USE WITH CAUTION: Vitamin E

INTRODUCTION

Retinitis pigmentosa (RP) is a group of inherited eye diseases that can lead to severe visual problems. This disorder is named for the irregular clumps of black pigment that occur in the retina.

In most forms of retinitis pigmentosa, cells in the retina called rods die. This leads to impaired night vision and decreased ability to see things to the side while looking ahead (peripheral vision). In some forms of RP, other retinal cells called cones die. This leads to a decrease in central and color vision. In all forms of RP, vision loss usually progresses with time. Loss of vision is usually first noted in childhood or early adulthood. Conventional medicine for retinitis pigmentosa is largely limited to vision aids.

PROPOSED NATURAL TREATMENTS

No natural treatments have been proven effective for retinitis pigmentosa, but some approaches have shown some promise. The substance lutein is an antioxidant that occurs in the retina. In a small, double-blind, placebo-controlled study, thirty-four adults with retinitis pigmentosa were given either placebo or lutein (10 milligrams [mg] per day for twelve weeks followed by 30 mg per day for twenty-four weeks). After this period, each group was switched to the opposite treatment and was followed for another twenty-four weeks. The results indicated that lutein supplementation improved visual field compared with placebo and also possibly improved visual acuity. However, a larger study is needed to verify whether these results are meaningful.

A large (more than six hundred-participant), double-blind, placebo-controlled trial found evidence that the use of vitamin A supplements at a potentially dangerous dose of 15,000 international units (IU) daily might slightly slow the progression of retinitis pigmentosa. However, the benefits seen in the four-to-six-year study period were modest at best. A subsequent study by the same researchers evaluated whether adding 1,200 mg daily of docosahexaenoic acid (a component of fish oil) with vitamin A produced better results. The results of this trial were largely negative. However, in another trial involving 225 adults, adding lutein (12 mg per day) to vitamin A for four years modestly slowed the rate of visual loss in the mid-peripheral field.

HERBS AND SUPPLEMENTS TO USE WITH CAUTION

In the large vitamin A study noted, some participants were given vitamin E at a dose of 400 IU daily. The results indicated that the use of vitamin E at this dosage might actually speed retinal damage rather than slow it. (The daily requirement for vitamin E is far lower than this: 33 IU daily for most adults.) Until these results are clarified, people with retinitis pigmentosa should avoid taking high dosages of vitamin E.

EBSCO CAM Review Board

FURTHER READING

Bahrami, H., M. Melia, and G. Dagnelie. "Lutein Supplementation in Retinitis Pigmentosa: PC-Based Vision Assessment in a Randomized Double-Masked Placebo-Controlled Clinical Trial." *BMC Ophthalmology* 6 (2006): 23.

Berson, E. L., B. Rosner, and M. A. Sandberg. "Clinical Trial of Lutein in Patients with Retinitis Pigmentosa Receiving Vitamin A." *Archives of Ophthalmology* 128 (2010): 403-411.

Berson, E. L., B. Rosner, and M. A. Sandberg, et al. "A Randomized Trial of Vitamin A and Vitamin E Supplementation for Retinitis Pigmentosa." *Archives of Ophthalmology* 111 (1993): 761-772.

_____. "Clinical Trial of Docosahexaenoic Acid in Patients with Retinitis Pigmentosa Receiving Vitamin A Treatment." *Archives of Ophthalmology* 122 (2004): 1297-1305.

See also: Cataracts; Diabetes, complications of; Glaucoma; Lutein; Macular degeneration; Night vision, impaired; Vitamin A.

Reverse transcriptase inhibitors

CATEGORY: Drug interactions
DEFINITION: Drugs used to interfere with actions of the human immunodeficiency virus.
INTERACTIONS: Coenzyme Q_{10}, St. John's wort
DRUGS IN THIS FAMILY: Lamivudine and zidovudine (Combivir), emtricitabine (Emtriva), lamivudine (Epivir), abacavir and lamivudine (Epzicom), zalcitabine (Hivid), delaviridine (Rescriptor), AZT (Retrovir), zidovudine (Retrovir), abacavir-lamivudine-zidovudine (Trizivir), emtricitabine-tenofovir (Truvada), didanosine (Videx), nevirapine (Viramune), tenofovir (Viread), stavudine (Zerit), abacavir (Ziagen)

COENZYME Q_{10} (CoQ_{10})
Effect: Possible Benefits and Risks

The reverse transcriptase inhibitors lamivudine and zidovudine can cause damage to the mitochondria, the energy-producing subunits of cells. This may lead to symptoms such as lactic acidosis (a dangerous metabolic derangement), peripheral neuropathy (injury to nerves in the extremities), and lipodystrophy (cosmetically undesirable rearrangement of fat in the body). The supplement CoQ_{10} has been tried for minimizing these side effects. In one double-blind, placebo-controlled study, use of CoQ_{10} improved general sense of well-being in people with human immunodeficiency virus (HIV) infection using reverse transcriptase inhibitors; however, for reasons that are unclear, it actually worsened symptoms of peripheral neuropathy. For this reason, people with HIV who have peripheral neuropathy symptoms should use CoQ_{10} only with caution.

ST. JOHN'S WORT
Effect: Dangerous Interaction

Use of the herb St. John's wort can lower blood levels of numerous medications, including protease inhibitors used for HIV. Case reports indicate St. John's wort also lowers blood levels of the non-nucleoside reverse transcriptase inhibitor nevirapine. If one has been stabilized on HIV medications while taking St. John's wort and stops taking the herb, one's blood levels of the drugs could rise, potentially leading to increased side effects.

EBSCO CAM Review Board

FURTHER READING
Christensen, E. R., et al. "Mitochondrial DNA Levels in Fat and Blood Cells from Patients with Lipodystrophy or Peripheral Neuropathy and the Effect of Ninety Days of High-Dose Coenzyme Q Treatment." *Clinical Infectious Diseases* 39 (2004): 1371-1379.

See also: Food and Drug Administration; Supplements: Introduction.

Rheumatoid arthritis

CATEGORY: Condition
DEFINITION: Treatment of the disease in which the immune system attacks tissues in the body, especially cartilage in the joints.
PRINCIPAL PROPOSED NATURAL TREATMENT: Fish oil
OTHER PROPOSED NATURAL TREATMENTS: Acupuncture, balneotherapy (spa therapy), boswellia, bromelain, cat's claw, curcumin (turmeric), deer velvet, devil's claw, folate, food allergen avoidance, gamma-linolenic acid, glucosamine, krill oil, magnet therapy, olive oil, relaxation therapies, rose hips, *Tripterygium wilfordii*, vegan diet, vitamin B_6, vitamin E, zinc

INTRODUCTION

Rheumatoid arthritis is an autoimmune disease in the general family of lupus. For reasons that are not understood, in rheumatoid arthritis the immune system goes awry and begins attacking tissues, especially cartilage in the joints. Various joints become red, hot, and swollen under the onslaught. The pattern of inflammation is usually symmetrical, occurring on both sides of the body. Other symptoms include inflammation of the eyes, nodules (or lumps) under the skin, and a general feeling of malaise.

Rheumatoid arthritis is more common in women than in men and typically begins between the ages of thirty-five and sixty. The diagnosis is made by matching the pattern of symptoms with certain characteristic laboratory results.

Medical treatment consists mainly of two categories of drugs: anti-inflammatory drugs in the ibuprofen family (nonsteroidal anti-inflammatory drugs, or NSAIDs) and drugs that may be able to put rheumatoid arthritis into full or partial remission (the disease-modifying antirheumatic drugs, or DMARDs).

Anti-inflammatory drugs relieve symptoms of rheumatoid arthritis but do not change the overall progression of the disease, whereas DMARDs seem to affect the disease itself. In rheumatoid arthritis, the drugs believed to alter the course of the disease (to slow it down or stop it) include antimalarials (hydroxychloroquine and chloroquine), sulfasalazine, TNF inhibitors (etanercept, infliximab, and adalimumab), interleukin-1 receptor antagonists, leflunomide methotrexate, gold compounds, D-penicillamine, and cytotoxic agents (azathioprine, cyclophosphamide, and cyclosporine). These drugs are unrelated to one another but work somewhat similarly in practice.

Most of the drugs in this category can cause severe side effects. Because of this toxicity, for years a so-called pyramid approach was taken with people with rheumatoid arthritis. Physicians started with NSAIDs to help with the pain and inflammation and progressed to successively stronger and more toxic medications only when the basic treatments failed. Natural treatments such as those described here might also be useful in early stages.

However, more recent research has found that severe joint damage occurs early in rheumatoid arthritis. This evidence has caused many authorities to suggest early, aggressive treatment with disease-modifying drugs to prevent joint damage. Nonetheless, this approach has not been universally adopted, and some physicians still prescribe NSAIDs for early stages of rheumatoid arthritis. The treatments described here may be reasonable alternative options.

PRINCIPAL PROPOSED NATURAL TREATMENTS

Rheumatoid arthritis is a difficult disease, and no alternative approach solves it easily. Even if one chooses

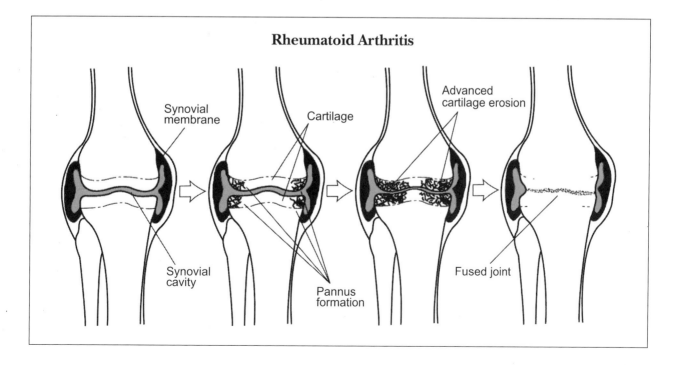

Rheumatoid Arthritis

Synovial membrane

Cartilage

Advanced cartilage erosion

Synovial cavity

Pannus formation

Fused joint

to use alternative methods, regular visits to a rheumatologist should be maintained to watch for serious complications. Medical treatment may be able to slow the progression of rheumatoid arthritis. It is not likely that any of the alternative options have the same ability.

Fish oil. Fish oil is the only natural treatment for rheumatoid arthritis with significant documentation. According to the results of about thirteen double-blind, placebo-controlled studies involving more than five hundred participants, supplementation with omega-3 fatty acids can significantly reduce the symptoms of rheumatoid arthritis. Also, at least one small study suggests that omega-3 fatty acids may help persons with rheumatoid arthritis lower their dose of nonsteroidal anti-inflammatory medication (such as ibuprofen).

However, unlike some of the standard treatments, fish oil has not been shown to slow the progression of rheumatoid arthritis. It has been suggested that omega-3 supplementation is more effective when omega-6 intake (particularly arachidonic acid) is kept low, as occurs with a vegetarian diet. The benefits of fish oil may also be enhanced by simultaneous use of olive oil. One badly designed human study hints that a relative of fish oil, krill oil, might be helpful as well. Flaxseed oil has been offered as a more palatable substitute for fish oil, but it does not seem to work.

OTHER PROPOSED TREATMENTS

Boswellia serrata is a shrublike tree that grows in the dry hills of the Indian subcontinent. It is the source of a resin called salai guggal, which has been used for thousands of years in Ayurvedic medicine, the traditional medicine of the region. It is very similar to a resin from a related tree, *B. carteri*, which is also known as frankincense. Both substances have been used historically for arthritis.

Research has identified boswellic acids as the likely active ingredients in boswellia. In animal studies, boswellic acids have shown anti-inflammatory effects, but their mechanism of action seems to be quite different from that of standard anti-inflammatory medications.

An issue of the journal *Phytomedicine* that was devoted to boswellia briefly reviewed previously unpublished studies on the herb. A pair of placebo-controlled trials involving eighty-one people with rheumatoid arthritis found significant reductions in swelling and pain over the course of three months. Furthermore, a comparative study of sixty people over six months found the boswellia extract relieved symptoms about as well as oral gold therapy. However, while gold shots can induce remission in rheumatoid arthritis, there is no evidence that boswellia can do the same.

Another double-blind study found no difference between boswellia and placebo. More research is needed to know whether boswellia is an effective treatment for rheumatoid arthritis.

Devil's claw. The herb devil's claw may be beneficial in rheumatoid arthritis. One double-blind study followed eighty-nine people with rheumatoid arthritis for two months. The group given devil's claw showed a significant decrease in pain intensity and an improvement in mobility. Another double-blind study of fifty people with various types of arthritis showed that ten days of treatment with devil's claw provided significant pain relief.

Other herbs and supplements. Glucosamine is best known as a proposed treatment for osteoarthritis, but it might also be helpful for rheumatoid arthritis. A double-blind, placebo-controlled study of fifty-one people with rheumatoid arthritis found that glucosamine at a dose of 1,500 milligrams (mg) daily significantly improved symptoms. Glucosamine did not, however, alter measures of inflammation as determined through blood tests.

Some evidence, including small double-blind trials, supports the use of the following herbs and supplements for the treatment of rheumatoid arthritis: gamma-linolenic acid (found in evening primrose oil and borage oil), cat's claw (*Uncaria tomentosa*), rose hip powder, and the Chinese herb *Tripterygium wilfordii* (applied topically or taken orally). *T. wilfordii* is believed to be unsafe for pregnant or nursing women and may present risks in other groups too.

Preliminary evidence suggests potential benefits with the following herbs and supplements: methyl sulfonyl methane, yucca, and a mixture of poplar, ash, and goldenrod.

Vitamin E may reduce pain in rheumatoid arthritis, but it does not seem to reduce inflammation. Some evidence suggests that adding vitamin E, or vitamin E plus other antioxidants, to standard rheumatoid arthritis therapy might improve results. However, an extremely large randomized trial involving more than 39,000 women found that taking 600 international units of vitamin E every other day did not reduce the risk of rheumatoid arthritis.

Persons taking the drug methotrexate for treatment of rheumatoid arthritis may benefit by taking folate supplements. Folate appears to reduce methotrexate side effects, including mouth sores, nausea, and liver inflammation. In addition, folate supplements may help reverse a more subtle methotrexate side effect: a rise in blood levels of homocysteine. Elevated levels of homocysteine are thought to increase risk of heart disease.

The following treatments are also sometimes proposed as effective for rheumatoid arthritis, but there is little to no scientific evidence for or against their use: adrenal extract, beta-carotene, betaine hydrochloride, boron, burdock, cayenne, chamomile, copper, feverfew, folate, ginger, L-histidine, horsetail, magnesium, manganese, molybdenum, pantothenic acid, D-phenylalanine, perilla frutescens, pregnenolone, proteolytic enzymes, sea cucumber, and vitamin C. Evidence regarding green-lipped mussel for rheumatoid arthritis is more negative than positive.

One study failed to find vitamin B_6 at a dose of 50 mg daily helpful for rheumatoid arthritis, despite a general vitamin B_6 deficiency seen in people with this condition. Zinc supplements have been evaluated as a treatment for rheumatoid arthritis, but overall, the study results have not been encouraging. Other treatments that have generally failed to prove effective in small double-blind trials include selenium, collagen, probiotics, white willow, and an Ayurvedic herbal mixture containing extracts of ashwagandha, boswellia, ginger, and turmeric. Two studies commonly cited as evidence that turmeric alone is useful for rheumatoid arthritis actually fail to provide any meaningful supporting evidence. A six-month, double-blind, placebo-controlled study of 168 people with rheumatoid arthritis failed to find that elk velvet antler enhanced the effectiveness of conventional treatment for rheumatoid arthritis.

Other alternative therapies. Adopting a vegan (pure vegetarian) diet might help mild rheumatoid arthritis, although the supporting evidence for this claim is weak. Identifying and avoiding food allergens has also been tried, but one controlled trial found no clear evidence of benefit with a low-saturated-fat, hypoallergenic diet.

Balneotherapy (hot baths), relaxation therapy, and magnet therapy have shown some promise for rheumatoid arthritis. Two separate groups of researchers conducting detailed reviews of eight randomized, controlled trials found some beneficial effects of acupuncture for rheumatoid arthritis, but they were not convinced that it was more beneficial than sham acupuncture or other standard treatments.

HERBS AND SUPPLEMENTS TO USE WITH CAUTION

Various herbs and supplements may interact adversely with drugs used to treat rheumatoid arthritis, so one should be cautious when considering the use of herbs and supplements.

EBSCO CAM Review Board

FURTHER READING

Allen, M., et al. "A Randomized Clinical Trial of Elk Velvet Antler in Rheumatoid Arthritis." *Biological Research for Nursing* 9 (2008): 254-261.

Berbert, A. A., et al. "Supplementation of Fish Oil and Olive Oil in Patients with Rheumatoid Arthritis." *Nutrition* 21 (2005): 131-136.

Biegert, C., et al. "Efficacy and Safety of Willow Bark Extract in the Treatment of Osteoarthritis and Rheumatoid Arthritis." *Journal of Rheumatology* 31 (2004): 2121-2130.

Canter, P. H., et al. "A Systematic Review of Randomised Clinical Trials of *Tripterygium wilfordii* for Rheumatoid Arthritis." *Phytomedicine* 13 (2006): 371-377.

Deutsch, L. "Evaluation of the Effect of Neptune Krill Oil on Chronic Inflammation and Arthritic Symptoms." *Journal of the American College of Nutrition* 26 (2007): 39-48.

Galarraga, B., et al. "Cod Liver Oil (N-3 Fatty Acids) as a Non-steroidal Anti-inflammatory Drug Sparing Agent in Rheumatoid Arthritis." *Rheumatology* 47 (2008): 665-669.

Karlson, E. W., et al. "Vitamin E in the Primary Prevention of Rheumatoid Arthritis: The Women's Health Study." *Arthritis and Rheumatism* 59 (2008): 1589-1595.

Lee, M. S., B. C. Shin, and E. Ernst. "Acupuncture for Rheumatoid Arthritis." *Rheumatology* (Oxford) 47 (2008): 1747-1753.

Nakamura, H., et al. "Effects of Glucosamine Administration on Patients with Rheumatoid Arthritis." *Rheumatology International* 27 (2007): 213-218.

Pradhan, E. K., et al. "Effect of Mindfulness-Based Stress Reduction in Rheumatoid Arthritis Patients." *Arthritis and Rheumatism* 57 (2007): 1134-1142.

Verhagen, A. P., et al. "Balneotherapy for Rheumatoid Arthritis." *Cochrane Database of Systematic Reviews* (2003): CD000518. Available through *EBSCO DynaMed Systematic Literature Surveillance* at http://www.ebscohost.com/dynamed.

Willich, S. N., et al. "Rose Hip Herbal Remedy in Patients with Rheumatoid Arthritis." *Phytomedicine* 17 (2010): 87-93.

See also: Bone and joint health; Boswellia; Devil's claw; Fish oil; Immune support; Lupus; Nonsteroidal anti-inflammatory drugs (NSAIDs); Osteoarthritis; Pain management; Rheumatoid arthritis: Homeopathic remedies; Soft tissue pain.

Rheumatoid arthritis: Homeopathic remedies

CATEGORY: Homeopathy

DEFINITION: The use of highly diluted remedies to treat disease in which the immune system attacks tissues in the body, especially cartilage in the joints.

STUDIED HOMEOPATHIC REMEDIES: *Apis mellifica; Calcarea carbonica; Causticum;* classical homeopathic remedy; combination homeopathic remedy containing *Rhus toxicodendron, Bryonia cretica, Strychnos nux vomica, Berberis vulgaris,* and *Ledum palustre*

SCIENTIFIC EVALUATIONS OF HOMEOPATHIC REMEDIES

Studies performed to evaluate the effectiveness of homeopathic remedies for rheumatoid arthritis have returned mixed results. A three-month, double-blind, placebo-controlled study of forty-six people evaluated the effectiveness of individualized homeopathic remedies for rheumatoid arthritis. At the beginning of the study, two homeopathic practitioners evaluated all of the participants and wrote out prescriptions. Participants were then randomly assigned to receive either the prescribed treatment or placebo; neither the researchers nor the participants knew who would receive treatment or placebo. The results showed significant improvement as compared with placebo among the participants receiving active treatment, most notably in pain and stiffness.

Another positive, double-blind, placebo-controlled trial of 111 people with rheumatoid arthritis evaluated the effectiveness of a fixed remedy containing *Rhus toxicodendron, Bryonia cretica, Strychnos nux vomica, Berberis vulgaris,* and *Ledum palustre.* The results showed that people in the treatment group experienced a significant decrease in the amount of analgesics required and in their perception of pain compared with those in the placebo group.

In a six-month double-blind study of 112 people with rheumatoid arthritis, treatment with individualized homeopathic remedies failed to prove more effective than placebo. Because of a high rate of dropouts, however, these results carry little weight. A high dropout rate also compromised the meaningfulness of an apparently negative six-month double-blind study enrolling forty-four people.

TRADITIONAL HOMEOPATHIC TREATMENTS

Classical homeopathy offers some possible homeopathic treatments for rheumatoid arthritis. These therapies are chosen based on various specific details of the person seeking treatment.

The symptom picture for *Calcarea carbonica* includes feeling extremely fatigued and depleted, having cold limbs and swelling in the joints, and having difficulty climbing stairs or even walking. These symptoms worsen with exposure to cold or dampness, are worse in the morning, and are worse with exertion.

For those with arthritic symptoms who are extremely sensitive to cold, the homeopathic remedy *Causticum* might be recommended. Other features of the symptom picture include feeling restless, while noticing that moving around does not make one feel better; preferring damp weather over dry conditions; and experiencing a dislike of wind.

If, however, one tends to feel better rather than worse in cool air, that person might fit the symptom picture of *Apis mellifica,* which is made from the venom of the honey bee. Other symptoms traditionally associated with this remedy include feeling restless and fidgety overall and noticing increased discomfort when exposed to heat from any source, when touch or pressure is applied to the joints, and when lying down.

EBSCO CAM Review Board

FURTHER READING

Andrade, L. E., et al. "A Randomized Controlled Trial to Evaluate the Effectiveness of Homeopathy in

Rheumatoid Arthritis." *Scandinavian Journal of Rheumatology* 20 (1991): 204-208.

Breuer, G. S., et al. "Perceived Efficacy Among Patients of Various Methods of Complementary Alternative Medicine for Rheumatologic Diseases." *Clinical and Experimental Rheumatology* 23 (2005): 693-696.

Brien, S., et al. "Homeopathy Has Clinical Benefits in Rheumatoid Arthritis Patients That Are Attributable to the Consultation Process but Not the Homeopathic Remedy." *Rheumatology* (November 13, 2010).

Fisher, P., and D. L. Scott. "A Randomized Controlled Trial of Homeopathy in Rheumatoid Arthritis." *Rheumatology* 40 (2001): 1052-1055.

See also: Aging; Bone and joint health; Homeopathy; Osteoarthritis; Rheumatoid arthritis.

Rhodiola rosea

CATEGORY: Herbs and supplements

DEFINITION: Natural plant product used to treat specific health conditions.

PRINCIPAL PROPOSED USES: Adaptogen, enhancement of mental function, fatigue, improvement of sports performance

OTHER PROPOSED USES: Altitude sickness, depression, female sexual function, liver protection, male sexual function

OVERVIEW

The herb *Rhodiola rosea* has been used traditionally in Iceland, Norway, Sweden, Russia, and other European countries as a "tonic herb" said to fight fatigue, aid convalescence from illness, prevent infections, and enhance sexual function. In the twentieth century, Soviet physicians classified rhodiola as an adaptogen. This invented term refers to a hypothetical treatment described as follows: An adaptogen helps the body adapt to stresses of various kinds, whether heat, cold, exertion, trauma, sleep deprivation, toxic exposure, radiation, infection, or psychological stress. Furthermore, an adaptogen supposedly causes no side effects, treats a wide variety of illnesses, and helps return an organism toward balance no matter what may have gone wrong.

Perhaps the only indisputable example of an adaptogen is a healthful lifestyle. By eating right, exercising regularly, and generally living a life of balance and moderation, individuals can increase their physical fitness and ability to resist illnesses of all types. Multivitamin/multimineral supplements could offer similarly general benefits, at least in people whose diets are deficient in basic nutrients. Whether there are any herbs that offer adaptogenic benefits, however, remains unproven (and somewhat unlikely). Nonetheless, advocates of the adaptogen concept believe that rhodiola (as well as ginseng, ashwagandha, reishi, suma, and several other herbs) have this property.

THERAPEUTIC DOSAGES

Rhodiola extracts are standardized to their content of salidroside (also called rhodioloside). A typical dosage of 170 to 185 milligrams (mg) daily supplies 4.5 mg of salidroside. When rhodiola is used as a one-time treatment, two to three times this dose is often used. Most published studies involved a single proprietary product. It is not clear that the results of these studies apply to products using different rhodiola sources or different methods of extraction.

THERAPEUTIC USES

Rhodiola is marketed as the new ginseng, said to fight fatigue, enhance mental function, increase general wellness, improve sports performance, and enhance sex drive in both men and women. A few double-blind studies involving a single proprietary product support the first two of these uses, finding that the use of a particular rhodiola extract by people in stressful, fatiguing circumstances may help maintain normal mental function.

SCIENTIFIC EVIDENCE

A double-blind, placebo-controlled study of fifty-six physicians on night duty evaluated the potential benefits of rhodiola for maintaining mental acuity. Participants received either placebo or rhodiola extract (170 mg daily) for a period of two weeks. The results showed that participants taking rhodiola retained a higher level of mental function as measured by tests, such as mental arithmetic.

Another double-blind, placebo-controlled study evaluated one-time use of the same rhodiola extract (at a dose of 370 mg or 555 mg) in 161 male military cadets undergoing sleep deprivation and stress. The results showed that rhodiola was more effective than placebo at fighting the effects of fatigue.

Finally, a third double-blind, placebo-controlled study examined the effects of a low dose of this rhodiola extract (100 mg daily for twenty days) in forty foreign students undergoing examinations (presumably a highly stressful situation). The results showed modest benefits on some measurements of fatigue and mental function, and no significant benefit on others. The study authors considered the outcome relatively unimpressive and blamed this on the dose chosen.

While these results may sound impressive overall, they were all performed in former Soviet republics, and studies from these sources must be viewed with caution. For reasons that are unclear, double-blind studies performed in the former Soviet Union (or China) almost always find the tested treatment effective. This consistent pattern of excessively positive results has made outside observers highly skeptical. For this reason, only if confirmation is obtained in a more reliable setting can rhodiola be considered to have real supporting evidence behind it.

One small double-blind trial performed in Belgium did find evidence that use of a different rhodiola extract at a dose of 200 mg one hour before endurance exercise may improve performance. However, another study failed to find benefit with a combination of cordyceps and rhodiola.

Weak evidence hints that rhodiola might be helpful for preventing altitude sickness and might aid in cancer chemotherapy (by protecting the liver). Rhodiola has also been studied as a treatment for depression. In a randomized trial, eighty-nine people with mild to moderate depression received rhodiola extract 340 mg, rhodiola extract 680 mg, or a placebo for six weeks. Those in both rhodiola groups experienced an improvement in most of their depression symptoms, whereas those in the placebo group experienced no such benefit.

SAFETY ISSUES

There are no known or suspected safety risks with rhodiola, and in clinical trials, no severe adverse effects have been reported. However, comprehensive safety studies have not been performed. Safety in young children, pregnant or nursing women, and people with severe liver or kidney disease has not been established.

EBSCO CAM Review Board

FURTHER READING

Colson, S. N., et al. "*Cordyceps sinensis*- and *Rhodiola rosea*-Based Supplementation in Male Cyclists and Its Effect on Muscle Tissue Oxygen Saturation." *Journal of Strength and Conditioning Research* 19 (2005): 358-363.

Darbinyan, V., et al. "*Rhodiola rosea* in Stress Induced Fatigue: A Double Blind Crossover Study of a Standardized Extract SHR-5 with a Repeated Low-Dose Regimen on the Mental Performance of Healthy Physicians During Night Duty." *Phytomedicine* 7 (2000): 365-371.

De Bock, K., et al. "Acute *Rhodiola rosea* Intake Can Improve Endurance Exercise Performance." *International Journal of Sport Nutrition and Exercise Metabolism* 14 (2004): 298-307.

Fintelmann, V., and J. Gruenwald. "Efficacy and Tolerability of a *Rhodiola rosea* Extract in Adults with Physical and Cognitive Deficiencies." *Advances in Therapy* 24 (2007): 929-939.

Shevtsov, V. A., et al. "A Randomized Trial of Two Different Doses of a SHR-5 *Rhodiola rosea* Extract Versus Placebo and Control of Capacity for Mental Work." *Phytomedicine* 10 (2003): 95-105.

Spasov, A. A., et al. "A Double-Blind, Placebo-Controlled Pilot Study of the Stimulating and Adaptogenic Effect of *Rhodiola rosea* SHR-5 Extract on the Fatigue of Students Caused by Stress During an Examination Period with a Repeated Low-Dose Regimen." *Phytomedicine* 7 (2000): 85-89.

Wing, S. L., et al. "Lack of Effect of Rhodiola or Oxygenated Water Supplementation on Hypoxemia and Oxidative Stress." *Wilderness and Environmental Medicine* 14 (2003): 9-16.

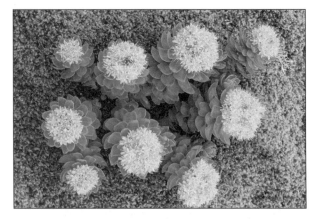

Extracts from the Rhodiola rosea *plant are used to fight fatigue.* (Rod Planck/Photo Researchers, Inc.)

See also: Altitude sickness; Depression, mild to moderate; Fatigue; Sports and fitness support: Enhancing performance.

Rhubarb

CATEGORY: Functional foods
RELATED TERM: *Rheum rhaponticum*
DEFINITION: Natural plant product promoted as a dietary supplement for specific health benefits.
PRINCIPAL PROPOSED USE: Menopausal symptoms
OTHER PROPOSED USES: Allergies, cancer treatment, diabetes, herpes (topical), kidney disease, liver disease, pancreatitis

OVERVIEW

The stalk of the intensely flavored rhubarb plant has been used in European cooking since the seventeenth century. Before this time, rhubarb species were utilized medicinally in traditional Chinese herbal medicine. Traditional uses include treatment of constipation, diarrhea, fever, menstrual problems, jaundice, sores (when applied topically), ulcers, and burns. Although there are many species of rhubarb, the one most studied is *Rheum rhaponticum*.

USES AND APPLICATIONS

Rhubarb root contains lindleyin, a substance with estrogen-like properties. On this basis, extracts of rhubarb have been tried for the control of menopausal symptoms. In a twelve-week, double-blind, placebo-controlled trial of 109 women with menopause-related symptoms, the use of a standardized *R. rhaponticum* extract significantly improved symptoms compared with placebo. Improvements were particularly seen in rate and severity of hot flashes. While this is meaningful supporting evidence, additional independent trials are necessary to establish that this rhubarb extract is a safe and effective treatment for menopause.

Other potential uses of rhubarb lack reliable supporting evidence. One human trial purportedly found evidence that rhubarb could reduce the impairment of lung function that may occur when people with lung cancer receive radiation therapy. However, this study had a number of significant flaws, and its results cannot be regarded as reliable.

In another human trial, this one using a cream containing sage and rhubarb, researchers failed to find more than modest benefits for the treatment of herpes. Additional proposed uses of rhubarb are supported only by test-tube studies. For example, various rhubarb species have shown hints of potential value for the treatment of diabetes, kidney disease, liver disease, allergies, and pancreatitis. However, the vast majority of effects seen in test-tube studies do not recur in human trials.

DOSAGE

A typical dosage of rhubarb root is one-half to one teaspoonful of the root boiled for ten minutes in a cup of water, three times daily. In the foregoing menopause study, a standardized extract was used. Such extracts should be used according to label instructions.

SAFETY ISSUES

As a widely consumed food, rhubarb is thought to be relatively safe if consumed in moderation. However, the plant contains high levels of oxalic acid, and rhubarb consumption can markedly increase oxalic acid levels in the urine. This could lead to increased risk of kidney stones and other problems. Rhubarb leaf contains the highest oxalic acid content. The roots and stems contain less oxalic acid but higher levels of anthraquinones, laxative substances similar to those found in senna or cascara. It is safest to use rhubarb standardized extracts that have been processed to remove oxalic acid.

Contrary to some reports, consumption of rhubarb probably does not impair calcium absorption. Weak evidence hints that excessive consumption of rhubarb could increase the risk of stomach or colon cancer. Maximum safe doses in pregnant or nursing women, young children, and people with severe liver or kidney disease have not been established.

EBSCO CAM Review Board

FURTHER READING

Choi, S. Z., et al. "Antidiabetic Stilbene and Anthraquinone Derivatives from *Rheum undulatum*." *Archives of Pharmacy Research* 28 (2005): 1027-1030.

Heger, M., et al. "Efficacy and Safety of a Special Extract of *Rheum rhaponticum* (ERr 731) in Perimenopausal Women with Climacteric Complaints." *Menopause* 13 (2006): 744-759.

Vollmer, G., A. Papke, and O. Zierau. "Treatment of Menopausal Symptoms by an Extract from the Roots of Rhapontic Rhubarb: The Role of Estrogen Receptors." *Chinese Medicine* 5 (2010): 7.

Yu, H. M., et al. "Effects of Rhubarb Extract on Radiation Induced Lung Toxicity via Decreasing Transforming Growth Factor-Beta-1 and Interleukin-6 in Lung Cancer Patients Treated with Radiotherapy." *Lung Cancer* 59 (2008): 219-226.

Zhao, Y. Q., et al. "Protective Effects of Rhubarb on Experimental Severe Acute Pancreatitis." *World Journal of Gastroenterology* 10 (2004): 1005-1009.

See also: Allergies; Cancer treatment support; Diabetes; Herpes; Kidney stones; Liver disease; Menopause; Pancreatitis.

Ribose

CATEGORY: Herbs and supplements

DEFINITION: Natural substance of the human body used as a supplement to treat specific health conditions.

PRINCIPAL PROPOSED USES: None

OTHER PROPOSED USES: Angina, congenital myoadenylate deaminase deficiency, congestive heart failure, enhancement of mental function

PROBABLY NOT EFFECTIVE USES: Duchenne muscular dystrophy, McArdle's disease, sports performance enhancement (high-intensity exercise)

OVERVIEW

Ribose is a carbohydrate vital for the body's manufacture of ATP (adenosine triphosphate), which is the major source of energy used by the cells. Quite a few studies have been done on ribose, mostly relating to its potential usefulness for individuals with heart disease. When the heart is starved for oxygen, as can occur with a heart attack or angina, it loses much of its ATP, and its ATP levels remain low for several days, even after blood flow is resumed. Scientists have found that supplying extra ribose in the blood helps restore the heart's normal ATP levels more quickly. This finding has raised hopes that ribose supplements might improve heart functioning and increase exercise capacity.

Ribose is best known as a sports supplement. However, current evidence indicates that it is not effective for this purpose.

REQUIREMENTS AND SOURCES

Ribose is not an essential nutrient. Although it is a common sugar present in the bodies of animals and plants, food sources do not supply recommended dosages.

THERAPEUTIC DOSAGES

Typical dosages of ribose recommended by sports supplement manufacturers are 1 to 10 grams (g) per day. However, researchers have used much higher dosages. For example, in a study focusing on coronary artery disease and exercise-induced ischemia (problems with blood supply to the heart), the participants took 15 g of ribose four times a day for three days.

Typically provided as a powder to be dissolved in water or in liquid form, ribose is also available commercially in capsules. The dissolved powder has a sweetish taste that some people find unpleasant.

THERAPEUTIC USES

Ribose may be of benefit in improving exercise tolerance in people with angina by helping the heart regenerate its ATP, but the evidence that it works remains highly preliminary. One small study found evidence that ribose supplements might improve heart function in people with congestive heart failure.

Sports enthusiasts are more interested in the effects of ATP on regular muscles than in its effects on the heart muscle. At least one animal study seems to show that skeletal muscle, like heart muscle, replenishes ATP more quickly when ribose is added to the blood. In theory, this could lead to enhanced performance in high-intensity anaerobic exercise, such as sprinting. However, six small double-blind, placebo-controlled trials in humans failed to find any benefit. In one of these studies, dextrose (a form of ordinary sugar) proved effective while ribose did not.

In one small double-blind study, ribose failed to prove effective for enhancing mental function. The researchers suggest that the dose they used (2 g daily) may have been insufficient.

In a few case reports, ribose apparently has produced an increase in exercise ability in people with a rare condition involving deficiency of the enzyme myoadenylate deaminase (AMPD). However, no double-blind studies of ribose in AMPD deficiency have been conducted. Small double-blind studies have failed to find ribose effective for another rare enzyme deficiency, called McArdle's disease, or for Duchenne's muscular dystrophy.

SCIENTIFIC EVIDENCE

Individuals with sufficiently severe coronary artery disease suffer reduced blood flow to the heart (ischemia) with exercise and experience angina pain. One small study examined whether giving ribose can improve exercise tolerance for people with angina. In the study, twenty men with severe coronary artery disease walked on a treadmill while researchers noted how long it took for signs of ischemia to develop. For the next three days, the men took either oral ribose (60 milligrams [mg] per day) or placebo, after which they repeated the treadmill test. Results of the final test showed that those taking ribose increased the time they were able to walk before developing EKG signs of ischemia, while those taking placebo had no such improvement. This preliminary study was too small to prove anything definitively, but it certainly suggests that further investigation would be worthwhile.

Another small placebo-controlled study enrolled people with coronary artery disease and congestive heart failure and found that use of ribose supplements improved objective measures of heart function and also enhanced subjective quality of life.

SAFETY ISSUES

There are no reports of lasting or damaging side effects from ribose, but formal safety studies have not been conducted. Reported minor side effects include diarrhea, gastrointestinal discomfort, nausea, and headache.

EBSCO CAM Review Board

FURTHER READING

Ataka, S., et al. "Effects of Oral Administration of Caffeine and D-Ribose on Mental Fatigue." *Nutrition,* January 4, 2008.

Berardi, J. M., and T. N. Ziegenfuss. "Effects of Ribose Supplementation on Repeated Sprint Performance in Men." *Journal of Strength and Conditioning Research* 17 (2003): 47-52.

Dunne, L., et al. "Ribose Versus Dextrose Supplementation, Association with Rowing Performance." *Clinical Journal of Sport Medicine* 16 (2005): 68-71.

Kerksick, C., et al. "Effects of Ribose Supplementation Prior to and During Intense Exercise on Anaerobic Capacity and Metabolic Markers." *International Journal of Sport Nutrition and Exercise Metabolism* 15 (2006): 653-664.

Kreider, R. B., et al. "Effects of Oral D-Ribose Supplementation on Anaerobic Capacity and Selected Metabolic Markers in Healthy Males." *International Journal of Sport Nutrition and Exercise Metabolism* 13 (2003): 87-96.

Omran, H., et al. "D-Ribose Improves Diastolic Function and Quality of Life in Congestive Heart Failure Patients." *European Journal of Heart Failure* 5 (2003): 615-619.

Peveler, W. W., P. A. Bishop, and E. J. Whitehorn. "Effects of Ribose as an Ergogenic Aid." *Journal of Strength and Conditioning Research* 20 (2006): 519-522.

See also: Sports and fitness support: Enhancing performance; Sports and fitness support: Enhancing recovery.

Rifampin

CATEGORY: Drug interactions
DEFINITION: A drug used with isoniazid for the treatment of tuberculosis.
INTERACTION: Vitamin D
TRADE NAMES: Rifadin, Rimactane

VITAMIN D

Effect: Supplementation Possibly Helpful

Rifampin, used with the antibiotic drug isoniazid in treating tuberculosis, might interfere with the metabolism of vitamin D. Although it is not clear whether this interaction actually causes vitamin D deficiency, one should be sure to consume adequate amounts of vitamin D on general principle.

EBSCO CAM Review Board

FURTHER READING

Bueno-Sánchez, J. G., et al. "Anti-tubercular Activity of Eleven Aromatic and Medicinal Plants Occurring in Colombia." *Biomedica* 29, no. 1 (2009): 51-60.

Lalloo, U. G., and A. Ambaram. "New Antituberculous Drugs in Development." *Current HIV/AIDS Reports* 7, no. 3 (2010): 143-151.

See also: Antibiotics, general; Food and Drug Administration; Vitamin D.

Rolfing

CATEGORY: Therapies and techniques
RELATED TERMS: Deep tissue massage therapy, manipulative therapy, postural relief, structural integration
DEFINITION: A vigorous deep tissue massage therapy designed to improve the body's overall skeletal structure and posture through collagen integration.
PRINCIPAL PROPOSED USES: Back pain, joint pain, knee pain, neck pain, posture improvement, sciatica, scoliosis, shoulder pain, repetitive strain injuries, spinal injuries, stress
OTHER PROPOSED USES: Anxiety, asthma, carpal tunnel syndrome, cerebral palsy, chronic constipation, chronic fatigue syndrome, digestive disorders, fibromyalgia, headache, ligament strain, osteoarthritis, premenstrual syndrome, relaxation, sports injuries

OVERVIEW

Rolfing is a method of deeply massaging all the connective tissue, known as fascia, between muscles, bones, ligaments, and tendons in the body in an effort to realign and restructure the overall skeletal composition. Rolfing therapy was invented in the 1930s by Ida Rolf, a biochemist, in an attempt to treat her own scoliosis and that of her two sons after being dissatisfied with the results of yoga, osteopathy, and homeopathy.

MECHANISM OF ACTION

Using hands, fingers, knuckles, elbows, and knees to apply intense pressure to inner collagen fiber, a rolfing therapist attempts to stretch and reshape the connective tissue, or fascia, between bones, tendons, muscles, and ligaments. On the theory that the skeletal structure follows the fascial makeup, rolfing therapy primarily seeks to establish increased fascial elasticity. Once tightened, fascia is unbound and lengthened through manipulation; the muscles, tendons, ligaments, and bones, which the fascia is attached to, may also then relax and realign after improper structure caused by gravity, inertia, sedentariness, repetitive movement, disease, or injury.

The first three sessions of rolfing therapy focus on massaging superficial tissue and improving breathing; the next four sessions involve deep manipulation of interior tissue structure; and the final three sessions integrate all parts of the body's skeleton through fascial redistribution and connection. After ten sessions of sixty to ninety minutes of rolfing using deep tissue reintegration, the practitioner can then rediscover proper skeletal balance, form, and posture and then release accumulated stress and energy.

USES AND APPLICATIONS

Rolfing is used primarily to reduce stress, alleviate pain, increase mobility, improve posture, and facilitate coordination. Rolfing is also frequently used in treating sports injuries and repetitive strain injuries, such as rotator cuff injuries.

SCIENTIFIC EVIDENCE

No double-blind, placebo-controlled studies of rolfing have been conducted, but there have been other scientific studies on the method. In 1963, the first major studies of rolfing being performed on children at the Foundation of Brain Injured Children concluded that after ten sessions, the impaired children improved in motor skills, muscle tone, posture, and coordination. In the 1970s, published scientific studies documented muscle tone, strength, and elasticity both before and after rolfing therapy, with empirical medical testing used to measure increased muscle performance. In 1981, a study was published that documented the improved lower body movement and mobility of persons with cerebral palsy who had been treated with rolfing therapy.

In 1988, a test revealed improved pelvic inclination in a group of women after rolfing therapy sessions,

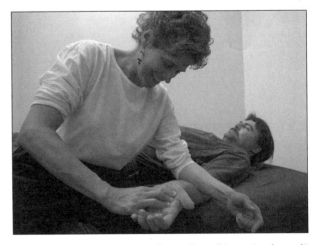

Rolfing therapy is being used to relieve this patient's tendinitis symptoms. (AP Photo)

and in 1997, a study documented the decrease of low back pain in persons who had received rolfing therapy. In the late 1990s, various studies looked at rolfing to treat repetitive strain injuries, such as carpal tunnel syndrome; all showed significant improvement after rolfing therapy. Also in the late 1990s, a study revealed that a group of elderly persons maintained improved balance after receiving rolfing therapy. Whether or not any of the above studies would have achieved the same positive results using any other therapy or technique is unknown, as no comparisons of dissimilar treatments were employed. Moreover, because no placebo or double-blind groups were implemented in any of the studies, there is no reliable scientific evidence to support these studies' claims, and the true efficacy of rolfing therapy remains unproven.

CHOOSING A PRACTITIONER

Ideally, one should choose a practitioner who is certified by the Rolf Institute of Structural Integration, headquartered in Boulder, Colorado. To achieve even basic rolfing certification, students must take advanced training of one to two years beyond traditional massage techniques. Many therapists claim to be well versed in the art of rolfing, yet these same therapists are often only superficially familiar with its specific techniques. Because rolfing involves deep tissue manipulation, treatment from a therapist who is not certified or licensed by the institute poses a risk of injury.

SAFETY ISSUES

Persons with rheumatoid arthritis and other serious inflammatory medical conditions should avoid rolfing because it may exacerbate or worsen these conditions. Likewise, all persons who are frail or fragile should abstain from rolfing, inasmuch as the intense nature of the treatments may result in subsequent bone fractures. Additionally, pregnant women, especially after the first trimester, should seek out only those certified in the use of milder, modified rolfing techniques especially designed for use during pregnancy, or they should avoid rolfing therapy altogether.

Mary E. Markland, M.A.

FURTHER READING

Anson, Briah. *Animal Healing: The Power of Rolfing.* Minneapolis: Mill City Press, 2011.

Brecklinghaus, Hans. *Rolfing Structural Integration: What It Achieves, How It Works, and Whom It Helps.* La Vergne, Tenn.: Lightning Source, 2002.

Rolf, Ida. *Rolfing: Reestablishing the Natural Alignment and Structural Integration of the Human Body for Vitality and Well-Being.* Rochester, Vt.: Healing Arts Press, 1989.

_____, and Rosemary Feitis. *Rolfing and Physical Reality.* 2d ed. Rochester, Vt.: Healing Arts Press, 1990.

Sise, Betsy. *The Rolfing Experience: Integration in the Gravity Field.* Prescott, Ariz.: Hohm Press, 2005.

See also: Alexander technique; Applied kinesiology; Aston-Patterning; Back pain; Bone and joint health; Feldenkrais method; Manipulative and body-based practices; Massage therapy; Neck pain; Osteopathic manipulation; Pain management; Progressive muscle relaxation; Reflexology; Scleroderma; Shiatsu; Soft tissue pain; Therapeutic touch.

Rosacea

RELATED TERM: Acne rosacea
CATEGORY: Condition
DEFINITION: Treatment of a chronic skin condition that primarily affects the face.
PRINCIPAL PROPOSED NATURAL TREATMENT: *Chrysanthemum indicum* (topical)
OTHER PROPOSED NATURAL TREATMENTS: Aloe, apple cider vinegar, aromatherapy, betaine hydrochloride, burdock, chamomile, Chinese herbal medicine, digestive enzymes, food allergen avoidance, green tea (topical), methylsulfonylmethane (topical), milk thistle (topical), niacinamide (topical), red clover, rose hips, selenium, vitamin B complex, vitamin C, vitamin D, vitamin E, yellow dock, zinc

INTRODUCTION

Rosacea is a chronic skin condition that affects the face (generally, to the greatest extent near the center), the eyelids, and, sometimes, the neck, upper back, and chest. Symptoms mostly occur in sun-exposed areas and consist of redness, acne-like pustules and papules (but not comedones, or blackheads), visible blood vessels (telangiectasias), and swelling of the

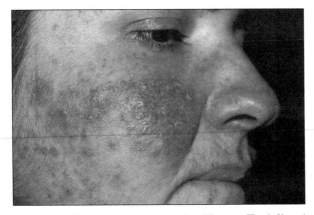

Woman with rosacea on her face. (Dr. Harout Tanielian/ Photo Researchers, Inc.)

skin. Dramatic facial flushing may occur after consuming alcohol, hot drinks, or spicy foods, or after exposure to excessive sunlight or extremes of hot or cold. In the eye, acne rosacea produces symptoms known as blepharitis. Over time, rosacea may cause the nose to become enlarged.

Treatment of rosacea involves avoiding stimuli that worsen the disease and using medications similar to those used for acne. Laser treatment can remove unsightly blood vessels and reduce flushing.

PROPOSED NATURAL TREATMENTS

A substantial (246-participant) twelve-week double-blind study found that a cream containing 1 percent *Chrysanthellum indicum* significantly improved rosacea symptoms compared with placebo. In another placebo-controlled study, a combination of milk thistle and methylsulfonylmethane topically applied by forty-six persons for one month appeared to be effective for rosacea. Weaker evidence hints that cream containing niacinamide might be helpful. One preliminary study found some evidence that a cream made from green tea may provide benefits as well.

Some alternative medicine practitioners believe that rosacea is caused by poor digestion and so recommend the use of betaine hydrochloride or apple cider vinegar to increase stomach acid. In addition, they may recommend digestive enzymes. However, there is no meaningful scientific evidence to indicate that using these treatments will reduce symptoms of rosacea.

Other natural treatments that are sometimes recommended for rosacea, but that also lack scientific sup-

port, include aloe, aromatherapy, burdock, chamomile, Chinese herbal medicine, food allergen avoidance, red clover, rose hips, selenium, vitamin B complex, vitamin C, vitamin D, vitamin E, yellow dock, and zinc. Some herbs and supplements should be used only with caution because they could interact adversely with drugs used to treat rosacea.

EBSCO CAM Review Board

FURTHER READING

Berardesca, E., et al. "Combined Effects of Silymarin and Methylsulfonylmethane in the Management of Rosacea: Clinical and Instrumental Evaluation." *Journal of Cosmetic Dermatology* 7 (2008): 8-14.

Draelos, Z. D., et al. "Niacinamide-Containing Facial Moisturizer Improves Skin Barrier and Benefits Subjects with Rosacea." *Cutis* 76 (2005): 135-141.

National Rosacea Society. http://www.rosacea.org.

Rigopoulos, D., et al. "Randomized Placebo-Controlled Trial of a Flavonoid-Rich Plant Extract-Based Cream in the Treatment of Rosacea." *Journal of the European Academy of Dermatology and Venereology* 19 (2005): 564-568.

Turkington, Carol, and Jeffrey S. Dover. *The Encyclopedia of Skin and Skin Disorders*. 3d ed. New York: Facts On File, 2007.

See also: Acne; Blepharitis; Scar tissue; Seborrheic dermatitis; Vitiligo.

Rose hips

CATEGORY: Herbs and supplements
RELATED TERM: *Rosa* species
DEFINITION: Natural plant product used to treat specific health conditions.
PRINCIPAL PROPOSED USE: Natural source of vitamin C and bioflavonoids
OTHER PROPOSED USES: Cancer prevention, kidney stones (prevention), osteoarthritis

OVERVIEW

A rose hip is the seed pod of a wild rose plant. Various wild rose species can be utilized as sources of rose hips. Traditionally, rose hips have been used to treat arthritis, colds and flu, indigestion, bladder stones, and gonorrhea.

THERAPEUTIC DOSAGES

Therapeutic dosages of rose hips products are generally adjusted to supply the desired amount of vitamin C and bioflavonoids.

THERAPEUTIC USES

Rose hips are used primarily as a natural source of vitamin C. There is no evidence that the vitamin C in rose hips is any better than synthetic vitamin C (the most common form of the vitamin), but those who prefer to use truly natural products can do so by using the herb instead of the chemical. Like other plant sources of vitamin C, rose hips also contain substances in the bioflavonoid family. Information on the potential benefits of these two rose hips constituents can be found in the respective articles.

SCIENTIFIC EVIDENCE

Some evidence from relatively small, double-blind, placebo-controlled studies suggests that rose hips might have value for osteoarthritis. More studies are needed to draw any reliable conclusions. In at least one placebo-controlled trial, rose hips powder appeared to have modest benefits for patients with rheumatoid arthritis.

Weak evidence hints that whole rose hips might be useful for prevention of cancer and, possibly, treatment or prevention of kidney stones.

SAFETY ISSUES

There are no known or suspected safety issues with rose hips.

EBSCO CAM Review Board

FURTHER READING

Christensen, R., et al. "Does the Hip Powder of *Rosa canina* (Rosehip) Reduce Pain in Osteoarthritis Patients?" *Osteoarthritis Cartilage* 16 (2008): 965-972.

Chrubasik, C., R. K. Duke, and S. Chrubasik. "The Evidence for Clinical Efficacy of Rose Hip and Seed." *Phytotherapy Research* 20 (2006): 1-3.

Rossnagel, K., S. Roll, and S. N. Willich. "The Clinical Effectiveness of Rosehip Powder in Patients with Osteoarthritis." *MMW Fortschritte der Medizin* 149 (2007): 51-56.

Willich, S. N., et al. "Rose Hip Herbal Remedy in Patients with Rheumatoid Arthritis." *Phytomedicine* 17, no. 2 (2010): 87-93.

See also: Citrus bioflavonoids; Vitamin C.

Rosemary

CATEGORY: Herbs and supplements
RELATED TERM: *Rosmarinus officinalis*

DEFINITION: Natural plant product used to treat specific health conditions.
PRINCIPAL PROPOSED USE: Dyspepsia
OTHER PROPOSED USES: Chemical dependency, muscle aches

OVERVIEW

The herb rosemary has been used as a food spice and as a medicine since ancient times. Traditional medicinal uses of rosemary leaf preparations taken internally include digestive distress, headaches, and anxiety. The fragrance of rosemary leaf has been said to enhance memory. Rosemary oil has been applied to the skin to treat muscle and joint pain and taken internally to promote abortions.

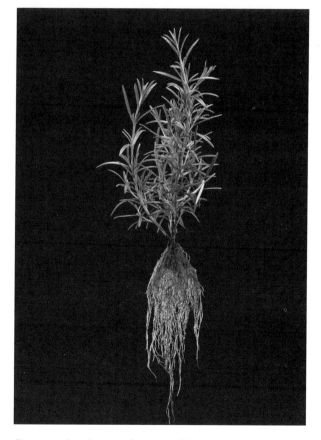

Rosemary has been used as a medicine since ancient times. (Stefan Diller/Photo Researchers, Inc.)

THERAPEUTIC DOSAGES

A typical dosage of rosemary leaf is 4 to 6 grams daily. Rosemary essential oil should not be used internally.

THERAPEUTIC USES

Germany's Commission E has approved rosemary leaf for treatment of dyspepsia (nonspecific digestive distress) and rosemary oil (used externally) for treatment of joint pain and poor circulation. However, there is no meaningful scientific evidence that rosemary is effective for any of these uses. Only double-blind, placebo-controlled studies can prove that a treatment really works, and no studies of this type have found rosemary effective.

Rosemary essential oil, like many essential oils, has antimicrobial properties when it comes in direct contact with bacteria and other microorganisms. Note, however, that this does not mean that rosemary oil is an antibiotic. Antibiotics are substances that can be taken internally to kill microorganisms throughout the body. Rosemary oil, rather, has shown potential antiseptic properties.

SCIENTIFIC EVIDENCE

One animal study found evidence that rosemary might help withdrawal from narcotics. Even weaker evidence hints that rosemary or its constituents may have antithrombotic (blood-thinning), anticancer, diuretic, liver-protective, and ulcer-protective effects.

Rosmarinic acid from rosemary has shown potential anti-inflammatory and antiallergic actions, but most published studies (including double-blind trials) have used a different plant source of the substance (the herb *Perilla frutescens*).

One controlled study failed to find rosemary cream protective against skin irritation caused by sodium lauryl sulfate (a common ingredient of cosmetic products).

Rosemary essential oil has been used in aromatherapy (treating conditions through scent). One controlled study evaluated rosemary aromatherapy for enhancing memory and found results that were mixed at best. Another study failed to find that rosemary aromatherapy reduced tension during an anxiety-provoking task; in fact, it appeared that the use of rosemary actually increased anxiety.

SAFETY ISSUES

Although rosemary's use in foods suggests a relatively low level of toxicity, rosemary has not undergone comprehensive safety testing. Rosemary essential oil can be toxic if taken even in fairly low doses, and the maximum safe dose is not known.

Based on its traditional use for abortion, as well as preliminary evidence showing embryotoxic effects, rosemary should not be used by pregnant women or women who wish to become pregnant.

One study suggests that rosemary may have diuretic effects. If it does, the herb could theoretically present risks in people taking the medication lithium.

Other weak evidence hints that rosemary may enhance the liver's rate of deactivating estrogen in the body. This suggests that rosemary might present risks for females as well as for anyone who uses medications containing estrogen. Additionally, one study hints that rosemary might worsen blood sugar control in people with diabetes.

Persons who are taking lithium should use rosemary only with caution. Persons taking medications containing estrogen should be aware that rosemary may decrease the effects of such medications.

EBSCO CAM Review Board

FURTHER READING

Lai, P. K., and J. Roy. "Antimicrobial and Chemopreventive Properties of Herbs and Spices." *Current Medicinal Chemistry* 11 (2004): 1451-1460.

Oluwatuyi, M., et al. "Antibacterial and Resistance Modifying Activity of *Rosmarinus officinalis*." *Phytochemistry* 65 (2004): 3249-3254.

Osakabe, N., et al. "Anti-inflammatory and Anti-allergic Effect of Rosmarinic Acid (RA): Inhibition of Seasonal Allergic Rhinoconjunctivitis (SAR) and Its Mechanism." *Biofactors* 21 (2005): 127-131.

Santoyo, S., et al. "Chemical Composition and Antimicrobial Activity of *Rosmarinus officinalis* L. Essential Oil Obtained via Supercritical Fluid Extraction." *Journal of Food Protection* 68 (2005): 790-795.

Slamenova, D., et al. "Rosemary-Stimulated Reduction of DNA Strand Breaks and FPG-Sensitive Sites in Mammalian Cells Treated with H2O2 or Visible Light-Excited Methylene Blue." *Cancer Letters* 177 (2002): 145-153.

Vitaglione, P., et al. "Dietary Antioxidant Compounds and Liver Health." *Critical Reviews in Food Science and Nutrition* 44 (2005): 575-586.

Yamamoto, J., et al. "Testing Various Herbs for Anti-thrombotic Effect." *Nutrition* 21 (2005): 580-587.

See also: Dyspepsia; Pain management.

Royal jelly

CATEGORY: Herbs and supplements

RELATED TERMS: Bee propolis, protein

DEFINITION: A medicine and nutritional supplement made of a thick, whitish substance that is secreted from a gland of the nurse bee, a young worker bee.

PRINCIPAL PROPOSED USE: General nutrition

OTHER PROPOSED USES: Antibacterial, antifungal, anxiety, asthma, blood pressure, diabetes, depression, fatigue, hair loss, hay fever, high cholesterol, hyperthyroidism, immunity, improving endurance, infertility, insomnia, kidney problems, life extension, liver problems, menopausal symptoms, sexual dysfunction, skin conditions, wounds, wrinkles

OVERVIEW

Royal jelly has been harvested for centuries along with honey and is used as a medicine in some Asian cultures; in Europe it is considered a food. The queen bee has the same genetic make-up as her worker bee sisters; however, the queen bee lives for up to six years, while her sisters live four to six weeks. This has led some to believe that royal jelly, the only food of queen bees, confers longevity.

MECHANISM OF ACTION

A number of theories exist on how royal jelly works, but its effectiveness is largely attributed to its chemical properties. Royal jelly is composed of proteins, amino acids, fatty acids, sugars, vitamins, and minerals. It has a high amount of nutrients, including pantothenic acid and vitamin B_6, and includes the compounds acetylcholine and gamma globulin. The components found in royal jelly (in percentages) are water (65), protein (13), sugars (11), and fatty acids (5).

Chemical studies of royal jelly have found flavonoids and a group of compounds called jelleins. Flavonoids reportedly have a variety of biologically active properties, including those that are antiallergic, antibacterial, and anti-inflammatory, and they have several effects, such as lipid oxidation, platelet aggregation, and vasodilation; flavonoids exert these effects through cyclo-oxygenase and lipoxygenase activity. Jelleins are purported to have antimicrobial activity.

USES AND APPLICATIONS

Royal jelly is used in a variety of forms. It can be taken in tablet form as a nutritional supplement, in typical doses of 50 to 200 milligrams per day. In its soluble-granule form, royal jelly also can be taken as a food additive; in the form of a paste, it can be taken as a component of a wound salve.

Royal jelly is commonly used as a nutritional supplement to treat the symptoms of menopause. It may also be helpful as an antimicrobial; it may mitigate fatigue; it may reduce anxiety, symptoms of asthma, high blood pressure, depression, hair loss, hay fever symptoms, symptoms of menopause, and wrinkles; it might control blood sugar levels in persons with diabetes; it may enhance immunity and wound healing; it might treat hyperthyroidism (Graves' disease), infertility, insomnia, kidney and liver problems, and skin conditions; and it may improve endurance and sexual function, lower cholesterol, and extend a person's life.

SCIENTIFIC EVIDENCE

Several scientific studies in the laboratory have proven the antimicrobial activity of royal jelly against such microbes as *Candida* species and *Staphylococcus aureus*. A few "uncontrolled" clinical trials have shown limited efficacy of royal jelly in lowering cholesterol and in controlling specific menopausal symptoms. One open-label clinical trial demonstrated that the oral ingestion of 20 grams of royal jelly could successfully reduce the blood glucose serum levels that are found in the blood during a standard glucose tolerance test.

SAFETY ISSUES

Royal jelly has been known to cause allergic reactions, especially in persons who are allergic to bee products.

Kecia Brown, M.P.H.

FURTHER READING

Boukraâ, L., et al. "Additive Action of Royal Jelly and Honey Against *Staphylococcus aureus.*" *Journal of Medicinal Food* 11, no. 1 (2008): 190-192.

Cherniak, E. P. "Bugs as Drugs, Part 1: Insects–The 'New' Alternative Medicine for the Twenty-first Century?" *Alternative Medicine Review* 15, no. 2 (2010): 124-135.

Chittka, A., and L. Chittka. "Epigenetics of Royalty." *PLoS Biology* 8, no. 11 (2010): e1000532.

Koc, A. N., et al. "Antifungal Activity of the Honeybee Products Against *Candida* spp. and *Trichosporon* spp." *Journal of Medicinal Food* 14, nos. 1/2 (2011): 128-134.

Münstedt, K., M. Bargello, and A. Hauenschild. "Royal Jelly Reduces the Serum Glucose Levels in Healthy Subjects." *Journal of Medicinal Food* 12, no. 5 (2009): 1170-1172.

Viuda-Martos, M., et al. "Functional Properties of Honey, Propolis, and Royal Jelly." *Journal of Food Science* 73, no. 9 (2008): R117-R124.

See also: Bee pollen; Bee propolis; Bee venom therapy; Functional foods: Introduction; Functional foods: Overview; Honey.